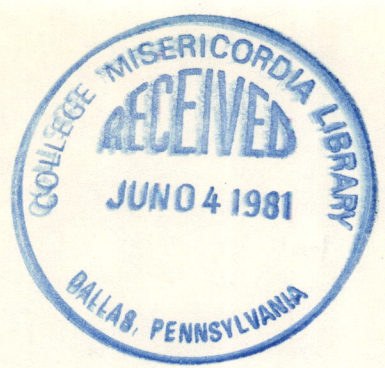

CONFUSION

6

CONFUSION
prevention and care

MARY OPAL WOLANIN, R.N., B.A., M.P.A.

Associate Professor Emeritus,
University of Arizona, College of Nursing,
Tucson, Arizona

LINDA REE FRAELICH PHILLIPS, R.N., Ph.D.

Assistant Professor,
Creighton University, School of Nursing,
Omaha, Nebraska

With 80 illustrations

Photographs by **Carol D. Falk, R.N., B.S.N.**

The C. V. Mosby Company

ST. LOUIS • TORONTO • LONDON   1981

Copyright © 1981 by The C. V. Mosby Company

All rights reserved. No part of this book may be reproduced in any manner without written permission of the publisher.

Printed in the United States of America

The C. V. Mosby Company
11830 Westline Industrial Drive, St. Louis, Missouri 63141

Library of Congress Cataloging in Publication Data

Wolanin, Mary Opal, 1910-
   Confusion, prevention and care.

   Bibliography: p.
   Includes index.
   1. Presenile dementia. 2. Presenile dementia—Nursing. I. Phillips, Linda Ree Fraelich, 1945- joint author. II. Title. [DNLM: 1. Cognition disorders—In old age. WT150 W848c]
RC394. P7W64   618.97′68983   80-18508
ISBN 0-8016-5629-X

AN/CB/CB 9 8 7 6 5 4 3 2 1   02/C/291

CONTRIBUTORS

DARLENE J. ANDERSON, R.N., G.N.P., Geriatric Nurse Practitioner, Hillside Manor Nursing Home, Missoula, Montana

PATRICIA KING, R.N., M.S., Instructor, University of Arizona, Tucson, Arizona

LEE MAXEY, M.S.W., Tucson, Arizona

FOREWORD

Mental impairment, by whatever name, is the most critical deterrent to the quality of life in the later years. Some 1 million elderly persons in the United States suffer from severe dementia to the extent that they are unable to carry out the normal tasks of daily living. An additional 3 million may be moderately affected.

Like "senility"—the word with which it is frequently linked—confusion in the elderly is often unjustifiably considered an inevitable consequence of growing old. The confused older person is the focus of stereotypic attitudes and may be unnecessarily institutionalized at considerable personal and financial cost.

While research continues to seek information on the mechanisms of the dementias of aging, the greatest inroads have been in the area of diagnosis. Sophisticated techniques such as computerized tomography, as well as changing attitudes toward aging among researchers and health professionals, have separated some 100 reversible causes of confusion in the elderly from the currently irreversible dementias. We have come to realize that the aging brain is particularly sensitive to a variety of insults occurring elsewhere in the body. A variety of conditions can compromise the mental integrity of an elderly patient, including sensory deprivation, both visual and auditory, the extreme vulnerability of the aged brain to a broad spectrum of medications, and even simple lack of routine hygiene practices or failure to treat minor illnesses. The mental disturbance that may occur when both eyes are covered following cataract surgery, for example, is a dramatic illustration of an effect of sensory deprivation.

Because of this, the National Institute on Aging initiated a special effort to develop guidelines for the diagnosis and treatment of mental impairment in the elderly. The report concluded that "it is crucial for health professionals, public planners, and lay persons to recognize that many curable physical and psychological diseases in the elderly produce intellectual impairment that may be hard to distinguish from irreversible brain disease," and that prompt diagnosis and treatment are imperative.

Nurses are frequently the front line of defense in contact with the elderly, whether in a clinic, a private physician's office, or a nursing home. The nurse may conduct a detailed screening before a visit with a doctor or may visit the elderly person at home to monitor his or her condition, provide routine care, and determine ways to improve general health and environment. Nurses are, therefore, often in a position to target very common reversible disorders by taking a social history of events that might have affected the patient's emotional status or by making an inventory of the prescription and over-the-counter drugs that the patient is taking. An inspection of the patient's medicine cabinet or other storage place may disclose that the patient is still taking drugs prescribed long ago or may have similar prescriptions from several physicians.

There is much that we do not know about Alzheimer's disease and the other so-called irreversible dementias of aging. We do know, however, that frequently much can be done to reduce the severity of their manifestations through symptomatic or supportive therapy, such as repeatedly supplying information on time, place, and person; structuring environments to make use of residual strengths; making changes as infrequently as possible; and treating the physical and emotional ailments that are liable to complicate the course of the primary disorder.

In the meantime, the National Institute on Aging is working with other federal agencies to make Alzheimer's disease a major research priority. We have also taken an active interest in the development of self-help groups of Alzheimer families seeking to promote education, services, and research in this area. Finally, we have published an information brochure answering the questions that families and friends of Alzheimer victims are likely to ask.

Confusion: Prevention and Care represents a comprehensive analysis of a woefully neglected issue for an audience that bears a vital responsibility for the care of the geriatric patient. It examines confusion, with its variety of definitions, the physical and psychological disorders that can result in confusion, the nursing diagnosis and treatment of the confused patient, and the role of the family.

Until recently, quality of life in the later years was subject to attitudes that typecast the elderly population and their needs. This volume goes far toward meeting an unfulfilled need that may lead to better health care for the 24.4 million Americans over age 65.

Robert N. Butler, M.D.
Director, National Institute on Aging

PREFACE

Reality, like beauty, is in the eye of the beholder. It can sometimes be difficult to determine whose reality is more valid, and who is confused.

Confusion occurs in persons of all ages and in every setting. Who has not become confused and disoriented in an unfamiliar hotel where the registration desk is located several stories above the entrance? Who has not felt confused by the noise, rush, crowds, and hubbub of a busy, multilevel shopping mall? A sense of instant confusion occurs as we try to make sense of an unexpected situation. Confusion occurs to all of us in varying degrees during our everyday life. In addition, confusional states are found at all levels of health care: home, community, and acute and long-term care settings. It is estimated that 50% of older patients in long-term care units are there because of confusion or will develop confusion during their stay.

This book is about confusion in the elderly—a highly subjective state recognized by the observer as behaviors that do not make sense in his context. The diagnosis of confusion, whether correct or incorrect, has tremendous implications for the treatment of a client from that point on. That single diagnosis affects the treatment he will receive socially, legally, medically, and psychologically. It affects the individual's life-style, living situation, and interpersonal relationships. It is imperative, therefore, that the label of confusion be used accurately, that interventions be directed toward treating a phenomenon that is often reversible, and that "true" confusion be prevented when at all possible.

Although this book is concerned primarily with the elderly client, the implications are by no means limited to that group. For example, the sensory alterations discussed, such as deficits, overload, and deprivation, can occur at any age. Confusion is universal, but it occurs more frequently and lasts longer in persons whose health is compromised and whose environmental patterns have been interrupted.

To a great extent, nursing literature has closely followed the medical model and has been organized around either disease entities and body systems or patient classifications, such as pediatric, medical, and surgical. One of the strengths of this book is its departure from the use of those traditional organizations; it begins with confusion as a nursing diagnosis and as a phenomenon that confronts the caregiver in the real world of working with elderly people. We believe that the diagnosis of confusion is not precise; we also believe that confusion and organic brain syndrome are not the same thing. We take the position that what practitioners call "confusion" is separate and distinct from the medical diagnosis "organic brain syndrome." Therefore, we will avoid all the controversies and contradictions about organic brain syndrome.

This book examines the physiologic, sensoriperceptual, and interactional factors that contribute to confusion. An entire chapter is devoted to analyzing the reasons for labeling nonconfused persons as confused. Since anything predictable should be preventable, prediction and prevention are emphasized throughout the book. Persons at high risk are identified, based on review of current literature and on our own experience.

A holistic approach to the phenomenon of confusion is developed in the first several chapters. The material in the clinical section that then follows is organized around standard assessment protocols, preventive measures, and interventions.

The clinical section begins with a taxonomic system of nursing diagnoses that identifies confusion as a manifestation secondary to an underlying and treatable set of circumstances. The assessment leading to those diagnoses is developed in a step-by-step process. Summaries at the end of the clinical chapters include charts for quick reference and as guidelines for care plans.

The final chapter in the clinical section describes the patient with Alzheimer's disease (senile dementia [AD-SD]) and outlines appropriate care for each stage of the disease.

The concluding section of the book comprises chapters dealing with the family of the confused client and the problems that confront caregivers who work with confused persons.

Others have written on the various theories of aging and social gerontology, so rather than address these topics, we refer our readers to such authors as Atchley, Brown, and Kalish, who have summarized and synthesized current thinking. Practitioners without such a background can certainly use our book, but previous basic knowledge would enrich their understanding of the elderly person and his environment and life history.

Undergraduate students will use this book as a supplemental text in educational programs preparing health caregivers to serve the elderly. Appropriate for expanding the knowledge of the graduate student in health care education, it can also serve as an important reference for caregivers in acute and long-term care settings that have a high percentage of elderly in their population. It is a resource for planners and workers in community programs for the elderly. Health professionals who work with the families of elderly people will find this book particularly helpful in interpreting to the younger person the context of the elderly person's behavior.

We have made some attempts to generalize in order to study the confused elderly person and establish some applicable principles and facts to replace commonly accepted ritualistic care and treatment. A body of knowledge is dependent on such generalizations. Humanity consists of people who defy neat categorizations and who refuse to conform to general rules. The elderly are no exception. Is it possible that caregivers have tried to force the unforceable into categoric molds? The answer to this question may be central to caring for the confused elderly person.

Throughout this text the pronoun *he* is used to refer to the client/patient, and the pronoun *she* usually has a caregiver as its antecedent. We tried various constructions to avoid this blatant sexism but found them awkward and distracting. The least disruptive grammar was chosen to suit our purpose.

The term used to describe the person receiving care also presented problems. We do not have a single word in our language to indicate the relationship of caregiver and person cared for in all settings, especially those outside the traditional walls of institutions. "Client" designates the elderly person who is ambulatory and fairly independent and for whom the "sick role" is clearly out of place. Emphasis on prevention and early detection has required frequent use of "client." "Patient" is reserved for the elderly person requiring the major caregiver resources of an acute or long-term care facility. The distinctions are not clear, and we regret the imprecision in such usage.

Confusion may be interpreted many ways. We have taken the liberty of placing our perspectives and interpretations before others. We acknowledge that these efforts are incomplete, but they stand as a first effort in interpreting confusion to caregivers. Our own knowledge comes from reviewing the "reporting back" of others and comparing this to our own research and experience.

Confusion cannot be understood vicariously outside the laboratory of day-to-day contact with the elderly person in his own world. Concepts presented here need to be broadened and the theories tested in the marketplace of ideas and in the clinical arena of "hands-on" experience. We challenge others to take our findings and debate, discuss, and pursue more research in order to expand the picture of confusion among the elderly, or for that matter, among persons of any age.

We wish to acknowledge the assistance of others who made it possible to put this book together, especially Major H. J. -Tiger Wolanin and Eileen McFeaters, who shared our lives and efforts and always encouraged us. Gladys E. Sorensen, Dean of the University of Arizona College of Nursing, backed up her interest with time and money when Mary Opal Wolanin began her research into confusion. WICHE, under a grant from U.S. Public Health Service, contributed to a second research project that gave Mary Opal the privilege of working with seven other nurses in the western region. Mary Kay Johns, formerly of the University of Pittsburgh and faculty advisor to Linda Phillips, and Evelyn Bold, a colleague, discussed and encouraged her interest in confusion. We are indebted to Cynthia Grant, who helped get us under way, and to Jo Lene Unruh, who prepared our manuscript and encouraged us. We extend special thanks to Carol Falk, whose photography lends additional humanity to the pages of this book, and to Handmaker Jewish Geriatric Center of Tucson, for allowing use of its facilities for that photography and for clinical research. Eleanor Johnson and Fred Heidenreich of the Arizona Health Sciences Library gave us every possible assistance. Mary Jane Hattstaedt and two anonymous critics gave positive feedback and constructive criticism throughout the development of the manuscript. We have been blessed with a wealth of support systems to bolster our egos and spirits when we doubted our own abilities.

Mary Opal Wolanin
Linda Ree Fraelich Phillips

CONTENTS

1 **What is confusion?** 1
2 **Conceptual perspectives,** 10
3 **The pathophysiology of confusion,** 25
4 **The nurse's role in the care of the confused client,** 39
5 **The four-level nursing diagnosis,** 47
6 **Process of holistic assessment,** 58
7 **Who's confused here?** 88
8 **Emergency care for clients who are acutely confused,** 101
9 **Care of the client with confusion secondary to compromised brain support,** 109
10 **Care of the client with sensoriperceptual problems,** 171
   LINDA REE FRAELICH PHILLIPS
11 **Care of the client whose confusion results from disruption of pattern and meaning,** 268
12 **Care of the client whose confusion results from alterations in normal physiologic states,** 308
13 **Care of the patient with a true dementia,** 319
14 **Therapeutic interaction with families of the confused elderly,** 350
   LEE B. MAXEY
15 **Summing it up: the caregiver's urgent needs,** 371

Appendix A Confusion in the elderly: a protocol to determine acute organic brain syndrome versus chronic organic brain syndrome, 376
   DARLENE J. ANDERSON
          B Educational programs offering specialization in geriatric/gerontologic nursing, 397
          C Nursing assessment of the geriatric lower extremity, 400
   PATRICIA KING
          D Relaxation as therapy for the elderly, 403

Tables and boxed material contents

Table 1-1 Terms used by physicians to describe confused behaviors of elderly clients according to social and cognitive inaccessibility categories, 4

Table 1-2 Terms used by nurses to describe confused behaviors of elderly clients according to social and cognitive inaccessibility categories, 5

Table 5-1 Taxonomic system of nursing diagnoses of confusional states in the elderly, 49

Table 9-1 Folacin content of some of the more common foods (recommended daily allowance is 400 μg), 115

Table 9-2 Foods containing calcium, 123

Table 9-3 Signs and symptoms of progressive hypothermia: the seven stages of hypothermia, 130

Table 9-4 Plasma half-life values for barbiturates and flurazepam in adults, 162

Table 11-1 Life change events that may occur with the death of a spouse, 269

Table 11-2 Common stressors that arise from the elderly individual's personal/interpersonal milieu, 272

Table 11-3 Stressors in both long-term and short-term care settings, 273

Table 11-4 Feeling states and processes commonly experienced by elderly individuals, 276

Fourth-level assessment for:

Hypoxia, 110
Gradual blood loss and iron deficiency, 111
Pernicious anemia, 113
Folic-acid deficiency, 115
Hemolytic anemias, 116
Dehydration, 118
Hypocalcemia, 122
Hypercalcemia, 126
Hypothermia, 130
Hyperthermia, 133
Uremia, 134
Hypoxemic hypoxia, 137
Cardiac failure, 140
Hypotension, 143

Intracranial pressure, 147
Hypothyroidism, 151
Hypoglycemia, 152
Hyperglycemia, 154
Digitalis toxicity, 158
Sensory alteration, 186
Tactile alteration, 205
Visual alteration, 227
Auditory alteration, 246
Stress, 283
Confusion related to social interaction, 302
Inability to empty bladder, 310
Constipation or impaction, 312
Incontinence, 313

Outcome criteria of successful nursing intervention against:

Gradual blood loss and
 iron deficiency, 113
Pernicious anemia, 114
Folic-acid deficiency, 116
Dehydration, 121
Hypocalcemia, 125
Hypercalcemia, 127
Hypothermia, 132
Hyperthermia, 134
Uremia, 136
Hypoxemic hypoxia, 139
Cardiac failure, 142
Hypotension, 145
Intracranial pressure, 148
NPH, 149
Hypothyroidism, 151
Hypoglycemia, 153
Hyperglycemia, 155
Digitalis toxicity, 159
Sensory alteration, 196
Tactile alteration, 215
Visual alteration, 238
Auditory alteration, 254
Stress, 295
Confusion related to social
 interaction, 303
Inability to empty bladder, 311
Constipation or impaction, 313
Incontinence, 314

More common drugs associated with confusion in the elderly, 156
Neuroleptics implicated in tardive dyskinesia, 163
Guidelines for providing a facilitative environment for the elderly patient
 with true dementia, 332

Chapter 5 summary: Nursing process with the confused elderly
 person, 57
Chapter 6 summary: Process of holistic assessment
  Tool 6-1: Assessment of mental status, 77
  Tool 6-2: Assessment of sensoriperceptual abilities, 78
  Tool 6-3: Assessment of structure and physiology, 81
  Tool 6-4: Assessment of life history and culture, 83
  Tool 6-5: Assessment of interaction with social environment, 84
  Tool 6-6: Assessment of interaction with physical environment, 85
Chapter 9 summary: Confusional states secondary to compromised brain
 support, 165
Chapter 10 summary: Sensory alteration among the elderly
  In general, 255
  Related to tactile problems, 258
  Related to visual problems, 259
  Related to hearing problems, 262
Chapter 11 summary: Disruption of pattern and meaning in the
 elderly, 304
  Confusion related to stressors, 304
  Confusion related to social interaction, 306
Chapter 13 summary: The true dementias, 346

1

WHAT IS CONFUSION?

Only two centuries ago we could explain everything about everything, out of pure reason, and now most of that elaborate and harmonious structure has come apart before our eyes. We are *dumb*.

This is, in a certain sense, a health problem after all. For as long as we are bewildered by the mystery of ourselves, and confused by the strangeness of our uncomfortable connection to all the rest of life, and dumbfounded by the incomprehensibility of our own minds, we cannot be said to be healthy animals in today's world.*

---

*Lewis Thomas in *Executive* **4** (3):47, 1978. Permission given by Graduate School of Business and Public Administration, Cornell University.

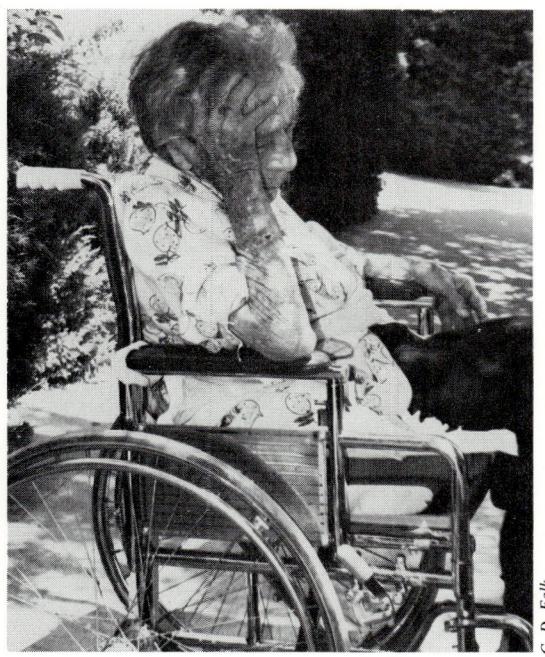

C. D. Falk

This book is concerned with confusional states in the elderly, their prediction, prevention, recognition, and treatment. The term *confusion*, while used freely by health professionals, is not clearly defined. It is a label for the behaviors that caregivers recognize as being deviant from those expected from the client in a certain place and at a certain time. The word *confusion* is entrenched in the language despite the efforts of health professionals to substitute a more descriptive and less subjective terminology.

Confusion can be categorized by etiology, type of onset (rapid or slow), duration of symptoms, degree of severity, prognosis for recovery, and the age of the client. This last classification is the central focus of this book. Confusion in the young is a temporary phenomenon. In the middle-aged it is a reversible event that has a definite etiology; when the cause is removed, the confusional state clears. Historically, the confusional state of the elderly is linked to "senility," which by definition is not reversible, or it is attributed to organic brain syndrome or disease, which has only recently been termed reversible, or to hopeless and permanent dementia. This book challenges the concept of irreversible senilities. A short time ago there were no reversible senilities or organic brain disease. Yesterday's irreversible senility is now known to be treatable, and today's irreversible senilities may yield to the newer knowledge that is being developed while this text is being written.

DEFINITION OF CONFUSION

This chapter defines confusion in the context in which professional caregivers use the word—the real world of relating to elderly clients and communicating with each other. Because communication takes place through shared meanings, it is necessary to establish a definition that is functional and also has a common meaning. A precise dictionary definition is desirable but not functional.

One of the more common definitions is based on use: "Behavior that is inappropriate to the occasion." This is an "Alice in Wonderland" definition that allows the observer to be completely subjective rather than objective, as required by a precise definition.

THE NURSE'S PERSPECTIVE

Confusion is a term used by nurses to describe a constellation of client behaviors, including inattention and memory deficits, inappropriate verbalizations, disruptive behavior, noncompliance, and failure to perform activities of daily living. Among many nurses, confusion of elderly people is invariably linked to certain medical diagnoses, such as organic brain disease, senile dementia, and senility. When the association is made, confusion is then viewed as a simple matter based on the following tacit assumptions:

1. Confusion is an expected and inevitable outcome of the normal aging process.
2. Confusion arises from pathology involving circulation, oxygenation, and metabolism of the brain tissue, and this pathology completely explains its existence.
3. Since confusion arises from a syndrome of the brain (organic brain syndrome), its effects are neither preventable nor reversible.

These three assumptions comprise the traditional medical model of senile dementia on which nurses base their own perspectives.

In addition to assuming that nursing diagnosis of confusion and the medical diagnosis of organic brain syndrome are synonymous, many nurses assume the term confusion has a precise meaning. Since the presence of confusion is determined by behavioral evidence, it is incorrectly assumed that the nursing diagnosis is objective and therefore has the same meaning for every nurse and for every client. However, Phillips (1973) reports that the definitions of confusion vary widely among nurses and have little relationship to consistent behavioral manifestations. In addition, Phillips (1976) reports that the client symptoms considered indicative of confusion appear to vary in relationship to other social and physical factors, including personal appearance, age, and the adoption of institutionally desirable behaviors such as compliance, motivation, and quiescence.

Gebbie and Lavin (1975), in the First National Conference on Classification of Nursing Diagnoses, identify the following as characteristics of confusion:

1. Disorientation to place, person, time, object, and purpose after reality information is given
2. Suspected impairment of attention span
3. Restlessness
4. Purposeless activity
5. Anxiety
6. Apprehension
7. Fright
8. Agitation

9. Verbosity
10. Confabulation
11. Rambling speech
12. Dependent and demanding attention-getting behavior
13. Withdrawal
14. Belligerence
15. Combativeness
16. Statements of confusion
17. Facial expression specific to confusion

The nurses who have identified these characteristics of confusion have described behaviors that lead to the general assumptions that the client is confused. With the exception of 1, 16, and 17, the behaviors are not exclusive and may be found in many conditions. The list gives no indication of whether one characteristic is more important than another or whether certain combinations of characteristics are more significant than others. From our viewpoint, *loss of memory* is a crucial omission. Goldfarb (1975) would have added this, for he believes that faulty memory and inability to learn are the most important signs of a confusional state. He thinks inability to learn is based on faulty memory, since memory is the link between the past and the present and the basis for problem solving and judgment. Goldfarb also believes memory is the part of adaptation that makes us sentient, responsive, and interactional. Consciousness, he says, is most likely a simple awareness of being aware and is therefore a memory.

Wolanin (1973) studied confusion in elderly clients by attempting to discover what behaviors caregivers saw, and what they recorded as having seen, in the clients they labeled confused. For the study, 30 elderly nursing home residents were chosen according to a planned sequence. All were consensually labeled as confused by the staff, and the diagnosis was confirmed by the head nurse. Seventy percent of the sample had been admitted with a diagnosis of organic brain syndrome or disease. All patients were English speaking, over the age of 65, and fully conscious. They had been residents of the facility at least 26 days in order to have been observed by the staff. Data were gathered from written records, such as nurses' records, physicians' examinations, histories, progress notes, nursing care plans, and referral forms, and from taped interviews with the staff. Clients in the study were also observed and interviewed by a standard protocol. The clinical records were well maintained, the staff very involved, and the clients cooperative.

The study emphasis was not on the client per se but on the caregiver's perception of the client's behavior. This is the reality of the caregiver/client situation. Textbook pictures and dictionary definitions fade out in the actual clinical situation where caregiver and client have their own perception of the same event. The perceptions dealt primarily with the nurse's interpretation of her observations, with the physician's records included since they influenced the nurse's observations.

The caregivers' backgrounds were extremely varied. Nursing personnel had changed frequently during the 2 years of record keeping. Their backgrounds included young nurses with associate degrees in nursing, middle-aged women with diplomas in nursing, and two nurses in their sixties who had bachelor degrees. Although data were collected from a large sample of caregivers who varied greatly by age, educational preparation, and experience, none of these variables appeared to affect the perspectives toward confusion. The physicians included a large number from a county hospital. There were no private physicians in the sample.

Data included adjectives, nouns, and verbs from the client's records or caregiver oral interviews that indicated behavior deviant enough to be recorded. The taped interviews contained any behavior the caregiver felt was significant to mention. If the term confused was used, the investigator asked, "What did you see that indicated confusion to you?" The caregivers were not told that the data were dependent on the terminology they used but were asked only about the client. Caregivers were understanding; nearly all began their reports concerning clients with "He isn't really responsible for his actions." Early in the study interviews, nurses attempted to guard their language. They prefaced their remarks about a client's behavior with statements such as "She is the sweetest old lady." They avoided gestures often used in describing confusion, such as the forefinger circling the ear. Later in the interviews, many became quite informal and relaxed. Information then included terms such as "zombie," "pack rat," and "screamer." Most of the time information given was simply "he is very confused" or "he is disoriented," with few explanations and the assumption that the investigator shared the meaning. There was an implicit understanding that everyone shared the highly subjective terms that were used.

Clients with behavior that disrupted the institution were reported as "agitated" or "wandering." Wandering is different from being lost. Being lost implies having a destination but losing direction. Wandering is an aimless moving from one place to another, especially to a forbidden area. The intent may be to move about and explore, but the connotation is that if the client were mentally intact, he would stay in one place and not explore. Wandering is institutionally disruptive because personnel and families are required to maintain constant vigilance.

The physicians' record frequently contained "confusion" and often "disoriented," but when the latter was used, it was described by time, place, or object. The physicians referred to memory gaps. "The patient is a poor historian" demonstrated their frustration in trying to obtain an adequate history. When they used another's observations, such as a family member's complaint about client behavior, they put the behaviors in quotation and named the source.

The observations by the caregivers fell into two categories, for which two descriptive terms were borrowed from Fisher and Pierce (1967): *cognitive accessibility* and *social accessibility*. These were positive terms denoting acceptable or expected behavior, which is socially productive as defined by our culture.

Cognitive accessibility includes those behaviors that indicate intellectual functioning, such as alertness, interest, idea association, thought quality, and memory. Because the behaviors of the confused person interfere with cognitive accessibility, the negative term, *cognitive inaccessibility,* was used by Wolanin to categorize the data describing behaviors that prevented the elderly person from interacting with his environment according to the caregiver's expectations.

"Social accessibility refers to those behaviors which enable one to produce intended effects on others: to make them love you, respond to you, help you, serve you and accept your love" (Fisher, 1973, p. 70). Because the behaviors observed and recorded by caregivers interfered with social accessibility, the negative form, *social inaccessibility,* is used for those institutionally disruptive activities recorded most frequently.

Table 1-1. Terms used by physicians to describe confused behaviors of elderly clients according to social and cognitive inaccessibility categories

Cognitive inaccessibility	Social inaccessibility
Poor memory	Unable to cooperate
No recent memory	Hostile
Unreliable memory	Belligerent
Unable to answer questions	Nuisance to staff
Lost when walking	Refuses to obey orders
Incoherent	Deviant behavoir
Poor time sense	Incontinent
Poor attention	
Agrees with all statements	

Table 1-2. Terms used by nurses to describe confused behaviors of elderly clients according to social and cognitive inaccessibility categories

Cognitive inaccessibility	Social inaccessibility
Written records	
Forgetful	Uncooperative
Not aware of surroundings	Combative
	Hostile
Cannot understand instructions	Belligerent
	Negligent
Incoherent	Suspicious
Uses wrong bed or drawer	Difficult to manage
	Noisy
Not sure where he belongs	Threatening to leave
Lost	Restless
Mixed up	Annoyed
	Wandering
	Runs Away
	Violent
	Agitated
	Excitable
Oral reports	
Forgetful	Agitated
Withdrawn	Violent
Cannot remember name	Critical
	Difficult to manage
Does not do as requested	Belligerent
	Antagonistic
Uses poor judgment	Not normal
Incoherent	Pack rat
Concentration poor	Combative
Delusional	Into others' possessions
Not accepting reality	Wanders
Not with us	
Loses room	
Mixed up	
Zombie	
Bland	
Not in contact	

Nurses noted behaviors that interfered with their instrumental function of caring for clients and maintaining a peaceful environment; physicians noted behaviors that interfered with their instrumental function of making a correct diagnosis (Tables 1-1 and 1-2).

Wolanin also looked for common elements in the condition of the 30 confused clients. All but one were hypotensive or normotensive (120/80 or below). There was a high correlation between sensory deficits and recorded antisocial behavior. Two of the confused elderly were almost blind; a number were deaf. The quality of information offered to the clients was diminished by sensory deficits alone. Seventy-five percent of the clients were receiving phenothiazine therapy, 51% were being given diuretics, and 20% were receiving some form of digitalis. All were confined to their rooms or to a long hallway leading to a dining room. None of these factors was considered in the records or reports concerning the confused patient.

This discussion should demonstrate the following points: (1) the diagnosis of confusion is made based as much on subjective feelings as objective observations; (2) there is a certain amount of imprecision in the use

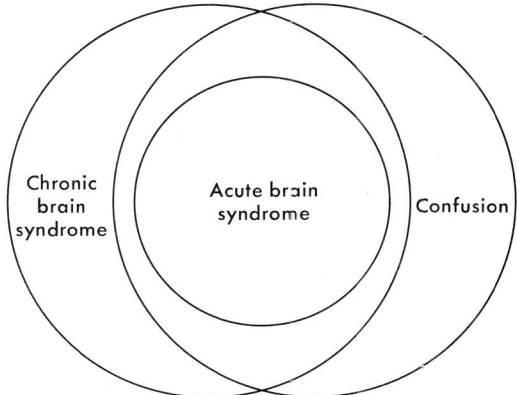

Fig. 1-1. The relationship between brain syndrome and confusion.

of the term confusion; and (3) the nursing diagnosis of confusion encompasses more patients and is different from the medical diagnosis of organic brain syndrome, although there are a certain number of clients who simultaneously receive both medical and nursing diagnoses on the basis of their behavior. Fig. 1-1 illustrates this point.

From our observations in nursing homes, it appears that those clients with acute brain syndrome are invariably seen by nurses as confused. Those with chronic brain syndrome may or may not be seen as confused. A third group is seen as confused, but they are not diagnosed as having a brain syndrome. Perhaps it is only for those clients for whom the diagnoses of *confusion* and *organic brain syndrome* overlap that a medical model is adequate as an explanatory base.

Phillips (1978) found that of the 110 residents in an extended care facility, approximately 80% had a diagnosis of organic brain syndrome. Of the 20% who did not have a diagnosis of organic brain syndrome, less than half were consistently referred to by nurses as unconfused.

THE MEDICAL DIAGNOSIS

Medical attitudes and beliefs about confused elderly can be traced through the evolution of medical diagnosis. The physician's diagnosis reflects personal culture and the scientific level of training received (Fig. 1-2). Diagnoses of senile dementia and organic brain syndrome were based on the presence of confused behavior, so the terminology used is a window into the physician's perspective. Giving anything a name helps to form a frame of reference; the medical diagnosis sets up expectancies and attitudes known as prognosis, which guides therapeutic action or inaction.

Senile dementia

Behavior leading to confusional states in younger clients is usually related to some disease entity. The addition of age, however, has led to a diagnosis of senile dementia if the elderly exhibit the same behavior. Dementia is derived from the Latin *demans*, or mad. It was a disorder that could be transmitted "by hand" and led to a hands-off attitude by caregivers. Today, dementia means an irreversible deterioration of intellectual faculties with concomitant emotional disturbances resulting from a brain disorder. Senile has a pejorative connotation, for it is always associated with the undesirable aspects and behaviors of the aged. Goldfarb (1975) studied a number of persons diagnosed as having either senile dementia or cerebral arteriosclerosis with psychosis. All diagnoses had been based on the client's disturbing behavior rather than on any physical findings denoting an impairment of cerebral function. The course of the disease and the longevity of the patient were poorest for those with a diagnosis of senile dementia, indicating a mental set that affected the physician's plan of treatment.

Cerebral arteriosclerotic disease

The first pathologic basis for the confusional states of the elderly was attributed to arteriosclerotic disease of the cerebral vessels. Goldfarb (1975) stated that this diagnosis had been based on the clinician's beliefs, convictions, and a procrustean* bed of diagnostic skills rather than on cause, onset, and prognosis. This reflected the state of the art of caring for the elderly person early in this century. Today, the diagnosis is still found on admission records in many institutions for the elderly.

Organic brain disease (OBD)

The first departure from cerebral arteriosclerotic disease and senile dementia as diagnoses was taken toward the middle of this century. Organic brain disease was used to describe the observations made by

---

*Procrustes was an innkeeper in Greek mythology who boasted that his beds fit everyone. He stretched the short and broke the bones of the tall to force them to fit the bed.

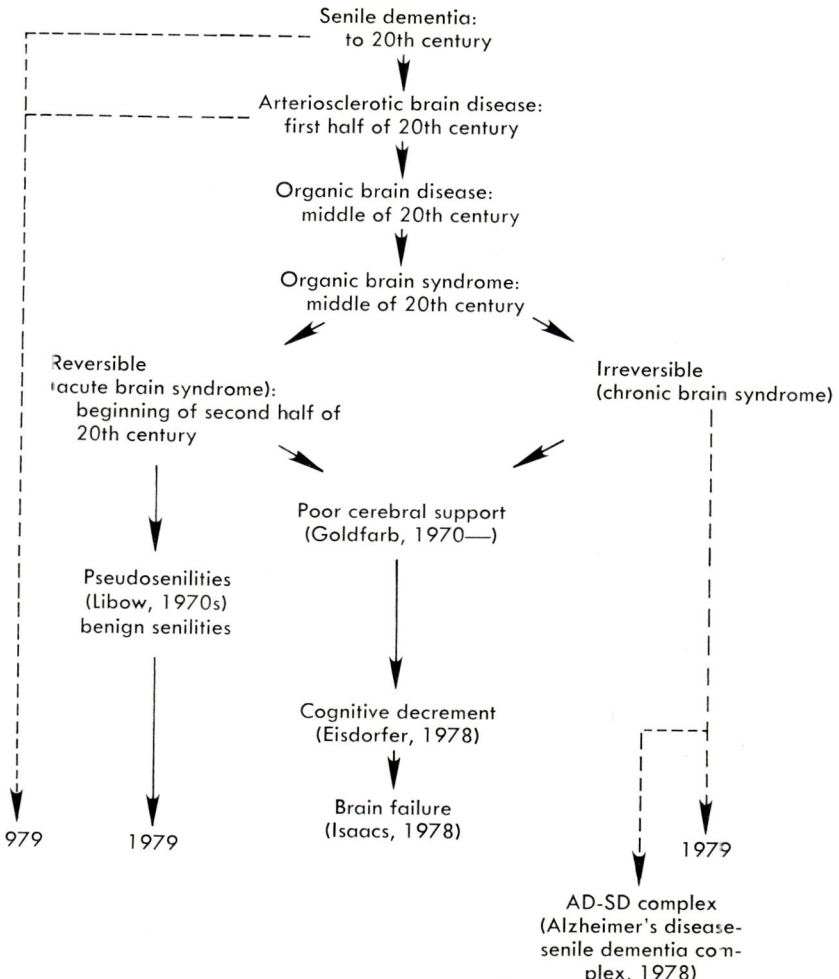

Fig. 1-2. The historic approach to diagnosis for the confused elderly patient.

physicians of the older people whose behaviors did not make sense in the context of their culture, and more particularly, in the culture of the caregivers. While used synonymously with cerebral arteriosclerotic disease (it was believed the underlying pathology was the same), this broader concept allowed for a defect in the brain and the blood vessels nourishing the brain.

Organic brain syndrome (OBS)

The diagnosis used to describe the observations of confused behavior is most likely to be organic brain syndrome at this time. With less certainty of the pathology to support the symptoms, *syndrome*, rather than *disease*, is used to indicate a constellation of signs and symptoms that collectively characterize an abnormal condition. Estimates are that 50% to 60% of the elderly who are segregated in nursing homes will have this diagnosis, and many ambulatory clients in their homes may have a mild and early form. While it is a major step beyond the hopelessness of senile dementia, the diagnosis has aroused dissatisfaction as more and more is learned about the treatment of the elderly with confusional states.

Present day terminology

Gerontologists and physicians who treat elderly people are suggesting the need for better terminology that follows the present concepts of cause and effect. Eisdorfer and Friedel (1978) prefer the term cognitive decrement to the term dementia and wish to drop the word senile. Isaacs (1978) proposes the use of brain failure, with the same meaning as cardiac or liver failure. He finds this more acceptable than the terms organic brain syndrome and cerebral arteriosclerotic disease, which had been based on clinical observations of client behavior rather than on any known lesion. Failure implies pathology and links it to a cause. The confusion becomes a medical entity rather than a psychiatric disease.

Goldfarb (1975) proposes "poor cerebral support," which implies brain failure from lack of essential elements to maintain normal function. Based on this dysfunction, etiology can be sought by evaluating pathophysiologic, neurologic, and structural abnormalities. Goldfarb agrees with Eisdorfer and Friedel in using cognitive decrement (memory losses) as the basis for much of what is seen in the confused state. Ability to remember the past and link it to the present or to the future are memory functions. In 5 years the term organic brain syndrome may be as obsolete as senile dementia is at present.

Reversible and irreversible

When organic brain syndrome was classified into reversible and irreversible, it allowed a whole new concept in the diagnosis and treatment of the elderly. For many years, the clearing of the mind after an illness was hampered by the idea of senile dementia. Libow (1978) suggested that the reversible types be termed "pseudosenilities" to differentiate them from true senility. Others have suggested the use of "benign senility," but this begs the question of what true senility is, or even if it is.

SUMMARY

We have attempted to establish an operational definition for confusion in the elderly that represents the caregivers' use of the term. A study of nurses' and physicians' spoken and written observations of confused clients has yielded behaviors that could be categorized under cognitive and social inaccessibility. Cognitively inaccessible behaviors refer to intellectual deficits, while socially inaccessible behaviors refer to institutionally disruptive behaviors and problems that prevent human interaction at a satisfying level. A study of physicians' attitudes through their medical diagnoses has shown the evolution from senile dementia to the recognition today that confusion results from treatable brain failure. This has resulted in confusion being recognized as a symptom of an underlying mental or physical pathology. For the purposes of this book, we define confusion as a condition characterized by the client's disorientation to time and place, incongruous conceptual boundaries, paranormal awareness, and seemingly inappropriate verbal statements that indicate memory defects.

REFERENCES

Eisdorfer, C., and Friedel, R. O.: Cognitive and emotional disease in the elderly, Chicago, 1978, Year Book Medical Publishers, Inc.

Fisher, J.: Competence, effectiveness, intellectual functioning and aging, Gerontologist 13:1, 1973.

Fisher, J., and Pierce, R. C.: Dimensions of intellectual functioning in the aged, J. Gerontol. 22:170, 1967.

Gebbie, K. M., and Lavin, M. A., editors: Classification of nursing diagnoses, St. Louis, 1975, The C. V. Mosby Co.

Goldfarb, A.: Memory and aging. In Goldman, R., and Rockstein, M., editors: The physiology and pathology of aging, New York, 1975, Academic Press, Inc.

Isaacs, B.: Comprehensive care of the cognitively impaired elderly. In Eisdorfer, C., and Friedel, R. O., editors: Cognitive and emotional disease in the elderly, Chicago, 1978, Year Book Medical Publishers, Inc.

Libow, L.: Senile dementia and the "pseudodementias": clinical diagnosis. In Eisdorfer, C., and Friedel, R. O., editors: Cognitive and emotional disease in the elderly, Chicago, 1978, Year Book Medical Publishers, Inc.

Phillips, L.: A word about confusion. Unpublished manuscript, School of Nursing, University of Pittsburgh, Pittsburgh, 1973.

Phillips, L.: The imprisonment model. Unpublished manuscript, College of Nursing, University of Arizona, Tucson, 1976.

Phillips, L.: Sensory deficits among the confused elderly. Unpublished study. 1978.

Wolanin, M. O.: Confusion in the elderly. Paper presented at Gerontological Research Conference, Blue Mountain Lake, N.Y., 1973.

2

CONCEPTUAL PERSPECTIVES

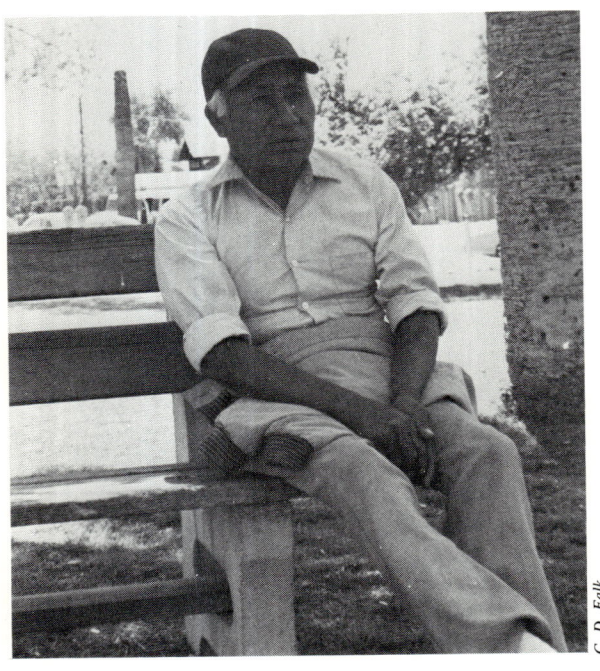

C. D. Falk

This chapter will develop a holistic model of confusion that will include biologic, perceptual, social, and cultural elements. Within this holistic framework, these elements will be viewed as stimuli that result in behavior responses and the need for adaptation. The cultural, perceptual, and social elements of confusion will be addressed most directly in this chapter. Although the biologic elements are viewed similarly, these elements will be considered in detail in Chapter 3. Based in part on the classic works of holists Goldstein and Angyal, this framework will be organized around several key concepts, which include the holistic nature of man and his reactions, individual organization, and the interaction process.

Fig. 2-1 illustrates our conceptualization of these concepts and their relationships to the cultural, perceptual, biologic, and social elements of man. In this figure, the central inner circle represents man's personal boundary across which the interaction process occurs. The shaded areas demonstrate the sphere of interaction, which extends beyond the individual into the environment to influence man's unique organization. It is impossible to separate the four elements of man from each other or from the individual and very difficult to portray the fluid nature of man's boundary and the relationships between elements. It is only for the purposes of discussion that man can be divided into boundaries and elements. A paradox exists in almost all of the writings about holism. The reader is first instructed to conceive of man as a whole, and then the authors proceed to divide man for discussion. To avoid this paradox, it might be helpful to look at Fig. 2-1 and to view the elements and concepts portrayed like facets of a gem stone. Like a gem, man has many facets, each of which can be identified and examined independently. However, as with the facets of a gem, man ceases to exist if even one facet is taken

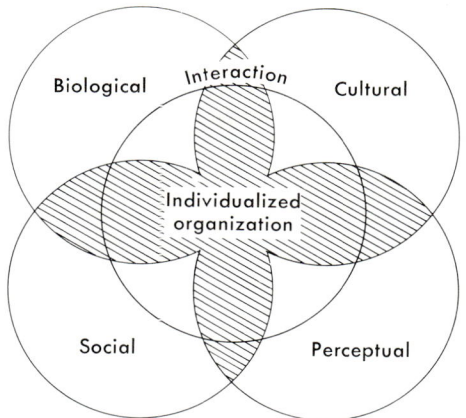

Fig. 2-1. Holistic nature of man.

away. Therefore, man is a whole being and reacts to the stimuli that impinge on one facet with the totality of all facets. Confusion is one example of this totality of reaction. As stated in Chapter 1, for the purposes of the conceptual framework, we will define confusion as a transient condition characterized by disorientation to time and place, incongruous conceptual boundaries, paranormal awareness, and seemingly inappropriate verbal statements.

Confusional states are seen among people who are not elderly or ill. For example, confusion in varying degrees is a reported symptom among prisoners of war (Bondy, 1943; Leighton, 1945; Vaughan, 1949), astronauts, explorers, and other types of prisoners (Shultz, 1967; Zubek, 1969; Brownfield, 1972). Healthy people report experiencing confusion in even more benign situations, such as during vacations and in shopping centers.

These people have certain factors in common with the others and also with many elderly people: (1) each is removed from his usual living situation that provides constant and predictable cues about the familiar world; (2) each is experiencing a certain amount of stress; (3) each has few means of escape from the situation; and (4) each is in a situation that has a certain amount of novelty associated with it. These similarities suggest that a holistic model of confusion can be based on the concepts of interaction, adaptation, and perception and how these are influenced in an environmental setting.

THE HOLISTIC NATURE OF MAN

Man is a unified being. As such, man interacts as a total individual with the total environment. This unity, as described by Tillich (1961), is the essence of the holistic position: "He (man) is a multidimensional unity: all dimensions distinguishable in experienced life, cross in him ... He does not consist of levels of being, but he is a unity which unites all dimensions" (p. 94).

The holistic model views behavior as a total expression of response to the stimuli that are impinging on man. If the organism perceives any stimulus as significant, that stimulus will produce a complex reaction involving the whole organism. Stimuli may arise out of the client's internal or external environment. From this perspective, physiologic, social, and cultural changes result in stimuli that necessitate new styles of adapting to and interacting with the environment. Failure to adopt new styles of adaptation results in many malfunctional behaviors, one of which is confusion.

The nurse is concerned with the client's reaction to what he perceives as total reality. Her task is to apprehend that reality as a holistic phenomenon and to help the client deal with it. As a 24-hour observer of human behavior, she has the opportunity to interact with people who are coping with all types of internal and external stimuli. Among elderly clients, confusion is one reaction to reality that the nurse and client must deal with frequently.

In 1939, Goldstein built one of the first theories of holism used in the field of medicine. From his work with brain-damaged patients, Goldstein recognized that no stimulus evoked a single or simple response. Rather, responses were exceedingly complex, involving the area stimulated and radiating to the whole organism. As a student of gestalt theory, Goldstein stated that not only is the perceptual field organized as an orderly whole, but the individual perceiving it "comes to terms" with the field or environment through interaction that is characterized by organized or preferred behavior. With this frame of reference, he formulated the following set of principles regarding the stimulus-response situation.

1. Since the total individual participates in any reaction, a change in any area results in simultaneous changes throughout the individual. A client experiencing pain provides an example of this totality of reaction. Even though the pain is confined to one part, a finger for example, the client's response to the pain is total. He will focus on the pain in his finger to the extent that all of his other behaviors will be influenced by this pain.
2. The total response of an individual to a stimulus depends on how significant the stimulus is to the individual. For example, the response of a client who believes that the pain in his abdomen is caused by appendicitis will probably be quite different from the client who believes that his pain is caused by cancer of the bowel.
3. A misconception of the environment at the sensory level will have consequences for the observable behavior of the whole individual. For example, if the client mistakes a shadow for an intruder, he will react as if the shadow really is an intruder. If he mistakes the pain of appendicitis for the pain of cancer of the bowel, he will react as if it really is cancer.
4. The effect of any stimulus can be evaluated correctly only if the observer is privy to knowledge concerning all of the other stimuli impinging on the individual as well as the total condition of the individual. The significance of appendicitis to a client, for example, can be judged accurately only if the observer is aware of all the implications that appendicitis has to that client within his social, cultural, biologic, economic, and historic setting.

Two terms coined by Goldstein are particularly useful to our discussion of confusion: ordered (preferred) behavior and disordered (catastrophic) behavior. Within man a dynamic relationship exists between excitation and constancy (Fig. 2-2.) It is as if a scale were present inside man, with constancy and excitation on two opposite ends of the pole. As stimulation impinges on man, from without or within, behavior is

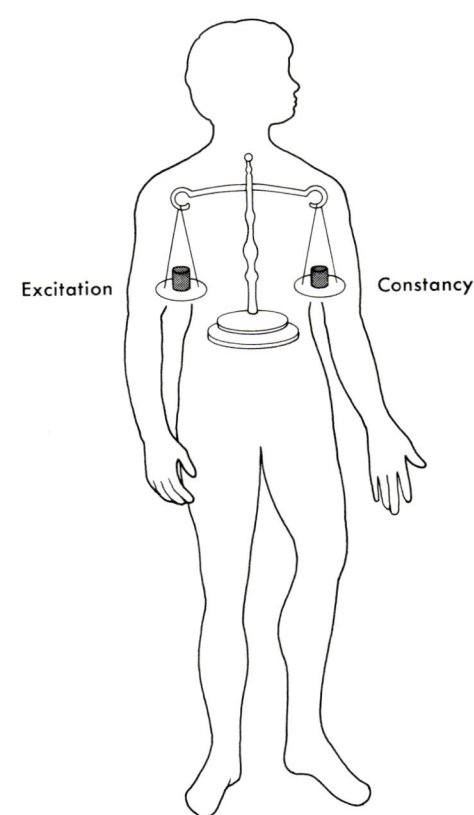

Fig. 2-2. Man in equilibrium. Excitation balances constancy equals ordered behavior.

ordered or balanced because man is able to maintain an equilibrium. To do this, as stimulation increases in one area (for example, in the work situation), man will attempt to block excitation in some other areas (for example, decreasing social engagements) and seek constancy in others (for example, organizing work space). The scale, then, remains in balance and behavior is ordered. In this model, adaptation occurs when the stimulus has effected a perceptual change and is either no longer perceived for its excitation qualities or man has learned to respond to the stimulus in a constant, successful manner.

In addition, according to Goldstein (1939), ordered behavior is the means by which the individual actualizes self. All ordered behavior, within all domains of the individual, is attributable to the ability of the individual to self-actualization through the media of internal and external environments. In short, ordered behavior is a testament to the individual's ability to adapt.

On the other hand, disordered or catastrophic behavior is evident whenever man is unable to equalize excitation and constancy (Fig. 2-3). Disordered behavior can result whenever the scale is tipped by either increased excitation or increased

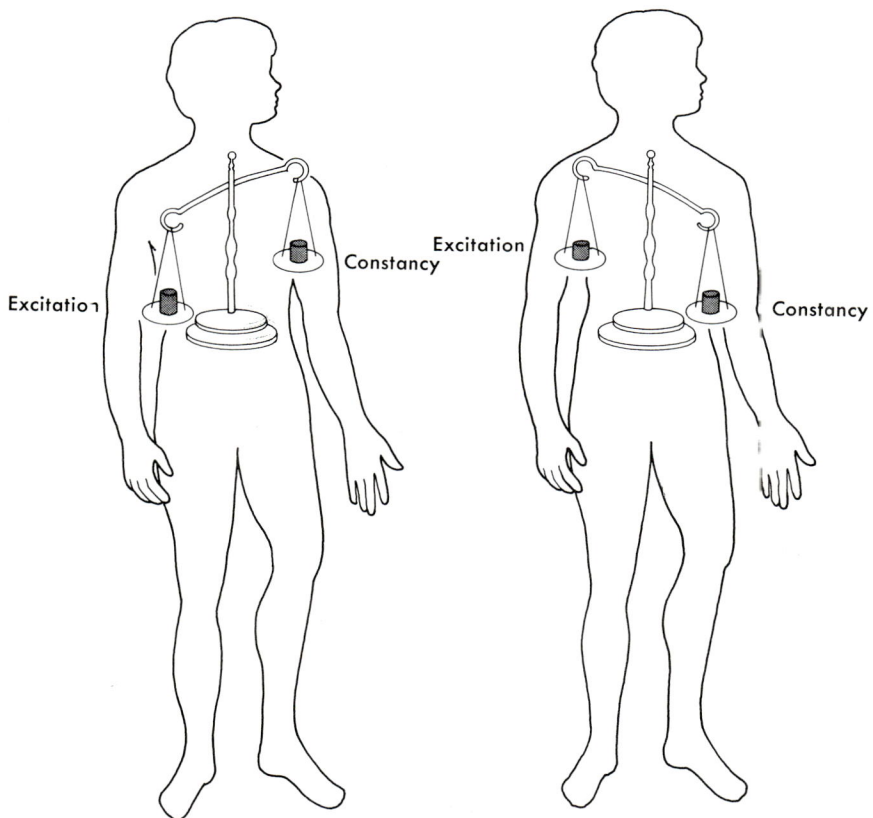

Fig. 2-3. Man in disequilibrium. Constancy overbalances excitation or excitation overbalances constancy equals disordered behavior.

constancy that is uncompensated in other areas. Catastrophic behavior is evident in both healthy and ill people. Under any circumstances, failure to "come to terms" with stimuli results in disordered or catastrophic behavior. Basically, catastrophe involves "... the danger of not being able to carry on even those performances which are essential ... for existence" (Goldstein, 1940, p. 89). The danger of catastrophic behavior lies not only in the situation or the task, but also in the fear of not reacting according to personal expectations and abilities. Catastrophic behavior is characterized by somatic and observable manifestations, such as sympathetic activation, apathy, anxiety, withdrawal, and confusion. It may progress to states of complete inability to cope. In catastrophe, the individual fails in those performances normally accomplished in an ordered state.

As with any age group, elderly people display catastrophic behavior. They are probably particularly vulnerable to catastrophe because of the nature of aging. "One of the most fundamental manifestations of aging is decreased homeostatic adaptation to environmental challenges" (Diamond, 1978, p. 66). For the aged, environmental challenges are superimposed on the primary physiologic changes of normal aging to produce a situation in which the aged have a compromised ability to interact with their environment and to effect ordered behavior. The elderly can become overwhelmed by the stimuli impinging on them and immobilized by the idea of not being able to react according to their expected capabilities. Whether young or old, however, it is the personal organization of the individual that determines whether a stimulus will produce ordered or catastrophic behavior.

INDIVIDUAL ORGANIZATION AND CONFUSION

"The person represents a dynamic organization of great fluidity.... Rearrangements and shifts of emphasis are continuously taking place in the process of living" (Angyal, 1948, p. 80). Although fluid and dynamic, man's personal organization is also governed by several principles that help explain behavior. Rogers (1970) identifies several of the principles that concern man's organization in general. They include: (1) "man is a unified whole possessing his own integrity and manifesting characteristics that are more than and different from the sum of his parts" (the holistic nature of man); (2) "man and environment are continously exchanging matter and energy with another" (the crucial relationship between man and his surroundings and its importance for the interaction process); and (3) "pattern and organization identify man and reflect his innovative wholeness" (organization as an essential quality of the human organism) (pp. 47, 54, 65).

In addition to general principles that explain man's organization, three principles have been identified that are of particular importance in a discussion of confusion.

1. *A part not functioning in accordance with the whole tends to be brought into harmonious function with the system.* Man does not comfortably tolerate a nonfunctioning or deviant part. To maintain organization and prevent catastrophe, compensatory function will be ascribed to the nonfunctioning part or to another part (Angyal, 1948). The following examples should help to illustrate this principle. If a client loses the use of one arm, he will most likely learn to function adequately in his environment by ascribing the functions of the lost arm to other parts of his body. If a client has aphasia, communication will become possible with him as he ascribes the function of communication to other means. The point at which compensatory function cannot be assigned to other parts is the point at which catastrophic behavior is displayed and catastrophe is experienced.

The implications of this principle for confusion are interesting. If, for example, a client loses the ability to remember recent events, he may compensate for the loss by any of the following means. He may (1) laugh about his inability to remember, (2) talk only about the remembered past in his remote memory, (3) withdraw completely, (4) deny the occurrence of the event in question, or (5) accuse those around him of lying about the event in question. Each of these five options is roughly comparable to the other, although the first is usually considered by caregivers to be a more "normal" response. None of the five necessarily indicates confusion. Rather, they all indicate an attempt to avert catastrophe by compensating for a loss of memory. Confusion enters the picture when the client is unable to compensate or has the uneasy subjective feeling of not being able to account for time.

Anosognosia is another interesting example of this principle. Anosognosia accompanies hemiplegia and is defined as the denial of ownership of a body part.

> The interplay of the patient's need to maintain his own sense of intactness and the altered way in which he perceives himself and can think about himself may lead to gross errors in identifying his environment, disorientation in time and space, mis-identification of those about him and elaborate confabulatory responses concerning his status (Ullman, 1964, p. 90).

The client displaying anosognosia may not be confused in the classic sense of the word but may be rather interpreting his body and his environment in a way that temporarily makes sense to him. He is averting catastrophe using his own frame of reference.

2. *If a position in the whole is perceived by the organism as unfilled, the organism will tend to fill it.* Disequilibrium experienced by the individual as the result of a deficit or need will be explained, even if this has to be accomplished by unconventional means (Angyal, 1948). For example, one night an elderly woman was admitted to the hospital and placed in a bed by the window. Below the window was the hospital emergency room, which had a red neon light flashing on and off that was reflected on the ceiling of the room. The woman began to cry and scream that the hospital was on fire. She was "filling" her perception of the unfamiliar stimulus of the flashing red light by naming it "flames on the ceiling." Confabulation is another example of the "filling" process, which is seen in many so-called confused patients. One elderly woman gave elaborate descriptions about her family members and the frequency with which they visited. She was filling her feelings of loneliness with stories about her family members who no longer existed. This filling process is the means by which many elderly people avert feelings of catastrophe and catastrophic behaviors. Unfortunately, as in the first example, often the familiar experiences used to fill in unexplained pieces can be more frightening than the reality.

3. *An open system will be perceived by the organism, will cause disquiet, and will be closed by the organism.* A person cannot tolerate the feeling of physiologic or psychologic incompleteness for long. The person will be motivated to seek completion or closure, even though completion is impossible and closure spells the end of the organism (Angyal, 1948). Hunger, for example, produces the feeling of incompleteness in the person. Even though the person will eat to fill the void, hunger again occurs. An example of this principle particularly evident among the elderly is the need for completing a life's work and the need for closure of affairs. It is often observed that upon completion, the person is then ready to die. Sometimes this almost compulsive need for closure is viewed by observers as evidence of confused behavior. In one nursing home, an elderly woman has been trying to finish a book for the past year. Although she is unable to see or hear adequately, she spends every day at her desk working. She sorts her papers and writes passages that she cannot even see to read. The staff views this behavior, which they openly call crazy, with amused tolerance. The need for closure and tasks that are seen to lead to closure help the person maintain a sense of order. Such tasks are seen by the person as displays of ordered behavior, even though others may not perceive the order and view the behavior as confused.

Thus, as stimuli impinge on an individual,

whether they will produce ordered behavior or catastrophe depends on certain principles of individual organization. If the stimulus can be interpreted and accounted for within the individual's knowledge, it is not likely to produce disordered behavior. And if the behavioral display is ordered, it will probably not be considered confused. For example, using a previous example, if the woman who was admitted during the night had been ambulatory and could have gotten from bed to determine the origin of the flashing light herself, the behavior she displayed probably would have been to go back to bed and fall asleep. Since, however, the stimulus could only be interpreted within her frame of reference—it looked like fire to her—her behavior became disordered. Under the first circumstance she would have been assessed as lucid; under the second, as confused.

To follow Angyal's work further, life is a dynamic and expanding process that involves the individual and the universe. There is no clear-cut boundary separating the environment from the individual. In fact, *it is impossible to separate the individual from the environment in space because both are entities in the total biologic process.* Angyal (1941) thought it would indeed be strange logic to classify food at one moment as a part of the environment and at the next as part of the individual, simply because of its physical location in the stomach cavity. Rather, the individual and the environment must be considered as one. Therefore, it is not only the internal organization of the individual that determines whether or not a stimulus will produce disordered behavior. It is also the organization of the interaction process between the individual and the environment.

THE INTERACTION PROCESS

The interaction between the individual and the environment occurs within a life space known as the biosphere (Angyal, 1941). The biosphere is an inseparable unit characterized by bipolar organization. The two poles of the biosphere are occupied by the subject (the individual), who is always striving for increased autonomy, and the object (the environment), which is constantly resisting the activity and energy of the subject. For the survival of both object and subject, a certain amount of tension must be maintained.

Essentially, the transactions within the biosphere are those of open systems. "Every living organism is essentially an open system. It maintains itself in a continuous inflow and outflow, a building up and breaking down of components, never being, so long as alive, in a state of chemical and thermodynamic equilibrium but maintained in a so-called steady state which is distinct from the latter" (Von Bertalanffy, 1968, p. 39). The exchanges within the biosphere are never chaotic because the organism possesses the capacity for self-regulation by which it maintains dynamic, rhythmic interaction (Hazzard, 1971).

Obviously, for survival, every individual takes in certain physical matter (oxygen, food, and water) and expels to the environment certain excreta (feces, urine, and carbon dioxide). However, other exchanges occur within the life space that are nonphysical and not so obvious. The individual could not survive without environmental cues taken in through sensory modalities, analyzed, and put out in the form of the appropriate action or inaction.

The idea of the interaction process is central to this discussion of confusion. How successful the client is in interacting determines whether or not he will be termed confused. Equally important, how successful the client is in interacting according to the expectations of others determines to a great extent if he will be judged as confused, whether he is or not. The interaction process has perceptual, sociologic, and cultural implications for the topic of confusion.

Perceptual implications

"Perception is an awareness of objects, persons, and situations. It is each individual's representation or image of reality" (King, 1971, p. 94). From birth to death, individuals are engaged in the business of perceptions. Through external stimulation they receive information via the sensory apparatus, through mentation they interpret the input, and through motor activity they act appropriately. By experience, individuals learn to deal with objects, and by remembering their experiences, they are able to acquire a store of information about the world (Ittleson, 1961). They begin to rely on constants in the world and learn to conform their reactions to their perceptions.

"We rely on things behaving reasonably, sensibly, and meaningfully... we can predict more or less correctly what will happen; and, more important still, we know what is the most effective way of reacting to it" (Vernon, 1971, p. 39). All human decisions and behaviors are based on the perceptions of the individual.

It is through perceptions that we begin to form concepts of reality. In essence, each of us expects the environment to behave in a certain predictable fashion. When we sense that it is not behaving appropriately, we are puzzled until we can resolve the incongruity. Our perception of reality is based primarily on our interpretation of the information our senses provide, as opposed to what society defines as reality. Therefore, any deficiency or distortion in the sensory mechanism can produce confusion.

"Knowledge of the identity of objects and features in the environment is obviously valuable to us. Not only does the apparent stability and permanence of most of them create a feeling of security; it also enables us to react to them rapidly and appropriately" (Vernon, 1971, p. 13). When our predictions about the world are incorrect and our reality is called into question, reaction time is slowed. And for the elderly, slowed reaction time itself is sometimes interpreted as confusion.

Essentially two important phenomena occur with aging that have implications for perceptions and for confusion. First, some of the most profound physiologic changes of aging occur to the sensory apparatus. Virtually every sense is in some way altered as the person ages. Therefore, the information about the world that the person receives is different and distorted (Chapter 10). Second, the constants in the world, on which the older person has based decisions and actions, change. Although the person expects to base present behaviors on the predictability of past experience, the world changes. The worlds of the person's childhood and adulthood are essentially gone. Each of us must learn daily about the new world in which we live. For the elderly, with preexisting difficulties with the sensory apparatus, learning becomes more and more challenging.

We may assume that since we each share overlapping life space (biospheres), the reality we experience is the same as the reality that everyone else experiences. Traditionally, reality has been divided into two domains: public data and private data. Public data consist of all items that are seen, heard, felt, tasted, and smelled by the general population. These data are symbolized and named in a way that is consistent for a culture, for example, chairs, tables, and clear days. Private data, on the other hand, include perceptions such as pain and fatigue. Although these are also named, they are experienced personally. The simplicity of these categories is deceptive. For example, it is extremely difficult with sensory experiences such as auditory, olfactory, and gustatory sensations to determine with any accuracy what is outside and what is inside the individual. The spatial location of these sensations is simply unclear (Von Bertalanffy, 1964). As a result, there is no assurance that our individual perceptions of these experiences are similar. It is the same with all of the objects in the public domain.

"Since the objects of the environment are formed under the influence of such highly variable factors as personal experience, one may say that every person has his own personal world consisting of objects... even if from the physical point of view the objects are identical" (Angyal, 1941, p. 159). We assume that we can make judgments about the degree to which someone else is perceiving "reality" and that our perceptions can be used as a yardstick against which to measure the perceptions of another. This is not true. Reality is a personal matter.

Although one presupposes that human beings live in the same world and thus perceive similar things, individuals differ in what they select to enter into their perceptual milieu. Their perceptual tools, sensory (functioning sense organs) and intellectual (brain process), vary from person to person. One's perception is related to past experience, self-concept, socioeconomic groups, biological inheritance, and educational background (King, 1971, p. 94).

At any given moment, the environment with which the individual interacts possesses a past, a present, and a future that enter into the interpretive process related to perceptions. In addition, the perceptual process is influenced by the person's physical and emotional needs at that moment. There are, therefore, no constant or universal realities.

Consider the concept of time as a universal reality. Often the extent of a person's confusion is judged based by his perception of time. For example, we say, "What day is it?" or "What month is it?" At the same time, we, the nonconfused ones, require clocks, calendars, and watches as constant reminders of the passage of time. Who has not had the experience of being on vacation, with no time reminders, and not being able to remember what day it is? Anyone who has moved to a sunny climate after having spent almost an entire life in parts of the country with seasonal changes has surely had the experience of being unable to remember what month it is. After all, December in Arizona looks very much like June in Illinois. Even time, a supposed universal reality, is only real to the extent that it is based on contextual landmarks. For the bored, time drags. For the busy, time flies.

Time is as variable and relative as each person's perception of it.

In addition, the passage of time has interesting consequences for the elderly. Wolanin (1978) uses the popular expression "time warp" to illustrate the peculiar consequences of time for the elderly. Time warp refers to the ability of any individual to "plug into" any period of the remembered past and relive it as if it were today. For the young person, the notion of time warp has limited implications; there are few years on which to draw. However, even for younger people, it is sometimes difficult to determine how much time has passed since an event. Hence, reunions and anniversaries hold significance. For the elderly client, 50 years may have passed since the event in question. He may, however, feel as if it occurred only recently. Time landmarks become blurred with the passage of time, particularly when the quality of today is colored by multiple losses and days that cannot be differentiated. Verb tense may be difficult to keep straight whenever "what was" is more personally significant than "what is."

Perception holds particular significance for confusion. If there is a change in the perceptual apparatus, the client experiences a distorted reality. Even if the perceptual apparatus is intact, the reality the client experiences is not identical to the reality of the nurse. To assume that the nurse's reality is the "true" reality and that the client's reality can be judged against this yardstick is essentially false. Rather, the "true" reality lies somewhere between the perceptions of the nurse and the perceptions of the client.

Sociologic implications

The nurse is an integral part of the biosphere of the clients for whom she cares. Her reactions and behaviors influence the behaviors of the client, just as every other person and feature of the environment does. Conversely, the client is part of the nurse's biosphere, and his reactions and behaviors influence her. Social scientists since Malinowski (1926) have recognized this "reciprocity of social interactions." Basically, reciprocity of social interactions means that in a social encounter, there is a fair exchange of sentiments, services, and behaviors that is approximately equal for each person involved. This is the law of distributive justice (Homans, 1961). In others words, during an exchange, each person will act in such a way that neither will be left with the feeling that he has given more or less than the other person. When a person feels he has given more than the other, anger is the result. When a person feels he has given less than the other, embarrassment results. People act to avoid these feelings. What the two people involved define as "fair exchange" is based on a number of factors, including the expectations and perceptions they each have of the other person's status, role, and capabilities. The following hypothetical examples should help to clarify this point.

Example 1. Ann Smith, age 34, is admitted to a hospital. She has had an automobile accident that has resulted in paraplegia. Although she cries frequently and is not making the progress expected, she is pleasant in her exchanges with the staff. She always says "thank you" and "please" and "I'm sorry you must do so much for me." She smiles gratefully when something is done for her. Although the staff expects she should be making more progress, based on their experiences with similar patients, they willingly do the things for her that she cannot do herself. Each of the people in this exchange defines the exchange as fair. Ann Smith is receiving the services she expects from the staff, and the staff is receiving the "payment" they expect from her in the form of positive sentiments (smiles and thanks). This exchange is operating according to the law of distributive justice.

Example 2. Ann Jones is admitted to a hospital. She is 34 and has had an automobile accident that has resulted in paraplegia. She cries and screams frequently. When the staff approach her to perform an activity, she refuses, swears, and orders them from her room. She is not making the progress the staff expects based on their experiences with other such patients. Beginning on day 2 of her admission, she is defined as "difficult." The nursing staff argue about who will care for her and express a great deal of anger about her to each other and occasionally to the patient herself. In this example, Ann Jones is violating the law of distributive justice. According to the staff's definition of the patient role and their expectations for certain types of payments (in the form of positive sentiments and progress), she is perceived as contributing nothing to the exchange. They are angry because they feel they are contributing more than she is.

Example 3. Ann Green, age 34, is admitted. She has had an automobile accident that has resulted in paraplegia. She cries and screams frequently. She swears at the staff and is unapproachable. However, she is making extraordinary progress. Within 2 weeks of admission she is performing all of her own activities of daily living. She is progressing so well that she will be discharged within the month. The staff's reaction to Ann is cautious. Although she can make them very angry, they tend to admire her progress. She is defined by the staff as difficult, but she is also said to be a "gutsy lady". In this example, the violation of the law of distributive justice is not so severe. Although the staff is not receiving the "payments" they expect in the form of positive sentiments, they are being rewarded by the rapid progress the patient is making. Based on their expectations, she is contributing as much to the relationship as they are, and her other behaviors can be tolerated.

Homans (1961) suggests that social exchange can be viewed as the chaining of behaviors in such a way that the behaviors of the participants are mutually stimulating and reinforcing to the other. Using a behaviorist's or operant model, Homans demonstrates that in a behavioral exchange between two people, the more positively reinforcing the behavior of one person is to the other, the more likely the reinforcing behavior is to stimulate further behavioral interaction. Conversely, the less reinforcing the behavior of one is to the other, the more likely the people are to initiate behaviors that will terminate or limit the amount of interaction. Homans is explicit that one of the most powerful reinforcement available in social exchange is sentiments, or those accepting signals that people send in the form of praise, smiles, and "open" body language. Hamans notes that the content of a behavioral exchange may not be nearly so important as the feeling, affect, and sentiment surrounding it.

The previous examples demonstrate that nurses and patients mutually reinforce and stimulate each other and that the notion of reciprocity and the chaining of behavior is in no way simple. The outcomes of interaction can be predicted or understood if the observer knows what each person in the exchange expects and perceives of the other person. The matter becomes even more complicated whenever the variable of chronologic age is considered. In the previous examples, the patient was 34 years old. Now consider the following example.

Example 4. Ann Smith, age 34, and Betty Jones, age 70, are both admitted to the hospital on the same day. Each has had an automobile accident that has resulted in paraplegia. All other things are equal, including their physiologic problems, social support systems, and previous life-styles (that is, both live alone and receive support from the government). Which woman will live independently again? Which has control in the situation? Which will become confused?

Of course, the answers to these questions are neither simple nor totally predictable. We can, however, for the purposes of illustration, follow the example to its conclusion. At least part of the answers to these questions lies within the interactional process and its reciprocity. Generally, the older the patient, the more likely he is expected to not make progress, to not be in control, and to not be lucid. The reinforcements that younger and older patients receive are, therefore, quite different.

To answer the first question, the younger Ann Smith is expected to make progress, and the staff's goals for the patient reflect this expectation. Even when she displays unpleasant behavior, as long as she progresses, her unpleasantness is tolerated, and her progress is reinforcing for both the staff and the patient. Betty Jones, on the other hand, is not expected to have such a high level of progress. Any progress that she makes is taken as a gift, and the staff's goals reflect this expectation. Undoubtedly, the progress itself is reinforcing to both the nurses and the patient, but so is lack of progress. Lack of progress confirms that the staff's expectations were accurate in the first place. As a result, we might expect that the younger patient is the more likely to again live independently.

Closely related to the expectations for progress are the expectations for control—the second question. Rehabilitation usually implies that control is gradually transferred to the individual being rehabilitated. The patient is expected to become more and more involved in his treatment plan and the decisions being made about his future. Ultimately, he becomes totally in control of his decisions and his life. Often, older people are viewed as incapable of being in control of their own affairs by simple virtue of their age. To protect them from their ineptness, decisions are made for them. An outsider often decides what is in their best interests, and their environment is shaped in accordance with the judgment. Consequently, in the institutional setting, more and more control is often taken from the older patient, unless he is capable of exerting his own authority or has an advocate to speak for him. Even then, the credibility of his judgment is often in question. For the younger person, however, more and more control is added in the name of rehabilitation; for the older person, it is taken away in the name of protection.

The idea of control is closely related to the idea of confusion—the third question. The older patient is expected, to some extent, to be or become confused. As opportunities for control and independent decision making are limited, situations in which he can demonstrate his capabilities are fewer. His credibility is first questioned by the nursing staff and later by himself. He becomes reinforced for passivity and dependence early in a hospitalization and is given few opportunities to act differently. For many institutionalized elderly, as the duration of hospitalization lengthens, the reinforcement cycle slips into a negative mode, whereby confused behaviors are positively reinforced and attempts at control and autonomy are negatively reinforced. For example, if he calls out or rings the bell too many times, he is segregated and ignored. If, however, he shrieks and lies on the floor, he is immediately reinforced by the attention of the nursing staff. The more bizarre the behavior, the more likely it is to bring attention (a form of reinforcement) from the staff. At other times, he is given attention for withdrawing behaviors. When he does not eat, the staff coaxes him. When he does not respond at all, the staff gives him attention to draw him out. The end result is positive reinforcement for behaviors that are both aberrant and withdrawn. Confusion can be viewed as withdrawal par excellence.

This process was demonstrated in a study by Phillips (1976) and will be discussed in more detail in Chapter 11. Generally, the study showed that through intermittent reinforcement, the nurse shaped confused behavior. The initial diagnosis of confusion was most often based on age, appearance, and language patterns and had little to do with behaviors. The patient was treated as confused, based on the preconceived notion that he was confused, and was consequently reinforced for inappropriate behaviors. The patient became confused as a response to a total social situation; his credibility was questioned before the nurse even met him. Socioligically speaking, a diagnosis of confusion can be made when no confusion exists, and confused behavior can be produced by reinforcement alone, all within the context of social interaction.

Cultural implications

Culture is assumed to be shared by all people who live in the same locale and share a common language. It is the ultimate of "public data." Culture is basically the frame of reference against which perceptions of reality are validated.

Culture has interesting implications for confusion. Jewell (1965), for example, presents an in-depth study of a Navaho Indian who was admitted to an Anglo psychiatric hospital with a diagnosis of catatonic schizophrenia. After investigating the Navaho culture, its code of social desirability, and the personality traits valued by the Navaho people, Jewell concluded that certain behaviors deemed by the medical personnel as symptomatic possibly arose because the diagnosticians were judging the man based on Anglo values. After breaking the language barrier, he found that the depression displayed by the patient was the result of an unfulfilled religious rite, which left the patient feeling vulnerable and unable to function. The withdrawal, which was considered symptomatic by the Anglos, was a socially desirable trait among the Navaho people. Even the flexibilitas cerea that was particularly diagnostic of catatonic schizophrenia seemed to result from the Indian believing that his "keepers" wanted him to hold grotesque positions for long periods, and he wanted to please. As a conclusion to this analysis of apparent pathologic confusion, Jewell states that "the cultural factor seems to be particularly important in reconciling overt behavior with covert personality dynamics" (p. 194).

The implications of this example are obvious. It is the conflict between Native American and Anglo culture and values. What about the more subtle difficulties that arise from cultural differences between aging people and their younger caregivers? These differences also give rise to many conflicts.

First, most elderly individuals alive today were not reared in technologic America. It is easy to forget that the culture and values of their youth were quite different from the culture and values of any other generation. Televisions were not common until the fifties, radios entered most homes in the late thirties, and even telephones were not a part of most people's lives until the thirties.

The 75-year-old learned about his body from 1902, when he was born, to the time he was a young adult in 1922. In all probability, the teachings of his mother persist in spite of a half a century of time. It is difficult in the 1970s to realize that while customs, manners, and morals have changed extensively, our older patients are more comfortable with the privacy and modesty they learned before sex was a three-letter word spoken freely (Phillips, 1977, p. 6).

The values, customs, manners, and morals learned in youth die hard. They continue to influence behaviors into adulthood and old age.

Sometimes, judgments that nurses make concerning an elderly person's "confused" behavior do not take into account the historic effects of aging. For example, elderly Americans who vividly remember the depression react differently to financial problems and the need to conserve personal resources than do their younger caregivers. One elderly woman was diagnosed as confused because she kept repeating that she needed to get up and clean out her refrigerator. Only by exploring her frame of reference did it come to light that she lived alone and had never before left her home for any period of time without first distributing her leftovers to her neighbors. She had been admitted to the hospital suddenly in the middle of the night with a fractured hip. Leaving food to spoil in her refrigerator was upsetting her to the point that she could speak of nothing else.

The historic influence on aging people has general implications for the aged. However, it is also a fallacy to consider the aged as a single homogeneous group that experienced historic events similarly. The person born in 1900 was 30 years old at the beginning of the depression. The person born in 1915, however, was 15 at the beginning of the depression. These people, although both over 65 today, belong to different generations and probably experienced this single historic event differently. For the person born in 1900, the depression probably meant financial disaster to him and his young family. For the person born in 1915, the depression probably had the most direct economic effect on his parents. However, the personal effect of the depression for the person born in 1915 probably influenced many of the important life decisions made in adolescence and young adulthood, such as educational options, career choice, and marriage. The *cohort effect* is often used to describe this differential effect of one historic event on a group of people who share an approximate birth year or generation. Generations are shaped by culture and usually span only about 10 years. The cohort effect has differential implications for people of different generations. The same standards cannot be used to judge the behavior of people belonging to different generations. All people between 65 and 95 cannot be lumped together as if they were a homogeneous group.

The relationship of a person to culture also has effects on observable behavior. One older woman in a nursing home was considered to be confused because she spent almost her entire day changing her clothing. Before every meal, she would retire to her room and change her clothes. Within her personal culture, a "lady" never appeared during the afternoon in "morning clothing." Nor would a lady appear for the evening meal dressed for afternoon visiting. She was simply living out the life-style to which she was accustomed and playing by the rules of the culture she knew. The nurses were judging her behavior based on their own cultural conceptualizations. Fig. 2-4 illustrates this point nicely. This photograph was taken by a newspaper photographer at a sporting event. The gentleman in the center of the picture is dressed in a white shirt, tie, and hat, as opposed to the younger people around him who are in shirt-sleeves. This gentleman is adhering to the culture he knows despite the informality that is currently the norm.

Culture is the underlying frame of reference that gives the meaning to words used in the culture (Spradley and McCurdy,

Conceptual perspectives 23

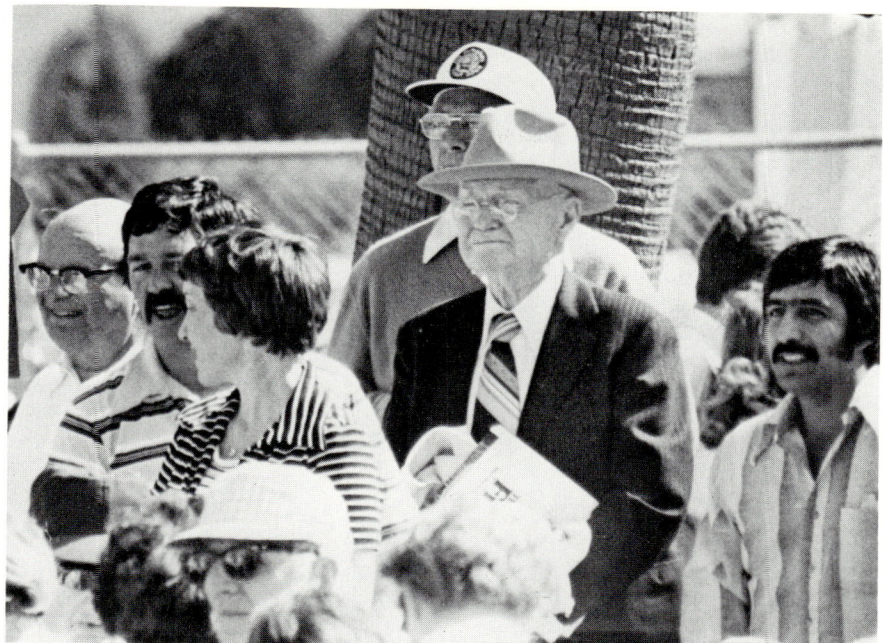

Fig. 2-4. An older gentleman at a sporting event. (Photo courtesy of the Tucson Citizen, Tucson, Arizona, 1979.)

1972). Therefore, even words have different meanings for the elderly individual. For the most part, elderly people do not share a common language of slang with their younger caregivers. Words can have very different meanings based on age and environment. The result is confusing for young and old. Even a 30-year-old can relate to not being a part of the word culture of today's 16-year-old.

Language and words have other interesting implications for elderly people. A phenomenon observed frequently in the sick elderly is the use of metaphoric or symbolic language. This phenomenon is often interpreted as confusion. For example, one patient of 86 spoke articulately on every subject except her family. If that topic was broached, she said, "They have poisoned me and now I am sick." The staff thought her to be quite paranoid and confused, not considering her history. She had cared for her own home and one grown son until 5 years before. At that time he decided to marry, quite late in life, and moved his mother into a small apartment of her own. The rest of the children had supported this move. The patient was terribly angry about the entire affair and had refused to speak to any of her children since. Hence, she was "poisoned by the children." Was she confused?

Another patient, who was quite ill and near death, responded frequently to the nurses with the following:

Thou go not, like a quarry-slave at night,
Scourged to his dungeon, but, sustained and
  soothed
By an unfaltering trust, approach thy grave
Like one that wraps the drapery of his couch
About him, and lies down to pleasant dreams.*

---
*William Cullen Bryant, *Thanatopsis*.

Sometimes she would say only part of the passage, and at other times she would recite the entire passage. She was originally considered to be confused until someone on the staff recognized this passage as *Thanatopsis*. Her words could then be interpreted as her statement regarding what she was experiencing and her impending death.

There is great variation, therefore, in the public domain in what is defined culturally as reality. A person's relationship to culture has historic and personal implications. The cohort effect of aging cannot be overlooked. It cannot be assumed that cultural reality is universally experienced and perceived in similar ways. In short, the degree to which one person can make a judgment about another person's reality is questionable.

SUMMARY

We have developed a holistic model of confusion that has focused on the perceptual, social, and cultural elements of man. The fourth element, biologic, will be discussed in Chapter 3. Man responds to stimuli as a total being. Confusion is one example of catastrophic behavior that arises whenever man cannot "come to terms" with the stimuli from without or within. Therefore, confusion cannot be viewed as a disease state but rather as a response that is secondary to some cause. Because man is ever changing and is faced with a constantly changing environment, confusion enters the picture whenever there is a problem with adaptation to stimuli and the responses of the past are inadequate for the demands of the present.

REFERENCES

Angyal, A.: Foundations for a science of personality, New York, 1941, The Commonwealth Fund.
Angyal, A.: The holistic approach to psychiatry, Am. J. Psychiatry **105**:178-182, 1948.
Bondy, C.: Problems of internment camps, J. Abnorm. Social Psychol. **39**:4-9, 1943.
Brownfield, C. A.: The brain benders, New York, 1972, Exposition Press.
Diamond, M. C.: The aging brain: some enlightening and optimistic results, Am. Sci. **66**:66-71, 1978.
Goldstein, K.: The organism, New York, 1939, American Book Co.
Goldstein, K.: Human nature in the light of psychopathology, Cambridge, 1940, Harvard University Press.
Hazzard, M. E.: An overview of systems theory, Nurs. Clin. North Am. **6**:385-393, 1971.
Homans, G.: Social behavior: its elementary forms, New York, 1961, Harcourt, Brace and World, Inc.
Ittleson, W. H., editor: Perceptual changes in psychopathology, New Brunswick, 1961, Rutgers University Press.
Jewell, D. P.: A case of psychotic Navaho Indian male. In Skipper, J. K., and Leonard, R. C., editors: Social interaction and patient care, Philadelphia, 1965, J. B. Lippincott Co.
King, I.: Toward a theory of nursing, New York, 1971, John Wiley & Sons, Inc.
Leighton, A.: The governing of men, Princeton, N. J., 1945, The Princeton University Press.
Malinowski, B.: Crime and custom in savage society, London, 1926, Harcourt.
Phillips, L. R.: The imprisonment model. Unpublished manuscript, 1976.
Phillips, L. R.: Assessment of the well elderly. Unpublished paper presented at the Gerontological Society Meeting, San Francisco, November 1977.
Rogers, M. E.: An introduction to the theoretical basis of nursing, Philadelphia, 1970, F. A. Davis Co.
Spradley, J. P., and McCurdy, D. W.: The cultural experience, Kingsport, 1972, Science Research Associates.
Schultz, D. P.: Sensory restriction: effects on behavior, New York, 1967, Academic Press, Inc.
Tillich, P.: The meaning of health perspectives in biology and medicine **5**:94, 1961.
Ullman, M.: Disorders of the body image after stroke, Am. J. Nurs. **64**:89-91, 1964.
Vaughan, E. H.: Community under stress: an internment camp culture, Princeton, N. J., 1949, The Princeton University Press.
Vernon, M. D.: The psychology of perception, ed. 2, Baltimore, 1971, Penguin Books, Inc. Reprinted by permission of Penguin Books, Ltd.
Von Bertalanffy, L.: The mind-body problem: a new view, Psychosom. Med. **26**:29-45, 1964.
Von Bertalanffy, L.: General systems theory foundations, development, applications, New York, 1968, George Braziller. Reprinted by permission of the publisher, George Braziller, Inc.
Wolanin, M. O.: Personal communication, 1978.
Zubek, J. P., editor: Sensory deprivation: fifteen years of research, New York, 1969, Appleton-Century-Crofts.

3

THE PATHOPHYSIOLOGY OF CONFUSION

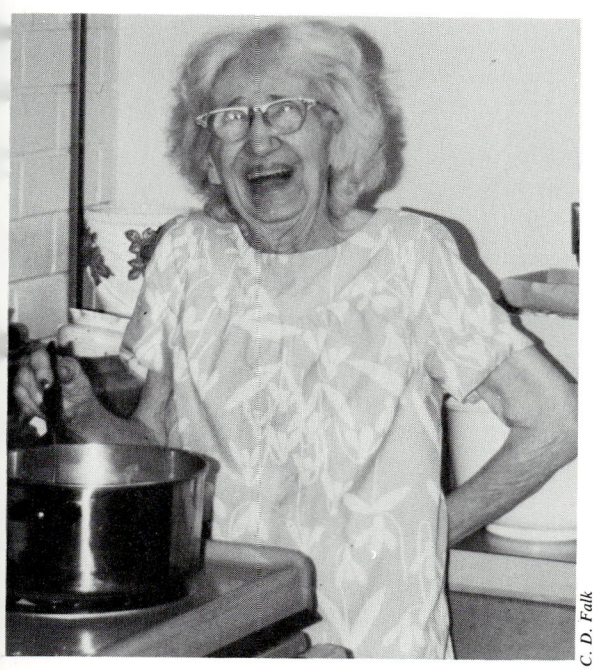

In this chapter we will review some of the more promising literature of pathologic conditons found in elderly persons exhibiting confusion. The underlying concept is brain failure (Isaacs, 1978) and Goldfarb's concept of poor cerebral support (1975), which results in brain failure. Brain failure may result from lack of nutrients, increased intracranial pressure, temperature changes, and fluid and electrolyte changes with dehydration and from drug toxicity. Mechanical problems may interfere with blood flow to the brain. Current researchers are reporting important studies of the brain hormones and slow-acting viral infections. However, findings in the whole field vary greatly; investigators reach conclusions that are diametrically different. Chapter 9 will be devoted to the nursing care of the client who is suffering from confusion secondary to problems that arise from pathology described in this chapter.

Goldfarb (1975) believes that normal decline in capacity for mental functioning progresses to the point of recognition only when accelerated by illness or physical impairment. His theory of poor cerebral support is based in part on Cannon's classic homeostasis theory, wherein the body strives to maintain physiologic equilibrium within narrow parameters. For the brain, as for other tissues of the body, a fairly narrow range of temperature, pressure, nutrients, fluid, and chemicals and minerals is required. Maintenance of the optimum internal environment to support the brain processes can be interrupted by three principal means:

1. Systemic problems that interfere with cerebral support (brain cell metabolism)
2. Mechanical problems, such as obstruc-

tion to flow in the vascular system, which deprives the brain of nutrients
3. Presenile irreversible dementias

SYSTEMIC PROBLEMS

The classification of systemic problems roughly follows a classification used by Verwoerdt (1976), in which he suggests that brain damage be broken into organic-cerebral factors and extracerebrosomatic factors. The latter include diseases that arise in adult years and have an adverse effect on the brain. Since these arise from outside the brain, they are treatable from outside. Etiology should be studied to determine which classification is being involved. Systemic disorders must be treated on the basis of the pathology, which is general, and not confined to the brain.

Hypoxia

The average healthy brain consumes oxygen at the rate of 3.5 cc/100 g of tissue/minute. This is equivalent to 20 percent of the total oxygen consumption of the whole body, or approximately 25 times as much as needed by a comparable unit of skeletal muscle tissue. There is no storage depot for oxygen in the brain, and it is dependent on a constant supply. Brain cells cannot survive longer than a few minutes without oxygen. The term hypoxia is used to describe an oxygenation abnormality, since it refers to an inadequate supply of oxygen to the brain tissue. It is often confused with hypoxemia, which is a decrease in the partial pressure of oxygen in arterial blood (Mitchell, 1977). Hypoxia may result from hypoxemia, for oxygen supply to the tissue is maintained both by cardiac output and by the amount of oxygen carried per unit of blood. Hypoxemia may result from low ambient oxygen, respiratory depression, various pulmonary disease states, and anemia. Hypoxia also results from inadequate perfusion of the brain tissue, ischemia secondary to hypotension, cardiac failure, and cerebrovascular insufficiency.

Timiras (1972) says that in a general sense the aging brain can be viewed as hypoxic. She compares the overt neurologic symptoms of hypoxia in the aged to symptoms resulting from high altitude sickness: impairment of memory, irritability, insomnia, and impairment of visual and motor performance. Rossen and others (1961) report that the healthy aged brain does not respond so acutely to abrupt decreases in arterial saturation as the young brain, a finding that may reflect the aging brain's adaptation to a relatively hypoxic state. The brain tissue may exist in a relatively hypoxic state, which is not clinically discernible until some event decreases the available oxygen supply either by increasing tissue demands or by limiting the supply.

Rossen and associates also report that brain impairment from hypoxia does not always have a poor prognosis, especially when the underlying systemic problem resulting in impairment is treated, controlling the mental deterioration. Contributing factors may be identified and measures taken to prevent further deterioration. Nutritional deficiencies, such as a lack of vitamin B_{12}, cardiac decompensation, hypotension (often secondary to prescribed medications), hypothyroidism, and respiratory disease, can all be treated with improvement in mental status when they are primary contributors to the hypoxia. Thirteen percent of acute myocardial infarctions come to medical attention primarly as confusional states (Butler and Lewis, 1977).

Hypoglycemia

In addition to a constant supply of oxygen, the brain cells require a constant supply of glucose. The "language" of the neurons in sensory, cognitive, and motor functions is primarily electrical. The energy for electrical activity is ultimately based on the oxidative phosphorylation of glucose in the mitochondria as a main substrate of cellular energy metabolism in the brain. There is no storage depot for glucose in brain tissue. Since the electrical activity of the brain is based on energy metabolism, it is possible that if blood flow, oxygen, or glucose to the brain is decreased or disrupted, the metabolism of the cell may cease, resulting in brain-cell death. Consequently, age-related decline in intracellular metabolism may also result from decreased rates of mitochondrial oxidative phosphorylation as a fundamental process of aging (Brody, Harman, and Ordy, 1975). Glucose is not only important for energy production, but also for the synthesis of vital proteins, amino acids, and the physiologically active amines of nerve cells.

Hypoglycemia may prove to be the ultimate disaster in the elderly (Riffkin and Ross, 1971). Diabetes in the elderly is more likely to be the adult-onset type, which is not usually treated with insulin. Many physicians use oral hypoglycemics such as tolbutamide and chlorpropamide as treatment. The long half-life of chlorpropamide may produce cumulative effects that result in prolonged hypoglycemia. Similar results may arise from tolbutamide. The onset of severe lowering of blood sugar may not be preceded by the neurologic signs resulting from increased epinephrine output, such as the nervousness, anxiety, and sweating found in the insulin-dependent person. Instead, the older person with hypoglycemia may show episodes of bizarre behavior, slurring of speech, disorientation, confusion, nightmares, crying out during sleep, and inability to be easily aroused. Chronic organic mental syndromes may result from repeated unrecognized episodes and may still be correctable if the cause is removed.

Hyperglycemia

Metabolic acidosis of the insulin-dependent diabetic person whose blood sugar is high may also be found in the elderly. Some elderly forget to inject their insulin, or with failing vision, inject the wrong dose or even air. Emotional or physical stress may trigger acidosis, or hyperglycemia may result from certain drugs that are frequently prescribed for the elderly: nicotinic acid, diuretic agents such as the benzothiazides, ethacrynic acid, and furosemide. Hyperglycemia and ketonemia result in an osmotic diuresis, with loss of body water and electrolytes (Riffkin and Ross, 1971). Change in mental status is one of the earlier symptoms of the interference with cerebral blood flow, which occurs with hypovolemia and hypotension of dehydration.

Hyperglycemic, nonketotic coma or a hyperosmolarity syndrome is more often found with the adult-onset type of diabetes found in the elderly. A profound impairment of awareness may be the first symptom. This is commonly followed by seizures. The blood sugar may be 1000 mg/100 ml, or over. Glycosuria may be present without the sign of ketosis (Alpers and Mancall, 1971). The dehydration that accompanies hyperosmolarity may be the origin of the neurologic abnormalities and may be associated with intracellular dehydration. There is a high mortality rate for elderly people with this syndrome, since treatment is complicated by their other physical problems. Fluids and electrolytes must be replaced without precipitating cardiac failure.

Also found in elderly diabetic patients is a confusional state with a nonketotic hyperosmolarity syndrome, which may be induced by drugs such as phenytoin (Libow, 1978).

Dehydration—fluid and electrolyte imbalance

Dehydration is a sign of lassitude and confusion in many older people, and conversely, confusion and lassitude are signs of dehydration. Thirst is often not recognized or is ignored by the elderly. Weakness and lack of accessibility to fluids may interfere with the normal channels of maintaining fluid intake, resulting in a dehydration that can be measured by the increased blood urea nitrogen. Normal values should not exceed 60 mg/100 ml of blood. If the sodium level is normal, simple oral fluid administration can restore hydration, but when electrolyte imbalance occurs, as with diuretic administration, hypokalemia may be present and weakness, lassitude, and even paralysis (Rossman, 1971). Dehydration should be suspected in any patient whose condition has a high degree of prostration, hazy mentation, and an unknown history.

Hypernatremia is another form of hyperosmolarity syndrome (Libow, 1978). It can result from inadequate fluid intake, overtranquilization, high protein mixtures used in tube feedings, or loss of fluid, as in excess of salt in sweating.

Not only can the elderly person who lives alone or who is not well cared for at home become dehydrated, but the institutionalized person may easily become the victim of iatrogenic dehydration during preparation for diagnostic tests or surgery. The elderly person who is marginally hydrated can pass into a state of dehydration rapidly if purged for gastrointestinal radiographic series. The laxative habit with large, loose stools or a short period of vomiting and diarrhea can lead to rapid dehydration. Dehydration cannot be understood without being aware of accompanying electrolyte losses and imbalances. The pathogenesis may not be clearly understood, but a dehydration encephalopathy may lead to mental changes that will cause an elderly person to be labeled "confused and disoriented." The lassitude can result in less than usual interest in the surrounding world and an indifference to events, which can be interpreted as confusion.

Hypercalcemia

Calcium acts as an alkaline buffer and helps to maintain a normal plasma pH (Wachman and Berstein, 1968). One hypothesis is that there is a continuous removal of small amounts of calcium from the bone throughout life to combat chronic acidosis. This is particularly true in advancing age. Libow (1978) finds that hypercalcemia may be present but not recognized until a confusional state results. It is found particularly in older people with an elevated serum calcium in metastatic carcinoma of the lung or breast, multiple myeloma, Paget's disease, and primary hyperparathyroidism. The immobile elderly person or the person on diuretic therapy are both vulnerable to confusion from hypercalcemia.

Hypocalcemia

Hypocalcemia is more frequently associated with malabsorption states and renal failure, but Libow (1978) states that the diagnosis of hypoparathyroidism may be overlooked in confusional states that are secondary to hypocalcemia.

Endocrine dysfunction

Timiras (1971) views the entire endocrine system as an integral functional unit rather than as an association of functionally independent structures. Therefore, an impairment of adaptive responses with aging could result from the failure of a specific function involved primarily with the control of homeostasis. The thyroid hormone has been more extensively studied than any other, even though much current research is being done on the adrenals and brain hormones. The thyroid hormones are important for their oxidative function.

The features of senescence are similar to the hypothyroid state: dryness of skin, diminished motor activity, impaired muscle strength, diminished resistance to cold, sparseness of hair, and lack of mental alertness. Rossman (1971) presents a picture of the elderly person with hypothyroidism as having grave neurologic signs and symptoms: cerebellar ataxia, auditory nerve degeneration, peripheral neuropathy, and mental sluggishness or torpor. Psychologic alterations are common in the person with myxedema and may range from apathy and depression to stupor and dementia (Schettler and Boyd, 1969). Other clinical signs may not accompany the psychosocial and mental alterations, so a thyroid evaluation is an important part of the diagnostic workup of the elderly person with progressive dementia. Unless treatment is initiated early, some degree of mental impairment may remain permanently.

Thyrotoxicosis is often not recognized in the elderly, because evidence of increased thyroid activity may be absent except for heart failure. Over the age of 50, even mild hyperthyroidism is likely to be associated with congestive heart failure and atrial fibrillation (Rodstein, 1971). The confusional states associated with hyperthyroidism may be based on hypoxia secondary to cardiac failure to perfuse the brain.

Accidental hypothermia

Lipton (1978) warns that older people may not sense cold as easily as younger people and that their ability to regulate body temperature is reduced. Some older people may feel comfortably warm although their bodies are cold. Lipton has studied accidental hypothermia of the elderly, which refers to events when a person falls and lies on the floor for some time in a room with low ambient temperature. British researchers who have studied accidental hypothermia for several years find that people over the age of 65 are vulnerable even in a mildly cool environment of 60° to 65° F (15.5° to 18.3° C). Heat loss from the body can occur rapidly. Allen (1974) gives the level of core temperature at which confusion begins as 93.2° to 95° F (34° to 35° C); however, sluggishness and lack of response is found at 96.8° F (36° C) core temperature.

Lipton is investigating the effects of alcohol, which accelerates loss of body heat, and of such drugs as imipramine, salicylates, pyrazolines, and related drugs that have an impact on body temperature control in warm-blooded animals. Exton-Smith and Windsor (1971) believe that phenothiazines in large doses have a direct influence on thermoregulation. Confused patients are often given this class of drugs for their confused state, but the drug tends to make them physically unstable and prone to falls.

Body functions take place within a very narrow range of temperature, with the normal person having a range of 97° to 104° F (36° to 40° C). The upper level is rarely reached, except in events that produce large amounts of body heat. American thermometers do not register body temperature below 94° to 96° F (34.4° to 35.5° C), so the core temperature at which the danger level is reached can only be inferred when the clinical thermometer does not register.

Sadakali and Owor (1974) studied hypothermic people in Uganda, where the ambient temperature was high, and immobility was not a cause for hypothermia. Their finding was that hypoproteinemia was associated with hypothermia in any age group. Older people, especially frail ones, are often malnourished and most likely to have hypoproteinemia. It is also related to poor economic conditions and inadequate dentition.

Hyperthermia

The range for hyperthermia with confusion begins at a body temperature 101.3° F (38.5° C) or higher. The older person exhibits confused behavior at a much lower temperature than the younger adult and will often display visual hallucinations. Thermoregulatory centers in the elderly do not offer the early warning signals of temperature change. Often the older person will not even be aware of higher or lower body temperature to remedy the situation. The sweat glands, which are reduced in number, may not act as an evaporative cooling system when the older person is subjected to higher ambient temperatures. When environmental temperatures rise above the body temperature, hyperthermia is most likely to occur in the elderly. Patients with cerebral atherosclerosis or with diabetes are more likely to be hyperthermic, which indicates that there are circulatory changes that involve the thermoregulatory centers of the brain (Agate, 1971). Destructive lesions in the hypothalmus generally produce hyperthermia (Alpers and Mancall, 1971).

Hypotension

Goldfarb (1975) states that a prophylactic measure for confusional states in the elderly requires guarding against periods of hypotension. Agate (1971) relates hypotension to circulatory disturbances, use of antihypertensive drugs, phenothiazines, diuretic therapy, and hypokalemia. Postural hypotension is found in one of ten elderly hospitalized patients (Wollner, 1966) and is associated with deficient baroceptor reflexes and serum sodim levels at or below normal limits. Hypotension is also found in the anesthetized or postsurgical elderly patient, and the length of the period of hypotension can be related to the postsurgical confusion.

Drug-related intoxications

The use of such drugs as barbiturates, tranquilizers, and compound analgesics containing phenacetin has been implicated in confusional states in the elderly. Exton-Smith and Windsor (1971) find that there are very few powerful drugs that do not affect the central nervous system. In the young with intact nervous systems this may not prove serious, but in old age the response is a confusional state. Exton-Smith and Windsor relate this drug action to the effect on the homeostatic mechanisms, so the physiologic balance becomes precarious. They cite the effect to the thermoregulatory mechanisms, through action on the autonomic nervous system, and to respiratory depression. Hurwitz (1969) found that patients over the age of 60 had 2.5 times the number of adverse drug reactions as those under 60. With reduced renal excretion one group of patients, with an average age of 70, exhibited a metabolic half-life for aminopyrine that was twice that of a group under the age of 30 (Jori, DiSalle, and Quadri, 1972). This may lead to prolonged drug action or toxic drug reactions.

Any consideration of drugs must include alcohol. Simon, Epstein, and Reynolds (1968) found that in a sample of 526 consecutive patients over 60 admitted to a psychiatric ward, 28% had a serious problem with alchoholism, although that was not the reason for admission. Rossman (1971) shows alcoholism as the most common cause of aneurin deficiency (thiamine) in the Western world. It is accompanied by neuropathy and encephalopathy, as demonstrated by Korsakoff's syndrome, with disorientation, amnesia, and confabulation, or by Wernicke's encephalopathy. Carlen and others (1978) demonstrated that chronic alcoholism is associated with cerebral atrophy (not from dehydration), as shown by computed tomography. Using brain scans of patients before and after abstaining from alcohol, they were able to demonstrate reversal of cortical atrophy by measuring the ventricular and sulcal size. On admission the patients had shown severe clinical mental impairment, but at the time of the second scan, 32 to 97 weeks later, they showed moderate to marked improvement. There was no improvement in those patients who continued drinking. This finding tends to associate cortical atrophy and mental impairment.

There is voluminous literature on the area of drug intoxication. We have reported only a few of the salient outcomes.

Pernicious anemia

Pernicious anemia (macrocytic-normochromic anemia) is almost exclusive to old age (Clifford, 1971). It is a disease of the entire hematopoietic apparatus and the general cellular metabolism. Intrinsic factor, which appears to be a glycoprotein substance formed in the fundus of the stomach, binds the vitamin B_{12} in the food that is eaten, protecting it from competitive binding with other substances. Receptor sites for vitamin B_{12} are in the terminal ilium, where it is liberated from the intrinsic factor and stored in the liver as vitamin B_{12} coenzyme. From there it is released to the bone marrow and other sites of metabolic activity. Vitamin B_{12} is essential for the maintenance of the integrity of the central nervous system; deficiency of this vitamin is related to demyelinization of the nerve cells (Clifford, 1971). The neurologic symptoms may occur before the anemia; these include changes in mental status, such as forgetfulness, confusion, depression, and irritability. Such symptoms are found in 60% to 65% of patients with pernicious anemia (Alpers and Mancall, 1971).

Pellagra

Pellagra, a dietary deficiency, is caused in part by a lack of nicotinic acid (niacin) in the diet, although lack of tryptophan and coexisting deficiencies of other vitamins cannot be ruled out (Alpers and Mancall, 1971). In addition to gastrointestinal and dermatologic symptoms, there is a polyneuropathy that is often accompanied by depression, confusion, and even frank dementia. The pathologic findings are changes in nerves, with patchy losses of myelin sheaths and axis cylinders. A syndrome that may be related to pellagra is nicotinic-acid–deficient encephalopathy, which involves mental confusion associated with cogwheeling rigidity. The precise nature of the syndrome is not known, and its presumed relationship to nicotinic acid is unsubstantiated at this time.

Butler and Lewis (1977) state that many elderly people are undernourished and that they develop reversible brain syndromes associated avitaminosis, pellagra, and other metabolic disorders. Even the middle- and upper-class elderly may be malnourished.

Terminal drop theory

Kleemeier (1962) noted that there were substantial declines in performance of dying people in relation to cognitive ability. He labeled the phenomenon "terminal drop." Psychologists have studied this influence on learning tasks and intelligence tests and determined that there are "nonintellective" variables such as physical health and motivation that may be responsible for the intellectual changes (Elias and others, 1977). The terminal drop hypothesis calls attention to the changes in intellectual function at the end of life and associates it with the physiologic changes that precede death. While age itself had been the variable in intellectual decline, this hypothesis denies time as a cause and puts the emphasis on the physiologic changes at the end of life.

Seigler (1975) suggests that study of cohort groups might better be based on time to death instead of time from birth, which is the present basis. His work in reviewing eight studies concludes that five of the eight supported a positive relationship between survivorship and a high level of cognitive performance at a given measurement point (Elias and associates, 1977). The studies indicate that some intervening disease process can usually be identified when individuals show a sharp decline in performance between testings (for example, 10 or more points on Wechsler Adult Intelligence Scale [WAIS] performance) (Seigler, 1975; Palmore and Cleveland, 1976).

Palmore and Cleveland (1976) suggest that rather than terminal drop, the terminology should be "terminal decline." Botwinick, West, and Storandt (1978) have described a battery of tests that correlated with measures of social activity and demographic characteristics in predicting who would die. Their classifications discriminated the differences correctly in 66% of the cases.

Intellectual decline associated with physical decline preceding death offers an important field for research in the future. At this time pathogenesis for intellectual decline has not been established, but the discussion of systemic causes of confusion can be enriched by this research, which crosses disciplinary lines and unites those who can relate clinical findings to intellectual declines. Caregivers of the dying patient have recognized that development of confusion is a prodromal sign of death.

Stress

The use of stress as a physiologic concept suffers from its many connotations, which tend to vary by discipline. However, the Selye construct described a reactive physiologic state. Stress, as used by behavioral scientists, connotes a certain amount of anxiety in its definition. It is recognized as a physiologic state that can be measured by heart rate, palm sweat, respiration, and vasomotor and galvanic skin reactions. Cross-disciplinary studies that focus on the effects of stress on the human organism are lacking in number and quality. Eisdorfer (1978) uses a more general approach, in which he defines stress as a reaction to physical, psychologic, and social stimuli, with responses that can be grouped into three categories: (1) physical response, (2) behavioral response, and (3) subjective states. Many researchers link stress to disease both as cause and as effect. The underlying assumption, according to Eisdorfer, which concerns relationship between life events and susceptibility to illness, is that life changes require adaptations. Adaptations are stressful depending on the magnitude of change.

Mason (1975) isolates the sympathetic adrenal medullary subsystem, which stimulates catecholamine secretion in response to psychosocial factors. This furnishes the link between the nonpathogenic stimulus and the pathophysiologic effect. It is a suggestion, rather than a cause-and-effect relationship, that explains the confusional state accompanying a high degree of stress in persons of any age. The well-known tunnel, even pinhole, vision of the person undergoing grave psychologic stress has been used to explain the confusional state that accompanies stress. Peplau (1963) described four levels of anxiety: mild, moderate, severe, and panic. In severe anxiety or panic, produced by a stressor that has either physical or ego threat, perceptual abilities are decreased. Cognitive processes are not used to gain relief; instead, some form of automatic relief behavior is used. This random behavior based on distorted perception can be interpreted as mental confusion, because it does not follow logical patterns.

Eisdorfer (1978) discusses the potential for discordance between socialized expressions of emotions, stating that neuroendocrine concomitants of emotion and psychomotor impulses likely to accompany physiologic states necessitate the control of emotions and aggressive motor activities. He concludes that the pathophysiologic and cognitive consequences of stress are complex, and present research findings have primarily been correlational in nature. A growing body of evidence is emerging that associates disease states with situational factors leading to stress. But at this time, the process by which stress leads to permanent destruction in physiologic processes, to the point of pathology, is not known.

Self-fulfilling prophecy

One way to ensure senility, according to Libow (1978), is to misdiagnose a case of reversible cognitive disorder and to treat the patient as a case of chronic brain syndrome. Libow feels that the medications and milieu experienced by the patients who are diagnosed as having chronic brain syndrome will certainly lead to fulfilling the prophecy. The clinical rule is to seek out and diagnose the "pseudosenilities" (Libow's term for reversible brain syndrome) with the expectation that effective therapy can be offered.

MECHANICAL PROBLEMS
Obstruction to cerebral blood flow

A large number of elderly people are admitted to acute hospitals with a secondary diagnosis of cerebral arteriosclerosis or cerebrovascular disease. Many older people living in their homes have this as one of several diagnoses. Elderly people admitted to nursing homes are likely to have the diagnosis of cerebrovascular disease of some type, although the term used may be organic brain disease. It is probably the most common diagnosis of the elderly population. The assumption is that there is an obstruction to the cerebral blood flow, or at times a cerebrovascular insufficiency, in which the arterial lumen is diminished. The vascular disease may take several forms: major ischemic lesions resulting from stenosis of the carotid, numerous microscopic infarcts in the cerebral cortex, or widespread subcortical ischemia, such as found in Binswanger's disease.

Stenosis (narrowing of vessel lumen) of blood vessels that feed the brain has been implicated in many confusional states. An atheromatous plaque, usually at the bifurcation of the carotid artery, which carries the major blood flow to the brain, can be visualized extracerebrally with angiography and treated with endarterectomy. Auscultation over the artery elicits a bruit, which can lead to further investigation. This accessible finding has led to widespread recognition and acceptance of this one etiology, although the treatment is to prevent the occurrence of stroke rather than to prevent organic brain syndrome. Atheromatous plaques can also be found in the vertebral arteries. Some investigators believe their data indicate that there is no hemodynamic change until the lumen is reduced by 50%, and others show that obstruction to flow does not occur until the transverse lumen is reduced by 70% to 90%.

Terry (1975) states that "observations on autopsied brains have proved that relatively few cases of senile dementia are accounted for by atheromatous changes in major arteries." Juul-Jensen (1970) affirms Terry's observations, stating that evidence to support cerebral arteriosclerosis is surprisingly meager or nonexistent. The records of 108 persons whose brains showed moderate to severe arteriosclerosis at autopsy were examined for evidence of dementia. The majority showed signs of dementia only if pathologic processes were found in the brain parenchyma, but the investigators concluded that arteriosclerosis of the basal arteries did not cause dementia in old age by itself (Goldfarb, 1975). Adams (1974) states that "belief in senility conditioned by faulty cerebral plumbing dies hard, but there is no pathological or physiological evidence to support the theory that widespread degeneration of nerve cells and tracts found in dementia in old age results from ischemia caused by atheromatosis" (p. 145). Terry and Wisniewski (1978) believe that arteriosclerosis is responsible for only 12% of cases of senile dementia.

These views, which leave room for controversy, represent the literature on arteriosclerotic disease. Older studies based on clinical findings as described in textbooks indicated widespread arteriosclerotic cerebral disease. More recent investigators, with improved technology for studying neuroanatomy, attribute confusional states to other reasons and deny the close association of confusional states (organic brain syndrome) to arterial disease.

The traditional belief that organic brain disease is the result of cerebrovascular disease has resulted in the erroneous belief that confusional states are untreatable. As long as cerebrovascular disease was accepted as one of the few etiologies, this belief was the basis for consigning the elderly patient with confusional states to the category of hopeless and untreatable patients.

Increased intracranial pressure

Increased intracranial pressure can cause confusional states, which can be rapidly followed by more acute signs such as stupor or unconsciousness. Older people are more subject than younger people to brain injuries from any kind of accident, even minor ones (Butler and Lewis, 1977). Seventy-two percent of all deaths caused by falls in the over-65 population result from head trauma. Thirty percent of all pedestrian fatalities are the result of brain injury. When the elderly person sustains a head injury in a fall, which leads to an extradural hematoma, the first symptom will be a change in mental status. With any rapidly developing change in mental status, an intracranial hematoma should be suspected.

A low-pressure hydrocephalus may first be recognized by increased irritability, difficulty in remembering, and ataxia from cerebellar pressure. Hydrocephalus, based on ventricular dilatation with diminished resorptive power by the arachnoid villi (obstruction to outflow), has been treated with ventricular shunts. Goldfarb (1975) concludes that these shunts have not produced good results, and there is no indication that these operations are of value in correcting memory loss in old age.

Libow (1978) notes that intracranial tumors present a picture of mental changes in approximately half the cases and that occurrence of signs and symptoms of intracranial pressure may be reduced or delayed because of cerebral atrophy of the aged. He says that papilledema occurs in only 11% of the elderly with intracranial tumor.

Death or loss of brain cells

Organic brain syndrome has traditionally been attributed to loss of brain cells with aging. Diamond (1978), in reviewing the literature on brain cell loss, points to the difficulties in counting cells in the brain and finds that reports about cell loss differ widely. The findings include (1) no cell loss, (2) cell loss early in life but not later, and (3) cell loss with aging. Several recent studies show no evidence of gross destruction of nerve cells or replacement by other types of cells. Work with DNA analysis of whole brains has shown no decrease in the brains of aged rats and mice. Diamond's own research in rat brains shows the greatest decrease in glial cells and astrocytes occurred in the first 108 days of life, then little more until after 650 days of life.

Terry and Wisniewski (1978), on the other hand, state that senile dementia is related to loss of neurons, diminished dendritic arborization, and tangles within the neuronal cell body. They further associate the neuronal loss with the shrunken cortex. Goldfarb (1975) associated the loss of memory to decrease in brain weight and neuronal loss. He related clinically measurable memory loss with a proportionately measurable loss of cortex and a dilatation of ventricles. He had postulated earlier that a loss of brain weight equivalent to 6% would be associated with a mild or moderate memory loss and that 20% brain weight loss was concordant with severe memory loss. Willanger and others (1968) concluded that psychologic testing could predict radiologic demonstration of cerebral atrophy. According to Brody (1973), a normal brain will have lost 25% of its cortical neurons by age 55 and another 25% by age 80.

Carlen and colleagues (1978) found that the shrunken brain cortex returned to its former size after alcoholics abstained for 6 months or more. Their work was done with serial computed tomography. Using an electron microscope examination of senescent human cortex, Cragg (1975) failed to find change in the number of synapses. Diamond (1978) concludes that there is good evidence that drastic structural changes do not occur in mammalian brains with aging. She further concludes that with an absence of disease, a stimulating environment, and good nutrition, the nervous system has the potential to oppose deterioration from aging. She quotes C. S. Minot (1908): "The period of old age, far from being the chief period of decline going on in each of us, will be the least." Based on her own research, Diamond agrees this is true, as long as the individual is exposed to a stimulating environment.

Summary

These mechanical problems may explain some of the cases of organic brain syndrome that do not yield to treatment and continue to deteriorate. However, our discussion indicates that this number is not a high percentage and that it remains with certainty only after all other causes have been explored.

Rarely mentioned in texts concerning organic brain syndrome is the association of confusional states with sensory deficits, sensory overload, or sensory deprivation. In addition, concern should be employed not to mistake depression for confusion.

It is important to remember that there are no longitudinal studies of the brain and that what is known about the aging brain is learned through postmortem examination. Healthy people do not have their brains studied, so findings are learned from the brains of people who have had some disease. There are no controls. This is not to cast doubt on traditional thinking, but it does encourage skepticism concerning the methodology of acquiring knowledge in this area, especially when people's rights may be jeopardized by misdiagnosis or improper treatment.

PRESENILE IRREVERSIBLE DEMENTIAS

Presenile dementias such as Alzheimer's disease, Jakob-Creutzfeldt disease, and Pick's disease are collectively named cerebral atrophy by neurologists. They may be more common than previously thought. The clinical abnormalities center around intellectual deterioration and failure of memory, especially recent memory. When the brain is examined grossly, atrophy of the cerebral cortex is obvious, with shrinking of the convolutions and widening of the sulci. There is a compensatory enlargement of the ventricles. Microscopically, there is a widespread patchy loss of nerve cells (Alpers and Mancall, 1971). There are two histologic changes: a neurofibrillary change and a senile plaque that is an extracellular accumulation of amorphous argentophilic material closely resembling amyloid. These same changes may be found in the brains of elderly people who have not exhibited any abnormal mental signs during life.

The senile plaques were found as early as the fourth decade of life in as many as 10% to 15% of brains examined, but this percentage rose until, in the tenth decade of life, they were found in 70% to 80% (Tomlinson, 1972).

Diagnosis is made by excluding other possible causes of dementia. The disease begins in middle life (presenile) and attacks more females than males. It progresses with complete disability in 4 to 5 years, and death follows. Presently, there is no treatment for these three presenile dementias except supportive care, which is a nursing responsibility. Terry (1978) believes that two thirds of patients with senile dementia are cases related to Alzheimer's disease, and he predicts that in the future the terms will be synonymous.

Terry and Wisniewski (1978) introduce the possibility that a new and abnormal protein may be synthesized in the cell by a slow virus that assists the entrance of new genetic material. The scrapie agent is similar to a slow virus. Found in sheep and goats, it can be transmitted to other species, causing spongy changes in the brain similar to that found in Jakob-Creutzfeldt disease and kuru, both of which are now known to be transmissible. Terry and Wisniewski suggest that because senile neuritic plaques are found only with scrapie agents acting on specific strains of mice, there is the possibility that senile dementia might be the result of a widespread slow virus infecting susceptible humans.

Pick's disease is also a progressive dementing disorder of middle and late life. The etiology is unknown, but the pathology is found not only in the cereral cortex, but also in the brainstem and basal ganglia. It is a very rare disease.

Jakob-Creutzfeldt disease begins with apathy, loss of memory, and abnormalities of behavior. Myoclonic jerks are a striking feature. The course of the disease is relatively short, with death occurring after 18 months or less.

ON THE HORIZON: NEW DEVELOPMENTS

The exciting discoveries of brain hormones have led to new developments that may initiate better treatment for the failing memory of the elderly person. In Belgium and Spain, brain specialists have recently given a pituitary gland peptide, vasopressin, to elderly people with failing memories and to traffic accident victims with head injuries that obliterated their recollection of the past. The treatment strikingly restored their ability to remember. Controlled studies are to begin in the United States using a synthetic vasopressin (Leff, 1978).

Kolata (1976) reported on findings that

showed normal diets could affect brain metabolism by furnishing precursors of neurotransmitters, acetylcholine, serotonin, and the catecholamines. The early work of Wortman, Fernstrom, and Cohen of the Massachusetts Institute of Technology and, independently, Haubrich of Merck, Sharp, and Dohme Laboratories, demonstrated that the rate at which the brain synthesizes acetylocholine can be increased by increasing the amount of choline in the diet. The intervening 2½ years has brought about newer knowledge at a rapid pace (Kolata, 1979). The research has included tryptophan as a precursor to serotonin and tyrosine as a precursor of the catecholamines (dopamine and norepinephrine). The idea of oxygen and glucose as sole suppliers of the metabolic needs of the brain has been shown to be in error. In addition, the blood-brain barrier is now known to be penetrated by other substances beside alcohol, tobacco, and narcotics.

The memory problems of the elderly may be based less on specific brain disease than on the combined effects of poor nutrition, loneliness, and social deprivation. Choline, a vitamin of the B complex, is part of a new strategy to treat the progressive senility known as Alzheimer's disease. A large body of scientific evidence links the nerve cells that use acetylcholine to memory formation in humans and animals. Christie and colleagues of Edinburgh tried choline supplements on patients with Alzheimer's disease and report a slowing of the mind-destroying disease process, though not to the degree hoped for. Etienne of the Allan Memorial Institute in Quebec believes the principal effect is achieved in the early stage of the disease (Kolata, 1979).

Davies and associates at the University of Edinburgh and Bowen and Perry in England have shown that Alzheimer's disease is associated with a partial loss of the neurons that make and use acetylcholine and with a reduction in activity of the brain enzymes that make acetylcholine. They believe senile dementia may be related to biochemical changes.

It is believed that as many as 15% of people over the age of 65 have severe memory problems that stem from Alzheimer's disease. The cause is unknown; the progress is insidious.

A 3-day symposium on the use of choline and related substances in nerve and mental disease was called in December 1978 in Tucson, Arizona. Organized by Wurtman of MIT, Growdon of Tufts New England Medical Center, and Barbeau of Institute of Researches Cliniques de Montreal, the symposium heard reports of choline's relationship to brain chemistry. The scientists' conclusions were guarded but hopeful. The use of choline in the treatment of tardive dyskinesia, which is thought to result from the failure of brain cells to release acetylcholine, appears to be reaching solid ground. The theoretic possibilities are much broader than just the use of choline, because the same basic strategy might conceivably be used to help the brain augment its supplies of other vitally needed nerve signal transmitters (Schmeck, 1979).

SUMMARY

The entire area of pathophysiology of confusion is developing but far from finished. Recent scientific discoveries and research now being conducted make this a fluid area of knowledge, and the reader is warned that the material may be outdated in the near future. The caregiver who keeps abreast of the literature should be encouraged to search widely in indices such as the *Index Medicus* and the *Cumulative Index of Nursing Literature* for additional information. The one definite conclusion is that confusional states in the elderly develop from many pathologic causes.

SUGGESTIONS FOR FURTHER READING

Eisdorfer, C., and Friedel, R. O., editors: Cognitive and emotional disturbance in the elderly, Chicago, 1978, Year Book Medical Publishers, Inc.

Rossman, I., editor: Clinical geriatrics, ed. 2, Philadelphia, 1979, J. B. Lippincott Co.

Verwoerdt, A.: Clinical geropsychiatry, Baltimore, 1976, The Williams & Wilkins Co.

REFERENCES

Adams, G. E.: Geriatric medicine, New York, 1974, Academic Press., Inc. Reprinted with permission. Copyright by Academic Press, Inc., (London) Ltd.

Agate, J.: Special hazards of later life. In Rossman, I. editor: Clinical geriatrics, Philadelphia, 1971, J. B. Lippincott Co.

Allen, E. T.: Prolonged immersion in cold water, Nurs. Times **70**:1928, 1974.

Alpers, B. J., and Mancall, E. L.: Clinical neurology, ed. 6, Philadelphia, 1971, F. A. Davis Co.

Botwinick, J., West, R., and Storandt, M.: Predicting death from behavioral test performance, J. Gerontol. **33**(5):755, 1978.

Brody, H.: In Rockstein, M., and Sussman, M. L., editors: Developing and aging in the nervous system, New York, 1973, Academic Press, Inc., pp. 123-133.

Brody, H., Harman, D., and Ordy, J. M.: Aging, vol. 1, New York, 1975, Raven Press.

Butler, R. N., and Lewis, M.: Aging and mental health, ed. 2, St. Louis, 1977, The C. V. Mosby Co.

Carlen, P. L., and others: Reversible cerebral atrophy in recently abstinent chronic alcoholics measured by computed tomography by scans, Science **200**:4345, 1978.

Clifford, G. O.: Hematological problems of the elderly. In Rossman, I., editor: Clinical geriatrics, Philadelphia, 1971, J. B. Lippincott Co.

Cragg, B. G.: The density of synapses and neurons in normal, mentally defective and aging human brains, Brain **98**:81-90, 1975.

Diamond, M. C.: The aging brain: some enlightening and optimistic results, Am. Sci. **66** (1):66-71, 1978.

Eisdorfer, C.: Stress, disease and cognitive disease. In Eisdorfer, C., and Friedel, R. O., editors: Cognitive and emotional disturbance in the elderly, Chicago, 1978, Year Book Medical Publishers, Inc.

Elias, M. F., Elias, P. K., and Elias, J. W.: Basic processes in adult developmental psychology, St. Louis, 1977, The C. V. Mosby Co.

Exton-Smith, A. N., and Windsor, C. M.: Principles of drug treatment in the aged. In Rossman, I., editor: Clinical geriatrics, Philadelphia, 1971, J. B. Lippincott Co.

Goldfarb, A. I.: Memory and aging. In Goldman, R., and Rockstein, M., editors: The physiology and pathology of aging, New York, 1975, Academic Press, Inc.

Hurwitz, N.: Predisposing factors in adverse reaction to drugs, Br. Med. J. **1**:536, 1969.

Isaacs, B.: Comprehensive care of the cognitively impaired elderly. In Eisdorfer, C., and Friedel, R. O., editors: Cognitive and emotional disturbance in the elderly, Chicago, 1978, Year Book Medical Publishers, Inc.

Jori, A., DiSalle, E., and Quadri, A.: Rate of aminopyrine disappearance form plasma in young and aged humans, Pharmacology **8**:273, 1972.

Juul-Jensen, P. A. R.: Aspects of pathology of presenile dementia, Acta Neurol. Scand. (supplement 43) **46**, 1970.

Kleemeir, R. W.: Intellectual changes in the senium, Proc. Am. Stat. Assoc. **1**:290, 1962.

Kolata, G. B.: Brain biochemistry: effects of diet, Science **192**:41, 1976.

Kolata, G. B.: Mental disorders: a new approach to treatment, Science **203**:4375, 1979.

Leff, D. N.: Brain chemistry may influence feelings, behavior, Smithsonian **9** (3):66-71, 1978.

Libow, L. S.: Senile dementia and "pseudodementias," clinical diagnosis. In Eisdorfer, C., and Friedel, R. O., editors: Cognitive and emotional disturbance in the elderly, Chicago, 1978, Year Book Medical Publishers, Inc.

Lipton, J.: Cold weather is especially hazardous for elderly, J. Gerontological Nurs. **4** (2):13, 1978.

Mason, J. W.: Organization of psychoendocrine mechanisms: a review and reconsideration of research. In Greenfield, N. S., and Sternbach, R. A., editors: Handbook of psychophysiology, New York, 1975, Holt, Rinehart & Winston.

Meyer, J. S., Lechner, H., and Eichorn, O.: Research on cerebral circulation, Third International Salzburg Conference, Springfield, Ill., 1969, Charles C Thomas, Publisher.

Minot, C. S.: The problem of age, growth and death, New York, 1908, G. P. Putnam.

Mitchell, P. H.: Concepts basic to nursing, ed. 2, New York, 1977, McGraw-Hill Book Co.

Palmore, E., and Cleveland, W.: Aging, terminal decline and terminal drop, J. Gerontol. **31**:76-81, 1976.

Peplau, H.: A working definition of anxiety. In Burd, S. F., and Marshall, M. A., editors: Some clinical approaches to psychiatric nursing, New York, 1963, Macmillan Publishing Co., Inc.

Riffkin, H., and Ross, H.: Diabetes in the elderly. In Rossman, I., editor: Clinical geriatrics, Philadelphia, 1971, J. B. Lippincott Co.

Rodstein, M.: Heart disease in the aged. In Rossman, I., editor: Clinical geriatrics, Philadelphia, 1971, J. B. Lippincott Co.

Rossen, R., Simenson, E., and Baker, J.: Electroencephalograms during hypoxia in healthy men: response characteristics of normal aging, Arch. Neurol. **5**:648-654, 1961.

Rossman, I., editor: Clinical geriatrics, ed. 2, Philadelphia, 1979, J. B. Lippincott Co.

Sadakali, F., and Owor, R.: Hypothermia in the tropics, Trop. Geogr. Med. **26**:265-270, 1974.

Schettler, F. G., and Boyd, G. S.: Atherosclerosis, New York, 1969, American Elsevier Publishing Co.

Schmeck, H. M.: Choline shows promise in treating memory impairment, New York, 1979, *New York Times,* reprinted in *Arizona Daily Star,* Jan. 31, 1979.

Seigler, I. S.: The terminal drop hypothesis: fact or artifact, Exp. Aging Res. **1**:169-185, 1975.

Simon, A., Epstein, L. J., and Reynolds, L.: Alcoholism in the geriatrically mentally ill, Geriatrics **23**:125, 1968.

Timiras, P. S.: Developmental physiology and aging, New York, 1972, Macmillan Publishing Co., Inc.

Terry, R. D.: Newsstory, Medical Tribune, June 18, 1975.

Terry, R. D., and Wisniewski, H. M.: Structural aspects of the aging brain. In Eisdorfer, C., and Friedel, R. O., editors: Cognitive and emotional disturbance in the elderly, Chicago, 1978, Year Book Medical Publishers, Inc.

Tomlinson, B. E.: Morphological brain changes in nondemented old people. In van Praag, H. M., and Kalverboer, A. F., editors: Ageing of the central nervous system, Haarlem, 1972, De Erven F. Bohn, N. V.

Verwoerdt, A.: Clinical geropsychiatry, Baltimore, 1976, The Williams & Wilkins Co.

Wachman, A., and Berstein, D. S.: Diet and osteoporosis, Lancet **1**:958, 1968.

Willanger, R. P., and others: Intellectual impairment and cerebral atrophy, a psychological, neurological and radiological investigation, Dan. Med. Bull. **15**:65, 1968.

Wollner, L.: Postural hypotension in the elderly. In Agate, J. N., editor: Medicine in old age, London, 1966, Pittman Medical Publishers.

4

THE NURSE'S ROLE IN THE CARE OF THE CONFUSED CLIENT

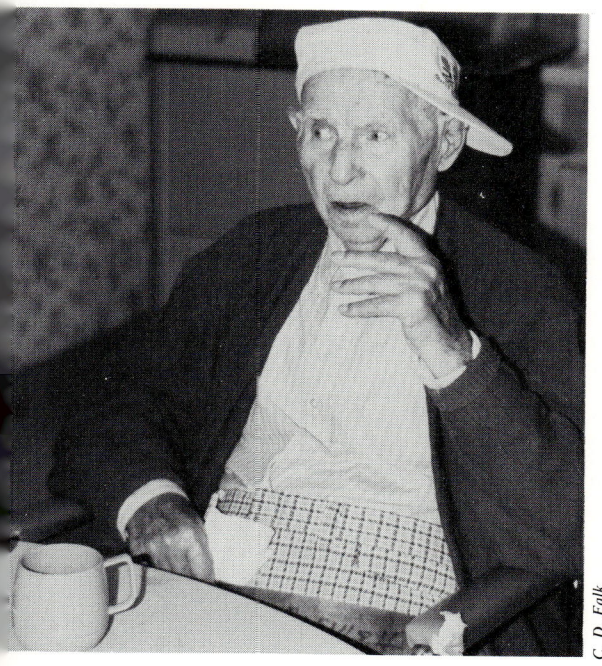

C. D. Falk

Nurses are in a position to offer the elderly a more hopeful environment and a chance to return to a more satisfying life. This can be accomplished by nursing the client through illnesses that contribute to confusional states, making good assessments and interpreting them to other caregivers, and adjusting the environment so the client can function more extensively. The nurse is often the one who predicts the client is in a position that will lead to confusion and who can make a preventive plan. As the group of health professionals who are most concerned with care of the elderly in the home, hospital, or long-term institutions, nurses can have a strong impact on the welfare of the elderly confused clients.

We take the position that confusion in the elderly is a nursing diagnosis, made by nurses and treated by nurses, with interdisciplinary assistance from other professionals in the health care field. And beyond the health care field, nurses recognize the importance of socioeconomic factors and family conditions as contributing to illness. Nursing's focus is not on disease and its treatment, but rather on the elderly person who has a life to live, a death to die, and a need to be sustained at his highest level of functioning during both processes. Confusion in the elderly is a symptom of environmental, social, sensory, and physiologic problems. If it is a prodromal sign of death, then to provide a good death is a nursing goal.

Since geriatrics/gerontology has been identified as a nursing specialty only in the past two decades, this chapter will also be concerned with preparation of nurses to serve the elderly.

CONFUSION: A LABEL FOR MEDICAL, SOCIAL, AND LEGAL ACTION

Confusional states in the elderly may result in a less than adequate diagnosis, which can lead to irresponsible labeling. This often becomes the basis for medical, nursing, and legal action. The medical action may be not to treat on the basis of hopeless prognosis, and the patient deteriorates as predicted. It may result in inappropriate relocation of the patient from his home to a situation in which he loses freedom to make his own decisions or to continue his previous life-style. This leads to behaviors that indicate to the caregivers that his confusional state is worsening and further safety measures must be taken.

Mrs. T., age 82, an independent woman engaged in community and church affairs, was admitted to the hospital with a fractured hip. She seemed alert on admission but soon became disoriented, then restless and noisy. After surgery, her restless fingers explored the tubes to her arm, to her bladder, and to the suction device that drained her operative site. She was restrained in the supine position. During the day, Mrs. T. could be brought into touch with reality, and she followed instructions fairly well, but at night she slept very little and called noisily for her mother. When the fifth day came, the plan to send her home to be cared for by her aged husband was considered and dismissed. The caregivers decided that Mrs. T. would have to go to a nursing home. The sixth postoperative day she was transferred to the nursing home by ambulance. She had not been told of the arrangements. When she reached the nursing home she was frightened, uncooperative, and belligerent. After consulting with the husband by telephone, the decision was made to send her to another city to the state hospital. At this time Mrs. T. became more anxious and refused to eat or cooperate in any way. She became more withdrawn each day. No family member was nearby, and she had no contact with the aged husband, who could not go to the hospital. Two weeks later she died.

The basis for all action taken with confused people is concern for the safety of the individual. The older person who lives alone or who has only an elderly spouse or family member to care for him should be protected. But community concern and legal action take place usually at the point where confusional states are diagnosed. Rarely are they treated as a life-threatening event that can be reversed; instead, they are viewed upon as permanent conditions. *Nurses are the intermediaries in making decisions, for their interpretations of behavior initiate action in many instances, especially in hospitals and institutions.* Legal action is required to place the older person in the "safe" place. This may require a conservatorship that removes control over property and business affairs. Guardianship may be sought. This involves the loss of the client's autonomy and decision making, which are legally vested in some responsible person. Protective services of the slightest degree require some surrender of autonomy. The confusional state is the critical determinant. An extremely ill patient with an alert mind does not have his legal status challenged or changed.

In some cases, placement in protective circumstances is desirable and obligatory. However, during the past 20 years the number of instances of reversible confusional states has increased to such a point that the elderly client must have the benefit of every doubt. He must be painstakingly diagnosed, and action should be postponed to a point of certainty. Nurses, who observe behavior, are often the critical caregivers who could call attention to hopeful signs. They are also the critical caregivers who can intervene at appropriate moments early in illness when there is time for prevention. Nursing caregivers, present around the clock in institutions or available for the home at regular intervals, can predict, prevent, and treat confusion.

In 1975, a group of gerontologists debated the prognosis of the confused elderly at a preconference colloquium of the European Social Research Committee of the International Association of Gerontology in Jerusalem. Wershow (1977) told of participants refusing to accept that, for the present and foreseeable future, there will be a large number of persons suffering from chronic brain syndrome, an irreversible disorder of memory and learning. He quoted various studies that place the severely senile in the United States between 360,000 and 925,000. He anticipated increasing numbers as the present aging population reaches the over-75 age group. When he asked that a realistic view be taken of the amount of care and money required for these people, whom he saw as hopeless, he enraged many of his colleagues. Cohen (1978) took issue, stating that Wershow did not distinguish between organic brain syndrome and senile dementia, but used the terms interchangeably. He pointed out that the high number of first admissions to nursing homes based on organic brain syndrome is not so much a matter of numbers as of inaccurate diagnosis and clinical perception. Armstrong (1978) denied the hopelessness of these individuals' ever again leading productive lives and insisted that even for senile patients, care can change the quality of their lives. Professionals in the field of gerontology are far from agreement concerning the confused elderly.

Nurses recognize that many persons will agree with both Wershow and Cohen. Their experience shows that confusional states in the elderly have multiple etiologies and varying prognoses. The existence of a syndrome that is progressive in its destruction of memory must be acknowledged. But the organic basis, usually linked to death of brain cells, leaves many unanswered questions. Nurses have seen hopelessly confused persons change and become alert and active. On the other hand, nurses who care for the lonely, isolated aged client in his home have watched successful efforts to maintain contact with reality change almost overnight upon transfer to another environment. Kerschner (1975), in speaking of the elderly persons who enter the hospital through the emergency room, states that "if one was not disoriented before, 10 minutes in most emergency rooms would complete the task" (p. 54). At this time it can be assumed that any confusional state that has such a sudden onset is also amenable to instant reversibility. The sudden death of brain cells does not seem to be at issue. Unfortunately, untrained and unaware health professionals, who are often unconcerned about the elderly, translate confusion and disorientation into organic brain disease or mental disease. The label thus becomes an entry point to the long-term state.

A 92-year-old woman demanded a great deal of the nursing home personnel and made trips into the nursing office at regular intervals to complain about mistreatment. She was called "that crazy old lady" by the staff. But when a nurse looked under the frowzy hair and into eyes that saw only with glasses, she also found a hearing problem, which was helped by putting new batteries in the hearing aid. The woman was facing her death. At her age, she was quite matter-of-fact, wanting to get ready for it, but she had one great task to complete. She had a book to finish—explaining her technique for teaching harmony. For the nurse who seemed to understand, the woman explained in writing: "The hazards of the last four years have robbed me of some material possessions, but worse still, the nervous tension of these experiences made me doubt the soundness of my judgment and even caused me to question my mental balance."

Diagnosis often becomes prognosis as health professionals use stereotypes for shaping their planning. Rowe of Harvard Medical School told the 1979 meeting of the American Association for the Advancement of Science that medical students base their image of the old on a number of myths, for they are not exposed to healthy older people. The students leave school with the idea that all old people are senile and sick all the time. Barely half of the medical schools have any programs on aging. The diagnosis may be erroneous, but it furnishes the blueprint for a plan of care. There is an implied prognosis, which becomes a fact as the older person becomes trapped in a system that closes down around him.

THE NURSE AS PRIMARY CAREGIVER
The nurse and the confused client

Wershow (1977) believes that the hopelessness of the older person, who has what he believes is irreversible brain disease, is a problem that should be turned over to the nurse practitioner. His negative approach implies that the physician is wasted on such patients. The role of the nurse is thus seen as custodial rather than therapeutic. He does not take into account those elderly clients who are reacting to environmental stresses, sensory impairment, or physiologic problems. The implication is that the physician is helpless or does not wish to be bothered, and the nurse should accept the responsibility by default.

In contrast, Kane and Kane (1978) believe the geriatric nurse practitioner is the appropriate caregiver for more positive reasons. They say the current lack of interest among physicians might be alleviated by upgrading the geriatric specialty, but an alternative is to use other forms of primary health care, such as the geriatric nurse practitioner.

The nurse's tendency to look at the client as a person in a community and as a product of his history, his family, and his culture has produced a holistic viewpoint that sees far beyond the body on the examining table. Instead of using the medical model of disease orientation, the nurse uses the perspective of the total client interacting with his social and physical environment. The traditions of nursing lie closer to the nurturing requirements of long-term care and to providing health promotion and supportive activities within the home. Nurses provide a valuable service in primary care, both in the community and in institutions.

The nurse as a primary caregiver is a relatively new concept that has developed along several lines. The setting contributes to the concept, as well as the qualifications and competency of the nurse. A director of nursing listened to the description of the duties of the geriatric nurse practitioner and laughed, "We do all those things in the nursing home, and not because we have special training, but because we are trained more than anyone else around."

Today a number of programs prepare the nurse to assume the role of primary caregiver in the home and long-term care unit. It is usually assumed that the primary caregiver is a physician and that anyone who assumes the role will practice as the physician does. Nursing's holistic view of health care takes a broader stance. This has led to several types of preparation.

Geriatric nurse practitioner

The geriatric nurse practitioner studies in a formal program, which emphasizes the skills of physical assessment, history taking, observation, and recording. After a prescribed curriculum in the classroom setting for 4 or more months, the nurse practices under the supervision and guidance of a preceptor physician in a clinical setting. These programs for the most part have been demonstration projects funded by the federal government or some foundation. One program, Mountain States Health Systems, prepared 21 nurses from nursing homes in the Rocky Mountain West to return to their original places of employment. Through a Kellogg Foundation grant, the agency-selected nurses were prepared through geriatric nurse practitioner programs at Cornell University, Syracuse University, and University of Colorado. They returned to their home communities for practice with a preceptor in their own nursing home. They have been most successful in early detection of illness in the elderly, such as congestive heart failure and pneumonia, and in initiation of early treatment. The ideal practice field for the geriatric nurse practitioner is still being explored, and nurses themselves are not in total agreement (Mauksch, 1975; Rogers, 1975). Ambulatory care settings seem to offer the best opportunities for evolving a nursing science and art in primary health care (Roy and Obloy, 1978). Two principal issues confront the geriatric nurse practitioner. The first is the need to be recognized for third-party payment. Since much of geriatric care is paid through Medicare and Medicaid, the regulations should include payment directly to the nurse for her services. The second issue concerns a number of states that are opening their nurse practice acts to give protection to the nurse practitioner. There is a great deal of opposition to expanding the nurse's role in health care, especially in primary health care. (See Appendix B for list of schools that provide courses for geriatric nurse practitioners.)

Certification of the geriatric nurse practitioner

The American Nurses' Association has a certification process by which nurses engaged in clinical geriatric and gerontologic nursing can be certified for excellence in practice. It recognizes professional growth in nursing care of the elderly. The certification process requires evidence of exemplary direct care given to the elderly clients. Written examinations, case studies, or research projects must be presented, and the nurse is judged by a committee of her peers. These nurses need not have studied in formal courses of instruction, nor have had preceptorships. Their practice is nursing as defined in present nurse practice acts. Nurses who have been certified use the initials C.A.N.A.-1 (Certified by the American Nurses' Association in the practice of geriatric nursing).

Geriatric clinical nurse specialist, geriatric nurse clinician, and gerontology nurse specialist

Graduate programs in geriatric or gerontologic nursing exist in a number of universities today (Appendix B). Gunter uses "gerontic" nursing to describe the dual aspects of the nursing role vis-a-vis the elderly. The graduate programs differ widely in their approach to the care of the elderly client, with some focusing on preventive care only, others on advocacy for the aging, and still others on preparing nurses for the care of the sick aged. The names given to the nurse vary as widely as types of preparation. Discussion concerning a standard terminology has still not resulted in a single descriptive name for the nurse who has a master's or doctoral degree in nursing care of the elderly. Some doctoral programs in nursing include a major clinical interest in the care of the elderly. Some programs prepare nurses as clinicians, while others prepare faculty to teach in nursing programs that are incorporating geriatric/gerontologic nursing content in their curricula. Some programs include physical assessment skills, and all emphasize health maintenance of the elderly client.

Geriatric nursing education at the baccalaureate level

Until the past few years little or no content on the elderly client has been included in the curricula of undergraduate schools. Efforts are now being made to satisfy the demands of providers of care that nurses be given a well-planned course in the care of the elderly as a distinct course of study rather than integrated in community health, mental health, and medical surgical nursing. For schools that use the life development approach or the holistic approach to teaching, this has caused some difficulty. Faculty members have expressed their dissatisfaction with their own preparation in this recent field of knowledge.

The Association of Gerontology in Higher Education (AGHE), with the Gerontological Society, has used a panel of 93 practitioners and educators in the fields of social work, nutrition, nursing, and clinical psychology to develop suggestions for a core curriculum in all four practice areas. The method used selected concepts, skills, and theoretical material that seemed most pertinent to those in practice. There was a high agreement among the panel that all content must be validated by field work or clinical practice with the elderly. (Foundation for Gerontological Education, 1980).

Continuing education in geriatric/gerontologic nursing

The use of continuing education courses has allowed the nurse to keep abreast of newer developments in giving care to the elderly. These programs are short term, usually workshop, conference, or symposium education, but some semester-length courses are offered by schools of nursing. Faculty for the courses are nurses who have risen to prominence in the field because of their experience, their publications, and research in nursing the aged. For those who find time or distance a hindrance, independent study is available. See Chapter 15.

The present trend toward tying mandatory continuing education to relicensure has led to a need for developing continuing education in specific areas of practice, in order that continuing education can be associated with improved patient care (Wolanin, 1979).

Present status of programs for nurses

Despite the wide range of educational programs already mentioned, there is still a shortage of well-prepared nurses to work with the elderly. In the field of specialized care, such as that needed by the confused elderly patient, the number is fewer still.

NURSING SETTINGS
Traditional

The traditional workplace of the nurse is in the hospital, where the nurse confronts a large increase in the number of elderly patients. The older person is sick more often and requires a longer hospital stay than other patients. They are found in the emergency room, intensive care unit, the operating suite, recovery room, and throughout the general nursing units. Estimates are that 35% to 50% of the patients in the general hospital are over age 65. For many older people without resources, the hospital is often the primary care unit they use, and only when care is imperative.

The nursing home, or extended care unit, is a phenomenon of the past two decades. Prior to 1960, there were few nursing homes. With the advent of Medicare and Medicaid, the number has grown rapidly. Nursing homes use nursing service as the major method of delivering care. During the early 1970s when state hospitals were emptied by sending their elderly patients back to the community, many older people went to nursing homes. The state hospital, which had formerly served as the final institution for elderly confused patients, changed its focus. The elderly client may not have received therapeutic care in the state hospital, but he went to nursing homes that also had no such care available. It is in this area that nurses have had an opportunity to fill a need, but they have not always been prepared to give appropriate care. The hospital and nursing home have been the settings in which most nurses have cared for the elderly.

Nontraditional
Home health care

Home health care is a system being developed to care for the elderly in their own homes. It is being recognized as an alternative to institutional care, but present day thinking also suggests that if home health services were available, institutional care would be the alternative rather than the rule. This community-based nursing requires a wide range of skills and knowledge. The focus is on rehabilitation and maintenance as well as prevention. Program funding has been sporadic and is one of the real obstacles to enlarging this type of care. Federal legislation is proposed for making payment possible through Medicare. Present research indicates that many elderly could stay in their homes if home health care services were available at a price they could pay.

Nursing clinics

One of the exciting outcomes of the past decade has been the nursing clinic, which cares for the elderly at a point accessible to their residence. Often, they are found in the high-rise apartment residences for the elderly. Others are operated in connection with nutrition centers. Nurses are the primary caregivers and refer to appropriate experts, including medical, social, housing, and economic specialists. The nursing clinic is not a medical clinic but a broad-based assessment center that offers treatment for nonmedical problems or refers to appropriate resources.

An elderly woman was insistent when she called the College of Nursing. "We need someone to take blood pressures here," she said, "for one of our people dropped dead with a stroke last night. Can't you send someone to help us?" The City Housing Authority arranged for a clinic room in the high-rise apartment building, and clinic hours were posted. Everyone wanted their blood pressure checked. Most clients were normotensive, but they stayed to discuss the real problems that brought them to the clinic. Some of the clients wanted to know how to penetrate the health care system and make it work for them. "How do you talk to the doctor and get him to listen?" "What does he mean by ... ?" "What is this medicine for?" But other health problems included replacing a light bulb for a nearly blind diabetic client, getting canes for people with unsteady gait, and crisis intervention for every possible kind of human tragedy.

Nursing care consultants

The role of the nursing care consultant is to make nursing expertise available outside regular health care institutions. A few nurses have opened offices where they receive ambulatory clients or from which they go into homes and give a wide range of services. The nurses make assessments, work with families, help with discharge planning, and serve as on-call nurses for their regular clients. Nursing care consultants are a knowledgeable group of nurses whose repertoire of skills allows them to be ready for any kind of crisis or just to reassure the elderly client that there is one person whom he can call. These nurses are paid by the client, which limits their services to those with adequate income, usually one who falls above the income limits for free community services. Eventually, it is hoped this service can be included in the health care policies that many older people carry to supplement Medicare.

The body of knowledge relating to the care of the elderly

The body of nursing knowledge that focuses on the special differences that aging brings to a person in today's society, or more especially, to being a person in today's health care system, is still limited. There is a little clinical research in the area of geriatric and gerontologic nursing. Textbooks are being produced to overcome some of the lag between the need and the solution, but the problem of caring for the confused elderly person has always been taken more or less for granted. Even with this gloomy picture, nurses should be encouraged that interest in the elderly is resulting at present in research applicable to nursing care. Nurses are reporting research in excellent articles as well. Two research awards are offered annually at the University of Arizona for excellence in research, enriching the knowledge of geriatric nursing. Mitchell (1977) says a review of the literature may reveal several causes of confusion other than those mentioned in texts (Luckman and Sorenson, 1974; Wintrobe and others, 1974).

SUMMARY

We have focused on the nurse's role as a primary caregiver, especially in relation to the health care of the confused elderly client. Confusion should be a nursing diagnosis made by nurses, and the clients should be treated by nurses with assistance from many other disciplines in the health care field, from the family, and from the resources of the community. For nurses to take this responsibility requires specialized preparation for the clinicians and faculty who will be educating students and those already in practice. Present approaches to filling this gap and the need for more research to develop a body of nursing knowledge have been emphasized. We hope to present an orderly body of knowledge about confusion of the elderly as a nursing problem.

REFERENCES

Armstrong, P. W.: More thoughts on senility, Gerontologist **18**(3):315-316, 1978.

Cohen, G. D.: Organic brain syndrome: reality orientation for critics of clinical intervention, Gerontologist **18**(3):313-314, 1978.

Foundation for Gerontological Education: A collaborative project of the Gerontological Society and the Association of Gerontalogy in Higher Education, Gerontologist (Part II) **20**(3): 1-61, 1980.

Kane, L., and Kane, R. A.: Care of the aged: old problems in need of new solutions, Science **200**:913-919, 1978.

Kerschner, P. A.: Recent innovations in the field of long term care. In Proceedings of the First North American Symposium on Long Term Care Administration, Toronto, July 27-31, 1975.

Luckman, J., and Sorenson, K. C.: Medical-surgical nursing: a psychophysiologic approach, Philadelphia, 1974, W. B. Saunders Co.

Mauksch, I. G.: Nursing is coming of age through the practitioner movement, Am. J. Nurs. **75**(10):1834-1843, 1975.

Mitchell, P. H.: Concepts basic to nursing, ed. 2, New York, 1977, McGraw-Hill Book Co.

Rogers, M. D.: Nursing is coming of age through the practitioner movement, Am. J. Nurs. **75**(8):1834-1843, 1975.

Roy, C., and Obloy, M.: The practitioner movement. Toward a science of nursing, Am. J. Nurs. **78**(10):1698-1703, 1978.

Wershow, H. J.: Comment: reality orientation for gerontologists, Gerontologist **17**(3):297-302, 1977.

Wintrobe, and others, editors: Harrison's principles of internal medicine, ed. 7, New York, 1974, McGraw-Hill Book Co.

5

THE FOUR-LEVEL NURSING DIAGNOSIS

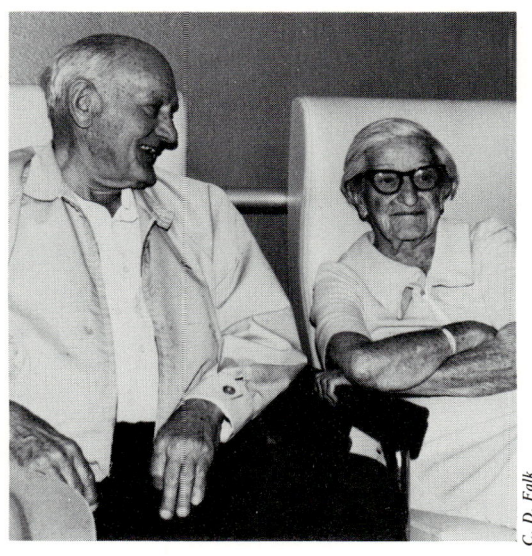

C. D. Falk

The clinical nursing section of this book is devoted to the care of the confused client, or patient, as he will be referred to when he is found in acute care settings. The confusional state will be referred to as a symptom of underlying or primary cause.

THE NURSING PROCESS

This chapter is based on the scientific approach to nursing care, often referred to as the nursing process. It is a logical and systematic method of recognizing a discordant event or change in a usual or expected state of an individual, a problem-solving process that uses data collection, analysis of data, and conclusions drawn from that analysis to formulate a statement called the nursing diagnosis. This is the basis for a plan of nursing care. Implementation and evaluation of nursing care follow. Outcomes of care are measured by criteria that predict what changes will occur as the result of care.

A nursing diagnosis states the client's need and problem in relation to nursing practice (Bower, 1977), and it is used to set goals for both nurse and client. If the nursing diagnosis reflects the client's inability to meet his needs, then this statement of the problem should illustrate what can be accomplished through nursing care.

The nursing process is restricted to problems the nurse recognizes and treats. Each discipline has its certain body of knowledge and skills that can be used to assist the client, and each uses its own form of assessment, reaching a diagnosis descriptive of the problem in terms of that discipline's capabilities. Nursing diagnosis differs from medical diagnosis, which is a description of pathology. The medical diagnosis offers direction to the physician for treatment in relation to altering the pathology. Nursing diagnosis attempts to define factors that impinge on the client from the social and physical environment, as well as from the pathology within the client. There is an assumption that pathology also exists in the social and physical environment or in the client's interaction with them.

The nursing diagnosis includes the physician's diagnosis, but goes further in describing how the client functions as a human being in his environment. It attempts to define causes of the confusional state in the elderly as they are related to such factors as relocation and other situational stresses, physiologic stresses, drug intoxications, and sensoriperceptual problems. The different set of professional boundaries permits the nurse to use the physician's diagnosis of organic brain syndrome in her diagnosis, but allows her to consider the client's external environment and to make a statement indicating that the client is confused secondary, for example, to a rapid change in living arrangements. The medical assessment takes place in the physician's office or in a formal examining area. The nurse's assessment occurs in many settings and will include the totality of the client's interactions with the social and physical environment; it reflects what interferes with function or contributes to dysfunction.

Nursing diagnosis is defined as the judgment or conclusion that occurs as a result of nursing assessment (Gebbie and Lavin, 1975). The nursing assessment is the first step in the nursing process, but it is also a continuous cyclic activity. Each datum observed calls forth subjective analysis by the observer and leads to further data collection. At some point the data yield a conclusion that is taken as a point for departure for the next step. Assessment is a highly subjective process on the part of the data collector. Decisions to include or discard data involve the client and the nurse, which makes every assessment a unique personal experience. The systematic assessment helps to neutralize some of the subjectivity, but it is still a human interaction and therefore differs with each pair who interact. The scientific method, or the nursing process, is an attempt to eliminate as much subjectivity as possible, but the nurse's background, attitudes, and skills determine what she will look for and what she will see. Even the most objective data varies according to the perceiver. A thermometer read by different people may have several readings.

Assessment enables the nurse to organize data into a relationship that can be analyzed against her normative expectations (Gebbie and Lavin, 1975). Normative expectations can be highly subjective, and it is the nurse's professional responsibility to take this into account when analyzing data.

A diagnosis is descriptive and prescriptive. Medical diagnoses have been codified to such an extent that the physician seeing the diagnosis can describe fairly accurately the signs and symptoms the patient will display without seeing him.

The etiology, prognosis, and treatment are equally well codified. The medical diagnosis is itself the description of a large number of cases from which generalizations have been drawn. The nursing diagnosis is particularized and specific to the individual. Generalizations may be drawn from the the nurse's experience, but the nursing diagnosis is a definitive statement pinpointing the events relating to a unique situation, for example, "confusion secondary to relocation to a nursing home complicated by decreased vision (cataracts in both eyes allowing blurred vision in good light only) and to inability to hear the human voice at 5 feet on the right side and 3 feet on the left." Such a diagnosis is descriptive, but it is also highly prescriptive. Its holistic approach points out nursing intervention that will eliminate or alleviate barriers to communication resulting from poor vision and hearing. It sets into motion a plan to accentuate the client's use of his remaining assets to maintain independence. This example prescribes:

1. Using good light, with no glare
2. Standing close to client when speaking and testing for comprehension

3. Using touch as a means of communication when appropriate
4. Teaching about environment: location of room, bathroom, and chair, then adding one new location daily
5. Assisting with activities of daily living until client can manage own feeding, bathing, dressing, and activity
6. Assessing hydration and nutrition daily to ensure fluid and nutrition needs are met during orientation to new environment
7. Using skills needed for nursing the blind and deaf
8. Reducing new experiences to a minimum and introducing gradually as tolerated

The nursing goal is to enable the client to become functional in the new environment as rapidly as possible without adding to the confusional state. The unwritten assumption is that if sensoriperceptual problems of the client are met appropriately, his confusion should be prevented and eliminated.

Specific nursing diagnoses have not been codified; an effort to do so is made through the use of standard care plans. The highly unique situation of each client may prevent the exact typologies found in medical diagnoses, although psychiatric diagnoses refer to a constantly evolving code as newer conceptualizations succeed old ones. A tentative taxonomy of nursing diagnoses based on confusional states of the elderly is offered in Table 5-1.

The nursing diagnosis requires assessment to determine qualities of confusion. Not all confusion is the same. In fact, it varies according to *degree*, from slight and momentary confusional states to those in which the client does not recognize his own name.

Confusion also varies with *time*, as in the "sundown syndrome" reported by staffs in nursing homes. Elderly clients, with clear mental status by day, suddenly become disoriented when night falls and institutional tempo changes. Confusion also varies with

Table 5-1. Taxonomic system of nursing diagnoses of confusional states in the elderly

1. **Confusional states in the elderly**
  1.1 *Acute or rapid-onset type of confusion (reversible)*
    1.11 The elderly person whose confusion is secondary to compromised brain support
      1.1101 Hypoxia
        1.11011 Anemic hypoxia
          1.110111 Blood loss (gradual)
          1.110112 Iron deficiency
          1.110113 Pernicious anemia
          1.110113 Folic-acid deficiency
          1.110114 Destruction of blood-forming organs
          1.110115 Other
        1.11012 Histotoxic hypoxia
          1.110121 Hypothermia (accidental)
          1.110122 Hyperthermia (high ambient temperature)
          1.110123 Hyperthermia (infection)
          1.110124 Dehydration
            1.1101241 Dehydration (diuretic induced)
            1.1101242 Dehydration (inability to get fluids)
            1.1101243 Dehydration (hyperglycemia)
            1.1101244 Dehydration (other)
          1.110125 Electrolyte imbalance
          1.110126 Hypocalcemia
          1.110127 Hypercalcemia
          1.110128 Uremia

Continued.

Table 5-1. Taxonomic system of nursing diagnoses of confusional states in the elderly—cont'd

        1.11013 Hypoxemia (ventilatory problems)
           1.110131 Emphysema
           1.110132 Black lung disease (pneumoconiosis)
           1.110133 Brown lung disease (byssinosis)
           1.110134 Obstructed airway
           1.110135 Other
        1.11014 Stagnant (ischemic) hypoxia
           1.110141 Cardiac failure (arrhythmias, congestive heart failure)
           1.110142 Increased intracranial pressure
           1.110143 Increased intracranial pressure (subdural hematoma)
           1.110144 Normal pressure hydrocephalus
           1.110145 Hypotension (circulatory failure)
           1.110146 Hypotension (drug reaction)
           1.110147 Hypotension (other)
           1.110148 Hypothyroidism
           1.110149 Other
    1.1102 Glucose excess or deficiency
        1.11021 Hyperglycemia (hyperosmolarity)
        1.11022 Hyperglycemia (nonketogenic)
        1.11023 Hypoglycemia (malnutrition)
        1.11024 Hypoglycemia (drug reaction)
    1.1103 Drug action, interaction, and reaction
        1.11031 Digitalis toxicity
        1.11032 Other drugs (name)
        1.11033 Alcohol and drugs (name)
        1.11034 Tardive dyskinesia
        1.11035 Other
    1.1104 Stress
    1.1105 Other
1.12 The elderly person whose confusion is secondary to sensoriperceptual (sensory alteration) problems
    1.1201 Visual deficits
        1.12011 Total blindness
        1.12012 Total blindness (new situation)
        1.12013 Diminished vision
        1.12014 Defects in visual field (hemianopia; no peripheral vision; loss of macular vision)
        1.12015 Diplopia
    1.1202 Hearing deficits
        1.12021 Total loss of hearing; no prosthesis
        1.12022 Total loss of hearing; prosthesis
        1.12023 Diminished hearing, bilateral
        1.12024 Diminished hearing, unilateral (state side)
        1.12025 Tinnitus
        1.12026 Other
    1.1203 Tactile deficits
        1.12031 Diminished ability to sense touch (hands)
        1.12032 Diminished ability to sense touch (feet)
        1.12033 Diminished ability to sense touch (trunk)

Table 5-1. Taxonomic system of nursing diagnoses of confusional states in the elderly—cont'd

        1.1204 Loss of propioceptive abilities
        1.1205 Sensory deprivation
            1.12051 Sensory deprivation from nonstimulating environment
            1.12052 Sensory deprivation from sensory deficit (name)
            1.12053 Sensory deprivation from other causes
        1.1206 Sensory overload
            1.12061 Relocation to new living arrangement
            1.12062 Too many people (crowds)
            1.12063 Too much information
            1.12064 Other
    1.13 The elderly person whose confusion is secondary to environmental (social and physical) factors
        1.1301 Interaction with environment without meaning; relocation
        1.1302 Helplessness, panic, or loss of control
        1.1303 Crisis or catastrophe
        1.1304 Situational depression
        1.1305 Loss of natural supports; grief, separation, rejection
        1.1306 Alterations in or modification of lifelong patterns of coping and adjusting
        1.1307 Abrupt cultural change
        1.1308 Perception of imprisonment
        1.1309 Other
    1.14 The elderly person whose confusion is secondary to altered physiologic states
        1.1401 Pain
        1.1402 Inability to feel pain (numbness)
        1.1403 Fatigue
        1.1404 Sleep deprivation
        1.1405 Inactivity
        1.1406 Interruptions in body rhythms
        1.1407 Problems with elimination
            1.14071 Full bladder (unable to empty)
            1.14072 Full bladder (temporary at night)
            1.14073 Indwelling ureteral catheter
            1.14074 Suprapubic drainage of bladder
            1.14075 Fecal impaction
            1.14076 Diarrhea
            1.14077 Colostomy or ileostomy
            1.14078 Other
        1.1408 Other
1.2 *Chronic or slow-onset type of confusion (irreversible)*
    1.21 AD-SD complex (Alzheimer's disease–senile dementia); arteriosclerotic cerebral disease; true dementias
        1.211 Able to function in community
        1.212 Able to function in protective surroundings
        1.213 Requires constant supervision
        1.214 Requires total care
        1.215 Terminally ill
    1.22 Alzheimer's disease
    1.23 Pick's disease
    1.24 Jakob-Creutzfeldt disease

physiologic status. Some clients react to weariness following activity, while others are rarely alert when first awakened in the morning or after a nap. These clients may be reacting to their circadian rhythms, to body temperature, to hormonal levels, or to the delayed action of hypnotics given the previous night. Confusion in the elderly must be described as behavior, but in the context of time, environment, human interactions, and preceding events.

Accuracy of nursing diagnosis is crude at best when compared with the accuracy of a calibrated glass tube or a metric tape. Skill in making nursing diagnoses may be refined as nurses increase their knowledge, skill, and experience. It is a judgment and a conclusion, and since the nursing plan depends on it, it must represent the best effort.

IMPLEMENTATION OF THE CARE PLAN

Nursing intervention logically follows the nursing diagnosis, which, if not explicit, exists at a subconscious level. Riehl and Roy (1974) say that interventions are devised by selecting the influential factors that can be manipulated, preferably the primary cause of the client's behavior. If that is impossible, then the contextual or residual areas should be manipulated by the nurse for the client's benefit. There are three kinds of nursing action: routine, ad hoc, and deliberative. The first two are given without planning; ad hoc responds to the exigencies of the moment only. Deliberative care takes into account factors identified in the assessment, weighing them carefully in making the diagnosis, then choosing the better alternative from several options for meeting individual goals. *Deliberative nursing is appropriate.* For example, group therapy will not be offered to the client whose confusion is secondary to pernicious anemia (deficiency of vitamin B_{12}). After replacement of the nutritional deficiency, group therapy might be considered.

Evaluation of the effectiveness of the nursing process used with confused clients begins with the nursing diagnosis of "confusion secondary to _____." It is based on determining if the primary problem has been met, while offering simultaneous treatment for the confusion. Confusion cannot be treated in isolation. Skills in nursing the confused client are important for preventing further deterioration and improving his present state. Evaluation is based on attainment of goals; it determines if nursing care has indeed contributed to change according to previously established criteria.

Riehl and Roy (1974) describe a two-level assessment, with the first level corresponding to the inference of a problem and the second level resulting in a more specific problem statement. In this text the nursing diagnosis takes place on four levels, the first of which is the recognition that the client's behavior is not that which is normally expected in this place and at this time.

The nature of confusion in the elderly poses a challenge to the nurse, similar to care of the premature infant or the comatose patient, where questions are not always answered. The nurse is dependent on her own observations, judgment, knowledge, and skills.

FIRST-LEVEL NURSING DIAGNOSIS

The nursing diagnosis of confusion in the elderly begins inductively from the observations listed in the characteristics of the state of confusion (Fig. 5.1). The first level of the nursing diagnosis of confusion is not one that demands professional knowledge or skills; anyone can make the inference and does. Families and neighbors describe the characteristics that form the basis for this first step. It is a reaction to behavior rather than a diagnosis based on assessment, analysis, and choice between alternatives. It meets Bower's (1977) assumptions, based on the holistic approach taken by nurses:

1. The behavior of the client is an outward sign of an inner experience
2. Until the client is free to disclose his

The four-level nursing diagnosis

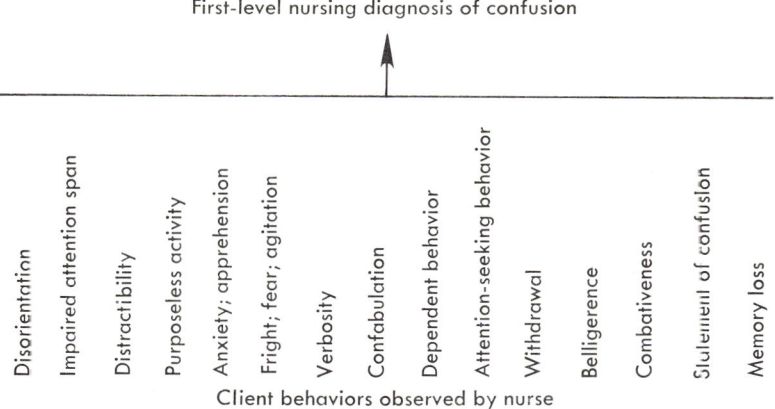

Fig. 5-1. Developing a first-level nursing diagnosis of confusion on basis of nurse's observation of client behaviors. (Adapted from Gebbie, K., and Lavin, M., editors: Classification of nursing diagnoses, St. Louis, 1975, The C. V. Mosby Co., p. 72.)

inner intent, an interpretation of his behavior is only guesswork
3. The client is free to disclose or not to disclose his interests, depending on the amount of trust

The first-level nursing diagnosis of confusion is so general that it gives no clue as to cause or to appropriate nursing action. It is a takeoff point that allows the nurse to assess for confusion rather than a fractured foot. The general term confusional state provides a conceptual framework for data gathering and analysis.

SECOND-LEVEL NURSING DIAGNOSIS

The first level is the subjective reaction to behaviors, which consensus of others deems inappropriate. The second-level diagnosis follows a short but excellent test for confusion based on:
1. Memory—recent and remote
2. Ability to follow instructions
3. Ability to use thinking processes and make a judgment

This test is by no means definitive; the nurse will be only one of several persons determining the amount and kinds of confu-

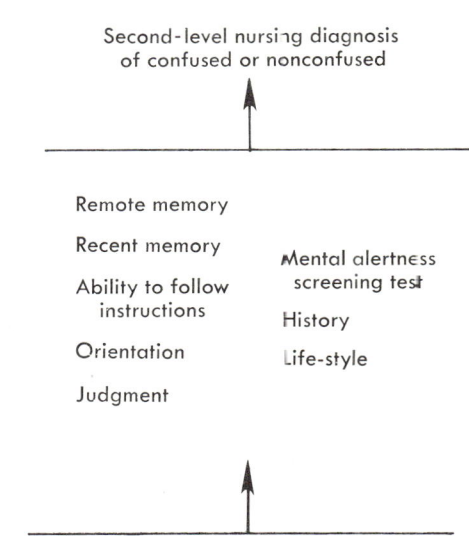

Fig. 5-2. Developing a second-level nursing diagnosis of confusion or nonconfusion on basis of mental alertness screening test.

sion. But this test is important for sorting the confused from the nonconfused. Unfortunately, there are many behaviors and conditions that lead to the erroneous conclusion that the client is confused, when really he is not (Chapter 7). Communication problems are especially found in this category, but apathy, depression, and lack of charm and attractiveness also lead to mistaken diagnoses. Often this is on a subconscious level, but the label of confused is a self-fulfilling prophecy for many. Fig. 5-2 shows the process leading to the second-level nursing diagnosis of confused or not confused. Diagnosis of the state of nonconfusion often must be defended, since stereotypes and attitudes are deep-seated. Confusion or nonconfusion, at this level of nursing diagnosis, is a general symptom that lacks an identified cause; therefore, it cannot be treated.

THIRD-LEVEL NURSING DIAGNOSIS

The third level of nursing diagnosis of confusion (Fig. 5-3) is never attempted without a complete general screening assessment. This comprehensive screening is performed to determine which of a number of differing broad categories may stand out as being important for the client. This includes assessment of the areas of:

1. Sensoriperceptual problems
2. Compromised brain support
3. Other physiologic causes
4. Brain damage
5. Exogenous causes

The screening assessment (Chapter 6) is quite comprehensive, and the elderly person should have no less than the full assessment. At the conclusion of the data gathering process and analysis, a third-level nursing diagnosis can be stated, for example, "confusion secondary to sensoriperceptual problems."

This assessment is much more specific than the first-level diagnosis of confusion, but it is still general. Planning and treatment are impossible until the sensoriperceptual

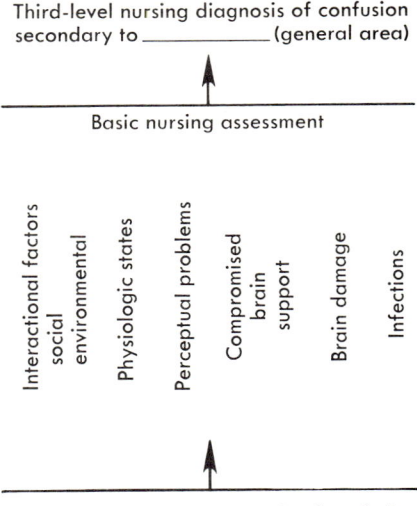

Fig. 5-3. Developing a third-level nursing diagnosis of confusion secondary to _____ (general area).

problem has been delimited to sensory deficit, sensory deprivation, or sensory overload. Specific intervention is dependent on a specific assessment of the indicated area. The third-level diagnosis is specific enough to point out the general direction for the next assessment, which should lead to the problem statement on which nursing care can be planned.

FOURTH-LEVEL NURSING DIAGNOSIS

If the screening assessment has delineated the physiologic factor of pain as the cause of confused behavior, the nurse uses her knowledge of pain assessment to determine the kind of pain, its frequency, onset, duration, location, and triggering mechanisms. She attempts to determine what, if anything, has controlled the pain. She adds to that her knowledge of the various ways the elderly deal with pain, knowing that absence of pain, or lack of feeling, is also significant when taken in context of other signs and symptoms. Then she can analyze

The four-level nursing diagnosis

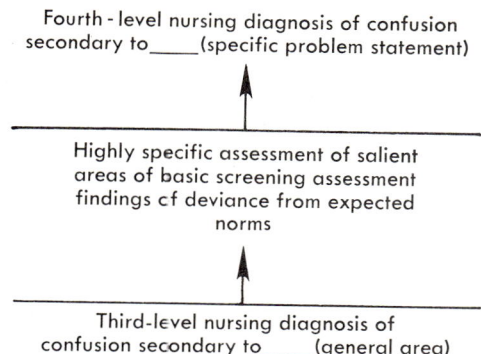

Fig. 5-4. Developing a highly specific fourth-level nursing diagnosis of confusion secondary to _____ (specific problem statement).

her findings to make a fourth-level nursing diagnosis, for example, "confusion secondary to pain in phantom limb (right below the knee amputation), particularly at night."

Intervention can now be highly specific. The primary problem is not confusion but the pain from the phantom limb, and confusion will not change until the pain is treated. These steps follow deliberative nursing. They prevent inappropriate intervention and allow positive action toward a goal that is no longer relief of confusion (Fig. 5-4). The goals now are relief of pain from a phantom limb and support of the patient in the confusional state, with constant validation of reality.

The content of each subsection of the clinical nursing portion of this book (Chapters 8 to 13) is devoted to specific assessments, identification of high-risk persons, prevention, exact statement of the problem, and appropriate nursing intervention. Outcome criteria are given for evaluation of successful nursing actions.

PREDICTABILITY—THE HIGH-RISK CLIENT

It is predictability that marks the truly deliberative nursing action. The development of confusion is rarely an unexpected event that no one could have predicted. Confusion follows an orderly sequence of events, but only recently have nurses become attuned to preventing this grave problem in their elderly clients.

A great, young, orthopedic surgeon dismissed the inquiries of the nurse researcher with a shrug, saying, "All hip-fractured patients become confused." He had a theory that his patient's confusion in connection with his hip repair was caused by mucous plugs in the airway. Today, caregivers can work with elderly clients to prevent mucous plugs in the crucial airway. A good nurse predicts and prevents on the basis of experience and research.

The little group of single women who met often to celebrate each other's birthdays and happy occasions included 90-year-old Alice K., who loved life and who was the creative spark in the group. When she suffered abdominal pain that required surgery one Sunday morning, Betty Spaulding, director of nursing, spent the rest of the day organizing a group of friends who would man every shift with Alice K. at the hospital day and night. She not only planned a tight schedule, but she planned their interactions. When Alice K. awakened she was to be greeted by name and her glasses put on. The friend would give her own name. There was to be no erroneous information. The friend would gently correct any disorientation or confusion. There was a program for varying the environment, and the morning paper was read to Alice as she could tolerate it.

The group supported Alice K. through her sudden relocation into pain and disability. At first Alice awakened confused after each period of sleep and especially after any analgesia. Sedation was held to a minimum. Her friends, who had been carefully coached by Miss Spaulding, kept her in touch with both the present and her life history. The story has a happy ending. Today, 4 years later, Alice K. is 94, still going to birthday parties, having her share of living and loving, and she has a mind that Miss Spaulding says is "clear as a bell."

This incident shows deliberative nursing in its highest form. The nurse rightfully predicted that unless appropriate action were taken, Alice K. was a high-risk candidate for confusion. According to Williams and others (1979), she would have had a low probability of returning to independent living. A careful plan of intervention, based on the nurse's assessment of the patient and her experience, knowledge, and judgment, led to the right action at the right time.

One of the major themes of this text focuses on prevention. *It is our position that much confusion in the elderly is predictable, and if predictable, then it can be prevented.*

Predictors of confusional states

Prevention of confusional states will be discussed with each clinical area in this book. We have defined certain predictors of confusion in the elderly. When nursing implements action at the primary care level of the confusional state, this will be prevention. Research has shown that certain conditions are prodromal. Unlike an infectious disease, confusion can be stopped before and during its incubation period. Predictors that are important and within the control of the nurse, who can manipulate the environment to decrease the threat, are (Wolanin, 1978; Wolanin and Holloway, 1980):

1. Loss of sense of self (depersonalization)
2. Loss of continuity with life history
3. Distortion of time and space cues (the hospital condition)
   a. Restricted space
   b. Lack of familiar objects
   c. Distortion of light and darkness
   d. Disruption of sleep cycle
   e. Period of amnesia (drugs and surgery)
4. Loss of control
   a. Sensory deficits
   b. Sensory overload
   c. Sensory deprivation
   d. Intubation (parenteral, suction, and oxygen)
   e. Urinary problems (bladder emptying, catheters, infection, and incontinence)
   f. Restraints
   g. Disruption of patterns of daily living (sleep, food intake, mobility, and orientation cues)
   h. Pain
5. Age (80 and over very vulnerable)
6. Sex (older men more prone to confusion)
7. Living alone
8. Physiologic problems that interfere with cerebral-support
   a. Hyperthermia
   b. Hypothermia
   c. Dehydration or excessive hydration (edema)
   d. Hypoxia
   e. Hypotension
9. Physiologic action of drugs

SUMMARY

Our summary for this chapter is contained in chart form, which takes the nursing process and the four-level nursing diagnosis through their various steps.

CHAPTER 5 SUMMARY
Nursing process with the confused elderly person

Nursing process	Nursing action
Define general problem	First-level nursing diagnosis of confusion. An inference based on client behaviors (Fig. 5-1)
	Mental alertness testing and history taking to determine
	Second-level nursing diagnosis of confused or not confused.
	Screening assessment to develop more specific
Develop a data base	Third-level nursing diagnosis of confusion secondary to fairly general areas.
	Specific assessment leading to refined
Problem stated in terms of client need for nursing action	Fourth-level nursing diagnosis of confusion secondary to very specific conditions.
Goal setting	Nurse uses knowledge, skills, and references to develop goals within nursing scope.
Plan for nursing intervention	Nurse selects nursing action from options available, with a reasonable prediction of achieving goal.
	Nurse develops a plan of nursing with specific actions and time frames.
Implementation of plan for nursing care	Treatment plan is placed into action with written guidelines (nursing orders), definite assignments, algorithms for recording progress, and coordination with other caregivers.
	Criteria are set that will indicate achievement of goals.
Evaluation of nursing action	Client progress toward goals is measured in relation to nursing care given and by use of criteria. Caregivers review effectiveness in relation to prevention, maintenance, and restoration, or prevention of further deterioration.
Reassess and plan	If care has been ineffective
	Were goals unrealistic? Was assessment thorough?
	Are there better courses of nursing action?

SUGGESTIONS FOR FURTHER READING
Bower, F. L.: The process of planning patient care, ed. 2, St. Louis, 1977, The C. V. Mosby Co.
Harrison, C.: Deliberative nursing process versus automatic nurse action, Nurs. Clin. North Am. **1**:387-397, 1966.
Henderson, V.: The nature of nursing: a definition and its implications for practice, research and education., New York, 1966 Macmillan Publishing, Inc.
Lamonica, E. L.: The nursing process: a humanistic approach, Menlo Park, Calif., 1979, Addison-Wesley Publishing Co.
Mitchell, P.: The process of diagnosis. in Mitchell,: P. H.: Concepts basic to nursing, ed. 2, New York, 1977, McGraw-Hill Book Co.
Zimmerman, D. S., and Gohrike, C.: The goal directed nursing approach: it does work, Am. J. Nurs. **70**:306-310, 1970.

REFERENCES
Bower, F. L.: The process of planning patient care, ed. 2, St. Louis, 1977, The C. V. Mosby Co.
Gebbie, K. and Lavin M. A., editors: Classification of nursing diagnoses, St. Louis, 1975, The C. V. Mosby Co.
Riehl, J. P., and Roy, C.: Conceptual models for nursing practice, New York, 1974, Appleton-Century-Crofts.
Williams, M. A., and others: Nursing activities and acute confusional states in elderly hip-fractured patients, Nurs. Res. **28** (1):25-35, 1979.
Wolanin, M. O.: Acute confusional states following traumatic relocation of the elderly: nursing intervention for prevention. Paper presented at the International Congress of Gerontology, Tokyo, Japan, Aug. 23, 1978.
Wolanin, M. O., and Holloway, J.: Relocation confusion: intervention for prevention. In Burnside, I. M., editor: Psychosocial aspects of nursing, ed. 2, New York, 1980, McGraw-Hill Book Co.

6

PROCESS OF HOLISTIC ASSESSMENT

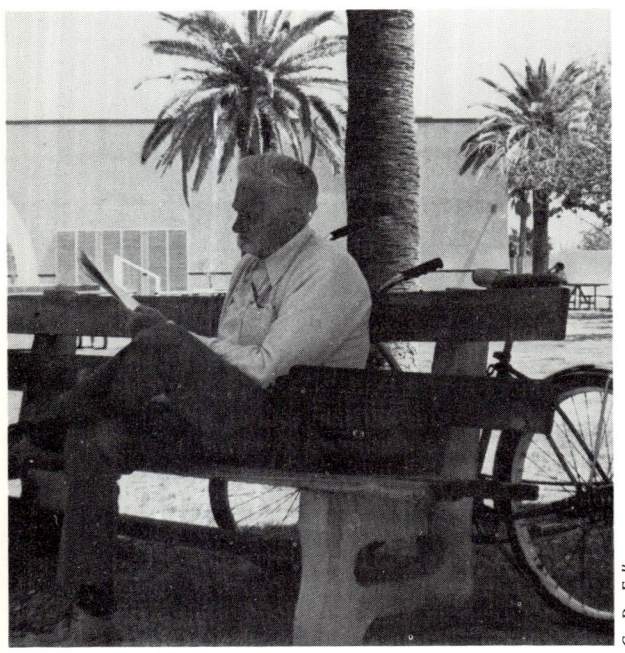

C. D. Falk

This chapter is concerned with the initial assessment of the elderly client. It can be adapted to the setting, for elderly clients are found in their homes or other residences, in acute care settings, and in long-term care units. Every elderly person deserves a full assessment from his primary health caregiver that describes his total functional ability and not just his physical body. For the health care provider, the major question is always to what extent the elderly person's health is at issue. For the elderly person, the answers lie in his total life experience. The assessment in this chapter attempts to take the holistic concept and apply it to the why and how of assessment.

WHAT IS ASSESSMENT?

Bloch (1974) found many uses of the word assessment, and some writers (Griffith, 1971; Weed, 1971) use assessment to refer to the process of analysis of findings and of drawing conclusions that comprise the problem statement (the SOAP approach, using subjective, and objective observations, analysis, and problem statement). Carrieri and Sitzman (1971) use assessment to describe the process through analysis. Mitchell (1977) uses the term assessment to "connote a critical appraisal of all factors past, present, and future" (p. 83). Wolanin (1980) believes that data collection involves concurrent analysis as the nurse constantly sifts through the findings to determine which are relevant. This interpretation determines which data will be studied more intensely, which will be discarded as not relevant, and which will be placed "on file" for future reference. Collection of data as an objective exercise is grounded in the subjectivity of the observer. In this text assessment refers to the process by which the nurse determines which data to seek, how she observes, and the decision that datum A indicates a need for observing datum B. Finally, the selective procedure of interpretation and analysis, which begins with the first observation and continues throughout the assessment, concludes with a statement of the nursing diagnosis. It is a dynamic intrapersonal activity by which the observations of the nurse and her total experience are brought together to explain and predict.

SECTIONS OF ASSESSMENT

The individual is a unity. The conceptual perspective of this text is based on a holistic approach to care of the client with confusional states. However, we find it difficult if not impossible to avoid the tendency to divide the assessment into smaller components. The fallacy in dividing the person is that he cannot be divided. He does not fit into neat compartments, and when the components are put together, the totality which is the individual still escapes. He is never the sum of the parts used by any systematic assessment. Nevertheless, assessment in this text will be divided into four areas that overlap and are far from mutually exclusive. This further emphasizes the unity of the person and the fallibility of caregivers who fail to acknowledge that assessment of the individual and his environment is only part of the whole. The assessment categories are:

1. The person as an organism—a part of life on this earth; an open system interacting with the biosphere (Putt, 1978)
2. The person as continuous in becoming, in space and in time; a product of his life history and his culture
3. The person in interaction with his social and physical environment; how he functions in his own world and in what ways this world affects his health status
4. Assessment of social and physical environment from the standpoint of being facilitative or obstructive

These four categories may seem highly abstract, but for the purposes of this text they will be formed into concrete observations. Assessment is subjective at best; therefore, we will be highly specific as to terminology and descriptions of behaviors.

The test of reality

The reality of the nurse is the basis for the first-level nursing diagnosis of confusion. The first three chapters of this text have emphasized that caregivers are measuring the client's reality by using their own as criterion. There must be further testing to determine if the first-level diagnosis is correct or if there is a difference between the reality of the client and the nurse, which can be explained by any number of other factors. In this text the second-level nursing diagnosis is made to determine if the client is confused, as measured by certain yardsticks. The result of such measurements should be recorded as behaviors instead of judgments. The judgment that must be made is: *Is the client acting appropriately in the situation as he perceives it? If not, what is preventing him from doing so?*

The answer may be that (1) the nurse needs to reconstruct her own point of view; (2) the client needs help with the areas of distorted reality (Chapters 8 to 13); or (3) the client may not be confused, and the nurse has the responsibility to identify why the mistake was made. For example, do the facial contortions and dysarthria of the client with tardive dyskinesia prevent the caregiver from knowing the person behind the mask? For the client who is not confused, but is one of the unfortunate group of people who are mislabeled, this text presents a special chapter on the nonconfused client (Chapter 7).

Assessing for confusion or nonconfusion

There are two concepts that should be considered when the caregiver is attempting to assess the state of confusion of a client. First, the assessment is based on the appropriateness of response. By itself, this presents an inborn margin for error. The concept of appropriateness is based on the premise that the nurse is in possession of certain information that endows her with the capability of comparing what the client says or does with some nebulous norm, thereby arriving at some judgment of what is appropriate. Just as the statistical concept of norms does not allow for individual difference, the concept of appropriateness does not allow for individual variability. Appropriateness is based on consensus of the masses, or what is traditionally normal, and who is to say that either the masses or tradition are always right?

Second, during the assessment process, in-depth baseline data are obtained on admission. Thus, changes can be compared to the baseline data on that client. With confusion, however, it is usually appropriate to conduct an intensive assessment of the state of consciousness only after the client begins to display peculiar behavior. It would be exhausting and time consuming to conduct the type of extensive assessment being proposed for every client who enters the health care system. There are no systematic baseline data with which to compare the results of the assessment, except those based on the initial intuitive notion that the client was lucid. It is, therefore, imperative that the nurse recognize high-risk clients and be alert to any indication of change in behavior. Data as a basis for comparisons of future behavioral changes that might indicate confusion should be obtained as early as possible. The nurse should not wait until confusion is full-blown before assessing the individual. By doing so she not only delays intervention but loses the valuable opportunity to collect longitudinal data that contribute to the understanding of the meaning of confusion for the client.

Methods of collecting data regarding confusion

The assessment of the confused client consists of two major phases: the *listening phase* and the *testing phase*.

The listening phase. This consists of a free-flowing type of interview or observation that focuses on the general aspects of the client's emotional state, his insight into his situation, his attitudes and feelings about himself and significant others, his attention span, and the general relevance of his response to conversational types of inquiry. The important action during this phase is listening, both to what the client says and to what he does not say. It is probably to the advantage of most nurses, unless they are very sophisticated in listening, to set down on paper what is said, by whom, and how, so that some form of formal analysis can be done.

The testing phase. One approach of testing is to divide behavior into four domains: cognitive, reality, perceptual, and interaction. By doing so, the assessor can evaluate those behaviors that comprise each domain and investigate each in depth.

COGNITIVE DOMAIN. Cognition implies all of those processes associated with mentation or intellectual functioning. It involves the ability to remember, reason, think abstractly, calculate, judge, and follow simple or complex commands. Of the important mechanisms of adaptation, the ability to learn may be paramount. The individual must store experience, retrieve the stored information, and use it in appropriate responses in terms of experience (McGaugh and Dawson, 1971).

One of the basic problems in assessing cognition is, that in order for a client to respond effectively and appropriately, the requested information must have relevance. The client must see some purpose for the asking; he must be interested in what is asked of him; and he must maintain that interest long enough to retrieve the information that is asked of him. If he perceives that the questions are nonsense, he might answer with nonsense, even if he has the capacity to answer appropriately. This is of particular significance for clients who are suffering from social deprivation or who are displaying depression or withdrawal. These clients tend to be suspicious or unaccepting of any interaction, especially when the questions seem to be aimed at making a fool of them. Relevancy is also important to the very ill, who must make an effort to comply with even the simplest request and who do not want to be bothered at that time. It takes a great deal of creative effort on the part of the assessor to obtain the kind of information that is needed to assess cognition and still keep the interaction meaningful.

Memory not only involves the recent and remote facets, but also the elements of *recall* and *recognition*. If a client can recall an event, he is capable of answering appropriately, with the only stimulus being the question itself. Recognition is a cruder form of memory testing in that the client may not be able to recall the correct answer from his own memory, but he is able to select the answer from a list of alternatives. It is advantageous to assess all four facets of memory. Simple, direct questions about the client's remote past, such as where he grew up, what school he attended, what jobs he held, and what significant items are in his past medical history, should come to mind. All give an indication of the capacity for remote memory, if this information can be verified. If there are no means available to verify the information, questions such as who bombed Pearl Harbor? and what president served during the Depression? can be used to assess remote memory. These questions, however, may be more threatening and irrelevant and should be approached carefully.

Recent memory can be assessed by asking the client the events that led to his hospitalization, where he lives, and what job he now holds. If the client is frankly unable to recall information, giving him three or four alternative answers and testing to see if he can choose the correct one gives an indication of whether his ability to recognize is intact. During the assessment of memory, the assessor should note whether the client admits he is unable to remember or fills in the gaps with confabulation. This gives an important clue to the kinds of dynamics operating to produce the symptoms.

Reasoning and the ability to calculate can be assessed by the use of a deck of cards, if the client is sighted. First, the client can be asked to sort the cards according to suits. This gives an indication of his ability to class items. Next, he can be asked why two cards, for example, the king of hearts and the king of spades, are alike and why they are different. This gives some indication of his ability to think abstractly. Next, he can be asked to add different numbers of the cards together, as well as to multiply and subtract them. Often, it is very revealing to engage the client in a simple card game, which also gives some indication of his ability to think abstractly. Somehow, the use of playing cards as a vehicle for assessment seems much less nonsensical than launching into a list of questions, such as asking the client to explain the meaning of "birds of a feather flock together." This, however, can be used if the client is sightless or responds negatively to the cards. Cards are of value also for the deaf. Another approach to the same kind of information might be done with environmental objects such as a spoon, fork, cup, glass, pen, pencil, Kleenex, and toilet tissue. The client could be asked to class these items, to tell the differences and similarities between the items in each class, and to give the use of each. With careful explanation, this could be done with blind as well as sighted individuals.

The client's ability to use *appropriate judgment* can best be assessed by long-term observation. If the client makes appropriate use of the objects in his environment, this is one facet of judgment. The client with hemiplegia who has had no training in ambulation but gets out of bed alone to go to the bathroom is using inappropriate judgment. Any demonstration by the client that shows an unawareness or unconcern for his safety and well-being is actually indicative of a deficiency in judgment.

The ability of a client to *follow simple and complex commands* is best assessed during the actual administration of care. During the course of a bath, for example, the client can be asked to perform increasingly more complex tasks, such as (1) wash your face, (2) pick up the soap and put the washcloth in the water, and (3) pull yourself up in bed using the side rails and turn on your left side. The acts that a client is asked to perform should be within his capabilities to respond. That is, if he has a left-sided hemiplegia, it is to no avail to request that he lift his left foot as a measure of his ability to follow commands.

For the ambulatory client in his home, following simple directions can be far more relevant. One of the best methods is to determine how the client keeps his medications and to help him construct a system that ensures compliance. Working together, the nurse and client can soon answer the question of whether the client is able to follow simple directions. Another relevant project is to make a shoe-box file for important letters or papers. The client's ability to use these projects effectively is tested on a return visit and will indicate his judgment. The client may be asked to keep a diary of his food intake for several days as a test for following longer instructions.

Distortions of cognition are so-called delusions. These are false beliefs "... that a person of similar education and experience would consider improbable or impossible and is not corrected in response to reason or logic" (Noyes and Kolb, 1963, p. 74). It is extremely important that if delusions are present, the nature of the delusional material be carefully noted. Delusions fulfill the general purpose of protecting the ego structure of an individual and maintaining a sense of integrity. Therefore, noting their content gives some indication of how to proceed when it is time to plan interventions to help the client cope with his cognitive disorders.

REALITY DOMAIN. Cultural reality is a consensus of what the majority of people in a society specify as real. The Yaqui sorcerer, Don Juan, in Castaneda's *Journey to Ixtlan* taught Castaneda that the world of everyday life is not real or *out there* as we believe it. Reality is a description of the world; "a description that had been pounded into me from the moment I was born" (Castaneda, 1971, p. 9). The sorcerer also explained that we know the world as it is described to us by our teachers, parents, and everyone who comes in contact with us, and we have no point of reference to compare it with anything else. Castaneda reaches the conclusion that the world we know is so taken for granted that no one realizes it is just a description and one of many descriptions.

The traditional medical approach to evaluate a person's reality has been to assess that person's orientation to time, place, and person. At one level this is a valid approach to the collection of reality-based data. However, on another level the emphasis has been on testing whether the client can remember these three things rather than understand these three concepts. Perhaps this will be clear if each is considered separately.

According to Feld (1967), "Time is defined as a relation or fact of continuous or successive existence, or the abstract conception of duration as limitless, capable of division into measurable portions, and essentially comprising the relations of present, past and future..." (p. 369). Time is externally compartmentalized by use of the apparatus known as a clock and calendar. However, we all hold within ourselves an internal clock that dictates the processes of our bodies. We also have the capacity to demonstrate personal time, which is a psychologic event, quite divorced from either the biologic phenomenon or the societally imposed measurement. Virginia Woolf wrote in *Orlando*, "that the human mind has the capacity to stretch an hour to a hundred times its clock length or to compress it into a second."* Somehow we caregivers have the ludicrous idea that by asking a client what time it is or what day it is, we are indicating the complexity that is time. It should be perfectly obvious that people

---

*Woolf, V.: Orlando: a biography, New York, 1973, Harcourt Brace Jovanovich, Inc.

need constant external reinforcement to be able to determine accurately what society defines as time. Rather than asking the person about time from the societal context, we should be considering the client's indication of his conception of time.

This is reflected in our language by the appropriate use of and response to verb tenses. For example, Mrs. H. answered all questions as though they were in the present, even when they referred to the past. Some languages do not have the verbs denoting past tense with all the variations found in the English language. The Indian in particular tends to see the past and present as continuous. It is necessary to ascertain whether the client conceives of the past as separate from the present and of the future as stemming from the present.

Where are you? is a valid question that is frequently asked of clients to ascertain their orientation to place. Perhaps, however, more information is needed in the assessment of a person's orientation to place. It may be necessary to ask the client to describe his impressions of the place, why he is there, and if the place is different from his home and how, in order to adequately assess his orientation to place.

Orientation to person presents another set of problems. Person implies more than name. A person, throughout his lifetime, assumes many roles that are as indicative of his conception of person as his name. It is imperative that nurses assess if the client can identify himself not only as a person but also as a role-player. This implies such questions as: who are you, what are you?, and what do you do?

Summary

Assessment is that process by which information for a data base is collected about the client and his situation for the purpose of planning nursing intervention. When dealing with a client who is suspected of being confused, it is imperative that the client be assessed on as many behavioral parameters as possible. Through assessment of complex factors the nurse can arrive at a more complete picture of the client and the status of his mental processes. Thus, those specific areas for which intervention is necessary or desirable may be more accurately delineated.

At the end of the assessment the nurse should be able to answer the questions of whether or not the client is confused and in what domains confusion exists. (See Tool 6-1 in the summary at the end of this chapter.)

Recording mental status assessment

Mental status is not easily described. Baseline information on mental status is necessary to make estimations of change or progress, but it must be described in qualitative rather than quantitative terms. Our yardsticks are not accurately calibrated; in order to share information with colleagues, or to store it for retrieval at a later date, precise recording is needed. A record should be made of questions asked and their answers. Quotations and described behaviors are the most precise methods of recording that we have at this time. The temptation to resort to numeric ratings or to use subjective adjectives should be resisted.

Assessing the client as a functioning organism

Nurses are quite skilled at assessing the structure and physiology of the client as an organism. Many nurses have added physical assessment skills to their repertoire although they have always done some physical assessment. The geriatric nurse practitioner and gerontologic or geriatric clinical nurse specialist have studied intensively to acquire knowledge and skills required to assess the client accurately and comprehensively (Appendix A). The baseline information that forms the data base will include careful reading of vital signs, reaction to effort, hydration, nutrition, mobility, elimination, and presence or absence of pain. Before proceeding with the examination, the nurse determines the client's sensoriperceptual abilities. If the client is found to have deficits on this cursory examination, the sensoriperceptual assessment is followed to the fourth level of nursing diagnosis, that is, confusion secondary to a specific sensoriperceptual problem, such as uncorrected myopia. In addition to the discussion which follows, Chapter 10 is devoted to identifying the high-risk clients with sensoriperceptual problems, preventing their confusion, and assessing and intervening for clients with sensory deficits, deprivation, or overload.

After determining what sensory deficits are present, if any, the nurse adjusts her approach to the client using skills needed for communicating with an impaired person, for example, facing the person in adequate light and speaking slowly and distinctly.

Perceptual domain

A client's perceptions represent the total of what he senses in the environment and how he interprets his senses. Basic to exploring the perceptions of the individual is the assessment of his sensory apparatus. It is true that the measures the nurse uses to assess the senses are crude at best. She measures deficit in terms of ability to function within the environment and does not offer the sophisticated ophthalmologic or audiologic testing that determines presence and type of impairment. However, the gross measurement provides information that can be used for making referral for more sophisticated testing. Some attempt should be made as early as possible to determine if the client is receiving sensory input and if that input is distorted or misleading.

Visual assessment. The sense of sight can be evaluated by the use of a set of pictures. These should be colorful, clear photographs of objects or animals the client should recognize. Suggestions are a baby, car, dog, flower, tree, or chair. These can be shown to him at varying measured distances, and he can be asked to identify the specific items and colors. Sight should be evaluated with the client's back to glare, with good light on the picture and an informal atmosphere. Evaluation should be made with and without glasses.

A simple vision test is offered at the end of this chapter on the short assessment form. Arrows diminishing in size are portrayed with varying intensity of black on white. The client is asked which way the arrow points as each smaller arrow is uncovered. This simple standardized test can be recorded on the nursing assessment so that all caregivers have an estimate of the visual capacity of the client.

In addition to determination of visual acuity, it is important to determine if the client has a normal field of vision and whether hemianopia is present. The field of vision can be assessed by having the client face the examiner, who is seated 2 to 3 feet away. The client is asked to cover one eye and fix his gaze on the examiner's nose. The nurse brings her finger from the outside of the client's visual arc in along the main axes of the visual field—nasal, temporal, superior, and inferior—with the client indicating when he first sees the wiggling finger. The nurse records the visual field in terms of 180 degrees of visual arc and estimates at what point in that arc the client first saw the finger. If during the examination it is ascertained that the client has hemianopia or loss of peripheral vision (loss of half the visual field, usually resulting from stroke), the information is followed with more exact testing.

Auditory assessment. The client's hearing can be evaluated by using a normal conversational tone in two ways: first, by asking a question that cannot be answered with a yes-or-no answer, and second, by asking the client to repeat some bisyllabic words, such as sunshine, raindrop, mailman, and postcard. The client should be seated directly in front of the tester, with the light on the tester's face. After successfully finishing this examination, he should be tested by the examiner standing behind him and repeating the process: a question without a yes-or-no answer and repetition of bisyllabic words. If there is a deficit in hearing, intensive study should be made to determine under what conditions the client has the best hearing. Referral for further testing may be indicated.

Tactile assessment. The sense of touch must be assessed on several levels. The first of these is soft touch. This is tested by using a wisp of cotton or the assessor's finger to touch, as lightly as possible, various skin surfaces to determine if the client is able to feel it. Pain sensation can be assessed by gentle pinpricks at various areas of the body. The client can also be asked to tell if the sensation is sharp or dull as the pin is applied by alternately using the point and the head. Heat and cold sensation is tested by the use of test tubes containing hot water and ice water applied to various areas of the body. Position sense can be examined by grasping the sides of the thumb and great toe and moving them. The client is asked whether the digit is pointed up or down.

Olfactory assessment. The sense of smell should be examined in clients who are suspected of being confused, because hallucinations of these clients may be of the olfactory variety. The client can be asked to identify several substances, such as tobacco, pine, and peppermint. The closely associated sense of taste is not too significant to a confused client and need not be assessed.

Body image assessment. Another important aspect of the perceptual domain is the client's image of his own body. This is a lifetime intrapersonal accumulation of sensations, both from the body and from those who react to the body. It includes the surface of the body, a feel for the space it occupies, internal sensations, and external posture, as well as attitudes about sexuality, emotional reactions, and personality of the individual. The body is compared with other bodies and with a previous body state, which may denote better or worse health. It is a composite of all the sensations arising from the body and includes a memory that enables the client to compare himself with his earlier, more comfortable, or more energetic self.

Through her interactions with the client and his family, the nurse will assess the client's perception of his present status and whether he sees himself as ill, the value he places on strength and energy, his past experience with illness and stress, how he has coped with stress previously, how he maintains his health, and what special strengths he has as a person (Murray, 1972).

Often it is easy to predict that a client will have a body image problem if he has an obvious defect or a body part loss. However, it should be kept in mind that any illness can severely alter the person's body image even when severe impairment is not apparent. Weakness, lack of energy, and change in sleeping or eating habits alter the body image. Clients measure their illnesses in terms of ability to function. Studies have shown older people with grave physical problems may evaluate their own health as good, while caregivers rated them as very impaired or ill. On the other hand, slight illnesses may be seen as threatening to the person who has always had a body that responded positively. The loss of a tooth may change the body image. The nurse should listen to the client for expressions of his feelings toward his body. (See Tool 6-2 in the summary at the end of this chapter.)

Assessing the client's structure and physiology

After the assessment of the integrity of the sensoriperceptual apparatus, the nurse continues with assessing the client as a functioning organism and an open system in his environment (Putt, 1978). She modifies her approach to take into consideration any sensory deficits discovered in the previous section of the assessment. This second part of the assessment should answer the following questions: (1) what structural or physiologic losses prevent normal function, (2) is there evidence of disease or impairment that should be referred to the physician, (3) what assets does the client have that can be augmented by the nurse's resources, and (4) what other points for referral are indicated. While assessing mental status and sensori-perceptual abilities, the nurse will have observed how the client interacts with his human and physical environments and how he compensates for any losses. Most nurses are quite comfortable with this part of the assessment. (See Tool 6-3 in the summary at the end of this chapter.)

Nursing assessment does not deal with the impairment but with the client who has an impairment. It is a description of the client as a functioning human being. This requires a wide assessment of the client interacting with his environment.

Wolanin (1974) used Abbey's FANCAP* (fluids, air, nutrition, communication, activity, and pain) approach to her functional assessment of the elderly, extending it to include elimination, socialization, and preparation for death. Appraising the whole client as he functions in his environment, this assessment assumes that the client has strengths that allow him to function adequately in many areas, but it also identifies those areas in which he needs nursing assistance to maintain a meaningful existence. The functional assessment stems from Henderson's (1964) definition of nursing as a process that assists the client who lacks the will, knowledge, or strength to return to health or independence or to face a peaceful death. This subsumes the nurse as a resource to the client and requires her to supplement or complement but never replace the client's own physical, social, or emotional assets. Offering nursing care of the appropriate quantity and quality depends on rigorous assessment of the client's assets and deficits.

The functional assessment is based on priorities in Maslow's hierarchy of human needs, which gives survival needs as basic. The primacy of air, fluids, and nutrition cannot be denied, but nurses have more difficulty accepting communication and socialization as primary needs of human beings. Perhaps it is because communication requires a personal commitment on the part of the nurse, which goes far beyond the technical interaction with oxygen, intravenous, and nasogastric tubing. When 200 nurses were asked which they preferred to care for, a comatose patient or a depressed patient, 99% indicated the comatose patient. The reason given by most was that the depressed patient was so difficult to communicate with. This nursing preference points to a blind spot that we, as nurses, may not recognize or admit. The comatose patient requires no interaction. In fact, some nurses said (Wolanin, 1975a):

"When you get them done up, they stay done up."

"I can daydream while I am caring for the comatose patient."

"I don't have to watch every little word."

Recognition of communication problems is basic to the assessment of the elderly confused client.

Place of assessment. The client is often observed in the artificial setting of the health professional's work place, where observations are made in terms of the present. This gives a one-dimensional view of the multidimensional client. Observation of his interaction with his social and physical environment is crucial in assessing the client with problems of mental status. If he is denied the advantage of his familiar and natural situation and placed in the strange environment of the health care unit, he reacts differently, becoming less observant and more anxious as he responds to questions and answers. His life history becomes obscured in the pressure of the immediate and may be forgotten.

Nurse as the primary caregiver. The nurse is often the primary caregiver for elderly persons, especially those in their own

---

*Used by June Abbey in her classes at the University of California.

homes or institutions. Elderly clients are loath "to bother the busy doctor." They turn to the nurse as someone who can spare the time and take the effort to help them.

The primary caregiver has the responsibility to make an interpretation to other involved members of the health care team. The nurse's systematic assessment of the older client's ability to function in his environment requires a concise statement, for it may be accepted as the only assessment. For example, a medication nurse mailed a list of a patient's drug orders to the physician to sign and mail back. This met the requirement that orders be updated monthly. She noted opposite the order for a hypnotic, "The patient does not sleep." When the orders were returned, the physician had crossed off the first hypnotic and written in the name and dose of another with a scrawled "Thank you" beside the discontinued order. More information would have helped the physician, but he did not ask for it. Wolanin (1975b) found that a telephone call to the physician was the most effective means (which include mailed order, physician's visit to patient, or physician's visit to desk or telephone) of getting a tranquilizer order changed. Rarely was the nurse's assessment questioned or challenged.

The vital signs. The most available indicators of the circulatory function, respiratory effectiveness, and ability to react to physical stressors are the vital signs. In the elderly, pulse and respiration are extremely sensitive indicators of change in the state of health. However, the admission vital signs can rarely be used as baseline information, for they are increased by the anxiety and stress of change and threat of illness. Serial readings under less stressful conditions are advised for vital signs. At some point the readings will show a stability, which is probably the baseline and can be accepted as the basis comparison. Serial readings should be continued until this point. The first blood pressure may give a reading reflecting the anxiety the client feels in the testing situation instead of his baseline blood pressure (Williams and others, 1979).

At the end of the assessment of the vital signs and the nurse's other evidence of the client's circulatory and respiratory health, the nurse should be able to answer the following questions:
1. Does this client's circulatory and respiratory status indicate adequacy to cope with the demands of his lifestyle?
2. Does it indicate disease?
3. What can he do to improve his status?
4. What, as a nurse, can I do to enable him to live more comfortably?

Body temperature response in the elderly is much different from the fast-reacting fever of the young. An elevation of temperature is usually significant and can reflect an infection, especially in the urinary tract, or an inability to lose body heat in a high ambient temperature. The pulse and respiration are more sensitive indicators of pneumonia or abdominal infections (Agate, 1971b). The slightest elevation of either may indicate a severe infection. When accompanied by a change in the physical condition or general malaise, it should be regarded with suspicion.

Even more important is the decrease in body temperature, which may indicate accidental hypothermia. This can be related to lack of body activity, low ambient temperature, conditions that lead to rapid heat loss, or drugs that affect the thermoregulatory system, such as the phenothiazines. The decrease in temperature may be so great as to be unmeasurable by the clinical thermometers used in most institutions. Changes in facial appearance and color and small changes in the respiratory rate are important observations to make with the temperature reading. Abnormal readings should include the contextual situation of the elderly person, including his activity, ambient temperature, movement of air, and drug intake.

Today, with electronic monitoring devices, taking the pulse is overlooked in favor of the more sophisticated sensors. The nurse who is in the home or the extended care unit, however, rarely has such equipment available and will still find the pulse a very sensitive indicator of change in the physiologic state. The rate may remain the same for the heart at rest during the life span, but the response to stress is altered with increased age. The quality of the pulse, its rate, rhythm, and change with effort are important baseline measurements.

Indicators of cardiac failure, such as the filling of hand veins when dropped below the level of the heart and the decreased or sluggish emptying when raised above the sternal notch, should be observed while taking the pulse. If the client has his body in a sitting position with 30 degrees of elevation, the neck veins should be collapsed. Increased central venous pressure will result in distention of the neck veins.

The lungs seldom perform for 60 to 70 years without changes in elasticity, and the chest itself undergoes changes that alter respiration. In elderly people the rigidity of the lung tends to expansion of the upper portion of the lung and may result in collapse of the basilar portion. The pattern of respiration changes, and the older person may have to move more air in and out of his chest to use a comparable amount of oxygen. Under any physiologic stress, tissue perfusion increases and oxygen demands are greater. Also, changes in the flow dynamics result from reduced propulsive force of the aging thorax. A decreased ability to cough results in the development of stasis in the supine position or in any enforced bed rest (Goldman, 1971). Respiration receives scant attention in taking vital signs, but it is a crucial measurement for the elderly client. The rate at rest, the depth, and the nature (short inspiration, long expiration, or any variation) are noted. Sounds of breathing should be noted even if the breathing is quiet. This offers a baseline against which later estimations can be compared. Change in respiration with effort should be observed, including the effort of speaking, of moving the body, or of any sustained effort. Additional stress is reflected in respiratory rate and is often the first sign of change in physiologic status.

The kyphotic elderly person with trunk shortening from loss of the intravertebral padding or compression fractures of the vertebrae will undergo increased respiration while sitting or after eating a large meal, resulting in extremely shallow breathing.

Blood pressure is also an important assessment of health in the elderly. The campaigns against hypertension in this country have resulted in a feeling that lack of hypertension is a good state. For the elderly, it is the hypotensive state that can lead to dizziness, syncope, and falls (Agate, 1971b). For the elderly, sudden hypotension is often the important sign of such grave disorders as coronary thrombosis instead of the classic symptom of chest pain. Hypotensive episodes may also occur as a response to medication.

With the publicity given blood pressure readings, the act of measuring produces a certain anxiety. The client should be told beforehand that his blood pressure will be taken six times: in both arms in the three positions of lying, sitting, and standing. He should be assured that this is a routine test, but it should be acknowledged that not everyone checks in all six positions. This process will indicate any postural hypotension and give information for some cardiac disorders that are manifested by differences in the blood pressure found in the arms.

The older person who is receiving antihypertensive, diuretic, or tranquilizing drugs should have this information noted in the nursing assessment in conjunction with the blood pressure readings.

Nutritional status. At the end of the nutritional assessment, the nurse should be able to answer the following questions:
1. Does the medical diagnosis indicate a problem that interferes with nutrition?
2. Does this client's nutritional status

appear adequate for a person in his situation?
3. Can he improve his nutritional status?
4. What assistance can I, as a nurse, give him to improve his nutritional status?
5. What drugs is the client taking that interfere with his nutrition?

To check the client's nutritional status, the admission weight is recorded and, where possible, checked against his normal weight or compared with his past weight. The general appearance of the body will offer evidence of recent rapid weight loss, as shown by skin folds over the skeleton. The girth should be measured with a tape measure to determine presence of abdominal edema and the dependent parts scrutinized for signs of edema. Color of the mucosa and nail beds may indicate anemia. Poorly healed lesions over the body may indicate poor nutritional status.

The mouth is an important part of the nutrition assessment, both from the standpoints of the past and for the future. The lips should be inspected for color, breaks in the mucosa, and lesions in the corner of the mouth, which may indicate avitaminosis. The number of teeth, state of repair, and approximation for chewing and biting or their replacement by well-fitting dentures should be noted. Bright red, bleeding, spongy gums indicating periodontal disease may also signal a nutritional deficiency. The tongue should respond with easy movement at command, but if there is a sluggish movement of the tongue, drooling, or dysarthria, ability to swallow should be tested. Nutritional status in the elderly is directly related to ability to chew and swallow. Chewing, swallowing, and talking are dependent on adequate saliva to moisten the food and lubricate mouth parts. Hydration can be checked by inspecting the saliva pool in the pocket under the tongue into which the sublingual glands empty.

Where possible, an estimate of the client's food intake should be obtained, noting protein and vitamin content and intake patterns. Some factors that give information when food histories are unavailable are the client's living condition (alone?); income for buying food; mechanical ability to buy, carry, and prepare food (muscular strength); and mental depression.

Hydration. At the end of this assessment the nurse should be able to answer these questions:
1. Does this client have enough fluid to carry on his life processes?
2. Can he supply the means to hydrate his own body (motor skills and alertness)?
3. What, as a nurse, is required of me to enable this client to have adequate hydration?
4. Does his medical regimen contribute to dehydration?

The skin of the client is rarely a reliable index of his hydration, for it is often dry and not related to the internal hydration. Hydration is assessed by the saliva-pool test already mentioned, but this test may be invalidated for the client who is being given drugs that dry mouth secretions. Hydration is also measured by the hematocrit, which may indicate hemoconcentration concurrent with hypovolemia.

Urinary output must be checked for relation of quantity to intake, time of excretion (as when the client is lying down at night), color, and specific gravity. The urinalysis is very important if available, but the nurse can use her other observations to make a preliminary check. The elderly may have renal impairment that prevents the dilution or concentration of urine.

The nurse will test her findings against the client's blood pressure and mental status to determine if hydration is adequate. She must interpret laboratory findings and add this data to her observations. She will note any drugs administered to the client that interfere with his hydration.

Elimination. At the end of this assessment the nurse should be able to answer the following questions:
1. Can this client eliminate his body wastes?

2. If not, what actions on the part of the client will establish satisfactory patterns of elimination?
3. What exercises, foods, medications, or other methods has the client used to regulate bowel activity during his life?
4. What nursing intervention is needed to assist the client to eliminate wastes from his body?

The elimination of wastes from the body is a survival need. Assessment of elimination is a continuation of the nutritional-hydration assessment. A high index of suspicion should lead the nurse to initiate the assessment for ability to empty bladder and bowel rather than waiting for any emergent signs and symptoms. Every relocated client (home to hospital or hospital to extended care unit or home) is vulnerable. The full bladder of the elderly client with a hypertrophic prostate is an emergency and can lead to bizarre and confused behavior. Fecal impaction is both a nursing and a client problem. The inactive or dehydrated client or the one who takes large doses of drugs will be a candidate for impaction.

Elimination may not be under the conscious control of the client. In such instances, incontinence of urine or feces is not only a physiologic problem, but a social one that will interfere with rehabilitation. There is a close association between incontinence and confusional states; which comes first is a point for debate. Incontinence is not an unsolvable problem. Its assessment requires a highly skilled nurse who is conscious of the many factors that contribute to incontinence—the possibility of infection, neoplasm, neurologic deficits, motor problems, communication problems, and drug effects.

Activity and motor ability. The questions to be asked at the end of this part of the assessment are not concerned with how impaired the client is but:
1. To what extent has he compensated for his impairments to negotiate his environment successfully?
2. To what extent does his limitation prevent his engaging in activity necessary to his physical being, such as relief of pressure, circulation, heat production, and sensory stimulation?
3. To what extent does his impairment result in loss of human contact?
4. What does this client need from me, as a nurse, to enable him to function as a whole person in his environment?

The older client's ability to use his body effectively must be judged by different criteria from those used for the younger person. Full range of joint motion and strength of muscles as well as coordination of muscle groups to enable the client to perform intended activities involve integrity of the neurologic and musculoskeletal system. Motor and neurologic losses are very common in the elderly; they range from joint stiffness to lack of coordination of muscle groups needed to execute the activities of daily living. There are widely varying degrees of loss, and the client may have compensated for much of this loss; others impose severe disability. The elderly client's motor ability is judged against his life history and adaptation to his present environment rather than against any standard for his age cohort. Various parts of the body have to be assessed separately, not as a whole. There may be good movement of the hands but poor shoulder movement and lack of strength in the biceps and triceps. The ability to comb one's hair, shave, dress, and feed oneself test the motor ability of the upper extremity in the most practical way.

An important part of the motor assessment for the older person is the inspection of his feet and lower legs, including the knee joint. To what extent are the quadriceps adequate to support the knee during standing and walking? Are the muscles of the lower leg wasted or weak? What circulatory problems are apparent on inspection of the leg —varicosities, ulcerations, or brown spots over the shin? Finally, what is the condition of the foot? Using King's assessment tool (Appendix C), the foot should be inspected carefully to include the sole. After the non–weight-bearing assessment the nurse must note the fit of the hose and shoes. Does the shoe enable the client to walk with a normal gait? The ability to walk should be judged by watching the client walk on a smooth but not slippery floor with a pair of hard-soled shoes that fit snugly.

Ability to move from bed to chair or from chair to standing position requires good hip and knee action. Many older persons have compensated for lack of strength by innovative means and assistive devices. Coordination of upper extremity and motor skill is required to effectively use the assistive devices.

The strength of the arm and shoulder muscles is important for the client who uses assistive devices, which become appendages of his body but require a totally different group of muscles to maintain mobility. The wheelchair may become a part of the body in the same way that a shoe is part of the foot, and it must be fitted just as closely. The client should be assessed in relation to his ability to be mobile with the use of the wheelchair. Do its dimensions correspond to the client's own in leg length, seat width and depth, and arm height? Does the height of the arm support allow leverage for getting in and out of the chair, and does the client use his braking system correctly? Motor ability of the wheelchair-bound or bedfast client requires an assessment of his ability to change position by himself. Can he shift his weight in the seat of the chair or move his knees from that constant angle of 90 degrees or less? Can the bedfast client shift position by pulling or pushing or rolling over from side to back?

Observation of the lack of ability to rotate the head from side to side can be crucial in planning for the safety of the individual. Many older people have cervical spondylitis that limits the neck movement for turning the head to see or hear.

Pain should be suspected when the elderly client restricts his activities and his world is reduced to smaller and smaller boundaries. In the home, prominence of over-the-counter analgesics should lead to further assessment for pain. The demobilization associated with pain becomes the cause of the client's own sensory deprivation.

Drug use. In the home the nurse must also assess whether the client can manage his own medication administration:
1. Can he be depended on to follow the regimen prescribed?
2. Does he understand the purpose of each drug?
3. Are his drugs kept in safe places (the kitchen window sill is often the storage place for a long line of drugs)?

All drugs assimilated into the client's body are part of his physiology. No assessment is complete without a full knowledge of all his medications and drugs, including prescription drugs, over-the-counter remedies, alcohol, folk remedies, and certain foods that interact with drugs in the body. It is important to know the state of hydration and, if known, any allergic reactions to foods or drugs. Not all of this information is available, and often it is acquired quite accidentally. But it should be considered an integral part of the assessment, and every effort made to complete the data base. For the confused elderly person two of the most important questions are:
1. What drugs does this client take?
2. What sudden changes have occurred in his life?

The two questions may seem unrelated, but a drug regimen that was satisfactory may be completely altered by exposure to excessive heat or cold, dehydration, or stress. The client is a unified whole interacting with his social and physical environment. Dividing him into compartments for assessment should never result in disregarding relationship between the elements that compose the total person and his environment. Drugs may be responsible for sudden changes, and sudden changes may alter the physiologic response to drugs.

Pain. Assessment of pain should answer the following questions.

1. Is this client having pain?
2. Is he able to feel the dangerous elements in his environment?
3. How does he perceive his discomfort?
4. What is his usual action to relieve pain and has it been effective?
5. What nursing intervention is required to relieve the cause of the client's pain or to prevent his lack of pain from threatening his safety?

Pain is such an important diagnostic tool that alteration in its occurrence in the elderly is a nursing problem. The existence of pain must be noted as to onset, type, severity, location, duration, context, what triggers its onset, and what relieves it. Pain is primary, leading to pinhole vision in which the client is unable to see his world except as it relates to the experience of pain. The elderly client in pain needs every possible mode of relief.

Also important in the elderly is the lack of pain, such as occurs with neurologic deficits. The inability to use pain as a warning signal results in pressure that can lead to ulceration. Agate (1971a) quotes one study in which only 19% of the elderly who had cardiac infarction or acute abdominal conditions felt pain. On the other hand, pain in the chest may indicate a gastric disorder or a hiatal hernia. The nurse must be on the alert for the other signs and symptoms of physical deterioration and not wait for pain as an indicator. (See Tool 6-3 at the end of this chapter).

The medical diagnosis

A medical diagnosis, when it exists, leads to an assessment designed around the known facts about the disease state and its signs and symptoms. The diagnosis and plan of treatment include the nurse as part of the plan for implementation. The confused client often is referred to the physician by the nurse, in which case she has the responsibility to make out a referral form listing her observations. Clients from nursing homes are frequently taken to the physician's office for diagnosis and treatment. The referral sheet should accompany the client. In turn, it is expected that the physician share pertinent information with the nurse to accompany the orders he gives for the client. Any referral to a community agency should have a summary of the assessment, which is pertinent to the receiving agency. The nurse is one of the few health professionals who makes estimates of the physiologic status.

The life history

The life history of the older person is important because of its extensive and cumulative nature. It may not be apparent and is often left behind at the door of an institution or home when the people who shared that history are gone. The demographic information gives some clues as to life history—age, race, marital status, nearest of kin, birthplace, income, work status, and place of residence. These data are all a part of one's life history but they are not *the* life history.

The health history also provides only a part of the life history. Education, religion, interests, cultural background, methods of coping with problems, and recent losses all contribute to understanding the present behaviors. The type of work experience can often give clues to health problems; for example, a high volume of noise in the place of work may lead to deafness. Presenting a totally different aspect, however, is the musician who has become deaf and loses his lifetime companion, the sound of music. What are the relationships that have been severed because of retirement or aging? Who are the significant people in the client's life, and are they also listed with the losses? The losses may have been physical, economic, status, privacy, or even the loss of the ability to control his own life. Were the losses recent? Was there enough time between losses for recovery, or were losses continuous and concentrated in a very short time? Whom does this client use as a confidant? What personal resources does he recognize? Is his religious faith a comfort?

The nurse may be dependent on family

for information about the culture of the older person. Myerhoff (1978) believes that generalizations cannot be made about the elderly, for they represent such a great variety of styles and forms in different cultural settings. She feels that the nonbiologic factors play a significant role, that is, "culture appears to explain more of the peculiarities and idiosyncrasies than do factors due to a common humanity" (p. 152). The nurse has not shared the culture or even the historic era of her elderly client, so she does not understand his world view. Her understanding of his life history is fleshed out with readings of authors who describe the aged, such as Curtin (1972), Sartin (1973), and Myerhoff (1979), and by listening to the elderly themselves as they reminisce.

Recording the information about the life history and culture of the client is a matter of synthesis and winnowing. The elderly would likely not talk if they knew what they were saying was a permanent record. Life history is shared with individuals who are trusted. The elderly have their little secrets and must be allowed to keep them. This means that gossip between caregivers is forbidden, and information should be shared only a basis of the need to know to give adequate care. A 56-year-old surgeon, after a 2-month hospital stay for a serious illness, wrote: "I am finally home and adapting very well. Friends call every day to check on my progress and are respecting my desire to have a whirl at taking care of myself. After 2 months of goldfish-bowl living day and night, I find my need for some privacy rather crucial."

As caregivers, we find the need for information as overwhelming as the client finds his need for privacy. The older person may cause conflict regarding assessment. The principle to be followed is the need to know. If information is really important, its value can be explained to the client. More often his need to have us know is the deciding factor. If we just offer a sincere interest and a willingness to listen, answers to our unasked questions are often forthcoming.

(See Tool 6-4 in the summary at the end of this chapter.)

Assessing the client's environment

Environments must be assessed to answer two questions:
1. What in this environment facilitates this client's ability to function as a person?
2. What in this environment prevents this client from functioning to the fullest extent of his abilities?

In order to assess the environment, it must be separated into its human (or social) and its physical components. The goldfish-bowl existence described in the previous section demonstrates the relationship of the two. The older client may complain that there is no place to hide, but he is actually saying, "I cannot hide from the people who invade my privacy."

Human or social environment. The human environment should be assessed for:
1. Members of a peer group, particularly a confidant
2. A natural support system—a reliable person the older person can depend on for help in a crisis
3. Affectional relationships—people or pets who give and receive love
4. Service personnel who can be trusted to provide goods and services, such as barbers, hairdressers, physicians, lawyers, nurses, and plumbers
5. People who have a negative influence and make the older client feel incompetent and tend to depersonalize him

The existence of a family is subsumed to take care of the first three of these human relationships. The quality of family relationships does not guarantee this, however; no assumptions should be made without some validation. When any of the three are missing, surrogates are needed to fill the gaps. Perhaps the gravest need is to have a continuity of caring people. The sudden loss of the human resources who have enriched one's life is a grave threat to life itself. Losses are readily discovered, but many interactions with the family and client may be required to identify supportive human resources to determine their real strength. *In some instances, where clients have outlived their family and peer group, there may be no one, absolutely no one to turn to, and the burden of the surrogate role falls to the caregivers.* (See Tool 6-5 in the summary at the end of this chapter.)

Physical environment. Assessment of the physical environment is accomplished by figuratively taking the position of the client and looking at the environment for obstacles to independent function. When the assessment is finished, it should have answered these questions:

1. What in the environment prevents the client's ability to function as a person?
2. How can a caregiver facilitate the client's ability to function by altering the environment or teaching the client to adapt to the unchangeable?

After assessment of the structural, physiologic, and sensoriperceptual abilities, the observer is better able to assess the physical environment in terms of the capabilities of the individual. Environments must be tailored to the special needs of the impaired individual, because our world is planned for young, strong, right-handed, medium-height people. Deviation from that norm has always required adaptation by the deviant individual. The healthy adaptive person rarely needs nursing assistance. The special needs of the client should be the basis for determining if the environment will serve as a barrier to function or facilitate the use of remaining assets. For the individual with problems of equilibrium and gait, the initial assessment is of the floor covering, railings, stairs, and lighting. The client with decreased vision requires color contrast, adequate lighting, stable furniture placement, and magnifying glasses to enlarge the small objects in his world. Any relocation requires a tactile orientation.

Interaction domain. Nursing intervention has two aspects: (1) helping the client to control or adapt, or (2) changing the environment to a more facilitative arrangement in which the client can interact at his own level. An assessment of the situation will determine which of the two interventions is appropriate, or if both are needed.

At the end of the assessment the nurse should be able to estimate to what extent the physical environment prevents interaction and to what extent the client needs the caregiver's assistance in restructuring his approach to deal with the obstructive elements of the environment.

Interaction with the human components of the environment is an important part of the assessment of the elderly client who may be confused. Interactions tend to be positive and negative rather than neutral. If the assumption is made that all behavior has meaning and reflects some inner experience, then interaction between humans takes on a constructive or destructive element, as well as being positive or negative. Interaction with others is a two-way process; the sending person is dependent on a receiver who is not a neutral part of the interaction but a force for action. While interactions are usually studied in relation to what the confused person says or does, the recipient is often an inciting factor of the reaction. Interaction of the confused person must be studied for its reactional component.

Observations of the interaction should include:

1. Does the client attempt to interact with others? Are his efforts met with an accepting response? To what extent is the recipient contributing to the attempt, either positively or negatively?
2. Is the interaction successful? If not, what appears to be the reason?
3. With whom does he interact most? Least?
4. To what kind of approach does he react best?
5. Is there any central or recurring theme in this reaction?

6. What defense mechanisms seem foremost in his interactions?
7. Does he use nonverbal forms of interaction? Why?
8. What emotional overtones are evoked by subjects? People?
9. Does everyone he contacts see him as confused? If not, where does the variation arise?
10. What interactions cause frustration? What actions on the part of caregivers reduce frustration?
11. Are certain people more successful in interactions with this client than others?
12. Is the client able to accept offers of friendship or love?
13. Does he demonstrate a need to give love?
14. Does the client seek privacy?

After making such observations, the caregiver should be able to pinpoint the most facilitative aspects of the social environment to keep the client involved as a human with other humans and to give him a chance to love and be loved.

The physical environment begins where the boundaries of our physical bodies end. However, as open systems, we remain part of our environment, and the very air we breathe is equivocal—is it part of us or our environment? Ambient temperature, adequate clothing, and air movement affect our reaction to that most constant part of our environment: the air that surrounds us. Much of our life is spent reacting to it, and this ability to react and control is an essential part of our being. We may use our environments to our advantage, or we may let them dictate our life-style.

Does the client have control over this essential part of the environment? Is he reacting to temperature, does he appear to be warm or cold, and can he adjust his clothing and activity or alter the temperature? The assessment of the client's interaction with his physical environment includes making an estimate of whether he alters and adapts to it or is passive and makes no attempt to change it for his greater benefit. The passive person may be trapped or imprisoned by the very environment that challenges another person to positive action. The trapped client may withdraw, or he may lash out in frustration at circumstances he cannot control. (See Tool 6-6 in the summary at the end of this chapter.)

THE TOTAL ASSESSMENT

For too many years the clients with mental health problems were compartmentalized as psychiatric patients. Their physiologic aspects were ignored, even though the physiology was being altered with drugs. For the elderly there can be no compartmentalization. Every elderly client deserves a full assessment; within the framework of this text it is essential.

Quinn and Ryan (1979) remind us that it is difficult to compress 80 years of living and life experience into 90 minutes of interview. It is not only difficult but inadvisable, unless the older person feels free to talk without being interrogated. For example, one 80-year-old said: "That young girl came in here and gave me the third degree—regular FBI interrogation."

The assessment of an older person never ends; new and important data are collected with each nursing transaction. The reader who has studied this chapter is wondering how time can be spared to make such an assessment. Time for this assessment is an administrative decision and should be part of the standard of care given by the agency. Several parts of the assessment can be made at the same time, and with practice, the caregiver economizes on effort.

Analyzing the data and drawing conclusions about the findings require some uninterrupted thinking if the assessment is to be a means to an end. Data that did not seem so important on the assessment loom large when considered vis-a-vis other data. An asset in one of the four areas (p. 59) may help in another. The total picture of the client must be brought into focus as he is reconstructed from the data. It is at this point that all the previous nursing experience is brought to the situation, and judgments are made. It takes time, but not that much time that it can be overlooked. The reader should think of this period of analysis and of the conclusions that follow as the central difference between *routine*, or *ad hoc*, nursing and *deliberative* nursing. The data should be analyzed as a whole instead of datum by datum as it was when collected. From the analysis and synthesis, conclusions can be drawn on which to base nursing action.

The result at the end is the third level of nursing diagnosis—a problem statement identifying general areas that need to be pursued by a specific assessment. There will be such statements as "confusion secondary to physiologic status (nutritional deficit)" or "confusion secondary to physiologic status (dyspnea with effort)." Either statement does not have enough specificity to prescribe nursing intervention. Nursing intervention for the one would be totally different from nursing intervention for the other. Specific assessments follow in Chapters 8 to 13, with the appropriate nursing intervention for prevention and treatment.

CHAPTER 6 SUMMARY
Process of holistic assessment
Tool 6-1. Assessment of mental status

Instructions
This examination overlaps with the sensoriperceptual examination; they may be done simultaneously.

Have client sit or lie in a comfortable, relaxed positon, with arms and hands resting on a table between you and him. Room should be well lighted, client should have back to any glare, and your face should be well lighted. If the test can be conducted in informal circumstances, the client is less likely to have stress alter his best response.

Cognitive domain
Recent memory: Introduce yourself and give a simple name to remember—first name, or one syllable last name. Ask client to repeat it to ensure he has heard it correctly. After 5 minutes ask client if he remembers name; if he is hesitant, repeat name. After 5 minutes ask name again, and if client hesitates, repeat name. At end of examination or after 15 minutes, ask if he remembers your name. If name is not remembered (recall), ask him which of three names it is (recognition). Record response of recent memory:
1. Correct after 5 minutes
2. Correct after 10 minutes (second)
3. Correct after two reminders (third)
4. Able to distinguish name from series of three
5. Unable to recall name with assistance

Remote memory (for person 60 years of age or older): Who dropped the bombs on Pearl Harbor? Who was president at the time of the Depression? If no immediate response, use recall: Germany, France, Japan? Coolidge, Wilson, Roosevelt?

Following instructions: Give one-step instruction, for example, will you take a sip of water? If successful give two-step instruction, for example, please take a Kleenex from the box and hand it to me. Three-part instruction—three relevant requests.

Reality domain
Orientation: Where do you live? Response? What is this place? Response? When is this (if evidence is available, such as clocks and calendars)? For the unsighted, ensure that access to time orientation is possible. Ask unsighted, which holiday have we just celebrated?

Computation: When were you born? How old are you now? Assist as needed. Record sequence of responses.

Tool 6-2. Assessment of sensoriperceptual abilities

Hearing test

Have client be seated across from you, about 4 feet distant. Your face should be well lighted; eliminate any glare. Use conversational tone. Ask client relevant questions that cannot be answered by yes or no, for example, what do you like to eat for breakfast?
Client response:
Ask client to repeat the following words spoken in conversational tone. Write answers given. Note carefully any turning of the head to hear and the need to speak more loudly or to speak more slowly before the client answers. Allow time between words and start by saying, "The next word is . . ."

Word given	Client's response
Beefsteak	
Mailman	
Staircase	
Floor mop	
Applesauce	
Postcard	

Stand about 4 feet behind client and repeat the examination using a different question and different words.
Question:
Client response:
Repeated words:
Client response:
Does the client have a hearing aid? If so, test again with hearing aid.

Vision test

Note how the client avoids obstacles in approaching the chair, how clothing is fastened, and whether the client "looks" at the situation.

In well-lighted room, ask the client to look at test objects and name them. If glasses are worn, test with and without glasses. Clean glasses. Stand in front of client. Place test sheet (p. 79) with smaller arrows covered on floor between you and the client. Ask which direction each arrow points, uncovering each smaller one as the client is successful. If he is unable to see all four, place on table in front of client at 3 feet and retest. Record as functional vision, partially functional vision in good light, very little functional vision, and nonfunctional vision. **A,** If client cannot see arrow direction, vision is nonfunctional. **B,** If client cannot see arrow direction, vision is not safe for function. Can see large objects only and in good light and with contrast. Unlikely to read signs or reality board, clock, or calendar. **C,** If client cannot see arrow direction, he can see little detail and walking may be unsafe. Can eat and care for self if light is adequate and contrast is used for detail. Test with clock and reality board. **D,** If client can see this arrow direction, probably has functional vision. Suggest for this client that a newspaper be used to determine ability to read signs and large headline print to smaller print. Indicate each response:

	Without glasses		With glasses	
A. Large arrow	Correct	Incorrect	Correct	Incorrect
B. Medium arrow	Correct	Incorrect	Correct	Incorrect
C. Small arrow	Correct	Incorrect	Correct	Incorrect
D. Smallest arrow	Correct	Incorrect	Correct	Incorrect

Check correct response for other test objects:
Cat
Clock
Cup

Continued.

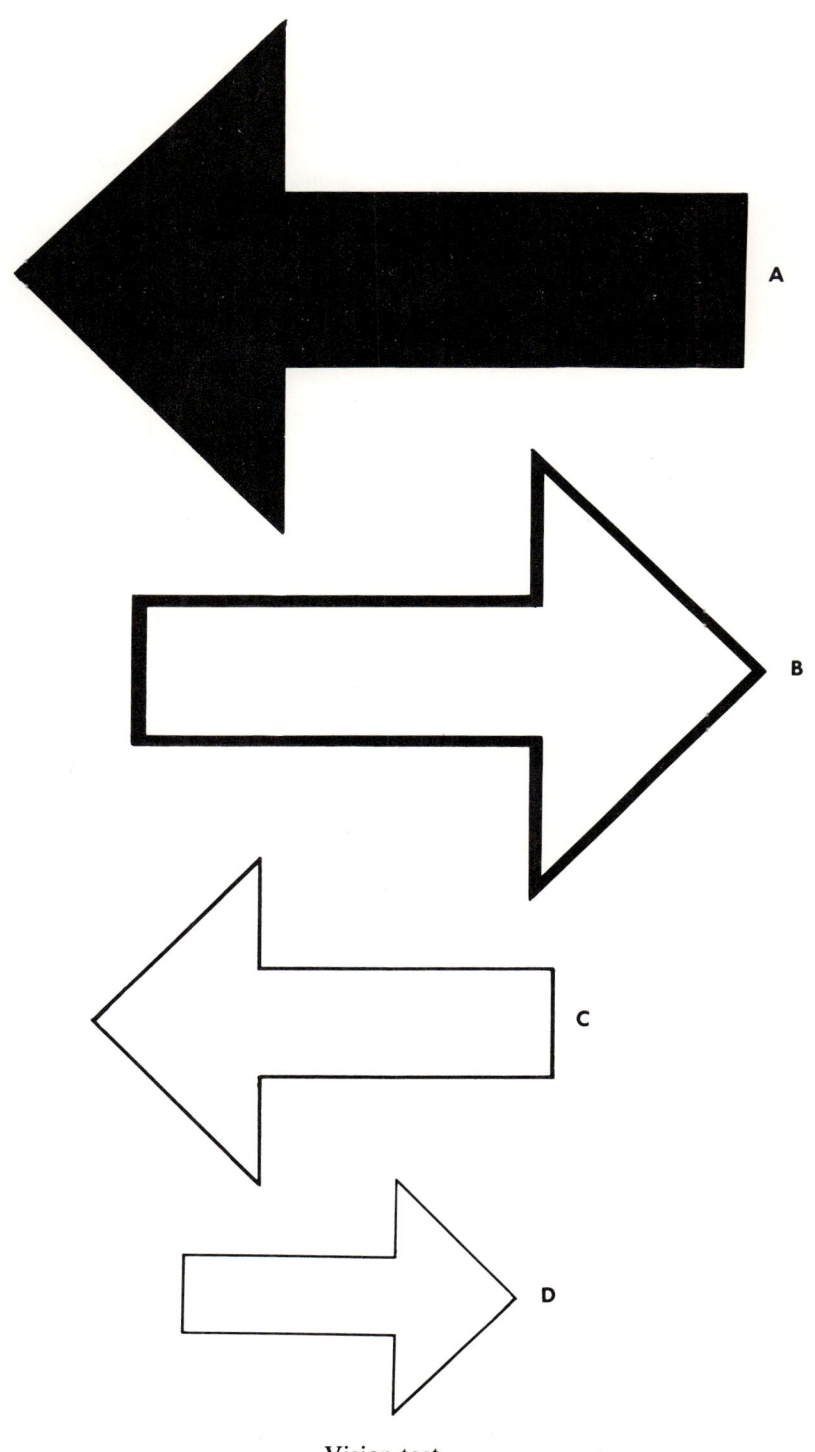

Vision test.

Tool 6-2. Assessment of sensoriperceptual abilities—cont'd

Touch test

Have client seated comfortably, preferably with a table on which to rest his arms and hands. Speak in conversational tone and wait for client to respond. Note responses.

Materials needed—wisp of cotton, pin, and two textures. With client still seated at the table, ask him to close his eyes and tell you if he feels anything and where he feels it. Touch exposed skin on arm with wisp of cotton; record response. Touch pads of fingers with cotton and note response. Touch skin at several points with blunt and sharp ends of pin, recording response.

Heat and cold: Materials needed—tube of warm water (115° to 120° F, or 46° to 49° C) and tube of cold water (40° F, or 4.5° C) or cold metal object. Touch skin in several places with hot and cold object and ask the client, who has his eyes closed, what the object feels like. Use the forearm, the shin, and if possible, the foot. Note accuracy of responses and record place and response.

Position in space: Ask client to close eyes, make a fist, and place hands on table. Grasp thumb and move up and down. Ask client to indicate what he feels, if anything, and prompt him if he needs to be reminded of up or down position. The great toe may be used.

Client's response:

Classification or abstraction test

Materials needed—pencil and pen, sheet of paper and envelope, Kleenex and handkerchief. Ask client to group scattered objects according to similar use. Offer an example—take metal coin and paper money and indicate that both are used to buy things. Record correct response. Writing instruments (client's response). Writing material (client's response). Handkerchiefs (client's response).

Smell test

Materials needed—three familiar, pungent-smelling substances that are in corked tube and can be released one by one. With client in same sitting position, uncork one tube of peppermint, coffee grounds, pine scent, cinnamon, and others. Allow a short interval between tests to provide restoration of ability to differentiate. Client may be allowed to open eyes if the substances are of similar colors. Ask client to tell what each scent is or of what it reminds him (woods instead of pine or apple pie instead of cinnamon are appropriate responses).

Tool 6-3. Assessment of structure and physiology

Basic body description
Weight: _____ Height: Arm span from fingertip to fingertip with arms outstretched.
Use as height measure for best height: _____
Actual height: _____
Temperature: Oral: _____ Rectal: _____ Time of day: _____
Pulse (sitting) (60 sec): Rate: _____ Rhythm: _____ Quality: _____
Respiration: Body position: ☐ Sitting ☐ Lying
    Rate (inactive): _____ Character: ☐ Abdominal ☐ Shallow
    Rate (after activity): _____ Character: ☐ Abdominal ☐ Shallow
Blood pressure: ☐ Lying ☐ Sitting ☐ Standing
    Right arm: _____ Left arm: _____
General appearance: _____

Nutritional assessment
Evidence of recent weight loss? _____
Girth measure at largest part of abdomen: _____
Saliva pool present under tongue? _____
Condition of lips: ☐ Cracked ☐ Fissures at corners
Gums: ☐ Pink and firm ☐ Red ☐ Bleeding ☐ Loose teeth
Teeth: ☐ Edentulous ☐ Two good molars opposite each other for chewing ☐ Two good incisors opposite each other for biting
Repair: _____
Tongue: Moves to right and left: _____
Swallowing ability (test with water): _____

Check after correct statement
Any evidence of edema—sacral area: Right: ☐ Leg ☐ Ankle ☐ Foot ☐ Left: ☐ Leg ☐ Ankle ☐ Foot
Skin: Ulcerations or discolorations (where): _____

Activity and pain:
    Walks: ☐ Without assistance ☐ With assistive device
    Combs hair: ☐ Without assistance ☐ Needs assistance
    Feeds self: ☐ Without assistance ☐ Needs assistance
    Bathes self: ☐ Without assistance ☐ Needs assistance
    Self-toileting: ☐ Without assistance ☐ Needs assistance
    Evidence of pain in any of above activities? _____ ☐ Wheelchair ☐ Ambulation ☐ Bedfast
Joints (normal range of motion?):
    Neck: _____
    Left: Shoulder _____ Elbow _____ Wrist _____ Hip _____
    Knee _____ Ankle _____
    Right: Shoulder _____ Elbow _____ Wrist _____ Hip _____
    Knee _____ Ankle _____
    Remarkable exceptions: _____

Structural changes which limit activity: ☐ Amputations ☐ Swelling ☐ Pain (location, onset, duration, character of pain): _____

Continued.

Tool 6-3. Assessment of structure and physiology—cont'd

Estimate of strength
Hand squeeze: _____ Lifts self from chair (arm or shoulder): _____
Walking strength: _____
For any person without the ability to walk freely, note gait. Use foot assessment in Appendix C.

Elimination
Ask for urine specimen. Give directions and materials. If unable to provide, examine abdomen for evidence of full bladder.
Indwelling catheter? _____ Suprapubic drainage? _____ Evidence of urinary incontinence? _____ 24-hour intake and output record: _____
Ask for bowel history. If any doubt, examine for impaction. Usual remedies taken for constipation: _____
Note hemorrhoids. Evidence of fecal incontinence? _____

Other
Eyes: Lid strength _____ Infection _____ Drainage _____
Conjunctiva _____
Female patient: ☐ Breast examination for tumor ☐ Vulva examination for irritation or discharge

General impression while examining
Ability to understand and follow instructions? _____
Weakness of musculoskeletal system _____
Evidence of bone loss (trunk shortening, kyphosis, or fractures)? _____

Drugs used
Drug: _____ Dose: _____ How taken: _____

Use of alcohol
Quantity and frequency: _____
Home remedies found useful? _____

Impression from laboratory reports, diagnosis, and other findings
_____
_____
_____
_____

Tool 6-4. Assessment of life history and culture

Instructions
This assessment should be made as an incidental process rather than a question-and-answer procedure. Some of the questions will be answered on the admission form. This forms a check, or when information is not available, it may offer the initial data.

Name: _____ Preferred name to be used in this agency: _____

Date of birth: _____ Age on admission: _____
Place of birth: _____
Childhood and school years spent in: _____
Parents: Ancestral background of mother: _____
         Ancestral background of father: _____
Religious background: _____
Residence prior to admission to agency (if relocated): _____
Living arrangements: ☐ alone ☐ with spouse ☐ with family member ☐ other: _____
Marital status: _____ Children: _____
Spouse's name: _____
Identification with the work world: What you think of yourself as being? _____

Retirement date: _____
Recent losses, with approximate dates: _____

Leisure activities enjoyed: _____

Outstanding accomplishments: What are things that make you proud? _____

What outstanding occurrence do you remember when you had to make a real effort to regain yourself as you had been? An illness, frightening experience, or loss? _____

What did you do that helped you overcome this? _____
Who have you been able to turn to for help in times past? _____
Who do you feel is your best friend or the one you can talk to about your troubles (confidant)? _____

What illnesses have you had that may affect your health now? _____

Is this (referral to present situation) going to make a difference in your life? (Effort to get client's perception of condition in relation to previous experiences.) _____

Tool 6-5. Assessment of interaction with social environment

Social ties
Can client use the telephone? _____ What arrangement is made to use it as a resource?
Is there a special list of telephone numbers to be called in emergency? _____
Is the telephone adapted for dim vision, hearing problem, or arthritic fingers? _____
Is there a friendly relationship with another person? Who, and does this person reciprocate?

Is there a pet? _____
Are there persons with whom client cannot communicate or cooperate in a helping relationship? _____
Does client initiate relationships with new or strange persons? _____
Are there continuing relationships from the past? _____
Is he curious about people and environment? _____

Communication
Are there any linguistic problems in communication? _____
    Language differences: _____
    Cultural differences/idiom differences: _____
    Does he forget words, especially nouns that can be recalled with help? _____
Are there mechanical problems in communication? _____
    Tongue or laryngeal problems or dyspnea? _____
    Aphasia, slurred speech, or lack of facial expression? _____
Can the client write his communication if speech is difficult? _____
Can the client read messages written to him? _____
Perceptual problems with communication:
    1. Decreased vision that prevents seeing facial expression? _____
    2. Hearing problem? _____
    3. Inability to use gestures? _____
    4. Lack of practice in communicating with others? _____
Is the client able to ask for help? _____
Does he recognize his need for help? _____
Is he suspicious of offers to help? _____
Can the client use social skills (courtesies or small talk)? _____
Assets: _____
Impression of interactional skills: _____

Tool 6-6. Assessment of interaction with physical environment

Client recognition of his special space:
1. Wanders
2. Unable to find own room
3. Able to direct another person to room

Client's use of cues in the environment to keep oriented:
1. Newspapers
2. Television or radio
3. Reality board
4. Asks questions
5. Writes notes to self
6. Receives mail

Ability to handle own nutritional needs:
1. Shops for groceries
2. Uses prepared foods
3. Seeks restaurants or nutrition centers
4. Prepares own food
5. Feeds self
6. Requires stimulation to self-feed
7. Needs assistance with food intake
8. Remembers to drink fluids; can care for own fluid intake
9. Needs to be reminded to give self-care for intake
10. Must have fluids offered with assistive device, such as tube
11. Requires fluids by special routes

Self-care toileting:
1. Self-care is sufficient
2. Needs help in getting to the toilet
3. Needs special type of toilet, such as raised seat, arms, or wheelchair space
4. Needs assistive devices, such as catheters and colostomy
5. Needs bowel or bladder rehabilitation program
6. Self-care requires special adaptive clothing
7. Unable to indicate toileting needs

Personal hygiene and grooming:
1. Able to care for own hygiene and grooming
2. Needs help with bathing, shampoo, and nails
3. Requires help with all aspects of hygiene and grooming
4. Unable to care for any of own hygienic needs

Dressing:
1. Able to choose appropriate clothing and dress self
2. Needs help with dressing
3. Unable to dress self

Independent living:
1. Able to maintain housekeeping, pay bills, and manage transportation and laundry
2. Unable to handle business affairs; housekeeping reduced to essentials; needs help with laundry; difficulty with transportation
3. Needs assistance with living arrangements
4. Unable to maintain independent living

Use of social service agencies:
1. Seeks appropriate help as needed
2. Uses help as offered
3. Unable to understand source of help or system

Continued.

86 *Confusion: prevention and care*

Tool 6-6. Assessment of interaction with physical environment—cont'd

Assessment of physical environment
The assessment of the physical environment is made in relation to the physical and mental abilities of the client.
Does environment present light barriers, furniture barriers, or floor-covering barriers?
Is there lack of contrast?
Is there individual space without crowding?
Are personal supplies marked?
Is there a reality board?
Is interior individually decorated?
Is there opportunity to handle money and buy small items?
Wheelchair and assistive walking devices: Have they been measured to fit the client?
Does he use assistive devices without strain?
Is there a place to rest during the day (nap time)?
Is there any privacy? Can families meet in private?
Impressions from data: _____
How can the environment be adjusted to facilitate independent and safe living for the client?
What adaptations will the client have to make?

SUGGESTIONS FOR FURTHER READING
Life history and culture
Curtin, S. R.: Nobody ever died of old age, Boston, 1972, Little, Brown & Co.
Myerhoff, B.: Number our days, New York, 1979, E. P. Dutton and Elsevier Book Operations.
Sarton, M.: As we are now, New York, 1973, W. W. Norton & Co., Inc.
Shakespeare, W.: King Lear.

Physiologic changes
Rossman, I., editor: Clinical geriatrics, ed. 2, Philadelphia, 1979, J. B. Lippincott Co.
Steinberg, F. U., editor: Cowdry's The care of the geriatric patient, ed. 5, St. Louis, 1976, The C. V. Mosby Co.

The environment
Butler, R. N., and Lewis, M. I.: Aging and mental health, ed. 2, St. Louis, 1977, The C. V. Mosby Co.

REFERENCES
Agate, J.: The natural history of disease in later life. In Rossman, I., editor: Clinical geriatrics, Philadelphia, 1971a, J. B. Lippincott Co., pp. 115-120.
Agate, J.: Common symptoms and complaints. In Rossman, I., editor: Clinical geriatrics, Philadelphia, 1971b, J. B. Lippincott Co., pp. 461-470.
Bloch, D.: Some crucial terms in nursing: what do they really mean, Nurs. Outlook **22**:689-694, 1974.
Carrieri, V., and Sitzman, J.: Components of the nursing process, Nurs. Clin. North Am. **6**(1):115-124, 1971.
Castaneda, C.: Journey to Ixtlan, New York, 1971, Simon & Schuster, Inc.
Curtin, S. R.: Nobody ever died of old age, Boston, 1972, Little, Brown & Co.
Feld, J.: Opening remarks, Ann. N.Y. Acad. Sci. **138**:369-370, 1967.
Goldman, R.: Decline in organ function with aging. In Rossman, I., editor: Clinical geriatrics, Philadelphia, 1971, J. B. Lippincott Co.
Griffin, E. W.: Nursing process: a patient with respiratory dysfunction, Nurs. Clin. North Am. **6**(1):145-154, 1971.
Henderson, V.: The nature of nursing, Am. J. Nurs. **64**(8):62-68, 1964.
McCain, R. F.: Nursing by assessment—not intuition, Am. J. Nurs. **65**:82-84, 1965.
McGaugh, J. L., and Dawson, R. G.: Modification of memory storage processes, Behav. Sci. **16**:45, 1971.
Mitchell, P. H.: Concepts basic to nursing, New York, 1977, McGraw-Hill Book Co.
Murray, R. L.: Principles of nursing intervention for the adult patient with body image changes, Nurs. Clin. North Am. **7**:701, 1972.
Myerhoff, B.: Aging and the aged in other cultures: an anthropological perspective. In Bauwens, E., editor: The anthropology of health, St. Louis, 1978, The C. V. Mosby Co.
Myerhoff, B.: Number our days, New York, 1979, E. P. Dutton and Elsevier Book Operations.

Noyes, A. P., and Kolb, L. C.: Modern clinical psychiatry, Philadelphia, 1963, W. B. Saunders Co.

Putt, A.: General systems theory applied to nursing, Boston, 1978, Little, Brown & Co.

Quinn, J. L., and Ryan, N.: Assessment of the older person: a holistic approach, J. Gerontol. Nurs. 5(2):13-18, 1979.

Sarton, M.: As we are now, New York, 1973, W. W. Norton & Co.

Weed, L. L.: Medical records, medical education and patient care, Chicago, 1971, Year Book Medical Publishers.

Williams, M., and others: Nursing activities and acute confusional states in elderly hip-fractured patients, Nurs. Res. 28(1):25-35, 1979.

Wolanin, M. O.: Registered nurses and the depressed patient. Unpublished study, 1975a.

Wolanin, M. O.: Process criterion versus impact criterion to measure quality of care in nursing homes, Proceedings of the First North American Symposium on Long Term Care. Toronto, Washington, D.C., 1975b, American College of Nursing Home Administrators.

Wolanin, M. O.: Nursing assessment. In Burnside, I., editor: Nursing and the aged, ed. 2, New York, 1980, McGraw-Hill Book Co.

7

WHO'S CONFUSED HERE?

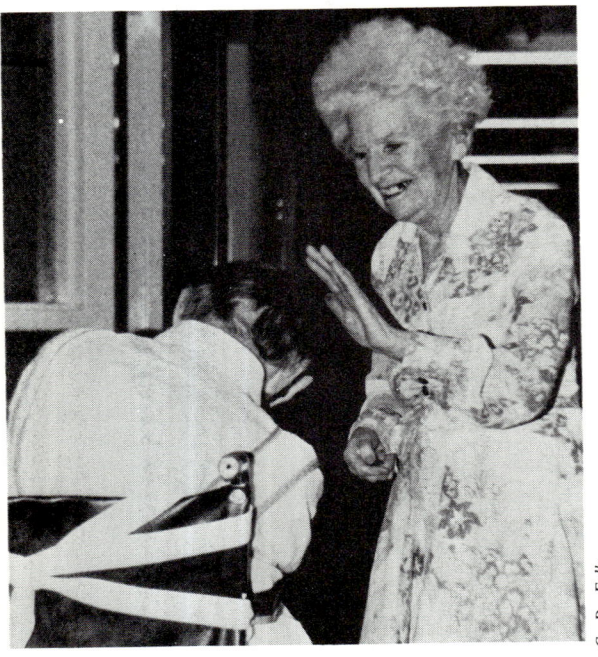

Making the diagnosis of confusion is a serious responsibility. If the word confusion had neutral connotations or made no difference in the treatment the person receives, it would not be particularly important whether it was associated with an individual or not. However, there is nothing neutral about "confusion" when used in reference to an elderly person. Once the diagnosis is made, it affects the subsequent nursing interventions, the quality of the patient's life at that moment, and often the future possibility of return to his normal life-style. After he is perceived as confused by the nursing staff, the judgment is conveyed to other health care workers. The nursing diagnosis of confusion is often a precursor to the medical diagnosis of organic brain syndrome. The confused patient may be confined, restrained, or eventually institutionalized. He may be suddenly deprived of decision-making powers and control, because those around him perceive him to be incompetent and incapable in even the simplest situation. The nonconfused elderly person who is mistakenly diagnosed as confused may subsequently become confused as his decision-making powers and social and sensory inputs are substantially reduced. A mistake in the other direction is not so crucial. To treat a person as competent can certainly do little harm. However, to treat a person as incompetent when he is not can do nothing but damage.

This chapter is intended to alert the reader to the responsibility and importance of assessing a situation to determine if the patient really is confused or if the nurse is so confused by the presenting patient behaviors that she thinks it is he, and not she, who is confused. Categories will be presented that represent the types of patients most likely to be diagnosed as confused, when actually they are not.

PROBLEMS WITH THE NURSING DIAGNOSIS OF CONFUSION

It is never easy to make a diagnosis of confusion. At times the nurse is faced with a plethora of patient statements and behaviors that appear "strange" and make the diagnosis seem easy. At other times, the cues are subtle, and it is difficult to decide exactly what is going on with the patient. In neither case is making the diagnosis easy. And, in either case, probably the only one who really has any idea about what is going on with the patient is the patient himself. The nurse's charge is to find out directly from him what he perceives to be happening, rather than make unjustified inferences based on her perceptions alone. The patient who displays confused behaviors and the nurse who diagnoses confused behaviors are both human. As a result, the margin for error and misinterpretation is large.

In addition, other concerns are crucial to the diagnostic process. These need to be considered every time the nurse entertains the idea of making a diagnosis of confusion. A first concern is that the diagnosis of confusion is based primarily on the appropriateness of a given response to a certain stimulus and the appropriateness of behavior within a certain context. Appropriateness assumes that the nurse is in possession of certain information that permits her to compare what the patient says and does to some behavioral norm, thereby arriving at some conclusion about what is appropriate. The concept of appropriateness is similar to the statistical concept of norms. To illustrate, Fig. 7-1 is a picture of the normal bell-shaped curve. For any normally distributed human characteristic (and there is every reason to believe that appropriateness of response is normally distributed), 68.2% or slightly more than two thirds of the people will fall under the widest part of the curve between $+1$ and -1 standard deviation from the mean or average. The way in which approximately two thirds of the people display any characteristic under consideration, therefore, determines what is considered to be average or normal. The characteristics of two thirds of the people, however, only indirectly tells us anything about the range of the distribution. The range is determined by the one third of the people who fall in the "tails" of the curve. People can deviate far from the mean and still be a part of the normal distribution. For example, if height is considered, the normal

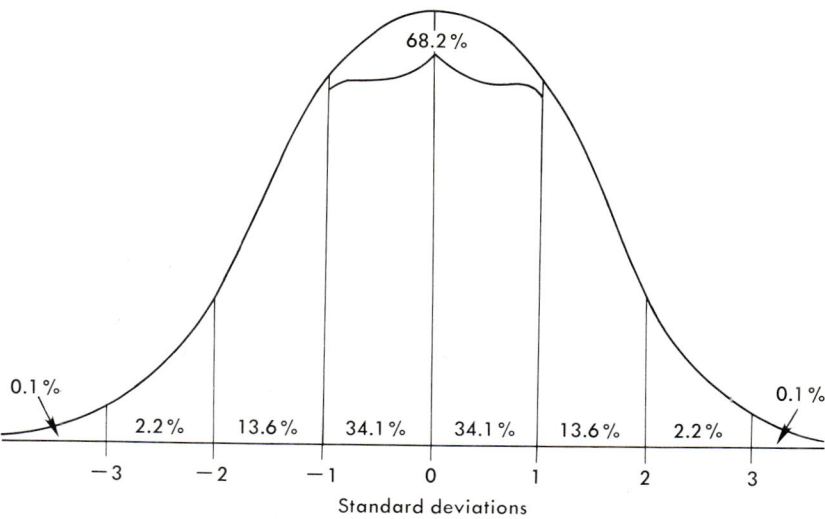

Fig. 7-1. The bell-shaped curve that demonstrates the normal distribution of behavioral characteristics.

or average height of women is between approximately 5 feet 4 inches and 5 feet 8 inches. Are the women who are 4 feet 10 inches or 6 feet 2 inches still normal? Of course, they probably are. The same principle applies to the determination of normal or appropriate behavior. That most people can perform certain cognitive gymnastics and behave in a certain way tells us nothing about the total *range* of human cognition or behavior that can still be considered normal. Norms indicate very little about individual variability. They only give us rough guidelines and indicate areas for further exploration. Determining appropriateness is more than identifying what is appropriate within the context of the observer or what most people would do under the same circumstances. The trick is determining the appropriateness that the patient attaches to his own behavior and what it means to him within his own framework. Does his behavior make sense to him? Does his behavior make sense to you within *his* framework? What stimuli is he responding to that may or may not be apparent to you? What meaning does the situation have for him?

This leads immediately to a second concern. How does the present behavioral response compare to past responses that this person has made under similar circumstances? Unfortunately, this is often an area about which the nurse has little information. For most other problems, an in-depth baseline assessment is performed during the admission procedure that can then be used for comparison purposes throughout the hospitalization. This is not usually true with mental status. Most clinicians become alerted to the need for a mental status assessment only after the patient is beginning to display behavioral changes or when the confusion is already full-blown. Therefore, in most cases there is no systematic baseline information with which to compare the results of an assessment, except perhaps an intuitive notion that the patient was "lucid" on admission. For most hospitalized people, caregivers simply do not know, for example, whether the patient is newly forgetful or whether he is a chronic forgetter or whether his attention span is becoming short or has always been short. It is, therefore, imperative that the nurse making the diagnosis of confusion gets this kind of information from the patient or his lifelong associates. The nurse needs to be alert to any changes in behavior that might be indicative of confusion as early as possible so that baseline information can be obtained for future comparisons. By not doing so, she delays instituting interventions that may prevent acute confusion from becoming chronic, loses the valuable opportunity to collect longitudinal data that would contribute to the understanding of confusion for this patient, and runs the risk of misdiagnosing confusion based on momentary impressions.

A third concern is with the precision, or rather, the lack of precision, involved in making the diagnosis of confusion. As indicated in Chapter 1, the First National Conference on Classification of Nursing Diagnoses (Gebbie and Lavin, 1975) identified seventeen separate characteristics of confused people. Goldfarb (1975) adds two more characteristics. Which of these are most indicative of confusion and which are most heavily weighted? We simply do not know. Probably "disorientation to place, person, time, object, and purpose after reality information is given" is more indicative of confusion than "anxiety." But is "combativeness" and "purposeless activity" more indicative of confusion than "suspected impairment of attention span"? In addition, does it take one characteristic to make the diagnosis of confusion, or does the diagnosis require the simultaneous presence of three or more characteristics? Again, we do not know. If the precision in describing confused behavior and the precision with which individual care providers use the word confusion were increased, the diagnostic process would be a whole lot easier. However, this is not currently the case.

A last concern falls under the category of "social desirability." Not every person, young or old, looks or acts exactly as we would like them. Older people come in all varieties and forms. Some are pretty and some are ugly. Some are immaculate and others are unkempt. Some are cute and some are despicable. Older people may be unkempt not because they are confused, but because they have never, in their entire life, considered personal hygiene to be very important. Some older people are hostile and strike out at any interference, because this is the way they have coped throughout their entire lifetime. This does not make them good or bad, but it does make some older people more socially desirable to us. And certainly, this does not make them confused. In the study of hip-fractured elderly (Williams and others, 1979; Phillips, 1976), it was apparent that the people most often called confused by the nursing staff were those who were socially undesirable or who presented problems that made the nurses' job harder. Behavioral displays that were indicative of confusion among the socially desirable subjects, for example, those who were considered to be cute, sweet, or lovely ladies, were either not perceived as confused at all by the staff or were excused. It seemed that just violating the stereotype of what the nurses considered to be acceptable behavior for an older person was sometimes enough to earn the diagnosis of confusion. This same finding appeared in the Phillips (1973) study of confusion. There seems to be a definite bias on the part of nurses toward diagnosing older people as confused, whether they are or not, if they do not meet the nurse's expectations.

There seem to be several categories of patients who are particularly vulnerable to being perceived as confused. These can best be considered using anecdotal accounts and case examples.

The problem patient or the nursing failure

This category includes those patients whom the nurse sees as particularly difficult to care for. They are people who require great skill, patience, creativity, and objectivity. They test the nurse's abilities to the utmost, often not responding to conventional treatments or approaches. They are often the people for whom the nurse believes she has tried everything and failed, making her feel inadequate and incompetent. Often, the nurse displays a great deal of anger and avoidance toward people in this category. Vera was one such patient.

Case study: Vera. Vera Z. was a 60-year-old woman who had been admitted to a university hospital for an acute reaction to radiation therapy following surgery. She had previously had an abdominal-perineal resection for colon and rectal cancer. She had a colostomy as a result of the surgery. She had multiple draining fistula and was in acute pain. Since her admission 3 months before, she had lost 75 pounds and had essentially refused to eat.

The nursing staff found it very difficult to care for Vera. They thought that her demands were incessant and that they could never provide her with comfort. The clinical specialist and nursing staff concurred that she was confused. They believed that she hallucinated freely, often incorporating the nursing staff into her hallucinations. The night before our first contact, she had gotten out of bed and was found wandering in the hall dragging her IV apparatus with her. She had described herself, at that time, as being "lost." She occasionally would tell the staff that she felt as if she and the nursing staff were in a dream together and that nothing seemed real.

The first day I interviewed Vera, she moaned and thrashed around on the bed constantly. She had received her pain medication about 30 minutes before our interview and complained about being "sleepy" and in "too much pain to talk." The clinical specialist and I had consulted on the best approach to this patient prior to my contact with her. The specialist indicated that Vera's pain behavior was constant. She advised that if I wanted to assess Vera's mental status, I had to be alert to being manipulated into discussing her pain, or I would obtain no other information. During our first contact, Vera did answer every question asked by referring to her pain. To this, I would give an empathic response, either verbally or nonverbally, and restate the question. Although she asked me to leave the room twice during this first contact, which I did, with a promise to return in one-half hour, and registered some disgust with my persistence, she correctly answered every question relative to her mental status. She knew where she was, what had happened to her, correctly identified me twice by name, related accurately much of her family history, and, when pressed, acted with social skill. During that contact, Vera was *not* confused, even though she could have easily led me to believe she was, based on her behavior, her nonresponsiveness, and her short attention span.

On leaving Vera's room, I interviewed the individual staff members about their perceptions of the patient. They reported that they felt helpless to relieve her pain and that they tried to avoid her at all costs. They said that they never went in her room unless they had to give her medication or to answer her call light. They estimated that 90% of their contacts with her centered on her pain. They registered anger, frustration, and despair. A conference was planned for the next day.

During the conference we shared our observations and feelings about Vera. The staff listed all of her tentative nursing diagnoses and then decided to actively intervene for pain, social isolation, and refusal to eat. They would attempt to ignore all other problems, including the possible confusion, deciding that if confusion really did exist, it arose from the three problems identified.

The approach the staff used with Vera was behavior modification, using the psychologic principles of positive reinforcement and shaping. The interventions planned were as follows:

1. Pain. The staff decided to try to separate Vera's pain behavior and the social interaction she received relative to pain from all other types of social interaction. No one on the unit would be permitted to relate to Vera about her pain, or even mention it to her, and would only report the problem to a specific "pain person." This person was to be the charge nurse on each shift. To assure that Vera would not be in pain, the pain person was to respond to Vera's requests for pain medication but was not to give social reinforcement during the process. That nurse was to assess the pain, administer the pain medication, and leave the room. She was to return later to evaluate if Vera had received relief and to reinforce the patient's "relief behavior."

2. Social isolation. The group felt that Vera had come to relate to others only in terms of pain because that was the basis on which most people related to her. This was resulting in social isolation and deprivation of other important sources of stimulation. As a result, a schedule was planned and posted on Vera's door. It provided for systematic and meaningful interactions with Vera about topics other than pain. Her family members were included in the scheduling of interaction. At specific times she would either be taken to the sun room, read to from the newspaper, the Bible, and other books, or talked to about social topics, such as the weather, current events, and her previous personal interests. The staff would attempt to elicit and reinforce appropriate responses from Vera on the focused items. A calendar was placed in her room, and part of the daily bath ritual included the marking off of the previous day. The emphasis of all interaction was to be sharing. For example, after a particular passage was read, the staff person was to stop reading and try to involve Vera in a conversation about what had been read. Each nurse who approached Vera was to introduce herself and tell how long she would be there. When she left, she would tell Vera what she was planning to do then. In other words, the staff was to try to make social interaction far more interesting and rewarding than pain behavior or pain interaction.

3. Refusal to eat. Before our conference, the physician had instructed the nurses to "force" Vera to eat. Consequently, meal time had become a battle time. We decided to quit making eating a "big deal." The nurses would bring the meal tray into the room, place it in an accessible place, and see that Vera was comfortable and could reach everything. The nurse and the family members would then leave. At the end of 15 minutes, everyone would return. If she had eaten *anything*, this was to be positively reinforced. If not, there was to be no comment made, and the tray would be removed.

We predicted, during the conference, that when the plan was instituted, Vera would be initially confused about how to react to the staff. We, therefore, felt that her behavior would become more erratic at first, but that this problem would be temporary.

In 1 week, we met again to evaluate the effects of the plan. The results were extremely positive. Vera had not gotten worse as predicted. Her behavior had begun to change in 2 days. Vera no longer moaned with every breath. She looked alert and interested in her surroundings, and the pained expression was gone from her face. One week previously, Vera had been taking pain medication six times daily and never appeared to be comfortable. Now, she was taking pain medication twice daily and rarely had uncomfortable episodes. The staff reported that caring for Vera was no longer the chore it had been. They also reported that Vera was no longer confused.

Even walking into Vera's room was different. Previously, she had been in a rather pleasant private room that was bare of her personal effects. Now the same walls were plastered with her get-well cards. There were books and papers on her bedside stand. Her family reported that she had requested her own clothing, her own books (which she was now reading by herself), crossword puzzles, and a ride in the car. In short, Vera acted like a person rather than an ill and difficult patient.

The treatment plan for Vera was not without its problems. As her behavior changed, her family's behavior became more difficult for the nurses to deal with. In addition, the eating problem went from bad to worse. Nonetheless, Vera's "confused behavior" and "pain behavior" completely disappeared, and she was eventually discharged.

Whether Vera was ever *really* confused is immaterial. When the staff ignored what appeared to be confusion and focused on the most important nursing problems, treating her as if she were not confused, her behavior improved measurably. Vera was a problem patient, a potential nursing failure. Like many other such patients, it is just possible that she was viewed by the staff as confused, and hence unmanageable, because it was easier to label her than to deal with the management problems she presented.

The patient with communication problems

All kinds of communication problems exist that can lead to the impression that the patient is confused when he is not. These problems range from simple problems involving the choice of words to very complex problems involving hesitancy and difficulties with self-expression that seem to indicate that the person probably is "not with it." For example, during an in-service session that was being conducted by a psychiatrist on the topic of managing the problem patient, a nursing assistant asked the following question: "What kinds of things can we do to help the family when the patient goes out?" The reply from the psychiatrist was: "Well, it seems to me that if the family feels we have acted promptly and called the police, that should help them a lot." The nursing assistant looked at the psychiatrist as if he had just gone mad and asked no more. To the nursing assistant, "goes out" was a slang expression for dying. In the psychiatrist's framework, "goes out" meant leaving the institution without being discharged. Who was confused in that interchange? This sort of difficulty occurs between professionals and between patients and caregivers all the time. These are the simple problems that involve a choice of words, without definitions, that are assumed to have shared meanings. In these situations, neither person is confused, but the person who misunderstands and replies on the basis of a misunderstanding appears to be.

What about the more complex problems? As people age, they require increasing amounts of information processing time. Hearing the information, understanding it, and formulating a response takes more time than it once did. Often, as the elderly patient concentrates intensely on the communication, he has a "blank" expression on his face. Hence, he may be said to look like a "zombie" by the nursing staff. This hesitancy, coupled with a blank facial expression, is often perceived by those around him as confusion. As McNamee (1978) notes, this problem is further compounded when the patient has a hearing difficulty: "He (the hearing impaired person) may be incorrectly labeled apathetic, goal-less, uninvolved, unmotivated, senile or even schizoid.... His self-respect may suffer when people regard him as *simple* because of his lack of comprehension" (p. 28). The need for increased processing time does not necessarily mean that the person involved is confused. Rather, the need for increased time may simply confuse the nurse about the patient's mental status.

Slurred speech, in our culture, is frequently associated with drunkenness or confusion. There are, however, people who have slurred speech who are neither confused nor drunk. For example, those people who have dysarthria may slur their words so badly that understanding is almost impossible. Dysarthria, however, is a muscular weakness that usually has nothing to do with mental processes. People with multiple sclerosis, parkinsonism, cerebrovascular accidents, and those who are edentulous (without teeth) may be dysarthric but have their mental processes completely intact. The presence of slurred speech makes an impression on everyone who has contact with the patient. For example, a drug salesman once reported to me that the discovery of L-dopa as a treatment for Parkinson's disease had caused significant alterations in the relationships between many patients and their families. Prior to the L-dopa therapy, the patients had slurred their words, drooled, and had a masked expression that had led their families to believe they were incompetent. After L-dopa therapy, however, the patients could finally express themselves about being wrongly treated as incompetent. Many families had needed intense counseling or had broken apart as a result of the anger that some patients felt toward their caretakers who had treated them like "idiots" for so long.

Cerebrovascular accidents result in many communication problems that can give the impression of confusion. Receptive dysphasia, expressive dysphasia, and agnosia are three examples of such communication problems. With stroke victims, the task of differentiating patient confusion from nurse confusion may be extremely difficult. With such patients, the nurse often finds that an alternate mode of communication, such as the written rather than the spoken word, reveals no confusion at all. It is therefore not the patient who is confused but the mode of communication that is confusing. Particularly deceptive are those patients who have the communication problems associated with a stroke but no other physical signs. If the communication deficit is mild, the patient himself and his family may not even realize that a stroke has occurred. With such patients, the nurse may forget to try alternate means of communication, assuming that the patient's behavior is indicative of senility and no more.

Communication problems in the elderly may be compounded by cultural differences if the person is in a nation or culture different from that of his birth. For example, around the time of World War II, thousands of people immigrated to the United States from Europe, many of whom were Jewish. Many of these people are now over 65 and are appearing with increasing frequency in our health care facilities. It is extremely difficult to make any kind of accurate assessment of a patient's mental status and ability to function competently when one does not understand his primary language, the impact of his life experiences, and his cultural ways. In these cases it is certainly best to err on the side of assuming competence and nonconfusion rather than the reverse.

The patient who challenges personal values

It is often difficult to understand and accept the behaviors and life-styles that patients display. As human beings, each of us has certain personal values that we consider to be inviolate. For example, each of us has certain values about what constitutes a crime. For some people stealing in any form is unacceptable, but for others minor pilfering from their place of employment or shoplifting small items is all right. Each of us has certain ideas about what constitutes appropriate expressions of sexuality. For some people any expression other than heterosexuality is inappropriate; others believe that bisexuality or homosexuality is appropriate. We also have certain standards regarding the amount of abuse the human body should be exposed to. Hence, there are those who abstain from all forms of stimulants, including coffee, and those who think drinking coffee and smoking cigarettes is acceptable but use of drugs is not. When our personal values are challenged, we are faced with discomfort and perplexity. We act in various ways to resolve the dilemma, and many of the behaviors we display have direct implications for our nursing care. Following is a case example that illustrates this point.

Case study: Paula and Anna. One Saturday, the supervisor on-call at a home health agency was contacted by an elderly woman who was quite distressed. The woman, who had just been discharged from the hospital with a cast on her broken leg, said that she had no food in the house, was the sole caregiver of her sick friend, and had to climb a flight of steps in order to give her friend, Anna, the care she needed. The woman, whose name was Paula, wanted the visiting nurse to stop by and help.

The nurse in the district was well acquainted with Paula. Her comment on receiving the referral was "Those two crazy old women can't live by themselves. We've tried for the last two months to get Anna into a nursing home, but she just won't go. You know, I think they have some sort of a 'sick relationship'." Although the nurse was insistent that the two should not be opened as active clients, because it would be "supporting a bad situation," she agreed to attend to the immediate problem. The rest of the story about Paula and Anna came out later.

Paula and Anna had lived together for over 25 years. They were lesbians. Anna was well over 70 and Paula was about 15 years younger. They lived in a poor section of the town in an area that was known as the black ghetto. Paula was white and Anna was black, and neither had close friends or family. Anna now had cancer of the larynx. She had a tracheostomy and required assistance for all of her activities of daily living.

The visiting nurse had initially visited the two after Anna had been discharged with the tracheostomy. She had attempted to teach Paula to give the physical care her partner required but had felt that her teaching attempts had been unsuccessful. Paula could not seem to learn. She was too emotionally labile; one minute she was attentive, and the next she was crying or screaming at the nurse. She forgot from lesson to lesson, and her attention span was short. The nurse described Paula as belligerent, confused at times, and "just too crazy to deal with." In the end, the nurse had discharged Anna from service because, in her opinion, the situation was totally undesirable, and Anna refused a nursing home placement. She felt that discharging Anna and not supporting the "bad situation" would precipitate a nursing home placement when Paula could not cope with the care that was needed. This seemed to her to be the only logical solution to the problem.

Instead of precipitating the nursing home placement, as predicted, Paula's broken leg provided an opportunity for another nurse to evaluate the situation. Her assessment was quite different. She described Paula as extremely anxious about the impending death of her partner and in need of a great deal of support. She set about providing that support by assigning a homemaker–home health aide to the home on a regular basis, by bereavement counseling with both Anna and Paula, and by scaling down the teaching sessions to small, manageable amounts. She did not perceive either Paula or Anna to be confused or "crazy," as confirmed by their behavior when they received the supports they needed. In the end, Anna did die. But she died at home, where she wanted to be, in the care of the person she loved.

As with the first nurse in this situation, when our personal values are challenged, it is all too easy to assume that the behaviors or life-styles we observe are the result of "mental instability" or "craziness." In fact, one of the ways we all handle the discomfort and perplexity that arise from behavior that is outside the boundaries of what we consider acceptable is to attach a label to it. By labeling the behavior, it is much easier for us to determine which of our roles is most appropriate to display toward the person we consider deviant. Depending on the label, we may choose any number of behaviors toward the person, ranging from complete avoidance to overt stigmatization. Our underlying intent is to convert our discomfort to feelings that we can more easily handle.

We all engage in this labeling process. Let

us, however, consider the assumptions that underlie any judgment that we make when labeling another person as deviant. Deviance is based on the idea that the societal norms (the value that the majority of people in a society are thought to ascribe to) and the modal behaviors (the acutal behaviors that the majority of people in the society display) are congruent. As the observer, we make the ethnocentric assumption that the value we hold dear is both normative and modal. Neither of these may be true. The value we consider normative may be held by only a small segment of a given society, and it just happens that we associate most frequently with those people who hold the same value. The value we consider to be normative may also be expressed by a majority of the patients, even though most people in the society do not act in such a way to uphold the value. Or it may be that the so-called normative value is in a state of change; that is, since a majority of the people do not act to uphold it, people's values are changing. This is called cultural lag, or the phenomenon that occurs when the rate at which values change lags behind the rate at which behaviors change. With cultural lag, it is not unusual for a majority of the people to espouse a value diametrically different from their behavior, simply because "it is the thing to do." In most cases, norms eventually catch up to actual behaviors.

It might be helpful to consider some examples. In Western culture, monogamy is both normative and modal. The majority of people still tell you that having one marriage partner is "right," and at the same time most people act in such a way that they only actually have one marriage partner at a time. Any other form of marital arrangement in Western culture is seen as deviant. In many eastern cultures, monogamy is modal but not normative. For economic reasons, most people in the culture have only one marriage partner at a time. However, the cultural norm espouses polygamy as desirable. In that culture, monogamy is actually deviant, even though a majority of people practice it. In Western culture, prior to the last 10 years, a bride's virginity was normative but probably not modal. A majority of the brides in Western culture were not virgins at the time of marriage, but society still espoused the norm. This is an example of cultural lag. More recently, the virginity of a bride is probably neither normative nor modal. Nonvirginity at marriage is no longer considered to be deviant. Attitudes toward divorce are another example of cultural lag. Although a majority of people enter into a marriage agreement with the idea of a lifelong partnership, it is becoming increasingly apparent that the majority of people does not actually practice lifelong unions with one partner. According to Bernard (1975), "It is not inconceivable that in the lives of today's teenagers the stable lifelong marriage may become 'deviant'" (p. 83). The point in all of this is, of course, that any number of things can be seen as deviant depending on where the observer is standing. In addition, instead of being carved in stone, norms and values change over time.

Our conception of deviance is variable and a label of deviant has implications for our behaviors; even more importantly, the whole idea of deviance has special implications for our assessment of the elderly. When people are young, it is not difficult for us to observe their behavior as unacceptable and assign a label to them, such as "junkie," "queer," "thief," or "alkie." But these labels are rarely applied to elderly people. Behavior outside of the boundaries of what we consider acceptable among the aged not only challenges our personal values but also challenges our ever-present stereotype of what "sweet old people" do. It is hard to reconcile the idea of being elderly with being deviant. With the old the tendency is to call any behavior that causes us personal discomfort "senility" or "confusion," because these labels do not have the evaluative impact that deviant labels do. If we consider a certain behavior as "bad," it is almost impossible to hang "badness" onto an elderly person. The result is that people whom we personally believe are deviant are very often called confused, which is, of course, not the case.

The patient who is physically unattractive

In Western culture, we value physical attractiveness almost above all else. As people age, we expect that they will maintain as much of their youthful attractiveness as possible. Unattractive old people conjure up certain associations in our minds that are unpleasant. How did Hollywood portray the wicked witch in *The Wizard of Oz*? She was old, and she was a hag. She was sharp featured, dressed in black, and had unruly hair and a crackling voice, all of which emphasized her wickedness. What is our reaction to a patient who looks like that? What does the proverbial dirty old man look like? Our picture of a "dirty old man" is never a short, round, white-haired gentleman with a smile on his face and a twinkle in his eye. Rather, that is our picture of Santa Claus, who is automatically assumed to be a "good guy." No, dirty old men are toothless, drooling, unkempt, and leering, with a sinister glint in their eyes. This is not to imply that women who look like witches or men who look like dirty old men are going to be immediately judged as confused. However, they are probably more likely to be than people who do not look ugly. Physical appearance simply has an effect on the judgments we make about people.

During Phillips' 1976 study of confusion, nurses were asked what about the patient led them to think that the patient was confused. Invariably, one of the things mentioned was appearance. "She looks like a zombie." "She just lays there and stares and I don't know what she is going to do." "She looks like a witch." Never were these expressions used as definitive indicators of confusion, but they would, nonetheless, enter into the description. It seems very difficult for some nurses to make judgments about mental status separate from physical appearance.

When an unpleasant physical appearance is coupled with an unpleasant or frightening physical deformity, the effects are even worse. Most people in the health care professions have gotten over their discomfort with understood handicaps, such as those produced by a stroke or arthritis. But when the nature of the deformity is poorly understood, it is difficult not to revert to old fears.

Example 1. Ms. W. is 95. She resides in a nursing home, where she spends most of her days in a wheelchair, mostly alone, on the front patio in the sun. Her face is mapped with lines and wrinkles. Her clothing is dowdy, too big, and covered with cigarette burn holes. Usually there is dried food on the front of her clothing. She sometimes smells of urine. When she speaks, she is difficult to understand, for she has no teeth and articulates very poorly. She is also almost blind and deaf, so that communication with her is extremely difficult. She taps her foot and moves her head as if she is listening to music that no one else hears. In addition to all of this, she has a neurologic deficit that causes her to fling her arms and legs around when she tries to move. The staff describes her with the following phrases: "She is like a fish out of water, always flopping," "She jumps and lurches like she will jump out of her chair at any moment," and "She is very confused and very crazy." Ms. W. is none of these things. She is simply very frightening. The nursing assistants do not seem to be able to get past her physical appearance long enough to realize that she is usually very lucid and simply cannot control her movements.

Example 2. Other kinds of patients have this same effect. Elderly Mr. J. suffered from chronic schizophrenia. After many years of phenothiazine therapy, he had tardive dyskinesia. He would writhe as he sat. His mouth, tongue, and limbs were in constant movement. Snake-like movements shuddered through his arms, shoulders, and neck. I found him one of the most terrifying men I had ever seen. It took another nurse, who talked to him long enough, ignoring his physical movements, to point out to me that he was neither confused nor actively psychotic. Patients with any of the choreas can give this same impression.

Example 3. Mr. B. has been in the nursing

home for over 2 years now and is in his seventies. The nursing staff, when pressed, admit that they are terrified by Mr. B. He is well over 6 feet tall, with extremely long limbs. His back is stooped and his arms dangle at his sides. The bones of his face and body are elongated, as if he had a growth disturbance in his youth. Mr. B. sits most of the time in his wheelchair with a blank expression on his face. He rarely smiles or initiates conversation himself. When he is spoken to, his voice is gruff, and he answers in only one or two words. The general impression Mr. B. gives is that of a Frankenstein-type monster of childhood nightmares. The nursing assistant staff state that he is "retarded," which he is not; he is "psychotic," which he has a history of but is not currently; and he is "dangerous," which is not true. From the staff's perspective, his physical appearance, which gives rise to and feeds into their fear of him, blocks any meaningful interaction through which they could judge his mental status.

It is difficult for all of us to rise above those fears carried from childhood of people who look grossly different or grotesque. If, however, we can acknowledge the possibility that physical appearance has an effect on our impressions about confusion, it may be more likely that we can sort our fear and confusion about such patients from the confusion that is the patient's alone.

The depressed patient

Making a differential diagnosis between depression and organic brain syndrome is one of the most difficult tasks of the geropsychiatrist. Drawing this fine distinction requires great skill and judgment and is the purview of medical personnel. Many elderly people, however, do not have the benefit of such skilled medical care. They receive their health care from nursing personnel and their medical care from physicians who are in family practice or who are general practitioners. It is, therefore, essential that both of these groups of practitioners realize that much of what passes for senility, chronic brain syndrome, and confusion among the elderly is actually depression. Cohen (1978) estimates that 10% to 20% of the elderly people who appear to be senile are actually depressed.

So closely associated are the symptoms of confusion and depression that many practitioners refer to depression as pseudosenility. Inability to concentrate, apathy, impaired attention span, and memory loss are signs of confusion among the elderly, but they are also signs of depression (Cohen, 1978). Disturbances of affect; seemingly inappropriate responses such as crying; changes in facial expression, posture, and grooming; and loss of interest in the surroundings may be signs of confusion, but they are also signs of depression among the elderly (Eisdorfer and Epstein, 1977). Agitation, hostility, and combativeness are associated with confusion and are signs of depression as well. Depression is the most common affective problem among the elderly. Cohen (1978) estimates its incidence at 25%. To even further complicate the situation, depression and changes in mental status often coexist. Anxiety and depression often appear in response to the patient's realization that he is having difficulty thinking clearly and remembering. Depression may exaggerate the mental status changes, making the patient appear more impaired than he really is.

There are certain symptoms that seem to be more indicative of depression than of confusion, and these may be helpful in determining which is present. For example, expressions of hopelessness, worthlessness, inferiority, inadequacy, helplessness, and suicidal thoughts are more indicative of depression than confusion. Suicidal attempts that are either active or passive (letting oneself die) are indicative of depression. Somatic complaints often accompany depression and not confusion. For example, disturbances in sleep or terminal insomnia (that is, awakening early in the morning), loss of appetite and weight, constipation, multiple physical complaints and high bodily concern, chronic pain of undetermined origin, and feelings of weakness and lack of energy often are associated with depression. The depressed patient may appear to be in slow motion. His general presentation, affect, and response may be slowed noticeably. With depression, it may be possible to identify with the patient or his associates the event or events that precipitated the depressive reaction, whereas with confusion, a precipitating event may not be identifiable. This is not always the case, but depression is usually associated with physical, cognitive, emotional, socioeconomic, or cultural stresses or losses.

Depressed elderly people often give the impression of being confused. Even though, theoretically, confusion and depression are distinct, the clinical picture of both is similar. Both confusion and depression may respond to therapy. However, signing the depressed patient off as being irreversibly confused leads to disaster. It is actually most desirable that a psychiatric consultation be considered every time a medical practitioner considers a diagnosis of chronic brain syndrome or a nursing practitioner considers a diagnosis of confusion. And, if psychiatric consultation is not possible, it is wise to follow Cohen's (1978) advice: when in doubt about whether the diagnosis is of senility or depression, treat it as if it were depression.

The troublemaker

Ms. Q. was one of the fractured hip patients in the 1976 confusion study (Williams and others, 1979). She argued with her daughter about where she was going to be placed after discharge, how the daughter should raise her children, and how often the daughter should visit, accusing the daughter of not caring about her. She argued loudly with the nursing staff about when and if she was going to ambulate, how she was to be transferred, how much she was going to eat, when and if she was going to physical therapy, if she would take medication, and when she was going to go to bed. During the course of her hospitalization, she was moved from two semi-private rooms because she disturbed the other patient: she had a total of four roommates. She was far from being the most favored patient on that orthopedic unit. The nurses thought she was disagreeable, nasty, hostile, and confused. According to the mental status tests used in that study, Ms. Q. was probably one of the least confused people in the study.

We have all cared for one or two Ms. Qs. Mine was a 92-year-old woman who was small and wiry. She spent most of her time in her bed chewing tobacco and spitting into a quart mayonnaise jar. She verbally abused the nurses and the other patients in her large, open ward. One day, after much argument, we gave her an enema. About halfway through the procedure, after screaming the entire time, she expelled the enema on me because she "couldn't hold it." That put her about as low as possible on my list of preferred people. We saw her, among other things, as confused. We thought that anyone who was lucid could never act the way she did.

Being nasty and difficult may mean many things, but it does not necessarily mean that the person is confused. For most nurses, it is extremely difficult to cope with the person who is nasty, causes trouble, and does not accept care. Since most of us have a bit of a "savior complex" anyway, we deal very poorly with people who reject our well-meant ministrations. The tendency is to find some reason to put the blame on, and among the elderly, that reason is often confusion. The fallacy in this is that when we call the behavior confusion, we no longer feel responsible to make any attempts at dealing with the behavior. We can encourage the use of all kinds of avoidance devices, such as restraints, tranquilizers, and simple force, with a clear conscience because, after all, the person is confused. Confusion and agitation often coexist, but often they do not. The distinction needs to be made clear so that specific interventions for each can be planned.

SUMMARY

The categories we presented of patients who give the impression of being confused when they are not are certainly not exhaustive. We hope, however, the point is clear. It is never easy to made a diagnosis of confusion. We find ourselves relying on our perceptions, which can be distorted, and our conceptions of what is appropriate behavior for another person. In addition, the tools we use to make our judgments and our conceptualization of confusion are imprecise. We have not studied the problem of confusion long enough or extensively enough to know for certain what behaviors are specific to it. And, the diagnostic process is flavored by our feelings about the patient, whether the feelings be pleasure and concern or anger and frustration. We can become easily confused ourselves, and the diagnosis may be more a display of our own confusion than the patient's. In many cases, as pointed out earlier in this book, it is not that seeing is believing, but rather that believing is seeing.

REFERENCES

Cohen, S.: Mental impairment in the aged: fable and fact. Presentation at the Gerontological Society's 31st Annual Scientific Meeting, Dallas, Nov. 16-20, 1978.

Eisdorfer, C., and Epstein, L.: Depression I and Depression II. In Workshop on aging, Educational Services Series of Sandoz Pharmaceuticals, East Hanover, N. J., 1977.

Gebbie, K. M. and Lavin, M. A., editors: Classification of nursing diagnoses, St. Louis, 1975, The C. V. Mosby Co.

Goldfarb, A.: Memory and aging. In Goldman, R., and Rockstein, M., editors: The physiology and pathology of aging, New York, 1975, Academic Press, Inc.

McNamee, C.: Communication, Can. Nurse 74:28-29, 1978.

Phillips, L.: A word about confusion. Unpublished manuscript, University of Pittsburgh, Pittsburgh, 1973.

Phillips, L.: The imprisonment model. Unpublished manuscript, University of Arizona, Tucson, 1976.

Williams, M. J., and others: Nursing activities and acute confusional states in elderly hip-fractured patients, Nurs. Res. 28(1):25-35, 1979.

8

EMERGENCY CARE FOR CLIENTS WHO ARE ACUTELY CONFUSED

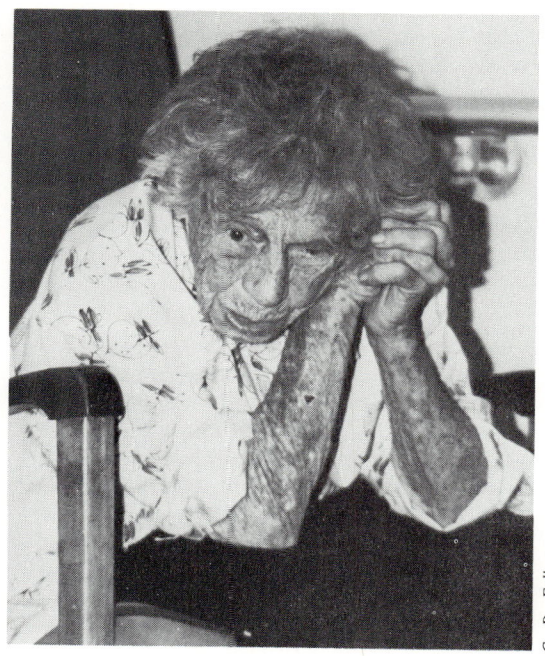

The need to make a precise nursing diagnosis of confusion makes it possible for the caregiver to prevent confusion and institute measures that treat the multiple underlying causes of confusional states. Our position is that unless confusion is viewed as secondary to some *other* cause and treated as such, the frequency, intensity, and amount of confusion that is seen will remain unchanged, and acute confusion will inevitably lead to irreversible confusional states.

However, in spite of this, it is legitimate to ask the questions: What does the caregiver do immediately with the elderly client who is displaying acute confusion, before she has time to assess and plan for the underlying cause? and What does the caregiver do in the emergency situation? This chapter will offer suggested treatments that will help in the immediate, emergency situation, while the nurse is making the second-level assessment. As a reminder, the areas to be screened during a second-level diagnosis appear in Tool 6-1. This chapter will be divided into three sections: (1) The signs and symptoms of acute confusion; (2) Anticipating or predicting confusion; and (3) Emergency treatment for confusion. When reading this chapter, the reader should remember that providing emergency treatment for confusion is similar to administering cardiopulmonary resuscitation; unless the underlying problem is identified and treated, the result is a kind of death, for socially the confused person becomes a nonperson.

SIGNS AND SYMPTOMS OF ACUTE CONFUSION

1. Disorientation to:
   a. A sense of time—as reflected by verb tense usage and verbal references to time sequences
   b. A sense of place—as reflected by inappropriate and incomprehensible references to location

101

c. A sense of person—as reflected by inappropriate references to self or calling oneself by a name from the past that is unexplainable
2. Inability to follow directions
3. Impairment of attention, perception, memory, and thinking, often with visual hallucinations, delusions, or illusions
4. Agitation and restlessness, particularly at night
5. Delirium or delirium tremens (associated with alcohol withdrawal)

A 67-year-old surgeon's firsthand account of his acute confusional state during a bacteremia with high fever follows. He says, "I don't know how to complete this list because somehow I seem to have a *fairly high degree of amnesia* for parts of the period."

1. "During a good part of the acute period my *memory was shot*. My son and friends kept reminding me that I had already told them whatever I had just restated. Obviously, I had forgotten what I had said or asked. That was most annoying—not the being told part but that I obviously didn't have all of my marbles. Is this part of the same process that one finds with the chronic brain syndrome? I believe that it was a transient problem (at least I hope so), because the memory seems all right again.
2. "I do recall having a *general lack of interest* in what was going on for a period of time, except as it caused pain. This seems to have been during the acute generalized phase of the bacteremia/toxemia, maybe the first 3 weeks. When it was all conquered, except in the shoulder, I redeveloped an interest in what was occurring to me. Being a surgeon, I was pleased to have left the medical-therapy-only approach and entered the 'cut-and-cure' phase of process.
3. "My cerebration was obviously affected during the acute phase. There seems to have been an *inability to concentrate* and carry on a logical thought process. I am certain my conversation was not always totally logical.
4. "I am impressed by the total *lethargy* that accompanied the whole episode. Just as one example, I recall on many occasions the need to urinate but would not quite get around to reaching for and placing the urinal for as long as 30 minutes. The same lapse of time between idea and action occurred in reaching for a magazine, telephone, or what-have-you.
5. "Finally, there was a decided *lack of insight* into the condition itself. While everyone else was seriously concerned with the problem and the possible outcome, it didn't bother me, except that it was an annoyance to be dependent on so many people, to be tied down and not productive, and generally not being the 'master of the fate' and the 'captain of my soul.' *Maybe that lack of insight is one of nature's protective measures.*"

Upon recovery nearly all victims of acute confusion can remember their state and tell about the illusions. Many say the memory is similar to remembering a television show, as if they were watching themselves acting on a stage.

ANTICIPATING OR PREDICTING CONFUSION

Among elderly people, certain factors make confusion predictable. The eye-patched patient was one of the first who helped the nurse recognize this possibility. Today, there are few patients who have their world blocked off by eye patches. The postoperative treatment for eye surgery has changed so that if the patient cannot see his environment, the caregiver now uses nursing measures that will maintain the patient's contact with reality. There are many similar factors that can be considered as "predictors of confusional states, such as (Wolanin and Holloway, 1980):

1. Age—those elderly individuals who are 80 years old or older are most vulnerable
2. Sex—men are more vulnerable than women
3. Living alone and lacking social supports—family members and familiar people help maintain contact with reality by helping "connect" the elderly person to his life history; lack of contact with one's life history helps to destroy one's identity and ability to react to the environment in a meaningful way

4. Relocation—particularly if the move is rapid, sudden, and unplanned
5. Confinement—to a restricted space where there is a lack of familiar objects
6. Disruption of the sleep cycle and distortion of light and darkness
7. Disruptions of patterns of daily living
8. Pain or discomfort from unmet physical needs
9. Drugs—such as sedatives, hypnotics, and analgesics
10. Lack of prostheses—including eyeglasses, hearing aids, and prostheses such as dentures or artificial limbs that enhance and complete the body image
11. Bed confinement—particularly in the horizontal position
12. Loss of control over body functions—including incontinence of bowel and bladder; impactions and diarrhea; and particularly, presence of tubes such as catheters, IV therapy lines, and nasogastric tubes
13. Restraints
14. Lack of contact with caring people and a stable environment—rapid change almost invariably leads to confusion, as does too much information presented too rapidly
15. Amnesia—as a result of drugs, surgery, or trauma

These predictors can be used for early identification of the clients who are most likely to become confused, so that emergency help can be given as soon and as aggressively as possible.

EMERGENCY TREATMENT FOR CONFUSION

The following emergency measures should be helpful in treating the confused client.

Establishing meaning in the environment

The environment should be inspected for normal living cues that the person can recognize. For example, is there an uncovered window near the client? Does the environment provide a means of differentiating night from day? Does the overhead light stay on all day? Does it need to? Is there a clock that is within visual reach and can the elderly client read the face on the clock? (This was quite important in the Williams and others [1979] study.) Is there a calendar? Does the client have objects around him that are familiar and associated with his life history, such as pictures or personal articles? Does he recognize that these things are his?

Exactly what the client perceives and what the world looks like from his vantage point should be determined. Many times what appear to be hallucinations are actually illusions that are created by the client's limited perspective of an unfamiliar environment because of sensory deficits. Many times, for example, an IV standard with a bag of blood hanging on it that is positioned slightly behind the client's line of vision appears to the client like a tall man. He may even give a name to the figure, thinking that it is someone who is quite familiar to him (Burnside, 1978). The environment must be adequately lighted. If the client uses a prosthesis, it should be in place and operational. Eye contact should be maintained. This means that the client's body position must be considered. People standing over the horizontal client may appear distorted, as shown in Fig. 8-1, A. This problem is even more pronounced, as seen in Fig. 8-1, B and C, when the client lacks his visual prosthesis and is able to focus only on either foreground or background. If the client cannot assume a sitting position, the caregiver should sit at the client's level, with the side rail down, in the client's direct line of vision. Many problems with confusion clear when the client is placed in a chair rather than in the horizontal position. The sedated client may see the caregiver who is standing over him as a fantastic monster with no counterpart in the real world and react accordingly. The following example illustrates sensitive nursing care for a potentially confused client:

An 84-year-old man had emergency surgery in the late evening. During the night, he opened his

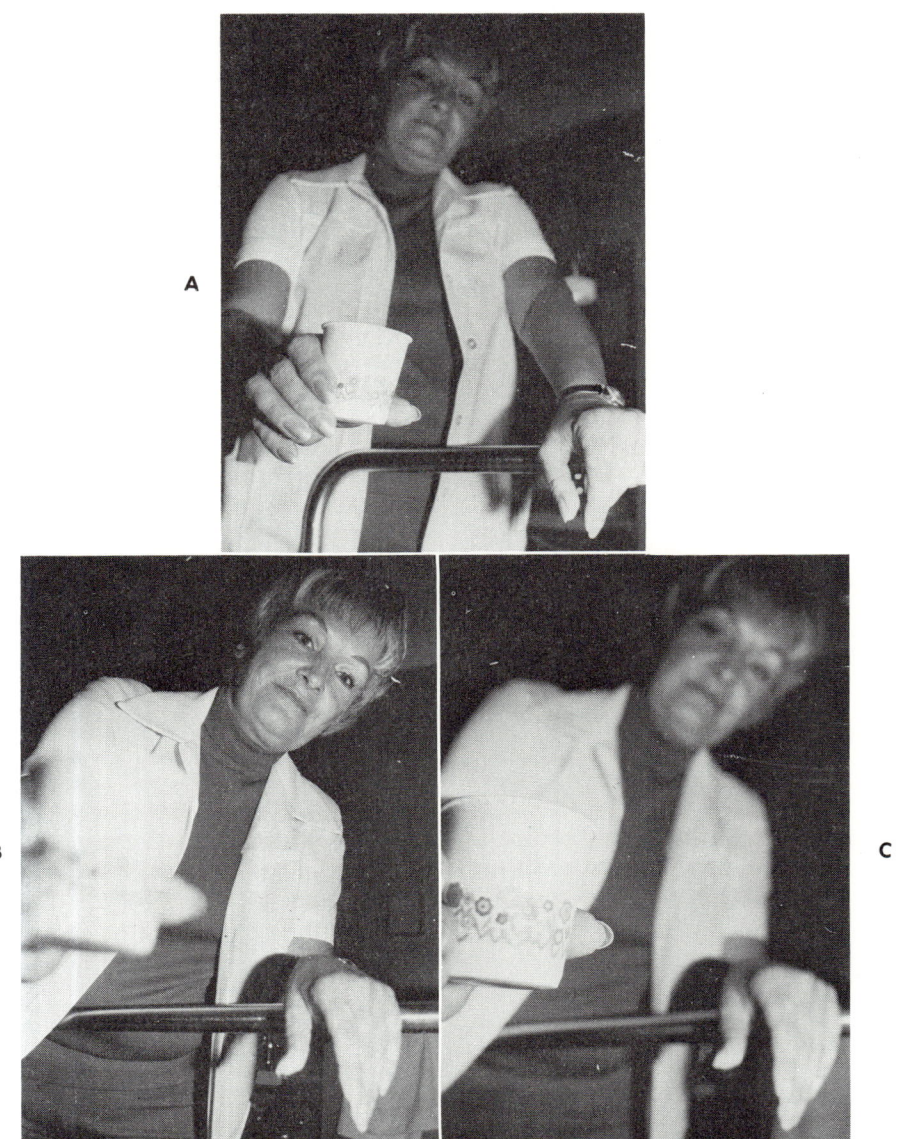

Fig. 8-1. Distortion of vision from the horizontal position. **A**, Fairly good focus and probably the best obtained by most elderly clients. **B**, The presbyopic eye is confronted with a confusing image of the huge and distorted paper cup against a white background. **C**, If the focus is on the cup, the background figures are blurred. (Photographs by C. D. Falk.)

eyes and saw the nurse sitting in his room. "Are you an angel?" he asked. Knowing that his vision was very poor, she turned on more light, sat by him with the side rail down, and spoke of their mutual acquaintances. He did not become confused, although it might have seemed inevitable because he had no family members to help him maintain contact with his life history.

The nurse who tries to perceive the environment through the client's eyes and ears will experiment with all kinds of orienting measures.

Explaining the setting, the equipment in the setting, and the rules is another means of establishing meaning in the environment. Simply describe the setting and the equipment in it. Let the client ask questions about any equipment that is unfamiliar. Explanations should be simple and straightforward. The more sense that can be involved in the explanation, the better. Let the client touch and smell and manipulate the things around him. Something that has been held in the hand lacks the mystery of the untouchable. Explain how the setting works and what the rules are. For example, how does he get help? How does he get a meal? How are drinks provided? Who are the people in the setting and what do they do? Probably nothing has more disturbing mystery in a strange setting than how to appropriately empty one's bladder or bowel. Most elderly people who get out of bed in a confused state are looking for the toilet. Even those people with indwelling catheters may not be able to comprehend that they no longer have the need to urinate, particularly when the catheter itself creates the feeling of this need. These problems can be foreseen and handled as the simple matters they really are.

Helping the client maintain a sense of his body (body image)

To grow old is to experience a number of body changes, but these happen gradually and can usually be incorporated into the present persona. The sudden change that may accompany fever, pain, stroke, or a fracture means that the adaptation period is reduced to hours instead of months or years. The person's competencies must be emphasized and used. The client should be helped to use his body in its normal or expected manner as much as possible. To discover that hands, arms or legs still function can reduce the sense of panic and create a sense of intactness. Remind the client about what he is able to do, no matter how little. Nursing care should complement and not supplant the elderly client's sense of who he is and what his body is. Active range of motion with quiet comment reinforces a sense of the body. Massage, bathing, and brisk toweling restores a sense of body integrity and boundary and can restore contact with a body that seems to be "floating off into space."

Providing continuity with the client's life history

Who we are now is determined by what we have been and by our ability to make this connection. The elderly person may not be able to make contact with his very identity during a confusional state. This may be compounded, in the institution, by various drugs, activities, and the vast number of hospital personnel. Reducing the total number of people the older sick client must come in contact with can reduce confusion. Primary nursing, that is, one person being held responsible for maintaining the identity and continuity with life history, should be as legitimate an assignment as responsibility for personal hygiene. Ascertaining the name the elderly person prefers to be called is important. Determining if there are family members to help make the link between the past and present, by means of visits or telephone calls, is essential. Reinforcing the objects in the environment from the client's past, such as taking out the pictures from his wallet or his personal toilet articles, can also be important. Show these to the client and encourage him to relate to them. Encourage life review as much as the person is able. If the caregiver knows of the client's past, specific incidents should be mentioned, all the while trying to get the client to relate to the incidents. Bringing the client's life history into the present reinforces areas of competence and the sense of self, while focusing away from the less comfortable present circumstances that are contributing to confusion.

Helping the client who shows agitation or unsafe behavior

Agitation is always related to fear or lack of control. The agitated person is begging for control. Unfortunately, the caregiver becomes alarmed when she finds an elderly person out of bed with tubes pulled out of proper orifices and trailing on the floor. Her annoyance is reflected in her words, actions, and the tone of her voice. One agitated person, the client, is enough in this situation. Even though the IV line that was anchored in the one accessible vein has been pulled out, agitation of the nurse changes nothing. Caregivers for the agitated elderly must have careful preparation in handling these kinds of situations. The caregiver's voice must never be raised. In fact, speaking softly allows the client the opportunity to lower his own voice. One person quietly taking command of the situation is natural; two frantic people arouse more fear and agitation.

The first question from the caregiver should be, "Are you looking for the bathroom?" The next question should be a quiet, calm inquiry into what help the client needs. The goal is to help the client regain control of his situation. The nurse can encourage the client to sit down by sitting down herself. A rocking chair is of great value, permitting the client to physically work off his agitation while rocking in one spot. As the client sits, the caregiver should never assume the threatening position of standing above him. Eye contact needs to be maintained. Offering a drink of water or some ice chips will engage hands that are flying. The nurse's offer of food may help.

Affectionately encircling the elderly person with her arms in a hugging fashion may be very soothing and offer control. The important principle is that the nurse must never show fear or agitation herself.

Giving attention to safety measures

The confused elderly client needs to be protected from harming himself by pulling out tubes or falling. Tubes present special problems because the human body reacts to tubes as foreign objects that alter body image and create discomfort and curiosity. Under any circumstances, the elderly person will attempt to explore his body to determine what is creating the sensations that arise from the tubes. Encouraging exploration under the guiding help of the caregiver is probably far more effective than trying to stop the exploration. The nurse should explain the tubes' purpose, taking the client's hand and allowing him to touch the tubes and determine where they enter his body. If he grabs the tube as if to pull, the caregiver should remain calm, speak to him gently, and maintain steady prohibiting pressure on his arm. Raising the voice or trying to wrestle with him will serve to increase his agitation and the likelihood that the tube will be pulled out. Even if the caregiver must remain talking to him and holding his arm for 15 minutes , he will eventually release the tube. Time should be allowed for this exploration to be repeated. If this approach proves to be ineffective, mittens applied to the hands are the next alternative. A third alternative is elbow restraints that are made from layers of soft, thick blankets and are wrapped and fastened around the client's elbows, thus prohibiting bending of the elbow. Each of these measures needs to be explained to the client, whether he seems to understand or not. At least once every hour each of these should be removed, the hands or elbows exercised, and the exploration process begun again.

Restraints, as a measure to prevent falls or the removal of tubes, are an absolutely last resort. Before applying restraints, there must be a careful evaluation of whose needs they serve. Serving the client's need to be protected differs from serving the caregiver's need to maintain control and order. If there is no need for the client to remain in bed, for example, why keep him there? Helping him to sit in a chair for awhile or bringing him out to the nurse's station in a chair is often soothing. Providing a sitter to be with him intermittently while he is up is preferable to restraints. Restraints can often be avoided by using more creative measures, such as making the environment more meaningful, providing more light, providing prostheses, or making a telephone call to a close friend and letting the client hear a familiar, reassuring voice.

Helping the client deal with illusions

What are usually thought of as hallucinations among elderly people are usually illusions, the difference being that illusions have a basis in fact and represent a misinterpretation of the environment. Thus, a rotating red light reflected on the ceiling is perceived as a fire and the TV repair cart outside the door makes the client think, "They have TVs watching me here." The nurse should listen to the "hallucination" and seek more information. Statements need to be verified and a basis in fact sought for the misperception. The nurse should never allow the client to think he is hallucinating by supporting his misperception. She should clear up the mistake and arrange the environment to preclude more errors. Older people know that they are "seeing things," but until they understand the things they "see," they will panic. Reality must be constantly and calmly described to the acutely confused client (Trockman, 1978).

Helping the client deal with confusion at night

The name "sundown syndrome" has been given to confusional displays that occur after dark. For the client who displays the sundown syndrome, the events that accompany the end of his day should be studied to determine precipitating factors, such as fatigue, unmet toileting needs, increased noise, decreased light, the effect of sedatives/hypnotics given after a day of activity, the effect of pain or pain medications (since pain is more common in the later part of the day), and the presence of fewer personnel. This last factor may be very important. The older person has more time alone and less with the nurse as she hurries on her visits. All of these add up to fear and strangeness without the support of another human being. Clients who have families sitting nearby are less likely to display sundown syndrome.

Helping the client deal with screaming at night

Nothing upsets night personnel like a screaming client who is confused and agitated from being afraid. Screaming is the only way he knows to get control, and it works. The fear should be the focus of the nursing interventions rather than the screaming. If the client's fear is reduced, quiet will follow. However, the need to have quiet in the night often results in nursing panic and frantic requests for sedation prescriptions. Instead, there should be answers obtained for the following questions: What does the client fear? Is it his pain? His loss of body competency? His lack of the familiar? His being alone? His fear of dying or of dying alone? A calm person by his side with adequate light in the room can often reduce the problem; helping him express his feelings may often resolve it.

SUMMARY

Acute confusion among the elderly does not occur without an underlying cause. There is always a reason for the confused behavior. Moreover, there are some measures that the caregiver can take during the immediacy of the situation to ameliorate the symptoms. It should be emphasized that these are palliative measures, however, and that the real treatment for confusion is treatment applied directly to the cause.

SUGGESTION FOR FURTHER READING

Working with the confused or delirious patient, Am. J. Nurs. **78**(9):1491-1512, 1978. (Self-study unit officially approved for 8 contact hours of continuing education.)

REFERENCES

Besdine, R. W.: Treatable dementia in the elderly—task force draft, May 1978, National Institute of Aging.

Burnside, I.: Personal communication, 1978.

Trockman, G.: Caring for the confused or delirious patient, Am. J. Nurs. **78**:1495-1499, 1978.

Wolanin, M. O.: Confusions in the elderly. In A sourcebook for nurses in geriatric settings, based on a continuing education offering of the College of Nursing, University of Arizona, Spring 1976, pp. 48-61.

Wolanin, M. O., and Holloway, J.: Relocation confusion: intervention for prevention. In Burnside, I., editor: Psychosocial aspects of nursing the elderly, ed. 2, New York, 1980, McGraw-Hill Book Co.

9

CARE OF THE CLIENT WITH CONFUSION SECONDARY TO COMPROMISED BRAIN SUPPORT

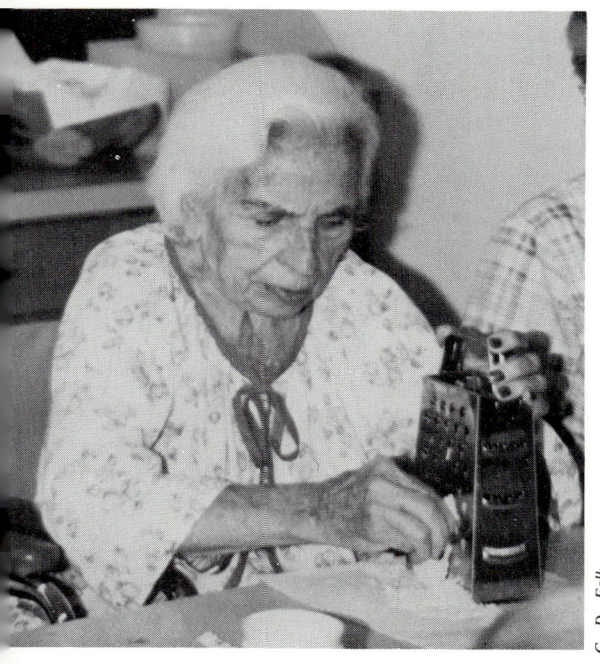

C. D. Falk

This chapter is concerned with nursing care of the elderly person with acute confusional states often known as "acute brain syndrome" or reversible brain syndromes. These are confusional states that are secondary to sudden changes in the brain physiology, which apparently interfere with the neurons as cells that metabolize oxygen, glucose, and other substrates. The aged brain is exquisitely sensitive to physiologic changes caused by a host of physical illnesses, and early in the development of such illnesses, the delicate function of the brain is easily disturbed (Besdine, 1978). The confusional state is often the first sign that the brain support is compromised. If the caregiver assumes that confusion in the elderly is ipso facto senility and untreatable, the primary disease may be overlooked, and the confusional state can lead to a permanent state.

Chapter 8 is based on the caregiver's interaction with the client who has an acute confusional state and applies to each section of this chapter. This chapter is concerned with treating the primary disease itself, which is outside the brain cells but exerts a detrimental effect on the brain. The strong client may muddle through his confusional state if his primary disease is recognized and treated promptly; but if he is treated as a senile person with irreversible changes, and his primary disease is not treated, he becomes another statistic among the elderly with chronic brain syndrome. Both confusion and the physiologic problem must be treated.

The confusional state is often a nursing

diagnosis, and as such should be dealt with by nursing personnel who are in frequent contact with the client. The underlying primary disease is often a very serious state that requires medical intervention and often emergency treatment.

Chapter 9 is divided into three major areas that deal with compromised brain support—hypoxia, hypoglycemia and hyperglycemia, and drug toxicity.

PART I
Hypoxia compromising brain support

Timiras' statement (1972, p. 509) that the aging brain in a general sense can be viewed as hypoxic should lead the nurse to the conclusion that any confused elderly client should be assessed for hypoxia that is neither slight nor easily accommodated by the client. Any stress condition can increase the need for oxygen and lead to a hypoxic state, which is recognizable by the symptoms of acute brain syndrome. These include the clinical observations of increased restlessness, inability to concentrate, apprehension, and a change from alertness to lethargy progressing to mild confusion and forgetfulness and eventually to unconsciousness (Groer and Shekleton, 1979).

Cyanosis is a late sign of hypoxia. It is based on observations dependent on environmental lighting, skin thickness, pigmentation, and the observer's subjective perception. Hemoglobin must be present in amounts large enough to interpret cyanosis meaningfully; a client with a hemoglobin deficiency must be very hypoxic before he appears cyanotic. The person with a large amount of hemoglobin may appear cyanotic even when not hypoxic. Cyanosis must be interpreted with other clinical signs (Groer and Shekleton, 1979). Air hunger is another symptom of hypoxia that represents the

---

Fourth-level general assessment for hypoxia

Behavior: confusion, restlessness, impaired memory, and distractability
Vital signs:
  Blood pressure: increased with early hypoxia but falls with prolonged hypoxia
  Respiratory rate, depth, and character: active expiration rather than passive process
  Cardiac function: rate, character of pulse, and presence of arrhythmias
Shape and elasticity of chest wall: kyphosis, scoliosis, concavity of chest front, movement with breath, and use of diaphragm and accessory muscles
Pupils: equality and response to light
Cough: ability to breath deeply and to cough; sounds of retained secretions
Secretions: character
Color
Air hunger

Past health history and work history for evidence of pulmonary disease infections, cardiac disease, and occupational hazards
Medications: drugs that affect the respiratory centers
Knowledge of laboratory reports:
  Red blood cell count: 4.5 million/cu mm
  Hemoglobin: normal 12 to 16 g/100 ml
  Normal arterial blood gas values (Phipps, Long, and Woods, 1979):

pH acidity of the blood	7.38 to 7.42
P_{CO_2} (Partial pressure of carbon dioxide in blood)	38 to 42 mm Hg
P_{O_2} (Partial pressure of oxygen in the blood)	80 to 100 mm Hg
Sa_{O_2} (Percentage of available hemoglobin saturated with oxygen)	95% to 98%

work of breathing. Dyspnea is the imbalance between need for air and the ability to meet that need. Lack of lung compliance, airway resistance, and the use of the accessory muscles (scalene, sternocleidomastoid, trapezius, and pectoral) contribute to the appearance of dyspnea.

This section on confusion secondary to hypoxia will be divided into four principal areas (Groer and Shekleton, 1979):

1. *Anemic hypoxia*, or hypoxia caused by reduction in amount of hemoglobin or blood available for oxygen transport; confusional states secondary to blood loss, iron deficiency, pernicious anemia (vitamin B_{12} deficiency), folic acid deficiency, and destruction of the blood-forming organs.

2. *Histotoxic hypoxia*, resulting from the cell's inability to utilize delivered oxygen due to impairment of the cell's enzyme system or electron transport chain; confusional states secondary to hypothermia, hyperthermia, dehydration with electrolyte imbalance, hypocalcemia and hypercalcemia, and uremia.

3. *Hypoxemic hypoxia*, caused by a reduction in the total amount of oxygen available in the blood—a ventilatory problem due to faulty blood-gas exchange; confusional states associated with emphysema and chronic obstructive lung disease.

4. *Stagnant (ischemic) hypoxia*, caused by poor tissue perfusion; the hemoglobin and oxygen content of the blood are normal or adequate, but oxygen is not delivered to the brain cells; confusion secondary to cardiac failure, increased intracranial pressure (subdural hematoma), normal pressure hydrocephalus, hypotension, and hypothyroidism.

CONFUSION SECONDARY TO ANEMIC HYPOXIA

The oxygen-carrying capacity of blood is dependent on the chemical combination of oxygen with hemoglobin in the erythrocyte. Anemic hypoxia can result from a lack of red blood cells, such as following a hemorrhage or a gradual but persistent loss of blood; from a lack of hemoglobin; from a lack of blood-forming components, such as vitamin B_{12} or folate; or from destruction of blood-forming organs, as in some drug reactions. Each of these will be discussed. In the aged, in the presence of frequent coronary disease, anemic hypoxia may precipitate cardiac arrhythmias or heart failure.

Confusion secondary to gradual blood loss (iron-deficiency anemia)

Signs and symptoms of anemia from gradual blood loss include pallor, especially of the mucosa, gradual loss of energy, a need to rest, and fatigue with minimal amount of exertion. There is usually an increased pulse rate. Depending on the area of the bleeding point, there should be some sign of bleeding, usually found in the stool if it is in the digestive tract. The small amount of bleeding may not be observable to the naked eye, but suspicion should lead to testing the feces for blood. Loss of blood with uterine bleeding may occur in the elderly woman with a tumor. There is no sudden onset that leads to immediate diagnosis, but the life-style often indicates a potential for bleeding, as in a frequent ingestion of aspirin.

Fourth-level assessment for gradual blood loss and iron deficiency

General fourth-level assessment for hypoxia

plus:

Drug history (aspirin; anticoagulants)
Note stools for frank blood or inspect for tarry appearance
Test for occult blood in stool
Evaluation of blood pressure in lying and standing position; there will be drop in blood pressure and an increase in pulse on standing
Awareness of any laboratory testing

Who is at risk to have confusion on the basis of hypoxia from gradual blood loss?

Clients with undetected bleeding from gastric ulcers, with gastrointestinal cancer, and with a long-standing history of aspirin ingestion for low-grade pain or arthritis are the most vulnerable.

Many elderly people depend on aspirin to prevent their next stroke, ease arthritic pain, relieve headaches, and be a general cure-all. Its inexpensiveness and accessibility preclude any policing, and often older people will have no idea how many aspirin tablets they have consumed in one day. Exton-Smith and Windsor (1971) estimate occult blood loss occurs in 50% to 70% of people taking aspirin. Gastrointestinal hemorrhages may also occur. The client who is self-medicating at home should have the proper information. The nurse, who assesses the environment of the elderly client, should know what drugs are available to him and should have an estimate of the frequency of dosage. A rectal examination should always include testing for occult blood.

Intervention has the following objectives:
1. Replace lost hemoglobin or iron and identify source of blood loss
2. Teach client dietary intervention
3. Monitor signs of gradual blood loss
4. Teach client to recognize signs of blood loss

The replacement of hemoglobin is the physician's first objective. This may require administration of packed red cells. The bleeding must be stopped; careful observation by the nurse may disclose the source of blood loss. Older people may have lost half of their normal erythrocyte count of 4.5 million/cu mm before symptoms appear, if the loss is gradual and the elderly person is accommodating. Transient ischemic attacks may occur if the elderly person stands in one position for any length of time, and this may be the first sign of anemia.

If the anemia is an iron-deficiency type, replacement of iron stores in the body is accomplished by administration of iron, often in the form of oral ferrous sulfate. It should be given after meals, because it can be so irritating to the gastrointestinal tract that the client may refuse to continue his medicaton. Adequate meals must be eaten —a problem for many elderly persons.

A dietary history should include food patterns. The client or caregiver must develop a sense of nutritional adequacy that recognizes quality and quantity of food. A cup of black coffee for breakfast, for example, is not a breakfast, and the tea, toast, and jam diet of many who live alone yields negative iron stores. There is a constant depletion of at least 1 mg daily through exfoliation of iron through skin cells, hair, nails, cells of the gastrointestinal tract, and urine.

In addition, 30% to 40% of the elderly develop an achlorhydria (deficiency of gastric acidity), which restricts absorption of dietary iron. Iron found in meat, for example, is rendered available through the proteolytic action of hydrochloric acid and pepsin. The major iron absorption takes place in the duodenum and upper jejunum. Surgery of the stomach, especially gastrectomy, leads to poor or no absorption of iron. When given with meals, iron may complex or bind with phytates and oxylates in milk and cheese, preventing absorption.

The usual diet of the client should be reviewed for iron content. Foods containing iron can be recommended on the basis of personal likes, ability to afford, and ability to chew. A change in diet must be realistic, or it will not be followed by the elderly person.

The nurse should observe the client carefully for continued blood loss. Urine should be examined for any bright blood or smokiness, which can indicate old blood. The stools of the client who is receiving iron are different from the tarry stools containing old blood. When the nurse is making her observation, she has an opportunity to teach the client or his caregiver the difference in consistency and color. When she makes her examination of the client's color, the client should be aware that the nurse is inspecting mucosa and should participate. The best teaching is done incidentally with the monitoring process and naturally, without producing anxiety. Ability to participate in self-care may lead to personal involvement that will produce a change in diet and medication patterns.

The elderly person in the home should be observed for signs of anemia and referred to medical supervision on its suspicion or recognition. On return home after treatment in a hospital, the environment must be adapted to include nutrition therapy. Often a refusal to take iron medication can be changed by helping the client adjust his meal patterns. If instruction on self-monitoring has not been given during the nurse's examination, it must be done before discharge.

Outcome criteria of successful nursing intervention against gradual blood loss and iron deficiency

1. The client is no longer confused.
2. The source of blood loss has been determined and treatment initiated.
3. The client or his caregiver recognizes signs of blood loss.
4. The client or his caregiver knows the more common foods that contain iron.
5. The client or his caregiver can give the reasons for giving oral iron after meals.
6. The client or his caregiver knows that oral iron produces dark or almost black stools.

CONFUSION SECONDARY TO LACK OF BLOOD-FORMING COMPONENTS (MACROCYTIC ANEMIA)
Pernicious anemia

Pernicious anemia (PA), a macrocytic anemia, is almost exclusive to old age. PA is normochromic, having adequate hemoglobin but a defect in the nucleus of the maturing cells. The ratio of DNA to RNA is reduced because of enzyme abnormalities in the pathway of DNA synthesis or a deficiency of vitamin B_{12} (cobalamin) or folic acid. The deficiency of vitamin B_{12} is usually not dietary in origin, but is rather the result of a lack of intrinsic factor or a disease of the terminal ileum, where absorption of vitamin B_{12} occurs (Groer and Shekleton, 1979).

Signs and symptoms of PA are generalized weakness; soreness and burning of the tongue (glossitis); smooth tongue (loss of papillae); numbness and tingling of extremities; a lemon yellow skin color; loss of coordination, particularly in the lower extremities; loss of fine hand movements; and confusion, as shown by irritability, memory loss, and mild depression.

Fourth-level assessment for pernicious anemia

Description of mouth and tongue
Assessment of gait and coordination
Disturbed position sense
Presence of Babinski's reflex (dorsiflexed toe)
Loss of vibration sense over toes
Loss of Achilles tendon and patellar reflexes
Blood-smear report

At greatest risk are those elderly people who have had total gastrectomy, or any surgery that interferes with ability of the stomach lining to produce intrinsic factor, or any condition that interferes with the ability of the lower ileum to absorb vitamin B_{12}. There seems to be a familial tendency for PA, and siblings should be watched when a family member suffers from it.

Today there is probably no prevention. However, early detection is possible.

Intervention is based on the following objectives:

1. Provide replacement of vitamin B_{12}
2. Act to relieve neurologic symptoms, including confusion
3. Teach family and client for restoration and adaption to disease

The nurse should provide for the replacement of vitamin B_{12} by assisting the client or a member of his family to administer the injections or by having him visit a clinic for injections the rest of his life.

Other care depends on the stage at which the condition is diagnosed. If there is confusion, the nurse should add to it as little as possible by introducing any changes very slowly until the acute symptoms subside.

The neurologic symptoms associated with PA are referred to by the names of subacute combined degeneration of the spinal cord, combined system disease, and posterolateral sclerosis. Malabsorption of vitamin B_{12} results in a myelopathy. Usually, the thoracic area of the cord is affected earliest and most severely (Alpers and Mancall, 1971), and the disturbance later spreads to include lumbar and cervical segments as well. The myelopathy may spread beyond the posterior and lateral compartments of the cord to the anterior aspects. Symptoms include paresthesias, more commonly found in the feet but also found in the hands. These are described as prickling, stinging, tickling, and numbness. They may be relieved by heat and aggravated by cold. Loss of position sense and ataxia are early symptoms. The difficulty in walking may range from slight lurching to extreme incoordination. Fatigue and weakness of the limbs involve the legs more than the arms. Spasticity of the legs usually develops, although a flaccid paralysis may result. Some sphincter disorder is invariably present (Alpers and Mancall, 1971). Mental symptoms occur in 60% to 65% of the clients with intellectual deficit, memory loss, and episodes of confusion. A prompt, positive response is often achieved with vitamin B_{12} treatment.

The family and client should be helped to anticipate restoration of function by noting each improvement of activity. Depression may have led to hopelessness, which may stand in the way of exploiting each improvement as it occurs. Inactivity may lead to ischemic ulcers that prevent restoration. Physical therapy should be obtained where available. If it is not available, the caregiver should be sensitive to each increment of change. The sphincter disorder may bring on the greatest amount of hopelessness, leading to confusion. The incontinence should be approached on an adult level, with avoidance of diapers-and-rubber-pants type of equipment. Bowel training can be achieved if the caregiver is willing to accept being trained as well as the client. The family should realize that this incontinence is a symptom of neurologic damage and usually yields to intervention.

Outcome criteria of successful nursing intervention against PA

1. The client and caregiver understand the importance of injection of vitamin B_{12} for remainder of life.
2. Arrangements have been made to provide vitamin B_{12} injections on a continuing basis.
3. The client or caregiver is given access to any physical therapy in the community to restore motor activity as the neurologic symptoms subside.
4. The mental confusion is treated as a symptom of the neurologic problem, and the caregiver understands the importance of introducing change gradually and maintaining accuracy in the environment.

Folic-acid deficiency

Lack of folic acid leads to development of a macrocytic anemia that is associated with arrest in red blood cell production, with symptoms similar to those of pernicious anemia. Among the elderly it may be more widespread than generally imagined. The body's stores of folic acid can be completely depleted after 3 to 4 months without adequate daily intake (a minimal amount of 100 μg daily). This deficiency is often found in conjunction with a deficiency of ascorbic acid, since the foods containing folate also contain ascorbic acid. Unlike pernicious anemia, the treatment need not be lifelong; however, good nutritional intake must be continuous, or recurrence is possible.

> **Fourth-level assessment for folic-acid deficiency**
>
> Include the general assessment for hypoxia
>
> plus:
>
> History of life-style
> Dietary intake, especially of fresh fruits and vegetables (institutional diets)
> History of alcoholism
> Does not respond to vitamin B_{12} therapy

Table 9-1. Folacin content of some of the more common foods (recommended daily allowance is 400 μg)

Food	Amount	Folate in micrograms
White beans	½ cup dry	132
Garbanzos	½ cup dry	125
Soybeans	½ cup dry	236
Beets	2 medium	93
Asparagus	5 to 6 stalks	64
Broccoli	1 medium stalk	72
Brussels sprouts	3 large	97
Cabbage	1 cup shredded	69
Lettuce, romaine	1 cup cut	102
Spinach	½ pound	463
Sweet potato	1 medium	84
White potato, fresh	1 medium	21
Apple	1 medium	10
Banana	1 medium	36
Cantaloupe	1 cup diced	49
Grapefruit juice	1 cup	52
Orange juice	1 cup	164
Strawberries	1 cup	24
Tangerine	1 medium	18
Whole wheat bread	1 slice	26
Oatmeal	¾ cup dry	34
Rice	¼ cup dry	37
Wheat germ	¼ cup	52
Milk, whole	1 cup	37
Egg yolk	1 large	50
Yogurt	1 cup	27
Brewer's yeast	1 tbsp.	286

The elderly people most vulnerable have malnutrition, such as is found in alcoholic cirrhosis, have little or no fresh fruit and vegetables in their diet, have a very low income, or are on institutional diets.

Prevention is dependent on recognizing those who are at risk and altering their dietary pattern. Many elderly who live alone are high risk in several categories. There is no storage depot for folate in the body. In several months the supply is exhausted unless it is replenished in the daily diet. The solution can range from referral to social agencies for income maintenance or counseling to treatment for alcoholism. The underlying essential fact in care and teaching is that a daily intake of folate is important. Often the problem is one of education; the older client has not realized how marginal his existence is until illness reveals how his life-style affects his health. He may have to redistribute his food dollar into more productive channels. Lonely, old people have been persuaded to spend the fresh fruit dollar on burial insurance policies or burial plots. Prevention is also a social problem.

Table 9-1 is to be used as a teaching tool. It provides a list of some of the richer sources of folate and is extensive enough to fall within the special dietary likes and dislikes of the elderly from many cultures.

Intervention is based on these objectives:
1. Assist with the medical regimen and give supportive care according to the client's dependency
2. Teach and prepare for discharge or for altering life-style within the present living arrangements

Assisting with the medical regimen during the acute phase will probably include giving some form of folic acid. The nursing care should be based on dependent needs, which may be extensive at first, and should always be focused on teaching and preparing the client for his reentry into independent living and food choices.

The client must be assessed in his particular setting and his life-style considered. Change must be introduced gradually. The nurse who works with this principle in mind can help the older person become independent and responsible.

> **Outcome criteria of successful nursing intervention against folic-acid deficiency**
>
> 1. The client or his caregiver knows the need for folic acid and ascorbic acid in the diet and can describe which foods offer the greatest amount.
> 2. The client or his caregiver is able to plan a diet that includes adequate amounts of folic acid.
> 3. The client recognizes symptoms of folic-acid deficiency.
> 4. Referral is made to follow-up agency if client desires.
> 5. Referral is made to community agency if financial problem is recognized.

Hemolytic anemias

The hemolytic anemias are not a single disease entity but the result of a number of conditions, characterized by the rate at which red blood cells are destroyed in relation to their production. Causes may be hemolysis from incompatible blood transfusion, malaria or streptococcal infection, spleen pathology, or reaction from drugs such as sulfonamides, phenacetin, and others. Hemolytic anemias may have a slow onset, during which the client makes adjustments to the gradual loss of red cells, or there may be a sudden onset, such as the transfusion reaction or infection with chills, fever, headache, irritability, and pain. Urinary output may be reduced.

> **Fourth-level assessment for hemolytic anemias**
>
> Include general assessment for hypoxia
>
> plus:
>
> Drug profile
> Recent treatment
> Diagnosis
> Onset
> Laboratory blood picture

The elderly who take many drugs, which may interact or act on the blood-forming organs, are vulnerable. Transfusion reactions are not uncommon among the elderly.

Prevention is best expressed by constant vigilance.

Intervention is based on giving supportive care according to dependency needs and assisting with the medical regimen. This covers a broad range of activities that could take place in intensive care, the renal dialysis unit, or the home. The hemolytic anemias require detective work at times, and the assessment of the client in his setting with his life-style is important.

CONFUSION SECONDARY TO HISTOTOXIC HYPOXIA

The brain cells have a relatively narrow range of conditions under which they function adequately. Temperature, fluid, electrolytes, and acid-base balance can vary little without upsetting the delicate environment in which the neuron does its work. This section suffers from the lack of knowledge of exactly how the brain works. Much of the information is based on the clinical picture that deficiency or excess provides. By the time this book is printed, the explanations may be available. For now, the theory is that the cell has an optimum environment for function and that it cannot metabolize its oxygen and glucose without these optimum conditions.

This section is devoted to the care of elderly persons who are confused because of body temperature imbalance, including hypothermia and hyperthermia; fluid and electrolyte imbalance, including dehydration; and calcium imbalance, with hypocalcemia and hypercalcemia.

Confusion secondary to fluid and electrolyte imbalance
Dehydration

Those who care for the elderly know that many are admitted to acute and long-term care units with severe dehydration. The basic illness may be less significant than the fact that older people are dehydrated during the illness because there is less intake of fluid than is lost by the kidneys, lungs, and skin, resulting in a fluid and electrolyte imbalance.

In a study at a Canadian hospital during a 12-month period, all patients over the age of 70 who were admitted as emergencies to the acute medical unit were seen within 4 hours of admission, and assessed for presence of mental confusion. Thirty (43%) of the total of 70 admissions showed evidence of confusion, as measured by the modified Roth questionnaire. Biochemical profiling and physical examination determined any evidence of dehydration. Of the confused group, 14 (47%) showed measurable improvement after a week of rehydration, and 7 (23%) showed definite reversal of the confused state. In this study, 70% of the elderly emergency admissions had been treated for their confusion by rehydration alone (Seymour and others, 1978). The gravity of the problem increases because fluid balance cannot be considered apart from the electrolyte balance.

While volume of body fluid can be a concern, hyperosmolarity, rather than fluid volume, is a critical issue. Sodium is the regulator of extracellular osmotic activity, and the serum sodium level indicate changes in water balance. Hypernatremia, or increased serum sodium level, indicates water depletion. In an effort to maintain a normal osmolarity, water is drawn from interstitial and intracellular compartments, including the cells of the brain itself. Signs of this fluid imbalance include mental confusion, lethargy, and profound weakness.

Dehydration becomes critical when water deficit is severe enough to compromise the vascular volume available for circulation or when hypovolemia occurs. Adequate perfusion of the cells requires sufficient volume to pump blood to all parts of the body. When the compensatory vasoconstriction of peripheral vessels can no longer maintain the blood pressure, it may drop to levels that will be recognized as shock. Scribner and associates (1969) consider a postural drop of 15 mm Hg systolic pressure and a diastolic fall of 10 mm Hg indicative of volume deficit, when the drop results from changing from the horizontal to the vertical position.

The signs and symptoms of hypovolemia are based on nerve and muscle function. The problem may include low total sodium content of the body, which cannot be measured by the serum sodium samples because the body makes an attempt to maintain a normal level by adjusting the fluid content. Therefore, the nurse must depend on her own observations and a history of the client's life-style and environmental conditions to create a high level of suspicion.

Smaller adults normally have less fluid in each body compartment, especially the extracellular compartment, so they become dehydrated more quickly and require fluid replacment sooner. The very old do not have the flexible regulatory systems by which the kidneys conserve fluid and sodium in times of stress. The younger person compensates for fluid loss by kidney action to maintain functional volume. The elderly client will require fluid and electrolyte studies and careful monitoring during replacement.

For many elderly persons, examination of the body will be misleading since they appear dehydrated under normal circumstances. Skin is dry, the mucous membranes appear dry, and when the skin is pinched into a fold, it returns to its previous state very, very slowly. Skin turgor in the elderly is best checked on the forehead. The mouth moisture, which should be a dependable gauge of hydration, may be altered by drugs that leave the mouth dry. However, if the axillary region is moist, the individual is probably sufficiently hydrated. The nursing history must include a drug profile: important drugs are diuretics, which are prescribed for many elderly; tranquilizers, which may produce indifference to food and fluids; and cathartics, which produce copious liquid stools.

118 Confusion: prevention and care

Fourth-level assessment for dehydration, with observable signs and symptoms

Assessment	Observations
Behavior	Change: confused; apathetic
Mouth	No saliva pool under tongue; brown furry tongue
	Thick, ropy saliva
Upper gastrointestinal	Anorexia; nausea; vomiting
Elimination	Oliguria
	Small, hard stools; constipation
Pulse	Pulse rate change: weak; arrhythmias
Blood pressure	Decreased; tend toward shock level with hypovolemia
Respiration	Rate change: breathing pattern shifts to deeper breathing
Eyeballs	Dehydration: soft; "mushy"
Skin and mucous membranes	Dry; decreased turgor
Nervous system	Muscle weakness: tingling; tetany (K^+ deficiency)
Abdomen	Distention (K^+ deficiency)
	Abdominal cramping (Na^+ deficiency)
Urine	Oliguria; concentrated

Other assessments
  Drug profile
  Mechanical problems preventing fluid intake
  Inability to swallow; dysarthria; motor disabilities of arthritis; parkinsonism; tardive dyskinesia; stroke
  Dependence on caregivers for fluids
  Dry weather; exposure to winds that rapidly dehydrate

Elderly people at risk are those who are taking diuretics, tranquilizers, or purgatives; who are depressed or grieving or whose mental status interferes with recognition of thirst; who are dependent on others to provide fluids; whose fluids are restricted for diagnostic or treatment procedures; whose bodies have been exposed to heat, particularly hot, dry winds; who are given highly concentrated liquids, such as nasogastric feedings; and who are losing fluid by vomiting, diarrhea, or excessive perspiration.

Prevention of dehydration is usually possible, except in the special cases in which the elderly seem to predominate.

1. The nurse should attend to fluid intake, teaching the elderly client in his home to give attention to fluid intake as an important part of his self-care and monitoring process. Either the client or his caregiver should be able to relate the association of certain drugs and dehydration and review the signs of dehydration. There should be an implicit contract for adequate fluid intake.

2. The institutionalized client is at the mercy of his caregivers. Many nursing homes do not have water at the bedside, and drinking fountains are not accessible from wheelchairs or to the trunk-shortened elderly woman. It is important to assess the client's intake instead of assuming that drinking fountains meet the need, especially where residents are slightly confused.

3. The hospitalized client may have fluids restricted for diagnostic or treatment reasons. Too many elderly persons are only marginally hydrated, and short-time restriction can lead to iatrogenic dehydration. Purging for radiographic studies of the bowel focuses on preparation of the client at the

expense of his human need for constant replacement of fluid. The elderly client who cannot take fluids by mouth or who is vomiting should have parenteral replacement before the fluid and electrolyte imbalance characterized by confusion occurs. Fluids are the second survival need after air (oxygen). *It is almost impossible to prevent someone from having air to breathe, but many mentally and physically disabled or sick persons are totally dependent on a caregiver for fluids.* The nurse who is responsible for the nursing actions of untrained personnel must teach and remind. The high-risk physical environment may have water, but not in a place that is accessible to the dependent person—examples are water on the wrong side of the stroke patient, water fountains and faucets that cannot be reached from a wheelchair, or simply no provision at all. The question should be asked, "How does this dependent client satisfy his thirst and need for fluids?" Adequate nursing demands a satisfactory answer.

Intervention is based on three major objectives:
1. Provide adequate fluids safely
2. Teach the elderly client to recognize his need for fluids and their importance when he is taking tranquilizers, diuretics, and cathartics
3. Plan for discharge

Good nursing demands constant attention to fluid intake. Prevention is much easier than a cure. For the elderly client who is dehydrated, nursing care is a highly individualized process based on one guiding principle: the composition and volume of body fluid may vary only within a narrow range if cells are to function optimally.

For the client who can take oral fluids, the need to rehydrate is imperative, but only within the reserve capacity of the circulatory system. Rapid replacement will tax this system and must be monitored carefully by (1) pulse rate, (2) blood pressure, and (3) thirst. Blood pressure is taken in the lying and sitting positions to determine when loss of fluid volume has been compensated. There should be little change in the two readings when hypovolemia is no longer present.

Fluids offered should contain electrolytes; warm broth, orange juice or other fruit juice, milk, and soups replace sodium and potassium. Ice-cold fluids should be served with caution since they may cause gastric discomfort, especially if given in quantity, and this serves to delay the fluid replacement. For the elderly person who rejects large amounts of fluids (and most do), the use of very small glasses or teacups lessens the distaste by diminishing the magnitude.

Fluids replaced by a nonoral route require that the physician determine the route and content of the fluid, as in nasogastric feedings. The nurse is responsible for reminding the physician when the client is in an institutional setting. The physician should know that fluid is being lost and replacement is necessary. The highly concentrated feedings usually chosen for nasogastric feeding often contain protein, which draws fluid from the body and causes diarrhea, compromising the purpose of the feeding. Water should be given between tube feedings in a normal pattern of thirst relief.

Frequency of feeding should be examined to determine if frequency is based on the institutional need to confine feedings to the fewest procedures possible or on the client's actual needs. Monitoring water intake is most important with nasogastric feedings. Large quantities of fluid given at once can produce vomiting. Frequent, small amounts of water between feedings replace fluid without upsetting the gastrointestinal tract.

Parenteral fluid replacement demands careful monitoring. The older person cannot tolerate rapid infusion. Most respond best to an infusion rate that is monitored and adjusted constantly to prevent circulatory overload. Giving "catch-up fluids" to meet a schedule is very dangerous in the elderly, who may have cardiac failure or renal disease. Because of the low cardiac reserve of the elderly, 2 ml/min or 120 ml/hr is a less dangerous rate and allows the body to readjust by shifting fluid from one compartment to another.

Signs of circulatory overload (pulmonary edema) include:
1. Bounding pulse
2. Engorged peripheral veins
3. Hoarseness
4. Dyspnea
5. Cough or pulmonary rales

The most likely candidates for circulatory overload are elderly clients with circulatory impairment, decompensated hearts, or any renal impairment. Renal failure is a contraindication for intravenous potassium.

The replacement fluid or any extraoral feedings should be distributed over the 24-hour period to allow for better electrolyte balance by the kidneys and to prevent overdilution of body fluids, with resultant fluid and electrolyte shifts.

Electrolyte replacement is required in fluid loss. The elderly client should be monitored by serum electrolyte and the acid-base balance studies. Electrolytes are lost when dehydration is caused by vomiting, diarrhea, catharsis, and excessive use of enemas. Not more than three enemas should be given on an order "enemas until clear" without consulting the physician and giving the clinical signs that indicate client tolerance.

Potassium is not well conserved at any age. Diuretics, vomiting, and diarrhea promote its loss. The nutritional intake may not contain the fruits, vegetables, and meats that normally furnish potassium. Potassium losses accompany conditions of stress or acidotic states. The most striking sign of potassium deficit is muscle weakness and apathy. For those 20% of the very old elderly who take some form of digitalis, potassium replacement is essential to prevent digitalis toxicity. If potassium is replaced intravenously, it must be done slowly, or cardiac arrest can occur.

Hyperkalemia can be anticipated in clients who have a significant decrease in renal output, especially if they are receiving any potassium supplement.

Replacement of sodium is rarely a problem in the elderly whose body regulatory processes bring about shifts in the body fluid compartments to effect optimum osmolarity. Often, half-strength saline is the greatest concentration given the elderly person; many elderly have a tendency to retain sodium. (For the nurse who needs to refresh her knowledge of fluid and electrolyte balance and acid-base balance, we recommend Soltis, 1979.)

The confused elderly client will require careful watching to prevent removal of the IV or nasogastric tubing. The veins of the elderly are fragile, often poorly anchored under the skin, and in the case of dehydration, quite likely to collapse with venipuncture. Venipuncture should take place under optimum conditions, with the informed client included in the team. Activity must be restricted during the time that as infusion is taking place. For the older person who may be at circulatory or pulmonary risk, this inactivity must be taken into account and provision made for maximum position change without compromising the IV line. Each elderly person is a candidate for pressure areas in as few as several hours in one position. One of the best plans for prevention of tube and needle removal is a frequent shift in position to avoid discomfort. The uncomfortable client will explore the probable causes of discomfort. The mouth should be rinsed frequently to prevent dryness and thick, ropy mucus, a by-product of dehydration. In addition, each nursing contact should include calling the client by name, identifying who the nurse is, and using touch on the hand to maintain identity and orientation.

The client must be taught to avoid fluid and electrolyte imbalances before he is discharged. The elderly client who has undergone any fluid or electrolyte imbalance is a candidate for a second episode unless he or his caregivers are taught prevention. The nurse must review the past event with the client or caregiver in terms of onset, signs and symptoms, and prevention. The reality of the situation should be studied—does the client have sufficient strength to take care of his fluid intake? Does he have the will? Is there money enough to include fresh fruit and meats in the diet? Does he realize which pills are diuretic?

Outcome criteria of successful nursing intervention against dehydration

1. The client has adequate fluid intake and output.
2. The client is no longer confused mentally.
3. The client or his caregiver understands the importance of adequate fluid intake.
4. The client's environmental constraints are reviewed and suggestions made for making fluids accessible.
5. The client or his caregiver understands the relationship of his medications, adequate fluid intake, and dietary modifications.

Confusion secondary to serum calcium imbalance

Disturbances of calcium metabolism include hypocalcemia and hypercalcemia. Calcuim is found in the plasma in bound (Ca^+) and ionized (Ca^{++}) forms. The free ionized form is the active form necessary for blood coagulation, skeletal and cardiac muscle contraction, and nerve function. It is this last function that is important in considering confusion secondary to calcium (Ca^{++}) imbalance.

Calcium and phosphate have a reciprocal relationship in plasma, with an elevation of one accompanying a decreased level of the other. Elevated phosphate levels lower the calcium level, which in turn stimulates the parathyroid hormone that increases serum Ca^{++} concentration, even if it is necessary to mobilize Ca^+ from the bone.

In renal disease, which many elderly clients have, the Ca^+ level is low because the kidneys retain phosphate. Calcitonin, a thyroid hormone, inhibits bone resorption and decreases Ca^{++}, while 1,25-dihydroxycholecalciferol, the active metabolite of vitamin D, increases the intestinal absorption of Ca^+ and helps to mobilize Ca^+ from the bone. Other hormones that may affect calcium balance include thyroxine, estrogen (if administered for long periods), adrenal steroids, and growth hormones (Groer and Shekleton, 1979).

Hypocalcemia

Like confusion, hypocalcemia is usually a symptom of a physiologic problem that requires medical treatment. A decrease in Ca^{++}, as found in the plasma, has an excitatory effect on nerve and muscle cells, resulting in a symptom complex known as tetany. The threshold of peripheral sensory nerve receptors to excitation is also lowered, and sensory changes may precede motor changes. Tetany can occur with low normal calcium levels if the serum pH is on the alkaline side, because more plasma protein becomes ionized and binds with calcium in the alkalotic state (Groer and Shekleton, 1979). Tetany is characterized by neuromuscular irritability, as shown by paresthesias; facial muscle spasm; carpopedal spasm; laryngospasm, which may obstruct the airway; bronchial spasm, which may resemble asthma; abdominal muscle spasm, which may mimic an acute abdomen; and convulsion, which is not relieved by anticonvulsant medications and is not accompanied by loss of consciousness. Tetany can be precipitated by exercise or emotional states because of hyperventilation and respiratory alkalosis.

Signs and symptoms of hypocalcemia include alkalosis, tetany, and a positive Chvostek's sign. The laboratory test for serum calcium is reported on the basis of total calcium. The ionized calcium (Ca^{++}) is estimated to be approximately half the serum calcium reported.

Changes in mental status can occur. These may be related to the negative feedback from the body as the result of uncontrollable neuromuscular irritability, or because hypocalcemia inhibits transmission of the impulse at the myoneural junction (Groer and Shekleton, 1979).

Fourth-level assessment for hypocalcemia

Life-style: pattern of food intake; foods containing calcium
Diagnosis of medical problem
Chvostek's sign
Observation for tetany
Laboratory tests:
  pH toward the alkalosis end serum calcium below 4.5 mEq/liter;
  electrocardiogram shows a prolonged Q-T interval due to lengthened S-T segment
Complaint of numbness or tingling in fingertips, nose, ears, and toes

---

Nursing attention should be directed toward early detection (Tripp, 1976). Part of the assessment should be testing for Chvostek's sign, which is elicited by tapping over the facial nerve immediately below the temporal bone and anterior to the ear. A positive sign is the spasmodic contraction of the facial muscles on the same side of the face.

Those elderly people who have interference with the feedback system by which the parathyroid hormone regulates the serum Ca^{++} level; who have loss of blood supply to the parathyroids by surgical removal or damage; and who have late-onset idiopathic hypoparathyroidism, which may be of autoimmune origin, are vulnerable. Also vulnerable are those elderly with a lack of calcium and vitamin D absorption from the intestinal tract, or those whose purging has resulted in rapid transit during which calcium is not absorbed. Those with acute pancreatitis, which causes calcium to be fixed by a fatty acid liberated from mesenteric fat (Groer and Shekleton, 1979); with neoplasms, such as tumors of the lung, breast, and prostate, including metastasis, which is associated with osteoblastic activity and skeletal uptake of calcium; and those who are transfused with large quantities of stored blood (calcium binds to excess citrate) are likely victims. Elderly people with a magnesium deficiency secondary to intestinal malabsorption, alcohol, or a restricted diet (hypocalcemia is a complication of magnesium deficiency) or who have a renal insufficiency are likely candidates for excessive calcium loss. Many who take large amounts of antacids are hypocalcemic, because calcium salts are best absorbed in an acid medium. Others vulnerable are the housebound who never receive sunlight.

The prevention of confusion secondary to hypocalcemia is dependent on preventing the calcium deficiency, which is the most common mineral deficiency in the diet of the elderly. It is lost through urine and feces. The recommended daily requirement is 800-1000 mg/day for adults. Calcium is most often taken into the body through some form of milk or milk products. When dietary instruction is given, milk intake should not be taken for granted. Dry milk substitutes for fresh milk when cost makes its use prohibitive. If the taste is offensive, it can be used in cooked foods such as soups or served ice cold. Some older people do not drink milk because of the discomfort from intestinal lactase deficiency. It is estimated that some 40% of adults have this deficiency, and many ethnic groups not reared with cow's milk, such as American Indians and blacks, have this intolerance. Intolerance is indicated by abdominal cramping and diarrhea and may be prevented by the use of a commercial preparation of lactase.

The dietary assessment should check that calcium-rich foods are eaten, such as turnip greens, Swiss chard, mustard leaves, dandelions and spinach, or almonds and pinyon nuts. Table 9-2 gives a list of commonly eaten foods with their calcium values. Leafy green vegetables are foreign to many diets, yet they can be tastily prepared, are

Table 9-2. Foods containing calcium*

Food, with approximate measure	Weight in grams (unless noted)	Calcium in milligrams
Milk and related products:		
Whole milk, 8 oz	240 ml	285
Dry, nonfat, 8 oz	80	1,040
Goat's milk, 8 oz	240 ml	315
Cheddar cheese, 1-inch cube	17	133
Cheddar cheese, 1-oz slice	28	163
Cottage cheese, 8 oz	225	207
Swiss cheese, 1-oz slice	28	271
Custard, 8 oz	248	278
Ice cream (factory pack), 3½ oz	62	76
Yogurt, 8 oz	246	295
Eggs:		
Egg yolk, 1	17	24
Fish and shellfood:		
Clams (canned solids and liquid), 3 oz	85	74
Canned mackerel, 3 oz	85	221
Oysters, 1 cup	240	226
Oyster stew, 1 cup		
(1 part oysters to 3 parts milk by volume)	230	269
Salmon (pink canned), 3 oz	85	159
Sardines, 3 oz	85	367
Shrimp, 3 oz	85	98
Nuts, beans, peas, lentils:		
Almonds, 1 cup	142	332
Beans (canned with pork), 1 cup	261	183
Brazil nuts, 1 cup	140	250
Peanuts, 1 cup	144	104
Green leafy vegetables		
Broccoli, 1 cup	150	195
Collards, cooked, 1 cup	190	473
Dandelions, cooked, 1 cup	180	337
Kale, cooked, 1 cup	110	248
Lettuce head, 1 lb	454	100
Mustard greens, cooked, 1 cup	140	308
Turnip greens, cooked, 1 cup	145	376
Spinach, cooked, 1 cup	180	223
Fruits:		
Pineapple, crushed, 1 cup	260	75
Raisins, dried, 1 cup	160	124
Rhubarb, cooked, 1 cup	272	112
Breads and miscellaneous:		
Cracked wheat, 1 loaf	454	399
Enriched French or Italian, 1 loaf	454	256
Rye, 1 loaf	454	236
Pumpernickel, 1 loaf	454	381
Enriched white, 1 loaf	454	381
per slice (20 to loaf)	23	19

*Quantities based on Home and Garden Bulletin No. 72, U.S. Department of Agriculture, September 1960.

Continued.

Table 9-2. Foods containing calcium—cont'd

Food, with approximate measure	Weight in grams (unless noted)	Calcium in milligrams
Breads and miscellaneous—cont'd		
Whole wheat, 1 loaf	454	449
Corn muffin, 2¾ inch diameter		79
Macaroni and cheese, baked, 1 cup	220	394
Custard pie, 4 inch	130	162
Pizza (cheese)l 5½-inch slice	75	157
Dark brown sugar, 1 cup	220	167
Canned creamed soup, 1 cup	255	217
Bean soup, 1 cup	250	95

inexpensive, and measure for measure, have more calcium than milk.

The older person who is housebound and deprived of natural vitamin D from the sun will require vitamin supplementation. Whether the client is in his own home or an institution, steps should be taken to correct his life-style without upsetting him. Constantly closed curtains can give the nurse an important message.

The elderly person's self-health care should include maintaining good bowel habits without purgatives and reducing the use of antacids to a minimum or to include low-phosphate antacids such as Amphojel.

Intervention is based on the following nursing objectives:
1. Facilitate calcium replacement
2. Provide safety and supportive care for person with demineralization
3. Teach and plan for discharge

The immediate treatment of hypocalcemia may be administration of intravenous calcium gluconate. This requires caution regarding the infusion site, because solution that leaks outside the vein can lead to sloughing of tissue. Calcium gluconate should not be added to any intravenous solution that contains sodium bicarbonate or phosphate, since calcium bicarbonate or a precipitate can be formed. A calcium infusion is contraindicated for the client who is receiving digitalis therapy. Under any circumstances, calcium must be administered very slowly and monitored carefully. Rapid changes are not tolerated well by the physiology of the elderly. The place of calcium in the cardiac cellular function should not be disturbed too rapidly, or there may be impaired intraventricular conduction, leading to cardiac arrest.

Oral calcium can be given but may be poorly absorbed by the elderly person whose gastric acidity has been reduced. A history will often reveal a calcium-deficient diet or the routine use of purgatives and antacids. This is a point that requires educational preparation for discharge. Every case of hypocalcemia demands follow-up to ensure that the previous condition has been remedied.

The hypocalcemic client may have a long-standing condition. If so, he will have demineralizaton of his bones. Women over the age of 60 particularly exhibit signs of bone loss, including brittle bones and fractures. All bones suffer, but the more commonly fractured are the ribs, radius and ulna (from reaching out to break the impact of falls), and the head and neck of the femur. Vertebrae tend toward compression fractures, especially in the thoracic and lumbar spine, resulting in kyphosis. Wachman and Bernstein (1968) hypothesize that bone loss results from continous removal of small amounts of calcium because of a "chronic acidosis" with advancing age. The calcium withdrawal is an attempt to maintain a normal plasma pH. A cane is helpful in preventing loss of equilibrium. Vision should be tested (see vision test in Chapter 6) to determine how well the older client can see objects on the floor or ground that would interfere with balance. Even a small stone can upset the equilibrium of a person with weakened knee ligaments or joints stiffened by arthritis. Floor coverings should be examined for looseness, color contrast, which may give the mistaken illusion of depth, and texture, such as shag rugs that make walking difficult for persons with gait problems. A foot and gait assessment should also be made (Appendix C).

Snugly fitting shoes can be an important aid to maintaining balance while walking. Laced oxfords are the best support shoe, even in the acute-care setting. If laces present a problem, a snugly fitting, hard-soled loafer is best. The elderly should avoid loose bedroom slippers.

The nurse in the acute-care unit includes referral to a community health agency for assessment of the client in the home, when possible. In the nursing home, one of the gravest problems is procuring well-fitted shoes. The loose, soft-soled house shoe can lead to foot problems that decrease mobility. Mineralization of the long bones is dependent on weight-bearing, while the entire well-being of the client is enhanced with mobility.

Outcome criteria of successful nursing intervention against hypocalcemia

1. The client no longer exhibits confusion secondary to hypocalcemia.
2. The hypocalcemic signs and symptoms are no longer present.
3. The client or caregiver understands the need for including calcium in the diet and has a list of major foods containing calcium; if needed, social service referral is made for financial or other assistance needed to maintain nutrition.
4. The client or caregiver understands the safety needs of the client with bone loss.
5. A home assessment has been made, or arrangements have been made for a home assessment through referral or by discussion with client or caregiver.

Hypercalcemia

Although there is individual variation, hypercalcemia is greater than the normal serum calcium concentration of 5.7 mEq/liter. It is associated with depression of nerve and muscle activity, including the cardiac muscle, leading to weakness and behavioral states, such as apathy, depression, changes in affect, drive, and coordination, which give the appearance of confusion to the observer. With high serum Ca^+ levels (over 15 mg/100 ml) acute psychosis may occur (Groer and Shekleton, 1979). Metastatic calcification (calcium deposition) in various body tissues tends to occur in the renal medulla, with internal hydronephrosis from hypercalcemic nephropathy. This favors formation of renal calculi (Groer and Shekleton, 1979). Glassy particles or conjunctival lesions that give a gritty sensation to the eye are another metastatic lesion. Extreme levels of serum calcium may create a crisis situation, with volume depletion and disturbances of acid-base balance. Death may occur in this state.

Hypercalcemia is associated with periods of immobility, when calcium leaves the bone and enters the extracellular fluid. Metastatic carcinoma, multiple myeloma, hyperthyroidism, and hypervitaminosis all lead to increased serum Ca^{++} (the ionized form that affects the nervous and muscular system).

Signs and symptoms of hypercalcemia are related to nerve and muscle inactivity and to an electrolyte imbalance. They include depression of nerve activity, with apathy and lethargy; change in affect, drive, and coordination, which gives the impression of confusion; decreased gastrointestinal activity, with anorexia, weight loss, nausea, constipation, and vomiting; skeletal muscle weakness; thirst; and polyuria. The serum Ca^+ level is over 5.8 mEq/liter.

Those elderly people who have prolonged immobilization (weight-bearing appears to affect normal retention of calcium in the bone); who have metastatic cancer or multiple myeloma; who have increased secretion of parathyroid hormone; who take excessive amounts of Vitamin D; or who have a high calcium diet, often exclusively milk, are prone to have hypercalcemia.

Fourth-level assessment for hypercalcemia

Fourth-level general assessment for hypoxia

plus:

History of dietary intake (large amounts of milk) with impaired renal function
Drug history, including excessive vitamin supplements
Medical diagnosis
Behavior: apathy, changes in affect and drive, and poor coordination
Gastrointestinal symptoms: anorexia, weight loss, and constipation
Skeletal muscle weakness: easy fatigability
Fluid intake and output: thirst and polyuria
Laboratory test results

Prevention includes the following:

1. Teach the client problems associated with excessive vitamin pill ingestion. The elderly person who depends on vitamins to supplement a poor diet can overdose with vitamin D. The administration of vitamins has been studied by the FDA as a matter for closer regulation. Until it is regulated, easy access to vitamins leads many older people to concentrate their preventive health measures in the magic of vitamin pillls. Education of the client and his family concerning the risks is important. Sunshine should be a part of the elderly person's life, but it should be taught to be used in moderation.

2. Promote mobilization. Mobilization is important to the fullest extent that is possible. Bed or wheelchair confinement may be needed at intervals, but these should not be prolonged a minute too long. As immobilization occurs, movement that requires use of skeletal muscles should be encouraged; a trapeze bar for moving in bed, side rails for turning, and pushing against a foot board may help to prevent demineralization of bone. Standing with support should be initiated as early as possible, if only for a few seconds.

3. Promote hydration for those prone to demineralization. When serum calcium exceeds normal, the excess is excreted by the kidneys. This requires large amounts of fluid to flush out the kidneys of the calcium. Without large amounts of fluid intake, dehydration of the body occurs as fluid is removed from the intravascular and interstitial compartments, leading to dehydration. There should be adequate fluid intake for any person who is immobilized.

4. Limit excessive calcium intake. The elderly person who lives on milk or other high-calcium foods and who takes antacids that contain absorbable calcium can precipitate a milk-alkali syndrome. The prevention requires an intimate knowledge of lifestyle and food habits. The older person in the home is particularly vulnerable, and prevention lies in a high index of suspicion and follow-up, with client and family education. The dairy industry has convinced us that milk is good for us, but its overconsumption and the underconsumption of other foods are not similarly stressed.

Intervention is based on the following nursing objectives:
1. Restore fluid volume and prevent renal calculi
2. Prevent fracture if hypercalcemia is from demineralization
3. Teach and plan for discharge

The renal effort to excrete excess calcium from the extracellular fluid results in polyuria and dehydration. Usually, there is sodium depletion from the polyuria, and saline and diuretics must be given to remove the Ca^+ excess. Three to 4 liters of fluid a day are required. Calcium precipitates out in alkaline urine, which is often excreted by the immobilized client or one with a kidney infection, and forms renal calculi. Foods promoting acidification of urine include cranberry juice, prune juice, and ascorbic acid. Urine should be maintained at an acid ph of 5 to 5.6. Urinary tract infection with urea-splitting organisms produces ammonia and increases urine alkalinity. Nursing measures to prevent urinary tract infection include adequate fluid intake, prevention of urine stasis in the bladder, frequent bladder emptying in the upright position, scrupulous asepsis during catheterization, and frequent perineal toilet.

Too often hypercalcemia results from bone demineralization, as in metastatic carcinoma. The brittle bones fracture easily when the client is moved. Turning must be done as often as with any immobilized client, but care will require more hands to prevent pathologic fractures, which often occur regardless of skill in giving care.

Client and family teaching is extremely important as a preventive measure. It is best done by example. The nurse who explains why fluids are being forced or why cranberry juice is given teaches indirectly. The mobilization of the client is a chance to emphasize the need for continued mobilization and how to accomplish it safely.

The place of milk in the diet should be part of the educational process, but the inadequacy of milk as a total diet should be discussed. It may lead to information about dental deficits, food economics, or insufficient strength to carry groceries and prepare meals. Often, distress from hiatal hernia leads to the use of milk and antacids for comfort. Such home remedies can lead to the milk-alkali syndrome. Prevention of recurrence may well be within the province of the nurse who does careful discharge planning and referral.

The nurse who visits the home can predict nutritional problems and has an opportunity to prevent a second occurrence of hypercalcemia, if the cause is not one of the disease states. The home should be assessed from the standpoint of safety measures to prevent fractures. The long-term care unit should have built-in features for safety, but the caregiver will need to be reminded of any special vulnerabilities of a particular client. In long-term care units the client cannot control his environment, so the caregiver must be conscious of such nursing care plan items as (1) continous assessment, (2) control over calcium intake, (3) mobilization to fullest extent of client's ability, (4) maintenance of an acidic urine, (5) adequate hydration, and (6) attention to nursing measures that prevent discomfort from hiatal hernia.

Outcome criteria of successful nursing intervention against hypercalcemia

1. The serum level of calcium has been reduced to normal levels by medical treatment.
2. The confusion secondary to the hypercalcemia is no longer present.
3. The client is adequately hydrated.
4. The client or his caregiver has reviewed with the nurse in discharge planning which factors in the environment or the client's life-style will contribute to further episodes, and planning has been made for prevention.
5. Safety measures have been discussed with the client or his caregiver regarding prevention of fractures.

Confusion secondary to body temperature imbalance

Body temperature is the amount of heat produced in the body through metabolism of food, exercise, shivering, and infection, minus the amount of heat loss produced through excretions, convection or loss of heat into the air, vaporization or evaporation, and conduction. Ordinarily, this heat production minus heat loss maintains a constant body temperature at or near 98.6°F (37°C). The narrow range of temperature is necessary for the adequate function of the nervous system and the action of enzymes.

Temperature regulation occurs in the hypothalamus, with production lowest during sleep and inactivity and highest with exercise of the skeletal muscles, especially with shivering. Myers (1970) suggests that the hypothalamus is dependent on a constant balance between sodium and calcium ions in the posterior hypothalamus to maintain temperature. Another theory is that the hypothalamus uses relative hypoxia as an indicator for heat conservation or production. Consciousness of cool, ambient air leads to the individual increasing protection from cold by more clothing and conserving the body heat by preventing its escape through convection or conduction.

This section deals with nursing care of the elderly client with confusion secondary to a problem in heat production or heat loss. Hyperthermia may result from producing more heat than can be lost, as in an infection, or an inability to lose heat by convection, as in a high ambient temperature. Hypothermia may be caused by a lack of heat production and by increased loss, as by inactivity or falling on a cold, drafty floor. The nursing action will depend on an accurate assessment of cause, resulting in efforts to increase or decrease heat production or heat loss. Hyperthermia is used instead of the usual term fever, and hypothermia is used to denote core temperature that is below normal.

Accidental hypothermia

Hypothermia may be intentional, as when it is used as a treatment or as an adjunct to treatment. The terms accidental, unintentional, or inadvertent hypothermia (Ozuna and Foster, 1979) describe the condition in which the core temperature (deep rectal) is below 95°F (35°C) (Green, 1975), which is not related to therapy. It is a condition usually found in the elderly or the extremely young (under 1 year), but it may occur at any age if there is prolonged exposure to cold. Accidental hypothermia has been recognized in the United States only recently but has been extensively studied in Great Britain, where the incidence is high (3.5% of patients over 65 admitted to the hospital in the United Kingdom in 1974 were hypothermic [Green 1975]). It is estimated that 10% of the British population over 65 are potential victims. No similar research has been done in the United States, but extrapolating these figures to the population of elderly in the United States would yield a figure of some 2 million (DHEW Pub. [NH] 78-1464). The human body needs to remain at or near 98.6°F (37°C) to continue functioning normally. The deep or core temperature is critical, for it governs the maintenance of normal cardiac, respiratory, cerebral, and renal function. Peripheral temperature may be cold—feet and hands may be quite cold, yet the deep body temperature remains normal; even the patient in shock may have a low peripheral temperature and maintain a normal core temperature.

Cold, wet weather tends to cool the body surface. Body heat is lost by radiation, conduction, convection, and evaporation. All of us have a thin capsule of air (air-skin or microclimate) around our bodies that is warmed by our own heat (radiation). In still air this persists and gives a feeling of warmth, especially if held in by clothing. However, a 5-mile-an-hour breeze will thin the quiet microclimate from 4 to 8 mm to 0.04 mm in thickness. At 22.5 miles per hour the microclimate or air-skin is reduced to 0.013 mm, or less than the width of a sheet of tissue. At an ambient temperature of 60°F (15.5°C), skin temperature will drop to 95°F (35°C) with no wind and to 72°F (22.2°C) when struck by a slight, 7-mile-an-hour breeze. Skin evaporation also increases with wind velocity, evaporating more internal water than the body can afford to lose. This is particularly important for older people, who may be thin and small with a large skin surface in proportion to body weight (Rosen, 1979).

Even mild ambient temperatures, such as 60° to 65°F (15.5° to 18.3°C), may contribute to hypothermia. However, there are risk factors that may determine who will be hypothermic in a certain temperature range and who will not. The greatest risk is to those who do not respond to cold normally (with shivering) and who cannot conserve their body warmth.

Clients with inability to respond to cold include elderly persons with vascular problems, such as diabetes or atherosclerosis; those whose thermal regulatory apparatus is disturbed by such drugs as phenothiazines, sedatives, hypotensives, and alcohol; those who do not generate heat, such as wheelchair and bedridden clients; and those with metabolic problems such as hypothyroidism. Hypoproteinemia was found to be a major cause in Uganda, where the mean low temperature is 60°F (15.5°C) and ambient temperature is not likely to be a cause (Sadikali and Owor, 1974). Irvine (1974) cites chronically ill persons with renal disease, anemia, arthritis, and malnutrition as those at risk. The most frequently given causes are falls and inability to get off the cold drafty floor, as with a stroke, a fractured hip, or Parkinson's syndrome.

Elderly clients may lose body heat during surgery from their inability to respond to cold because of such factors as muscle relaxants, narcotics, and sedatives; vasodilating drugs (narcotics), which increase heat loss; anesthetics, particularly halothane, which depress the heat-regulating system; spinal blocks, which cause vasodilatation below the level of the block with loss of heat by radiation; room-temperature parenteral fluids; and exposure of skin to cold cleansing solutions that cool by evaporation (Ozuma and Foster, 1979).

Abbey (1974) describes the typical posture of the cold, elderly client in a wheelchair—immobile and "hugging" himself to maintain body heat in the trunk (Fig. 9-1). This is hypothermia at the lower border of normal temperature; it is a normal state seen as apathy and listlessness, which can be relieved by raising the ambient temperature to 75° to 80°F (23.8° to 26.6°C). When the elderly clients were warmed, they became active and alert. At this marginal state, if the elderly person cannot respond with shivering, the first signs are confusion,

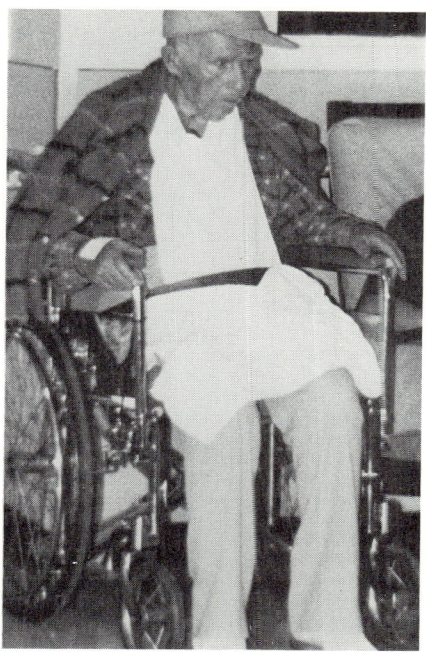

Fig. 9-1. The elderly, who may chill easily, take measures to protect themselves. This man, in August with the temperature at 80°F, wears three shirts, a knee covering, and a baseball cap to protect his bald head. (Photograph by C. D. Falk.)

disorientation, and apathy. Pinel (1975) is concerned because the caregiver may treat the confusion with phenothiazines, which contribute to a greater degree of hypothermia. At this marginal state and below, the skin becomes waxy and feels cool to the touch, including the skin of the abdomen, which is usually warm. Restlessness occurs with hypoxia, and there is a risk of falling. Slurred speech, muscular rigidity, bradycardia, and a slow, shallow respiratory rate are characteristic. Cardiac arrest may occur at core temperatures below 90°F (32°C).

Many older people will not slip to the critical stages that threaten life but will linger in the marginal state of confusion and disorientation. It is our experience that elderly clients tend to become apathetic, with-

Table 9-3. Signs and symptoms of progressive hypothermia: the seven stages of hypothermia*

Signs and symptoms	Temperature range
Shivering	95°-96.8°F (35°-36°C)
Confusion and disorientation	93.2°-95°F (34°-35°C)
Amnesia	91.4°-93.2°F (33°-34°C)

Cardiac arrhythmias
  Muscular rigidity
  Cardiac arrest
	91.4°F (33°C)

Semiconsciousness
  Dilated pupils
  No tendon reflexes
	86°-91.4°F (30°-33°C)

Ventricular fibrillation	82.4°F (28°C)
Irreversible coma Death	75.2°-82.4°F (24°-28°F)

*Adapted from Allen, E. T.: Prolonged immersion in cold water, Nurs. Times **70:**1928, 1974.

drawn, and confused at a higher core temperature than indicated in Table 9-3, which is based on a study of younger people (Allen, 1928).

Signs and symptoms have been discussed already, but the reader is referred to Table 9-3 for a more extensive and systematic coverage.

Fourth-level assessment for hypothermia

Vital signs (see Table 9-3 for signs and symptoms of hypothermia stages)
Blood pressure: for severe hypotension
Behavior (see signs and symptoms, Table 9-3)
History of drugs, chronic disease, and falls
Sleep patterns
Environment: ambient temperature and movement of air near floor
Appearance of prostration

The elderly people at risk have circulatory problems; take drugs that interfere with heat regulation, such as sedatives, phenothiazines, or vasodilators; have problems that interfere with vasoconstriction; or have the inability to recognize cold (abnormal temperature response). The elderly person who undergoes surgery is also vulnerable, as is the one with debilitating chronic disease or lack of mobility. Social problems, such as living alone with no one to detect falls or coldness, poorly heated housing, lack of bed covering, and lack of money to pay for heating costs place the individual at high risk. Others who have a high risk of falling and remaining on the floor without warmth include those with visual problems, insomnia, nocturia, incontinence, or who take bedtime hypnotics.

Prevention of hypothermia is everyone's job—a politicosocial problem in general and one for the caregiver in a direct sense.

The nurse making an assessment of the elderly person in his home should have a suspicious nature. The physical condition (vital signs), amount of clothing, drug regime, and ambient temperature should be assessed in relation to causes of hypothermia. If the client lives alone, frequency of visits by others or telephone reassurance programs should be noted. A health history as part of the assessment should include sleep patterns, nocturia, hypnotics and sedatives taken at night, night lighting, drug profile (with time of day for dosage) and, finally, ingestion of alcohol. The occurrence of postural hypotension and any evidence of circulatory disorders should also be noted.

Medication review often reveals that the high-risk client is taking drugs that lead to impaired thermoregulation. The physician as gatekeeper to prescriptions has the responsibility to evaluate carefully the role of his prescriptions in accentuating conditions that lead to hypothermia.

Intervention is based on the following nursing objectives:
1. Restore the body warmth
2. Provide safety with careful monitoring

The treatment of confusion secondary to hypothermia is the treatment of the hypothermia. Depending on the stage of the hypothermia, the client can be treated at home or moved to a hospital as an emergency. The client at home with a core temperature of 93.2° to 95°F (34° to 35°C), without a drop in blood pressure and with a pulse that is not irregular or in bradycardia, can be restored to warmth by such nursing measures as raising the ambient temperature to 80°F (26.6°C), conserving body temperature by preventing convection (with adequate covering), and, if the client is responsive, oral intake of warm fluids. The body temperature should not be raised more than 1°F (0.6°C) an hour. If the warming occurs at a more rapid rate or if the blood pressure is unstable, the room temperature should be gradually dropped a few degrees. Rapid rewarming causes vasodilatation, which will lead to hypotension that could be fatal. It also forces the cold blood from the periphery to the body core, worsening the hypothermia. The client must be under the supervision of a physician who understands hypothermia as a stress.

Nurses visited a former school teacher who was dying of cancer in her apartment. She was fiercely independent and asked only that Meals-on-Wheels bring the small amount of food she was able to eat; that she get a decent night's sleep; and that a nurse check her daily. When making her bed, the nurse noted the one thin blanket and asked if she was warm at night. The client cried as she admitted her cold nights. That night she had extra warm blankets on her bed.

That everyone has warm shelter, warm clothing, and a warm bed is too often taken for granted. Socioeconomic reasons may prevent the elderly person from self-protection against the cold. It may be necessary to refer to community agencies to change the environment.

The nurse in the acute-care hospital surgical department should be aware that the elderly client is approaching an experience potentially dangerous for hypothermia. Ozuma (1979) found that of the 10 patients she studied, all experienced a greater fall in oral temperature before the surgical incision was made than during the operation. Medications had depressed the heat regulating system, the sedated patient could not ask for more warmth, and the trip through drafty halls to surgery reduced the microclimate around the client and led to loss of body heat by convection. Finally, the cold solutions the skin was prepared with led to heat loss by evaporation. Prevention should include warm blankets, a head cover for the trip through the halls to surgery, and warmed solutions for preparing the skin. Following surgery, the patient's temperature should be watched as closely as his blood pressure. The recovery room nurse should be aware of the elderly person's heat loss. Ozuma (1979) found that it was not unusual for patients with spinal blocks to have a temperature of 94°F (34.5°C) on admission to the recovery room because of vasodilatation of the blood vessels below the block.

McLean and others (1974) studied 70 patients, aged 28 to 97 with a mean average age of 70.4 (but including six over 90), with rectal temperatures from 72°F (22.2°C) to 95°F (35°C). They were allowed to rewarm spontaneously under medical and nursing supervision. There was no correlation between age, rewarming, and severity and duration of the hypothermia. Thirty-two (45.7%) of the 70 patients died, most on the first day of admission but a few between 2 to 5 days and one on day 28. Of the six who were 90 or over, one died and five recovered, including a 97-year-old.

The study leads to the conclusion that the aged client can suffer severe hypothermia and still recover if given good care. However, once he has recovered, he is no longer a high-risk client but a known hypothermia victim, and his life must be built around the need to maintain normal core temperature.

Excessive handling and energetic resuscitation can lead to shock or cardiac arrest. Unless the client's condition improves as indicated, with very gradual warming, he should be hospitalized as an emergency.

Metabolic functions in hypothermia are reduced, the liver does not function normally, insulin is inactive at a low body temperature but may become active on rewarming, and the client will require dextrose intravenously, but only at replacement levels. Oxygen can be given to avoid carbon dioxide retention. With the rewarming, hyperventilation may occur, which can reduce the amount of carbon dioxide in the blood to below normal levels, possibly depressing the respiration rate (Pinel, 1975).

Aspiration of vomitus is a common complication. Endotracheal intubation and gastric lavage can be helpful if the temperature is not too low, but with very low temperatures (90°F, or 32.2°C) there is a danger of cardiac dysrhythmias with intubation.

The ordinary glass clinical thermometer is not calibrated below 95°F (35°C) and is often at 96.0°F (35.5°C). English thermometers are calibrated to a lower temperature, and such thermometers would be produced in the United States if there were a demand. The need is obvious. Methods of taking the temperature are not standardized. Oral and axillary temperatures are useless for this kind of measurement, and only the deep rectal temperature is dependable. The British measure the temperature of freshly voided urine as an exact measurement. This assumes that the client is able to cooperate, which is not always true.

The highest-risk personnel are those who unwittingly or unknowingly subject the older person to conditions that cause hypothermia. The physician who prescribes drugs should be reminded of the potential consequences of drugs for hypothermia. The nurse who enters the home or who is responsible for the elderly person in an institution must be aware of the potential hazards in inadequate clothing or bedding and a low thermostat reading. The surgical nurse who does not appreciate the surgical experience as a heat-losing event is an accomplice to hypothermia. The political system, which does not generally afford income maintenance to pay utility bills, also contributes to hypothermia in the elderly. (An extra energy-bill payment was made to certain elderly people during the winter of 1980.)

The gravest risk for the elderly person is exposure to cold. Poor housing, lack of heat, lack of clothing, outdoor toilets, all are hazards for the elderly.

Outcome criteria of successful nursing intervention against hypothermia

1. The client is no longer confused secondary to hypothermia.
2. The client has been rewarmed to a normal body temperature.
3. There are no complications from pressure or excessive handling.
4. The physiologic status is stable.
5. Contributing environmental factors have been discussed in the plan for prevention of further episodes.

Hyperthermia

There is no clear-cut definition of hyperthermia for the elderly. Normal temperatures seem to differ for various people, but for the purposes of this discussion, hyperthermia will be considered as a core temperature of 100°F (37.7°C) or over.

Hyperthermia in the elderly comes from two principal sources: (1) reaction of the body's immune system to infection, and (2) ambient temperatures above the body's own temperature, whereby the loss of heat by convection becomes impossible. Further, among the elderly, the loss of many sweat glands deprives the body of evaporative cooling.

Signs and symptoms differ with the degree of fever. With the onset of a temperature of 100°F (37.7°C), the individual shows premonitory symptoms of apathy, weakness, faintness, and headache. With further elevation of core temperature, tachycardia is observed, with weakness, dry mouth, and increased respiration. There is a clouded sensorium, with shortened attention span, inability to focus on an idea, forgetfulness of events in the immediate time/space, and an inability to note the full extent of the happenings in the immediate environment. Often there is irritability. These symptoms are usually related to confusion. With higher elevations of temperature, sounds or visual objects are turned into hallucinations, for example, a motor buzzing may be heard as a bomber flying through the room.

Fourth-level assessment for hyperthermia

Mental status
Vital signs
Hydration
History of exposure to high temperatures or evidence of infection
Chest sounds and cough
Abdominal tenderness
Signs and symptoms of lower urinary tract infection

The high-risk elderly who may have hyperthermia are those with an infection, often of the lower urinary tract. Jaffe (1971) divides urinary tract infections into two categories: the dramatic ones, with hematuria, fever, and acute retention; and the silent, insidious ones. The elderly who have circulatory problems (diabetes or atherosclerosis), in which the protective mechanism of vasodilatation does not respond to high ambient temperatures; who are in a high ambient temperature where the body cannot lose heat by convection; or are dehydrated are also at high risk.

Prevention of hyperthermia requires the following:
1. Act to prevent infection. Any intubation carries a risk of infection, particularly the urinary catheter, and risk is related to length of time in the bladder. Adequate fluids for maintaining urinary output are important if an indwelling catheter is necessary.
2. Teach client or caregiver to protect body from high ambient temperatures by avoiding direct sunlight in summer, wearing light clothing, using fans, drinking cool drinks, eating a light diet, having adequate rest and sleep, and reducing physical activity.

Intervention is based on the following nursing objectives:
1. Reduce temperature
2. Observe source of temperature
3. Give support for experiences during hyperthermic events

Nursing the elderly client involves a titration of care. Slight hyperthermia may yield to cool drinks (iced water is not recommended unless the client specifically asks for it). Lightweight clothing should be held to the minimum that meets the client's modesty needs. If the elderly person is in bed, the bed linen should be very light. Tepid sponging of the face and hands will make the client more comfortable. Activity should be reduced. Cooler ambient temperature and movement of air are needed.

If the core temperature is elevated over 103°F (39.4°C), body cooling should be assisted by such measures as cold packs to the head or back of the neck. Sponging with alcohol can be done with tepid water containing half alcohol for rapid evaporation. One body part is sponged with the alcohol-tepid water solution and allowed to air-dry. The client's face should be protected from the alcohol fumes and should not be washed with the alcohol solution. Before attempting to reduce the hyperthermia, the vital signs should be carefully checked, and rechecked often during the alcohol sponge to ensure that no rapid change occurs in the blood pressure or pulse. If the client starts to shiver, the cooling process is stopped, because shivering will raise the temperature back to its previous level. Hydration should be reestablished as tolerated by the client. Aspirin is given cautiously if the client is taking anticoagulants. The decreased number of sweat glands found in the elderly reduce the effectiveness of evaporation.

If the ambient temperature is not over

80°F (26.6°C), infection should be suspected, and observation for signs of urinary tract infection should be made. A urine specimen should be examined as soon as possible for pyuria and concentration, while the voiding pattern is observed for changes toward frequent small amounts, often with a distinct odor. The chest should be examined for signs of pulmonary consolidation. The signs and symptoms should be reported to the physician for specific therapy.

With reduction of temperature to normal, the client usually is able to tell of the bizarre events and thoughts he had during the hyperthermic period. The nurse listens carefully, and helps to bring about an understanding of the hallucinations or delusions occurring with fever. Unless the client explores the experience with someone, he may tell himself that he is on the verge of insanity. The association of the visual and auditory events, which do not make sense, to his fever, which does make sense, helps the elderly client find meaning and comfort in what may be a frightening experience.

Outcome criteria of successful nursing intervention against hyperthermia

1. The client is no longer hyperthermic or confused.
2. The contributing factor has been corrected, ambient temperature cooled, and infection treated.
3. The client or caregiver knows the contributing factors and can discuss recognition of them.

Confusion secondary to renal failure (uremia, azotemia, and uremic encephalopathy)

Brocklehurst (1971) finds that renal failure is a common terminal phenomenon in older people. Renal failure means the kidneys are unable to excrete the normal load of metabolites produced in the body. For the elderly client, the metabolites include those drugs given to treat many of his multiple disorders. This results in longer half-life for many drugs and an accumulation of their effect in the body. It also means azotemia, which is an increase of the end products of protein metabolism in the blood, namely urea, creatinine, and uric acid. Azotemia is the chief biochemical sign of uremia (Roberts, 1976). The encephalopathy which results may be based on several mechanisms, the most important being the acidosis and the possibility of water intoxication as the urea in the brain sets up an osmotic gradient. As urea is pulled out of the brain area with treatment, the neurologic symptoms subside. With terminal illness the treatment may not be successful.

The changes of aging include the decreased functional capacity of the kidneys; the glomerular filtration rate falls from 140 ml per minute per 1.73 sq m of body surface at age 21 to approximately 97 ml at age 80 (Rockstein and Sussman, 1979). Diseases such as pyelonephritis or other kidney infections further reduce the kidney function through chronic disease. Kidney infection is one of the most frequent infections for which elderly people are hospitalized.

Fourth-level assessment for uremia

History of earlier kidney disease
Laboratory test results
Edema
Behavior—mental status
Urinary output

Signs and symptoms of uremia are the result of altered fluid and electrolyte balance. The mental state is seen as confused because of lethargy, shortened attention span, inappropiate behavior, irritability, depressions, and overtly psychotic behavior. There are complaints of headache, weight loss, anorexia, shortness of breath (fluid in the chest), pitting edema, hypertension, numbness of feet and legs, muscle twitching, and itching. The urinary volume may be increased or decreased; there may be bleeding from any mucosa; and laboratory tests will indicate azotemia and electrolyte imbalance.

Prevention of uremia in the elderly of today presents problems. Since uremia is an end point of many years of kidney infections, prevention may be impossible. The 65-year-old person of 1980 lived nearly 25 years before the sulfonamides were available to treat streptococcal infections and another 5 years before penicillin was available. Many had scarlet fever and other streptococcal infections including glomerulonephritis in their early years. Prevention of the present generations from future uremias may be underway, but the kidneys of those mentioned carry lasting scars. The use of intrusive measures such as catheterization may introduce infection in the elderly who are hospitalized for unrelated illness, for example, "prophylactic retention catheters" for the client with hip fracture.

The elderly man with prostate problems is especially vulnerable, but any elderly person who is immobile or on bed rest has a likelihood of developing kidney infections. Fluids and asepsis are very important, especially since the hospital environment contains the potential for nosocomial infections.

Intervention is based on the following nursing objectives:
1. Restore fluid and electrolyte balance
2. Monitor and observe response to treatment and care
3. Give supportive care
4. Teach and prepare the client and his family for discharge or a peaceful death

Care of the elderly person with chronic uremia is focused on restoration of the fluid and electrolyte balance. Edema, which is present in many cases, may be caused by sodium and water retention, congestive heart failure, or decrease in serum protein (Roberts, 1976). This is a grave medical problem that will require careful treatment, much of which is delegated to the nurse. The use of renal dialysis for the elderly with terminal uremia is seldom considered. Therefore, the nurse's goals are directed toward providing as stable an internal environment as possible through control of fluids and nutrition. The client is frequently uncomfortable, with headache and pruritus. He has a potential for increased physical injury with his blurred vision, lack of mental alertness, and inability to maintain normal sleep and rest patterns. If fluids are restricted, the mouth must have special care, for ulceration is a possibility and infecton with *Candida albicans* is frequent. Administered fluids are assessed in relation to the client's serum potassium levels, which may be high. Ice, crushed from measured cubes for estimating intake, may be the most comforting fluid, especially if the mouth is sore.

Monitoring and observing response to treatment of the client with uremia requires constant vigilance and a background of up-to-date pharmacology. Medications should be prescribed and administered with caution to the elderly person with uremia, but the likelihood of digitalis preparations, antihypertensives, antibotics, and antacids being ordered is almost inevitable. Toxic effects develop rapidly, for excretion by the kidney is impaired. Digoxin is particularly dangerous because of the client's inability to excrete potassium and the possibility of dangerously high levels of serum potassium. Anemia accompanies the chronic uremic state, but treatment for anemia (iron and folate) is rarely tolerated by the client.

Nursing care must be planned to save the client's energy and to provide rest periods. Discomfort from pruritus can be controlled somewhat by reducing levels of serum phosphorus with an aluminum hydroxide antacid, keeping the skin moist and supple, reducing room temperature, and avoiding emotional tension. Foods and fluids are rarely enjoyed by the client whose mouth is often sore. Mouth care is very important, and foods should be served as attractively as possible. Food or fruit juice should not be left in the room if not eaten but preserved to maintain freshness. This means very small servings are offered frequently.

The family should be given attention and teaching. The reduced accuracy with which the uremic client views his environment make his judgments questionable. If the client goes to his home, his family should have a fair picture of the future and access to frequent nursing consultation. Warnings concerning use of over-the-counter drugs that contain sodium will have to be given. And they must be prepared for the physical changes that will take place: sickly appearance, weakness, and lack of color.

The outcome for the elderly client with uremia may well be death. If this is the way to his death, then the nurse has an opportunity to assist the client and his family in making preparation for this event.

Outcome criteria of successful nursing intervention against uremia

1. The client or caregiver understands and can explain the measurement of intake and output and the observation of edema.
2. He can describe the comfort measures used to ease mouth infection, pruritus, and insomnia.
3. He understands preventive measures for mouth infection.
4. He knows the name, dosage, frequency, purpose, and side effects of medications.
5. He can describe the foods that should be eliminated from the diet and is able to plan for more suitable foods.
6. He participates in a plan for follow-up care (adapted from Miller, 1979, p. 1333).
7. If death occurs, the client and his family are supported emotionally and physically through the dying process.

SUGGESTIONS FOR FURTHER READING

Miller, P. L.: Problems of the urinary system. In Phipps, W. J., Long, B. C., and Woods, N. F., editors: Medical-surgical nursing: concepts and clinical practice, St. Louis, 1979, The C. V. Mosby Co.

Roberts, S. L.: Renal abnormalities. In Burnside, I. editor: Nursing and the aged, ed. 2, New York, 1980, McGraw-Hill Book Co.

CONFUSION SECONDARY TO HYPOXEMIC HYPOXIA (VENTILATORY PROBLEMS)

Hypoxemic hypoxia refers to the condition in which the total amount of oxygen in the blood is inadequate. It is a ventilation problem based on blood/gas exchange at the alveolar level where the oxygen content of the blood is renewed. The aging process affects the ventilatory system, but in today's industrial society it is difficult to know what ventilatory decrements are from aging and which are from exposure to pulmonary insults, such as smoke, fumes, dust, and industrial air pollution (black lung disease of miners and brown lung disease of the textile workers). In addition, there are the infections that few older persons have escaped in life. The result is a reduced reserve capacity for dealing with stress and added demands for oxygen.

There are ventilatory problems associated with normal aging. Age-related anatomic changes include kyphosis, or forward curvature of the spine resulting from the loss of cushioning cartilage between the vertebral bodies, especially in the thoracic area, and demineralization or thinning of the bone. Compression fractures of the vertebral bodies add to the deformity, which results in a pushing forward of the neck and shoulders, a shortening of the vertical dimension of the chest, and a general trunk shortening that forces the viscera against the diaphragm. This limits the excursion of the diaphragm and decreases lung expansion in the lower chest. It also limits the ability to cough effectively or to breathe deeply.

The cartilage that connects the rib cage with the sternum calcifies and stiffens with age, and chest expansion is decreased with the diminution of the intercostal muscles. The lung has less room for expansion as well.

The lung shows many changes with time. Calcification of the cartilage in the trachea and bronchi causes rigidity. The bronchioles are less distensible, and with the more rigid rib cage, the decrease in breathing capacity is from 60% at age 55 to 25% at age 85. Epithelial cells atrophy or degenerate with normal aging, a process accelerated by air pollution. There may be increased viscous mucus that is more difficult to raise, particularly since coughing is less effective. The lungs decrease in weight and their color changes from pink to charcoal gray as carbon particles from the air collect on the surface. The walls of the air sacs (alveoli) show destruction, decreasing the functional respiratory surface of the lung by about 2.9 feet (0.27 sq m) from young adulthood to old age (Klocke, 1977). Capillaries supplying lungs undergo the same degenerative changes that occur in other organs of the body.

The decreased chest cavity and distensibility of the bronchioles and alveoli cause a decreased vital capacity. The maximum breathing capacity or amount of air that a person can exchange with the outside air falls from about 165 liters per minute at age 25 to less than 75 liters per minute at 85 (Rockstein and Sussman, 1979). Respiratory rate and tidal volume change little throughout life, but with a larger dead space, less of the air taken in is used effectively in aging since the tidal air is in contact with a less functional alveolar surface. The efficiency of gas exchange is also diminished.

Environmental factors such as air pollution and infections result in such pulmonary diseases as emphysema, bronchiectasis, and chronic bronchial disease. Tuberculosis in our time is age-related, because the person who reaches age 65 in 1980 was 30 before the age of specific drug therapy for tuberculosis was discovered. It was a common disease then, and the person may well have been exposed.

Signs and symptoms of hypoxemic hypoxia include all the signs of hypoxia found in the preceding sections (note especially the general signs of hypoxia in the introduction to part I). The principal difference is the effort in breathing: the use of the accessory muscles, extreme dyspnea with very little exertion, production of thick, heavy sputum, and the mental symptoms leading to the label confused, with indifference to surroundings, distractibility, and total attention focused on breathing.

Fourth-level assessment for hypoxemic hypoxia

Vital signs—describe the breathing process as to rate, chest movement, sounds, effort, distress, and position
History of respiratory disease or a medical diagnosis of respiratory disease
Cough—depth and production of sputum
Medication profile
Life-style
General appearance—is life built around process of breathing?
Abdominal versus chest breathing, especially with use of the accessory muscles
Mental status

Those elderly with diminished gas exchange are those who have obstructive lung disease or emphysema, chest infections, or an accumulation of secretions, as found in postsurgical patients with a depressed cough reflex, prior anticholinergic drug therapy or with upper abdominal incisions or abdominal distention. Also at risk are those elderly with restrictive disorders that reduce the size of the intrathoracic space, such as kyphosis or scoliosis, neuromuscular disease of the chest wall, such as Guillain-Barré syndrome and stroke, or chest pain causing splinting, as from pleurisy. Abdominal distention from gas or fluid (cirrhosis or ascites) or from obesity limits chest excursions, especially with a person in a recumbent position. Any person who must be immobilized in a recumbent position is at risk over time. Others at risk include those who change altitude too rapidly, who have worked in industries with air pollution, such as mines, cotton mills, agriculture, and asbestos mining and manufacture, or who have smoked tobacco over years.

Prevention begins now for everyone; but for the elderly, the damage is long-standing, and prevention is not retroactive.

The aging process leads to an impaired respiratory apparatus; therefore, the goal of prevention is directed toward decreasing the possibility of additional stresses or demands on the system. Sudden physical or emotional change is the most important factor to avoid. The main objectives are maintenance of adequate cardiac function, good nutrition, balance of exercise and rest, and freedom from air pollutants. Exercise that promotes deep breathing to avoid dead air space at the base of the lungs, laughter (belly laughs involve deep breathing), avoidance of the supine position when ill, and avoidance of smoking (either one's own or that of others), contribute to good hygiene of the lung.

When the older client is admitted to a general hospital, the nursing care plan must include measures to prevent accumulation of secretions: deep breathing, coughing unless contraindicated, as by eye surgery, and frequent change of position, with chair rest preferred and bed rest an alternative. When blood gas values are available, the nurse must be aware of them. Prevention is the key to intervention.

Intervention is based on the following objectives:
1. Prevent hypoventilation
2. Assist in removal of secretions
3. Assist the client to live within his limitations

Preventing hypoventilation demands a recognition of the factors causing it. Any condition that prevents the free interchange of gases across the alveolar membrane is a threat. Some measures under the nurse's control are the teaching of deep breathing, positioning the client, helping him to his feet and assisting him to walk, and encouraging his voluntary effort to cough up secretions. The use of analgesics for pain is important. No one will cough if it hurts too much; the pain relief must do just that, while not depressing the cough reflex. Adequate hydration to thin the viscous secretions, allowing them to be brought up with a cough, is important.

Deep breathing must be taught to the elderly, who may not have consciously or unconsciously made the effort for some time. A deep sigh or a yawn is as effective and often is easier to achieve. Conscious deep breathing is almost invariably followed by a cough. It is the cough that forces secretions out, while the forced inspiration helps to prevent atelectasis.

Coughing may have to be taught to the surgical patient who has an upper abdominal incision. It is necessary for him to take a deep breath and hold it. He should use the diaphragm and the contracted abdominal muscles to forcibly push the air against a closed glottis. An elderly person with an abdominal incision will need splinting, with a pillow held firmly over the area when he coughs or the nurse's hands supporting the abdomen to reduce pain or discomfort.

Position is conducive to easier breathing. The sitting position, in which the client bends forward at the hips and rests his arms on an over-the-bed table, usually offers a larger intrathoracic space than a semi-Fowler's position. Many people with ventilatory problems prefer to sit by their bed and rest their arms on the bed, which gives a longer length to the posterior chest.

Assisting with the removal of secretions has been discussed under prevention; adequate hydration, easing pain, and promotion of deep breathing and coughing are the principal means available. However, mechanical means may have to be used, and the nurse must be prepared to aspirate or to care for a tracheostomy, with removal of secretions by a catheter with suction if necessary.

Assisting the client to live within his limitations requires ingenuity. Most older people with breathing difficulties have long since learned how to compensate for their disabilities if they are given the resources. The older person must be assessed within his customary environment to determine what his limitations are and what conditions tax his respiratory capacities. What are the activities of daily living that must be surrendered to another person? To whom can they be given? The answers are highly individualized and require on-the-spot assessment, a knowledge of community and family resources, and finally, an imagination that puts known factors together in new combinations.

Outcome criteria of successful nursing intervention against hypoxemic hypoxia

1. The client is no longer confused secondary to hypoxia.
2. The client or his caregiver has been taught and can discuss preventive measures for hypoventilation.
3. The residential environment and lifestyle have been reviewed or discussed with the client or caregiver and modifications planned to prevent the stressors resulting in hypoventilation.
4. The client shows improvement on the basis of specific criteria that evaluate postoperative respiratory status developed by Johnson (1975, p. 1474-1475):
   a. Temperature within normal limits
   b. Lungs clear or clearing in regard to rales, rhonchi, or decreased breath sounds that indicated atelectasis
   c. Productive cough
   d. Respiratory rate below 30 and lower lobes expanding with deep breathing, or normal breathing pattern resumed

---

SUGGESTIONS FOR FURTHER READING

Rokosky, J. S.: Respiratory status. In Mitchell, P. H., editor: Concepts basic to nursing, ed. 2, New York, 1977, McGraw-Hill Book Co.

Phipps, W. J., and Daly, B. J.: Problems of the lower airway. In Phipps, W. J., Long, B. C., and Woods, N. F.: Medical-surgical nursing: concepts and clinical practice, St. Louis, 1979, The C. V. Mosby Co.

Phipps, W. J., Long, B. C., and Woods, N. F., editors: Medical-surgical nursing: concepts and clinical practice; Unit VII, Gas transport problems, St. Louis, 1979, The C. V. Mosby Co.

CONFUSION SECONDARY TO STAGNANT (ISCHEMIC) HYPOXIA (POOR PERFUSION OF BRAIN CELLS)

Although the ventilatory apparatus is satisfactory and there is no anemia, hypoxia may occur as a result of poor perfusion of the brain cells due to failure of the circulatory system. This section is divided into the care of the patient with cardiac failure and hypotension, and because it does affect the circulatory system, hypothyroidism is included in this area, although this placement can justly be questioned. In addition, perfusion may be hindered by increased intracranial pressure, and by normal pressure hydrocephalus. The hypoxia resulting from mechanical failure of the perfusion system is often first noted by the symptom of disordered mentation: confusion and lack of memory are the clinical signs. Treatment of the hypoxia is dependent on treatment of the underlying cause.

Cardiac failure

Cardiac output is basic to the subject of perfusion. Cardiac output decreases linearly from about 5.0 liters per minute at age 20 to 3.5 liters per minute at age 75 because of the reduction in stroke volume and decrease in heart rate. Heart rate decreases from the 140 beats per minute at birth to 70 in the young adult. In the older male it varies from 60 to 84. Characteristic EKG changes indicate conduction system alterations with age, and anatomists find many changes in the aging heart (Rockstein and Sussman, 1979). Clinically, this is noted as reduced reserve to meet added body requirements because of stress. Valvular disease, ischemic heart disease, and coronary thromboses are factors that reduce the cardiac reserve of the elderly person. The generation reaching age 65 were in their 20s when the sulfa drugs were first used against streptococcal disease, and they were in their 30s when penicillin became available for rheumatic fever. Therefore, these elderly people were exposed to the streptococcal infections that caused heart damage, which greatly reduces pumping capacity of the heart in later years.

Cardiac failure, or the inability of the heart to perfuse the body at a level at which it can function effectively, is found in older people who have no previous history of disease. The problem seems to be myocardial failure related to normal aging alone. Studies of admissions to geriatric units find congestive heart failure as the diagnosis in 14% of the elderly. Caird and Dall (1973) estimated that 40% of the elderly living at home had definite evidence of heart disease, and of those age 75 or over, 50% were affected.

Harris (1970) found normal EKGs in 26% of the residents of an old-age home who were over the age of 75 and 29.3% normal EKGs in the group who were 60 to 69. This gives an indication of the overwhelming number of institutionalized elderly who have cardiac problems. Rodstein (1971) finds that history is often unreliable, because cardiac failure and drug toxicity exacerbate the confusion, agitation, and depression. He believes pulmonary symptoms such as wheezing, coughs, and dyspnea may result from cardiac failure. Insomnia and nocturnal wandering may be caused by heart failure and diuretic-induced nocturia.

The diagnosis may be difficult for the medical practitioner to make, because the symptoms overlap those of many other conditions. Many older clients may have anemia or vitamin deficiency, which can be mistaken for congestive heart failure.

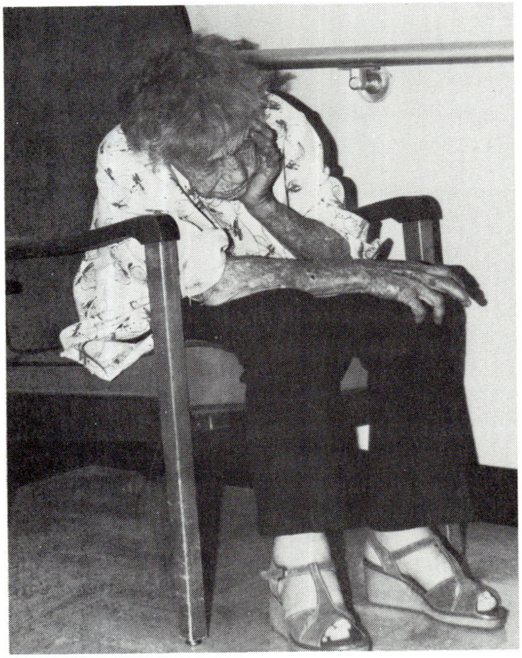

Fig. 9-2. The elderly patient with congestive heart failure can be exhausted easily. Note edematous feet. (Photograph by C. D. Falk.)

Fourth-level assessment for cardiac failure

Vital signs, with descriptions of findings
Signs of right-sided failure and fluid retention:
  engorged neck veins (test in sitting position at 30 to 45 degree angle; veins should be collapsed above suprasternal notch)
  engorged veins on dorsum of hand when held below the level of the heart (note whether veins collapse when hand is raised to level of sternal notch)
Ascites or pitting edema of dependent body areas
Dyspnea on exertion; talking, walking, moving in bed
Cough—character and sputum raised, chest rales, and position; frothy sputum with left-sided failure (orthopnea or cough when lying down)
Weight gain (fluid retention)
Oliguria
Behavior—restlessness, agitation, confusion
Drug profile—digitalis preparations and diuretics

Signs and symptoms of cardiac failure include confusion, disorientation, agitation, and restlessness, on the basis of the hypoxia; dyspnea on exertion, or even talking in severe cases of left-sided failure with fluid in the alveoli; a persistent and hacking cough, with mucoid expectoration; edema of the dependent parts and abdominal ascites; weakness and fatigue (Fig. 9-2); orthopnea; basal pulmonary rales; liver engorgement with tenderness in right-sided failure; and distended neck veins, also found in right-sided failure.

Prevention should focus on minimizing physical and mental stress, with the assumption that all elderly people have lost some or much of their cardiac reserve and with these objectives:
1. Conserve cardiac strength
2. Restore oxygen to cells and tissues
3. Reduce accumulated fluid
4. Teach and plan discharge for prevention of further episodes

The elderly person with no cardiac reserve uses the strength of the nurse to supplement his own. Chair or bed rest is prescribed. Chair rest is best for the orthopneic patient and produces less confusion than a bed with side rails. The arms must be supported so no weight hangs from the shoulder, and the position must be altered often to prevent pitting edema over the dependent areas (feet and buttocks can break down if pressure is exerted too long). Elevating the feet can be very tiring. Personal hygiene is important and must be planned to prevent overexertion. Needs of the patient should be anticipated and met to reduce the agitation that can arise from worrying about being cared for. Sedatives may be needed.

Therapeutic self-care cannot be achieved by the sick patient and will require assistance from the nurse. Administration of digitalis preparations is usually necessary, often initiating the therapeutic plan. The nurse must know the difference between digitalization and the maintenance plan, (part III of this chapter). Accurate observation of vital signs is important while digitalization is being achieved.

The elderly person who is hospitalized for the first time may not understand the use of oxygen. Whatever form of equipment is used, the procedure should be quietly and efficiently performed after a simple explanation. The confused patient will often react to the process of putting equipment together, and the nurse should expect to remain with the patient until the oxygen has relieved the hypoxia and the confusion. The anxiety caused by the process of being attached to a strange apparatus can undo the value of the oxygen itself. The response to the oxygen should be noted in relation to vital signs, restlessness, and confusion.

Oxygen need is frightening to the patient, and often some form of sedation is given to allay some of the anxiety. If drugs are used, the effect on the respiratory center must be considered so that minimal doses are given: enough to achieve the objective of decreasing anxiety, without depressing respiration.

The fluid accumulates in the tissues, then in the abdominal cavity and the chest. The body weight, as it changes from day to day, and the measurement of the abdominal girth are two signs of increased fluid accumulation. Finally, the chest rales and cough indicate the level at which hypoxia becomes crucial.

Fluid reduction is usually accomplished by powerful diuretics. The patient's response must be carefully monitored to prevent electrolyte imbalance. Elderly individuals do not handle rapid change well; rapid diuresis may cause hypotension. Salt retention is minimized by a low-salt diet. Frequently, the elderly patient with congestive failure refuses food and asks only that his mouth be kept wet with ice chips. The mouth must be cleaned thoroughly and often during the period when food and fluid intake are minimal. Output is carefully measured and balanced against the fluid ingested. Body weight is the best indicator of reduction in fluid.

The elderly patient who has one episode

of congestive heart failure will be a candidate for more unless a careful rearrangement of his life-style is followed. He will need to be under medical supervision, which will supplement his own living habits. Rest and activity patterns should be studied; energy requirements of the living situation may have to be altered to meet energy tolerances. Dietary intake should be assessed for adequacy of vitamin, protein, and caloric intake and for salt restriction. The situation should be studied to determine if the diet prescription is realistic in terms of financial, social, and energy requirements. Referral may be needed. The patient will need to understand the uses of his medications and the the signs and symptoms that warn of toxicity. He should be visited in his living quarters to determine adaptation.

Outcome criteria of successful nursing intervention against cardiac failure

1. The patient is recovered from the acute episode without problems from immobilization.
2. The patient is no longer confused.
3. The patient or his caregiver recognizes the signs of fluid retention and dyspnea and relates them to heart disease.
4. The patient or his caregiver has assessed the life-style and residence and determined what areas have to be altered to prevent further occurrences.
5. The patient or his caregiver knows the signs of digitalis toxicity.
6. The patient or his caregiver has a plan for taking action on the early warning signals of congestive heart failure.

This subsection has not included many cardiac problems, such as the patient with cardiac arrhythmias, a pacemaker, and many more that are important. These will be found in any good medical nursing textbook, and we recommend staying abreast of this area through nursing periodicals such as the *American Journal of Nursing, Nursing,* and *Nursing Clinics of North America.*

SUGGESTION FOR FURTHER READING

Roberts, S. L.: Cardiopulmonary abnormalities. In Burnside, I., editor: Nursing and the aged, New York, 1980, McGraw-Hill Book Co.

Hypotension (hypoperfusion of the brain; cerebral insufficiency)

Perfusing the brain with blood and transporting oxygen to the brain cells is dependent on adequate heart pump action and a vascular system capable of maintaining blood pressure necessary to perfuse distant tissues (Daly and Norman, 1979). Changes in behavior may be one of the early signs of hypotension or hypoperfusion. This includes the sudden loss of strength and changes in sensorium, which are most marked when hypoperfusion is present.

The causes are many, as indicated in the list of those persons who are high risk. The underlying mechanisms are the same—a failure of cardiac output from such diverse causes as cardiac disease, compromised vasculature (atherosclerosis), postural changes with inadequate baroceptor sensitivity, and overvigorous use of drugs and drug interaction with alcohol. Bed rest or immobilization is instrumental in hypotension, as learned in the experiments and actual experiences of the astronauts. Any process that leads to extensive peripheral dilatation, for example, vasodilators or hot baths, may lead to hypotension. The vast amount of publicity given hypertension may distract the nurse from realizing the very old are often not hypertensive, else they may not have survived to old age. The many occurrences in the elderly client's life that can cause hypotension, either as a sudden episode or for a prolonged period, should be part of his daily nursing assessment. Standing in line, especially in a hot room, can be dangerous, as can hypothermia.

Hypotension is not only dangerous from the standpoint of lack of cerebral perfusion with loss of ability to react appropriately with reality (confusion), but it may also be the cause of falls, which result in hip fracture or head injury that can lead to subdural hematomas. It often is the early sign of atypical or silent myocardial infarction of the elderly. Rodstein (1971) reports that of 51 consecutive nonfatal myocardial infarctions in one home for the aged, 15 were atypical with pain: 21 were atypical with dizziness, weakness, vertigo, confusion, dyspnea, syncope, and abdominal distress; and 16 were silent. Painless myocardial infarctions are not infrequent during or shortly after surgery.

Duncalf and Kepes (1971) find that 33% of elderly patients with heart failure or coronary insufficiency have postoperative cardiac complications with surgery. Those who receive diuretics, which may lead to a depletion of extracellular fluid and a loss of electrolytes, may develop a severe hypotension resistant to vasopressors during anesthesia. Halothane, a popular anesthetic agent, may lead to bradycardia, hypotension, and cardiac arrhythmias. Duncalf and Kepes warn that in the recovery room, the elderly surgical patient's restlessness may be a sign of cerebral hypoxia, and it is important to distinguish this from restlessness due to pain. Narcotics given for pain relief, which depress the respiratory center, could have fatal consequences. They recommend oxygen to prevent hypoxia. The maintenance of proper blood pressure is also necessary.

Signs and symptoms of hypotension include a drop in systolic and diastolic blood pressure to levels that do not support cerebral perfusion, usually evidenced by dizziness or even fainting when standing, confusion, and the sensation of "blacking out." The heart rate may be unchanged. Postural hypotension is noted on switching from a lying to a sitting or standing position. The first sign may be limpness or weakness of the entire body. The carotid sinus syndrome occurs with fainting preceded by giddiness, dizziness, and fading of vision (sometimes with scintillating scotomas); confusion with amnesia and hallucinosis; convulsions, which are not found in all patients; and by symptoms of an unstable nervous system, such as palpitations, moist palms, emotional instability, and skin sensitivity.

Gradual onset signs are sudden falls, often from a standing position (drop attacks), weakness and fatigue on effort with a lack of energy, postural hypotension, and confusion and lethargy.

Fourth-level assessment for hypotension

Blood pressure readings in three positions (lying, sitting, and standing); pulse
History of onset: drug history and recent immobilization
History of combining alcohol with drug regimen
Carotid sinus syndrome: turning of head, tight collars, or pressure on neck
Electrolyte studies
Nutritional pattern
History of malignancy
Observation of behavior, strength; sudden changes in cardiac status
Signs of cardiac insufficiency

Those elderly people most at risk have cardiac failure or low cardiac output, myocardial infarction, Stokes-Adams syndrome, cardiac arrhythmias, or carotid sinus sensitivity. Others at risk are the ones who receive overvigorous treatment of hypertension with drugs that cause hypotension or with tranquilizers, especially in the phenothiazine family, or who have alcohol interacting with antianginal or antihypertensive drugs, such as reserpine, methyldopa, hydralazine, guanethidine, ganglionic blocking agents, nitroglycerin, and peripheral vasodilators.

Also at risk are individuals immobilized at bed rest or with postural (orthostatic) hypotension, hypovolemia, carotid sinus syndrome, and micturition syncope. Elderly people with electrolyte disturbances, such as hypokalemia from dietary deficiency or diuretics, or with hyponatremia, as is found in Addison's disease from metastasis of malignancy to the adrenal glands, are also vulnerable.

Prevention of hypotension depends on treating the cause. For the person with postural hypotension, changing from the horizontal to the standing position must be done in three stages: sitting up until the head clears, dangling the feet over the side of the bed while supporting oneself with one's hands on either side against the mattress, and gradually standing to guard against dizziness. For the person with micturition syncope, rapid emptying of the bladder can result in a peripheral vascular collapse and systemic hypotension (Alpers and Mancall, 1971). Men should sit on the toilet while urinating and remain sitting if they are prone to dizziness. This is particularly important at night and in the early morning when the bladder may be full and the blood pressure at its lowest. For older people alone, this is important for prevention of falls in the bathroom during the night.

The history of alcoholic intake should be considered carefully when drugs are prescribed for the elderly who live alone or have little contact with others. Phenothiazines' side effect of hypotension can be exacerbated by alcohol. The metabolites of flurazepam (Dalmane) may remain in the body for several days and interact with alcohol. The tricyclic antidepressants produce hypotension, and their use by the person who takes alcohol should be carefully monitored. Alcohol and the antidiabetic agents or hypoglycemics interact by multiple mechanisms and cause unpredictable fluctuations in serum glucose levels (FDA drug bulletin, 1979). Alcohol may increase the blood pressure, lowering capability of antianginal and antihypertensive agents such as reserpine, methyldopa (Aldomet), hydralazine (Apresoline, Dralzine), guanethidine (Esimil, Ismelin), ganglionic blockers, nitroglycerin, and peripheral dilators. Propanolol may mask the signs and symptoms of alcohol hypoglycemia (Coleman and Evans, 1975).

Adequate hydration and nutrition to prevent hypovolemia or electrolyte imbalances and anemia are important preventive measures.

Causes of hypotension require medical workups for diagnosis and treatment. The institutionalized or homebound elderly often do not have access to the medical supervision that is available to the ambulatory. *The caregiver is often held responsible for the observation and reporting of the signs, symptoms, and history for the elderly person who is confused and who is a "poor historian."* Prevention means accepting one's role in this event and taking appropriate action to secure medical services.

Elderly individuals taking antihypertensive drugs should be monitored carefully. A history of dizziness on arising in the morning should be reported to the doctor prescribing drugs. Known cardiac patients should be watched carefully for signs of cardiac insufficiency or sudden change in vital signs. Rodstein (1971) states that coronary artery disease is present in almost all individuals over the age of 70.

Intervention is based on the following nursing objectives:
1. Relieve the emergency situation
2. Prevent further attacks by assisting in the medical regime
3. Teach prevention and prepare for discharge

The elderly person who is hypotensive requires cerebral perfusion, and the horizontal position is the first requirement. Observation of the vital signs and ascertaining what preceded the attack of syncope (if the hypotension has resulted in this emergency) is important. If hypovolemia is the cause, fluids may be given to replace the needed blood volume. Drug intake should be carefully reviewed. The use of alcohol in connection with hypotension should be noted. Where falls have occurred, the nurse should be alert for fractures of hip, forearm, and ribs.

Relief of confusion secondary to hypotension is dependent on relieving the cause. Finding causes and preventing episodes of hypotension are nursing concerns that ultimately make the difference. The nurse is referred to the introduction to this subsection in relation to the care of the elderly surgical patient.

For those persons whose drug regimen is leading to hypotension, a high index of suspicion should lead to monitoring at frequent intervals. For the institutionalized elderly person on a high number of drugs, the vital signs should be checked at regular intervals and at once when any sudden change occurs. Behavioral changes such as confusion and forgetting should lead to a serial blood pressure monitoring in three positions. All falls should be investigated for hypotension.

The client who has dizziness or giddiness should be reviewed for possible causes and should be referred to the physician with the nurse's observations and findings. The status of the heart as an efficient pump should be observed and the fluid and electrolyte status reviewed.

After the possibility of hypotension is observed or after treatment for hypotension, the nurse should teach the client. If postural hypotension is the problem, the cause (drugs, hypovolemia, or malnutrition) should be dealt with, but first, the client should be taught the three-step method of arising from a horizontal position. Telling is not enough; demonstration should be given and returned. The nurse should be present the next three times the client attempts to arise and patiently review the steps as the client himself goes through the process. The reasons for each step should be given as the client arises the first time; after that he should be able to give them to the nurse. If possible, a padded chair should be alongside the bed as an additional stabilizer.

The client with carotid sinus syndrome will need to practice turning his body instead of his head when looking to the side. If the elderly client is still driving and the problem is on the left side, he will have to arrange for assistance with backing and checking on the left or may have to restructure his mode of transportation.

The client who has a metastasis to the adrenal gland may have Addison's disease with sodium deficiency. The resulting weakness and hypotension can lead to falls; the caregiver should be on the alert for changes that indicate electrolyte imbalance. Sodium replacement in the elderly is not simple. Hormone therapy will be needed for the remainder of life. Caregiver and client will need to appreciate that the good feeling that comes after electrolyte balance is restored can be lost if treatment is not continuous.

The nurse, as one of the persons responsible for administering drugs, must be constantly vigilant. The pharmacist who fills and refills prescriptions for many drugs should ask the ambulatory client about himself. The physician should have access to complete lists of the drugs his patient is taking—those he orders, those ordered by others, over-the-counter drugs, and other self-care medications and preparations (see part III of this chapter).

Outcome criteria of successful nursing intervention against hypotension

1. The discharge plan contains elements of prevention of further hypotensive episodes.
2. The client or caregiver is able to demonstrate preventive care.
3. The client or caregiver recognizes the side effects of hypotensive drugs.
4. The client is no longer confused.

No episode of hypotension is a single, isolated event. It is a signal, a warning that the nurse should see as a challenge. It demands follow-up in the client's future. If the hypotension is part of a circulatory problem, a heart block, or congestive heart failure, the nurse must be aware of the dynamics of the heart as a pump, the nursing care for restoration of function, supportive care, maintenance care, and terminal care.

SUGGESTION FOR FURTHER READING
Ebersole, P., and Hess, P.: Care of the aged: nursing roles and functions, St. Louis, 1981, The C. V. Mosby Co., Chapter 8.

Increased intracranial pressure (subdural hematoma)

The older person may have increased intracranial pressure, just as people of any age, and from the same causes; there may be space-occupying lesions, such as tumors or subdural hematomas, or cerebral edema following loss of blood supply. The lesions displace the normal brain and vascular tissues. The subdural hematoma may result from a head injury after a fall when a small capillary is ruptured. The bleeding and hematoma formation may take a day or a month. For the person with a tumor, the change will be gradual. The ability to assess accurately and detect early is an important observational skill of the nurse. It is essential to have baseline information for comparison. As intracranial pressure increases, there is hypoxia of the ascending reticular activating system—the seat of consciousness. As the increased intracranial pressure compresses the contents of the skull against the foramen, the brainstem herniates into the narrow space, threatening the respiratory center in the brain. This pressure is sometimes not recognized until it is far advanced.

Alpers and Mancall (1971), in various studies of head injury, give the incidence of subdural hematoma as 1% to 10%, with the higher figures in the very young, the very old, and the chronic alcoholic. For many of the aged the prescribed drugs can have the same effect as alcohol, while still other clients ingest both drugs and alcohol (see part III of this chapter). In the three high-risk groups the subdural space is real rather than potential, and the bridging corticodural veins are less well cushioned and more liable to injury. The injury may be a direct injury to the head or it may be a fall, with a tearing of a bridging vein across the dural space from the jolt rather than from the blow. The fall may be slight and often forgotten, but enough to shear the vein as the brain moves within the skull. It may be associated with blood diseases, such as pernicious anemia, leukemia, metastatic tumor, and syphilis.

If a history of a fall is present, the diagnosis may be simple. Too often the subdural hematoma is found by the observation of gradual deterioration of personality, confusion, forgetfulness, and loss of judgment (Carter, 1971). There may be a symptom-free period of a day to several weeks. Bleeding is slow, and a clot tends to form. The clot will gradually be enclosed completely. Most are bilateral. During this time the elderly person may have a dull headache and mild vertigo. Signs of increased pressure are present in some cases but may be absent. Convulsions may occur, and there may be hemiparesis and homonymous hemianopia.

The history of head injury and periods of somnolence and confusion alternating with normal awareness are important (Alpers and Mancall, 1971).

Signs and symptoms of increased intracranial pressure include headache, which increases with such strain as vomiting, coughing, straining at stool, or stooping; and changes in behavior, such as drowsiness, lack of concentration, a fluctuating state of consciousness, or a loss of consciousness, all often mistaken for confusion. Pupillary signs may also be present, resulting from compression of the oculomotor nerve on the same side as the pressure; as pressure increases, the pupil eventually remains dilated (Wilson, 1979). There may be a previous sluggish reaction to light. Baseline information is important; some older persons have permanently dilated pupils from past injuries. Visual acuity is lessened by increased pressure on the optic nerve; however, papilledema is not always found in the elderly because the skull has increased room from diminished brain cortex. Great pressure is possible before it transmits along the optic nerve. Vital signs show blood pressure rising as cerebral pressure rises, but the pulse slows reflexly as the blood pressure rises. Slowing pulse in conjunction with a rising systolic pressure is a significant observation (Kinney, 1979). Pressure on the brainstem with herniation produces respiratory change, resulting in deep and stertorous breathing. Focal motor signs include weakened extremities on the opposite side of the swelling and loss of reflexes, such as Babinski's. *Any change should be noted.*

Fourth-level assessment for increased intracranial pressure

Good baseline data for comparison: vital signs, pupils, and strength
History of change in behavior, motor ability, or visual acuity
History of fall or falls
Drug or alcohol consumption
Signs and symptoms of increased intracranial pressure

Those elderly people with brain tumor or metastasis to the brain; who have a history of falls when the head may have been struck or jolted; who have hypotension resulting from phenothiazines or antihypertensives; or who have limited vision, stiff joints, weakened muscles, impaired equilibrium, dizziness, or vertigo, all are prone to falling. The alcoholic or the person who lives alone and has no one to notice changes in status are also potential risks.

Prevention is limited to minimizing falling by protecting the high-risk persons.

One study showed that of all falls in a retirement residence, more than half took place during the daytime and in the bedroom (Feist, 1978). This probably results from instability, hypotension, or stiff joints on arising from sleep. Delayed action of bedtime sedatives may leave a hangover effect. The blood pressure, lowest at night, is further decreased by venous pooling with postural hypotension. The elderly should be taught to rise from the horizontal position in easy stages (see hypotension section in this chapter).

Drug intake is probably more responsible for falls in the elderly than any one other factor. Prevention may require a drug holiday, including abstinence from alcohol.

The environment should be assessed for uneven or glaring surfaces, impeding objects, and adequacy of light. Furniture must be replaced only one piece at a time. Nightlights should throw a lighted pathway from the bed to the bathroom. For the unstable, walking aids such as a cane or walker are essential.

Intervention is based on the following objectives:
1. Maintain the patient's status as a person during the surgical event
2. Plan discharge for prevention of further episodes

The treatment for increased intracranial pressure resulting from tumors and subdural hematoma is to surgically relieve pressure. The elderly person goes from a confused, preoperative state to being a neurosurgical patient experiencing many relocations, new faces and voices, confusing activities, and a high degree of environmental stress. He will be traumatized by having his head shaved, and his body image will be affected in addition to his loss of identity. Nurses who care for the preoperative and postoperative patient need to be experts in neurosurgical nursing, but they also must be aware of the special physiologic needs of the elderly, their sensory deficits, and their potential for sensory overload.

To avoid creating or increasing confusion, the nurse is urged to see the broader picture of the elderly person as one with a personal life history, a unique culture, and an age-altered physiology that must be maintained. Family members can help maintain identity and link to life history by using visiting hours for reorientation of the patient and giving information and physical contact. Their role may prevent further loss of contact with reality. Primary nursing is the best staffing strategy for nursing care, which includes restorative measures and prevents immobilization hazards such as circulatory problems.

Discharge planning is very important for the relocated client. The home situation should be reviewed carefully to remove hazards such as architectural barriers. Falls because of oversedation require re-education regarding drugs and alcohol use. No patient should be released from the neurologic unit if he cannot return to a safer environment than the one that contributed to his admission.

Outcome criteria of successful nursing intervention against increased intracranial pressure

1. The client is no longer confused secondary to increased intracranial pressure if a subdural hematoma has been the cause.
2. A family member has reviewed the home environment, including medications and alcohol, and has removed hazards.
3. The client has been taught how to arise from a horizontal position to prevent hypotension.
4. If no family member is available, referral is made to a caring agency; if necessary social services should be sought to send the client to a protective environment until he can resume his independent care.

Normal pressure hydrocephalus

In 1965, Adams and others described "occult hydrocephalus" with "normal cerebro-spinal fluid pressure," more frequently known as normal pressure hydrocephalus (NPH), or communicating hydrocephalus, and in some instances, idiopathic hydrocephalus.

Signs and symptoms are related to those for intracranial pressure. NPH is a syndrome with enlargement of the ventricles, compression of the cerebral tissue, and normal levels of pressure for the spinal fluid in lumbar puncture (below 200 mm H_2O pressure). The classic symptoms are confusion, progressive dementia with memory deficit, incontinence, and an unsteady gait (Alpers and Mancall, 1971). Signs of increased intracranial pressure (headache and papilledema) are usually absent, and the onset is recent, usually within a year (Lancet, 1977). The gait is not ataxic or that of proprioceptive deficit, but rather unsteady with a widened base and zigzag steps (Stone, 1974). The upper extremities are not involved. As the disease progresses, the gait disturbance may lead to inability to walk or stand. Incontinence is a late symptom, but is out of proportion to the confusional status.

The age of the patient distinguishes this hydrocephalus from that of the child with the skull that can be expanded against the internal pressure. The hardened skull of the adult allows no external signs other than those symptoms already listed. In a study of 54 patients with NPH (Katzman, 1976), 20 were in the 55 to 59 age group, 15 were 60 to 64, and 7 were 65 to 70. Incidence peaks in the late fifties. Diagnosis is made by radiography or computerized tomography. Visualization reveals the anterior horns of the lateral ventricles to be enlarged, followed later by enlargement of the remainder of the ventricles. History is extremely important. The differentiation must be made between NPH and Alzheimer's disease. Careful observations by the caregiver are crucial (see Chapter 13).

The treatment is surgical. A shunt is made to the peritoneal area, to the right atrium via the superior vena cava and jugular vein, or, rarely, to the ureter. There is a high rate of shunt failure, with complications such as obstruction of the ventricular catheter, thrombosis of the jugular vein, septicemia, meningitis, subdural hematoma, thrombophlebitis, pulmonary emboli, and pneumonia.

The cause has not been established to determine who is vulnerable. The only clue is that thickened meninges seem to be found in cases examined at autopsy.

Prevention of NPH at the present level of knowledge is undefined. Early detection is the best hope. The family member or nurse should be aware of the onset of unsteady gait, confusional problems, and incontinence. However, this resembles so many other problems of the aged that the only distinguishing characteristic may be the suddenness of onset. Differential diagnosis requires skill in neurologic assessment and the use of careful medical testing.

Intervention is based on the following objectives:

1. For the patient who is benefited by surgery, restore contact with previous life history
2. For the patient who does not benefit from surgery, plan discharge with the family for care during his deterioration and death

The treatment for NPH is surgical and resembles the nursing care needed by the client with increased intracranial pressure who requires surgery (see section on subdural hematoma in this chapter). In three studies (Lancet, 1977) improvement for confusion and mental status were given as 25%, 70%, and 23% after surgery. This leaves a large number who will not improve and will have progressive deterioration and a shortened life span. At this time there is no diagnostic test that indicates which person will benefit from shunting.

For the client who does benefit, restoration of function is a process that must be aided by family, caregivers, and all professional personnel. The client has undergone relocation not once, but many times; he has been subjected to environments and people with varying potentials for diminishing the human spirit. He has lost contact with his life history, even his present, and his reunion with reality will have to be regained over time as he takes the physiologic steps to recovery. Constant testing will be needed to determine to what extent he is of the fortunate percentage who make improvements. Caregivers will have to deal with their own feelings of disappointment if the surgery does not yield return to normal function. There is always risk of abandonment of the client when he needs help to return or to face his own loss of mental and physical function.

Discharge planning takes all this into consideration; the family must be brought into each step of the process and involved completely. For some families—and this may mean only an aging spouse—the future will deal with predeath bereavement. The need for hope is never greater and yet seldom so unrealistic. Miracles can be hoped for but not really expected; attainable goals have to be set. The goal of a peaceful death may demand the fullest skills and resources of the caregivers in supporting both the client and the family to the best recovery possible. Discharge planning is facing the facts and going beyond the neurosurgical event to allow for a completed life.

Outcome criteria of successful nursing intervention against NPH

1. The patient's physiology is supported during the surgical procedure.
2. The surgical event does not add iatrogenic confusion to the patient's own state.
3. The family is involved and supported throughout the surgical event; they have a discharge plan that includes their psychosocial and physiologic functions in recovery or in the terminal phase of the patient's life.
4. Referral has been made to community agencies that can assist the family and client during the postoperative period.

SUGGESTIONS FOR FURTHER READING

The following are programmed self-instructional units that the nurse can pursue at her own pace. They can be obtained by using a library that has past volumes of the *American Journal of Nursing* or by writing to the American Journal of Nursing, 555 West 57th Street, New York, N.Y. 10019.

Patient assessment; neurological examination, Part I, Am. J. Nurs. **75**:1511-1535, 1975.

Patient assessment; neurological examination, Part II, Am. J. Nurs. **76**:2037-2057, 1975.

Patient assessment; neurological examination, Part III, Am. J. Nurs. **76**:609-633, 1976.

Kinney, M.: Neurologic assessment, Management of the person with neurologic manifestations, and Problems of the nervous system. In Phipps, W. J., Long, B. C., and Woods, N. F., editors: Medical-surgical nursing: concepts and clinical practice, St. Louis, 1979, The C.V. Mosby Co.

Stone, M.H.: Normal pressure hydrocephalus, Nurs. Clin. North Am. **9**(4):667-676, 1974.

Hypothyroidism

Decrease in the production of thyroid-stimulating hormone by the pituitary and of the thyroid hormone by the thyroid gland is shown by a decline of the basic metabolic rate from age 30 to age 70 by as much as 20% (Rockstein, 1975). Distinct structural changes, such as replacement of normal connective tissue with dense collagenous material, take place. Myxedema (hypothyroidism) is more often found than hyperthyroidism in the aged (Rodstein, 1971) and may be caused by atrophy, pituitary disturbance, and surgical removal of the thyroid gland. The cohort of women reaching 65 at this time were the subject of numerous thyroidectomies during the 1930s through 1960s, which may be one of the reasons that myxedema is more often found in the middle-aged and aging woman.

The most characteristic finding of hypothyroidism is the puffy face of the victim whose speech is slurred and whose motor reaction is extremely sluggish. The mental status can easily be mistaken for confusion, for reactions are slow and forgetfulness is common. About 12% of persons with hypothyroidism have pernicious anemia (Cassmeyer, 1979).

The tendency toward chilling, or the inability to maintain a constant body temperature, is partly from the falling metabolic rate. The elderly person may have no complaints but is brought to the physician by the family because of sluggishness, mental torpor, and sleepiness. Protein and electrolytes accumulate in the interstitial space, resulting in a puffy, nonpitting edema in the periorbital space, the hands, and the feet. Pleural effusion may be present, along with ascites at times. Vital signs are depressed with slow pulse rate, elevated diastolic blood pressure, and slowed respiration.

Depression of hepatic function leads to carotenemia because of reduced conversion of carotene to vitamin A, which causes a yellowish discoloration of the skin (Groer and Shekleton, 1979). Plasma lipids, especially serum cholesterol levels, are increased.

There are degrees of hypothyroidism, but added stress, especially infection from pneumonia, pyelonephritis, or cellulitis, may precipitate a myxedemic coma (Cassmeyer, 1979), in which there is decreased blood flow to the brain.

Treatment is replacement of the thyroid hormone, which must be carefully monitored because of cardiac insufficiency.

Signs and symptoms of hypothyroidism include change in mental status, with apathy, forgetfulness, and sleepiness, often mistaken for confusion; metabolic signs such as cold intolerance, weakness, lassitude, low energy, and low body temperature; circulatory signs such as decreased cardiac output and rate, decreased blood pressure, decreased respiratory rate, and dyspnea on exertion; increased cholesterol level with a high incidence of atherosclerosis and coronary disease; nonpitting edema, shown in the puffy face, hands, and feet; gastrointestinal manifestations such as weight gain, constipation, and poor appetite; motor activity that is sluggish, slow, and accompanied by slow reflexes; and finally, the general appearance: thickened, dry skin, sparse dry hair, dry brittle nails, anemia, and easy bruising resulting from capillary fragility.

> **Fourth-level assessment for hypothyroidism**
>
> Behavior: sluggish motor and mental reactions, forgetfulness, lethargy, and sleepiness
> Appearance: yellowish discoloration of skin and puffy edema of eyes, hands, and feet
> No change in intellect
> Inability to keep warm
> Skin: dry; hair: sparse and dry
> Speech: slurred (thickened tongue)

Those elderly people who have been overtreated for hyperthyroidism, who have had removal of thyroid tissue, who have a hypopituitary disorder preventing thyroid gland stimulation, or whose thyroid gland has atrophied with aging are all at risk.

Prevention is carried out by ensuring that high-risk persons appreciate the necessity of continued hormone replacement. For those who are aging, early detection and referral to medical treatment are essential. The nurse should be fully aware of the hypothyroid signs and symptoms and carry a high degree of suspicion when assessing the sluggish, drowsy, but intellectually intact elderly person.

Intervention is based on the following objectives:

1. Monitor replacement therapy
2. Prepare the client for self-care

The mental status of the person with hypothyroidism is misinterpreted as confusion because it differs from the previous condition and the change is in the direction that uncritical onlookers can attribute to confusion. The signs and symptoms include the appearance and motor activity representative of the stereotype of aging to many people, and it is easy to associate the slowing down of hypothyroidism with the slowing down of aging. They are not the same. Aging is not the loss of engagement with life that the elderly person with hypothyroidism shows; this can be proved by the change that occurs with treatment.

Treatment must be cautiously initiated with monitoring. The cardiac muscle is flabby and weak. When treatment is pushed, cardiac arrest is possible, and any signs of coronary insufficiency or congestive failure resulting from increased metabolic demands call for a reduction of dosage. The elderly client may respond to very small doses; often the change may be dramatic as he actively and alertly takes part in life again.

The nurse may monitor the progress of the elderly person in the home. In the institution, she will be held responsible for recognizing any danger signs of treatment. Monitoring is often done by measuring protein-bound iodine, but clinical signs can occur and must be noted while waiting for laboratory confirmation.

Teaching the client or his caregiver the importance of continued treatment and medical supervision is important. Often, recovery to the premorbid state is falsely reassuring, and treatment will be neglected. Abrupt withdrawal of the replacement therapy can precipitate a myxedemic coma, characterized by loss of consciousness, hypotension, vasomotor collapse, bradycardia, and seizures (Groer and Shekleton, 1979). The client must recognize the signs of oxygen need, tachycardia, and overactivity as signals to seek medical help.

> **Outcome criteria of successful nursing intervention against hypothyroidism**
>
> 1. The client is regaining his former motor and interactional abilities.
> 2. The client or his caregiver knows the signs and symptoms of replacement hormone overdose and the hazards of abrupt withdrawal.
> 3. The client or his caregiver can explain the need for lifetime replacement therapy.

During the period while replacement therapy is being instituted, the nurse can help the hypothyroid client. A warm environment and adequate clothing are needed.

Activity should be geared to the potential of the client, which is often extremely low. A high-protein, low-calorie diet with roughage is needed for the nutritional needs and tendency toward constipation. The dry skin may need lotions (Barber, Stokes, and Billinings, 1977).

PART II
Glucose imbalance compromising brain support

CONFUSION SECONDARY TO HYPOGLYCEMIA

Nerve cells are dependent on a constant supply of glucose for normal metabolic activities to produce the electrical potential that is the function of the nervous system. Hypoglycemia is a lowering of the blood glucose to a commonly accepted standard of below 50 mg/100 ml. This cannot be measured by urinalysis, which can only show that sugar is not spilling into the urine. It does not show the degree to which the glucose content of the blood is below the point of triggering a negative response to a urine test. Severity of symptoms is related not only to the blood glucose level, but more especially is a reflection of the rate of the fall of the level. More severe symptoms occur with a higher level of blood glucose that falls abruptly.

Many older diabetic clients do not show the signs of increased epinephrine output that occur in hypoglycemic attacks of the young; that is, they may not experience the sweating, anxiety, nervousness, and tachycardia. The elderly may develop loss of consciousness without warning. Rifkin and Ross (1971) warn that cerebrovascular accident with temporary or permanent neurologic deficits or myocardial infarction may occur with attacks of hypoglycemia. Alpers and Mancall (1971) find that where there are neurologic residuals, the damage resembles hypoxic encephalopathy.

Signs and symptoms of mild hypoglycemia are neurologic manifestations such as confusion, nervousness, apprehension, hyperactivity, diplopia, generalized weakness, palpitation tachycardia, sweating, nocturnal headache, diplopia or blurred vision, bizarre and psychotic behavior, nightmares, somnolence, crying out during sleep, and an unusual sleep posture (Rifkin and Ross, 1971; Alpers and Mancall, 1971).

Signs and symptoms of severe hypoglycemia also include stupor, seizures, and coma.

Fourth-level assessment for hypoglycemia

Observation of behavior
History of diabetes
Drug history (including alcoholism, insulin, and antidiabetics)
Recent food intake
History of onset, life-style, and recent losses or changes
Reports of any urine or blood tests
Vital signs

The vulnerable elderly are those who have hyperinsulinism from a pancreatic tumor, liver disease, or disease of the pituitary, adrenal, or thyroid glands. Also at risk are the elderly with leucine sensitivity; who are starved; or who take antidiabetic drugs (hypoglycemics) with little food intake or with diarrhea. The potentiation of the antidiabetic drugs such as tolbutamide, chlorpropamide, and tolazamide put the alcoholic diabetic at risk (FDA drug bulletin, 1979).

Prevention is much easier than treatment. Hypoglycemia frequently proves to be the ultimate disaster in the elderly. Insulin-dependent diabetic persons have rarely reached the age of 65 without recurrent episodes of hypoglycemia, many of which were sudden in onset. They and their families are prepared for hypoglycemic attacks. Precautions must be taken for the elderly person, who is more likely to have the late-onset, noninsulin-dependent type of diabetes. The oral antidiabetic medications also lower blood glucose levels, and when conditions exist that do not renew the body's supply of glucose, such as lack of food, nausea and vomiting, overdose of the drug and especially ingestion of alcohol with little or no food intake, the blood level can drop.

Families should exercise the same precautions with the less dramatic oral medication as with parenteral insulin. There must be awareness of the relationship of food and drug. The drug should be discontinued until the physician can be consulted if the elderly person is unable or unwilling to eat his usual allowance of food. Early detection in the mild phase is important, and the family should be the first to note the signs and symptoms of mild hypoglycemia. Behavior change is the first clue, and since this resembles the changes traditionally associated with cerebroarteriosclerotic disease, the elderly person can easily be diagnosed as having chronic brain syndrome. Early detection is extremely important, for with each episode involving neurologic signs and symptoms, there is neurologic loss (death of cells).

Prevention means separating alcohol ingestion from drug taking. This is a family problem if the older person is unable or unwilling to accept the dangers involved in combining the two.

The elderly insulin-dependent diabetic client with diabetic retinopathy should have his drug measurement and injection technique monitored at frequent intervals to ensure the correct dose is given. He should have access to quickly assimilated sugars, such as orange juice or candy. If he lives alone, there must be some person who is in daily contact, perhaps through the telephone reassurance program. If he is institutionalized, caregivers should be aware of the neurologic signs of reduced glucose to the cells of the brain.

Intervention is based on the following objectives:
1. Restore blood glucose level
2. Teach and plan discharge

The first aid for the elderly person who has hypoglycemia is restoration of the blood glucose level to the point where neurologic signs disappear. If oral glucose can be taken, this is relatively simple; a glass of orange juice or some concentrated form of sugar should suffice. If the elderly person is uncooperative or unwilling to take oral sugar (alcoholism may cause stubbornness or a stuporous condition), use of parenteral injection should be promptly instituted. Hypoglycemia is an emergency even in the mild form.

Hypoglycemia should be viewed as a call for help. The discharge planning may require looking at the life-style of the elderly client and teaching him what parts of it will require change to prevent recurrence. The physician will want to rule out endocrine problems. The community should be concerned with the possibility of starvation, which may be from social, psychologic or economic causes. The elderly person should not be discharged from care until these efforts are made and follow-up arranged. Prevention of the next attack may require such drastic measures as relocating the elderly person to an environment where he has proper care and food. No hypoglycemic episode is a single event; it becomes one of a series unless the client and his caregiver recognize their role in prevention.

Outcome criteria of successful nursing intervention against hypoglycemia

1. There are no longer neurologic signs of hypoglycemia, including confusion.
2. The client or his caregiver can relate the lack of blood glucose to:
   a. lack of food intake
   b. antidiabetic drug ingestion
   c. alcohol and antidiabetic drug ingestion together
3. The client's life-style and environment have been reviewed for contributing factors, and problem solving initiated to reduce the hazards.
4. Appropriate community referrals have been made for continued care.

The high-risk environment is one where the elderly person is alone and lonely, where he takes alcohol to relieve his loneliness or for social reasons, or where the retirement income does not stretch to cover food.

CONFUSION SECONDARY TO HYPERGLYCEMIA

Arguments over strict control for the adult-onset type of diabetes has led to careful questioning of information learned on the basis of juvenile-type or insulin-dependent diabetes. The elderly person with adult-onset diabetes does not have the same threatening kinds of ketoacidosis that haunt the younger diabetic person. Hyperglycemia may lead to quite different events that cannot be predicted by the presence of acetone in the urine: hyperosmolar nonketonic coma and lactic acidosis. The adult-onset diabetic elderly may suffer from complications of overutilization of glucose by the cells. Fat and muscle cells cannot utilize glucose without insulin, but glucose can enter nerve cells and the lens of the eye in the absence of insulin (Kolata, 1979) and can be present in such high concentrations that they are damaged. Hyperosmolar nonketonic coma occurs in elderly persons with blood sugar of 1,000 mg or more per 100 ml, along with a hypernatremia. Neurologic manifestations reflect intracellular dehydration on the basis of the increased osmolarity of the extracellular fluid (Alpers and Mancall, 1971). It may occur in the mild diabetic client after burns, hypothermia, use of steroids, immunosuppressive drugs, anticonvulsants, or after peritoneal dialysis or hemodialysis (Riffkin and Ross, 1971). Blood sugars may rise to 2,700 mg/100 ml. Serum osmolarity is usually above 350 mOsm/liter. There may be mild to severe acidosis.

Signs and symptoms of hyperosmolar nonketonic coma include dehydration, signs of thirst, polyuria, progressive lethargy, confusion and mental obtundation, and hypotension. There is often aphasia, hemiplegia, and seizures, indicating neurologic involvement. Blood studies indicate hyperglycemia of 1,000-2,700 mg/100 ml and serum osmolarity of 350 mOsm/liter or more.

Fourth-level assessment for hyperglycemia

History of diabetes
History of recent stress
Signs of dehydration: mushy eyeballs, scant urine output, hypotension, and shock
Progressive mental changes from lethargy to lack of response (coma)
Signs and symptoms of hyperosmolar nonketonic coma

The mild adult-onset type of diabetes leads to greater risk for the elderly client controlled by diet or oral hypoglycemics, if he is subjected to stress such as hypothermia and drugs and conditions leading to dehydration.

Prevention often means early detection. The hyperosmolarity type of coma can be predicted if there is added stress in the situation. The elderly diabetic client with the adult-onset type of disease does not have the classic signs of thirst and polyuria. When these occur, it is a warning sign that the body is trying to restore the blood glucose to its normal state, which results in dehydration. The warning signs can slip by the vigilant caregiver because less is expected with the milder symptoms; the ease of control makes the disease seem less dramatic than insulin dependence.

Intervention is based on the following objectives:

1. Restore physiologic status
2. Prevent permanent confusion and immobilization complications
3. Teach for prevention of recurrence

The care of the elderly patient with hyperosmolar nonketonic coma is emergency and must be conducted in an acute-care setting where laboratories are available to monitor the rehydration, electrolyte restoration, and pH of the blood serum. Usually, half-strength normal saline solution and insulin are given. The mortality rate is very high because of age, the likelihood of vascular disease, and severity of the condition when recognized. Renal involvement may prevent recovery (Mitten and Phipps, 1979).

During the acute illness, the pulmonary condition of the aged person will require attention directed toward prevention of pneumonia. The impaired peripheral-vascular system will demand constant attention to prevent complications that occur with immobilization; the earlier the condition is recognized, the higher the probability that treatment will be effective in preventing such complications.

Outcome criteria of successful nursing intervention against hyperglycemia

1. The blood sugar has been reduced to normal levels; the client is rehydrated and mentally aware of who and where he is.
2. The caregiver and client have discussed early warning signs of hyperglycemia.
3. The caregiver and client can participate in the therapeutic self-care.
4. Referral to community agencies has been made where appropriate.

As soon as mental function returns, restoration of orientation should begin. Usually, the emergency condition has resulted in relocation with strange faces and voices. When the acute condition has lessened, discharge planning should begin with the patient and family. Conditions that led to the hyperglycemia should be discussed, and the early warning signs (thirst, polyuria, and dehydration) should be combined with a plan for action. For the elderly person who lives alone, the names and numbers of persons to call should be posted in large letters on the wall beside the phone. Referral should be made to community agencies such as the diabetic association and home health care nursing services for follow-up. A discharge plan in large type should be sent home with the client with poor vision.

Ketoacidosis of the elderly diabetic client will not be discussed here because it is well known. Its onset can be better recognized, urine testing can usually predict the onset, and nurses are acquainted with the emergency measures.

PART III
Drug toxicity compromising brain support

CONFUSION SECONDARY TO DRUG TOXICITY

The problem of drug toxicity in the aged arises from a number of causes. The first and most easily recognized is the significant variation in physiologic response of the aged to a drug or to polypharmacy (many drugs). It is understood that the changes occuring with aging tend to cause the abnormal handling of a drug. The study by Hurwitz (1969) showed that patients over the age of 60 had two and a half times the number of adverse drug reactions as those admitted to the hospital under the age of 60. Another study (Caranasos and others, 1974) found that adverse drug reactions doubled in the period from the fifth to the eighth decades of life. Both studies indicate that women have twice as many incidents of adverse drug reactions as men and that this is increased in white women over the age of 50. The assumption can be made that polypharmacy increased with polypathology (Ritchey, 1975), increasing the sheer number of drugs that can interact at any one time. The Hurwitz study showed that there was a 3.4% incidence of altered drug reactions in patients taking 1 to 5 drugs and 24.8% in those taking 6 or more and as high as 50% in those taking 20 drugs. Adverse drug reactions and drug interactions are the

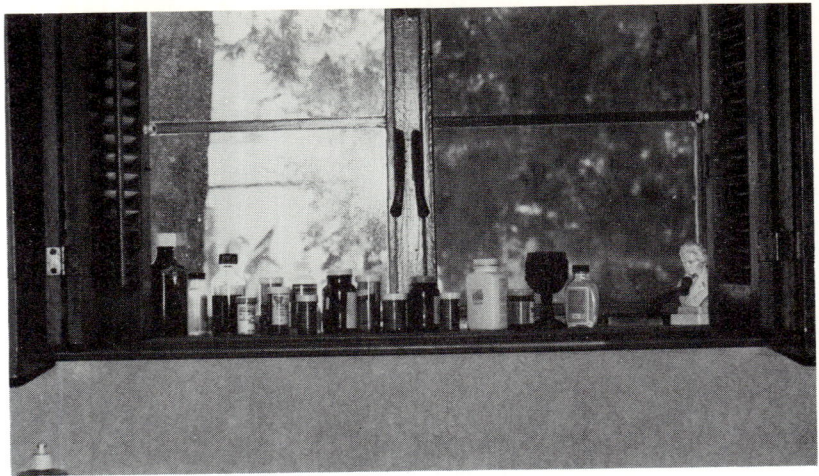

Fig. 9-3. Kitchen windowsills in the homes of the elderly are the storage place for drugs. Easily accessible, near water, and seen when preparing meals, this is the likely place to find drugs, although sunlight may lead to their deterioration. (Photograph by C. D. Falk.)

More common drugs associated with confusion in the elderly (adapted from Kayne, 1976)

Central nervous system depressants
  Barbiturates
  Chlordiazepoxide (Librium); diazepam (Valium); flurazepam (Dalmane); pentazocine (Talwin); salicylates and the narcotic analgesics; and the nonnarcotic drugs such as propoxyphene (Darvon)
  Alcohol, alone, or in conjunction with any of the above (the lethal dose for barbiturates is nearly 50% lower in the presence of alcohol than when used alone [Bogan and Smith, 1967])
  Signs of confusional state: bizarre perceptual disturbances, delusions, thought disorders, panic, and memory disorders
Hypotensives
  The phenothiazines; chlorpromazine (Thorazine); thioridazine (Mellaril); haloperidol (Haldol)
  The tricyclic antidepressants: amitriptyline (Elavil); imipramine hydrochloride (Tofranil)
    Sympatholytic antihypertensive drugs: guanethidine (Ismelin); reserpine (Sandril, Serpasil, Raudixin); methyldopa (Aldomet)
    Hypotension produces impaired mentation that can lead to syncope if blood pressure drops below level required for perfusion of brain
Anticholinergic or atropine-like drugs
  Belladonna alkaloids: atropine and scopolamine (scopolamine is found in many over-the-counter sleep-producing preparations)
  Antipsychotic drugs (also known as the major tranquilizers): chlorpromazine (Thorazine); thioridazine; haloperidol
  Tricyclic antidepressants (see hypotensives: amitriptyline and imipramine)
  Antiparkinsonism agents: diphenhydramine (Benadryl); trihexyphenidyl (Artane); benztropine mesylate (Cogentin)
  Propantheline bromide (Pro-banthine), a synthetic used for ulcers
  Signs of confusion include disorientation, impairment of recent memory, agitation, delusions, and picking at dressings, tubings, and catheters

penalty exacted for the availability of so many potent therapeutic agents (Ritchey, 1975) and are multiplied with ingestion of increased numbers of drugs (Brown, 1977).

A social factor that cannot be ignored in considering the place of drugs in the aged is that drugs, especially tranquilizers, are substituted for human understanding. The elderly client with many problems seeks help from the physician who may not have any time to listen to the real problem the client is trying to communicate, which is often loneliness, depression, and despair. *A social problem is converted to a medical problem.* Drugs are prescribed, so drug interaction replaces human interaction. Listening to the elderly would decrease adverse drug actions through decreasing the sheer number of drugs taken by a single individual. Prescriptions are often renewed for years without a critical review of whether the drug is proving beneficial or not, let alone whether it is toxic.

The result has been collections of drugs on kitchen windowsills throughout the homes of the elderly in America (Fig. 9-3). Medicine cabinets are full of old prescriptions.

Drugs and confusion

Mental disturbances related to drug use are not uncommon and are not age-related. In clients over the age of 60 who have a higher incidence of drug reactions, the first sign often is a change in mental status. Too often, changes in behavior or confusion are attributed to the client's age, senility, or a functional disorder such as depression, while the adverse drug reaction goes unrecognized.

"My mother is a junkie. She pops pills all the time. She was a strong woman until my father's final illness and death. Then she started taking his prescriptions, and the pharmacists renewed them. She was so bad that she couldn't handle her own affairs—confused! I had to bring her into my home, and then we put her in a nursing home where they stopped all her drugs. She cleared up at once, and mentally, she was the same organizing person she had always been. We got her an apartment and she lived independently again. Then she began slipping, and I found out she was back on all those prescriptions again. I put her in a nursing home to get over her confusion, and she hid pills in those little sachet pillows and took her supply with her. Again, she cleared up when taken off the pills. But what am I going to do with her?"

It is obvious in this incident that mother is applying a maladaptive solution to her problem, which no one has recognized. Grief and depression demand strong medicine if there is no human interaction to share the burden of loss. If agitation is present, the tendency to prescribe tranquilizers is particularly strong. Epstein and Simon (1967) found that of the elderly patients admitted to a psychiatric ward, 13% had reversible brain syndromes, and 33% had reversible brain syndrome superimposed on chronic brain syndrome. That is a total of 46% who should have been treated for acute brain syndrome.

Drugs used as tranquilizers form only a small number of those that cause confusion in the elderly. Antibiotics used to treat pneumonia or kidney infections, digitalis preparations for the heart, and other drugs that are given for a target site far removed from the central nervous system may still result in confusion. The following mechanisms may be involved, although the exact action is still not known:

1. Drugs that alter the metabolic environment of the brain cells secondary to fluid and electrolyte imbalances (diuretics), acidosis (alcohol), and hormonal disturbances (deficient or excessive thyroid)
2. Drugs that interfere with the cerebral blood flow (hypotensives, such as phenothiazines) or reduce the cardiac output
3. Drugs that reduce the blood glucose ((hypoglycemics)
4. Drugs that interfere with oxygen supply to the brain by depressing the respiratory center (many narcotics)

5. Drugs that alter the brain hormones, such as anticholinergics and antidepressants
6. Drugs that alter or compete with the amount of needed substances of the brain, such as vitamins or amino acids

These common drugs associated with confusion in the elderly do not exhaust the possibilities, which seem to equal the drugs in use. One of the gravest problems in the elderly is the action of digitalis products; another is the widespread use of alcohol in our society. Each will be discussed in greater depth.

Digitalis toxicity

The sheer number of the elderly who have cardiac problems and who are being treated with digitalis preparations make this a critical drug to be observed. Rodstein (1971) reports congestive heart failure in a home for the aged at 48% for the ambulatory residents and 58% for the incapacitated.

Signs and symptoms of digitalis toxicity include the confusion resulting from the poor perfusion of the brain associated with congestive heart failure. Digitalis toxicity exacerbates the confusion, agitation, and depression. Other manifestations include headache, dizziness, visual disturbances, disorientation, hallucinations, apathy, fatigue, and weakness. These neurologic signs and symptoms accompany the more commonly described gastrointestinal symptoms of nausea and vomiting. The cardiac signs and symptoms are found by electrocardiogram, which points out the interference with the conduction system: atrial, atrioventricular node and ventricular arrhythmias; atrioventricular block (premature beats and bigeminy); atrial tachycardia with block; artrial fibrillation; ventricular tachycardia; and nodal rhythm. There is an isoelectric or inversion of the T wave, depression of the S-T segment, and an increased P-R interval.

Any person taking digitalis preparations is a candidate for toxicity, but those who have renal failure or conditions leading to a serum potassium imbalance are especially susceptible. Toxic effects may take place with no dosage change if the intramyocardial potassium level is depleted by use of diuretics, if there is no potassium intake for reasons of nausea or vomiting, for iatrogenic reasons such as preparation for diagnostic tests, or when potassium depletion is caused by diarrhea.

Fourth-level assessment for digitalis toxicity

Change in rate, rhythm, and quality of pulse
Behavior changes: mental status
Gastrointestinal symptoms: appetite loss, nausea, and vomiting
Neurologic signs: headache, visual disturbances, fatigue, and weakness
Laboratory studies: serum digitalis level, urinalysis, and other studies indicating renal failure and serum K^+
Electrocardiogram (EKG) for electroconduction changes
Drugs that lead to K^+ depletion

Prevention is vigilance. Digitalis is one of the few very toxic drugs with a narrow range between maintenance dose and toxic dose, and toxic dose and lethal dose. The client who takes a digitalis drug or his caregiver should know the circumstances that lead to toxicity. Any illness may change the status of the body in such a way that the maintenance dose becomes toxic. The highly refined glycosides do not have the early warning signs of toxicity.

Intervention is based on the following objectives:
1. Observe for toxicity of the client who is taking digitalis
2. Teach client or caregiver prevention

Nursing action requires vigilance in observing the client who is administered digitalis and the events that will precipitate hypokalemia. The treatment is discontinuing the digitalis product. The half-life of some preparations is long (digitoxin and powdered digitalis); while for others it is moderate (digoxin and gitalin); and the toxicity may persist for as long as 10 days after the drug is discontinued (Rodstein, 1971). If potassium is given by intravenous infusion, it must be given very slowly and monitored by electrocardiography. The elderly person who has liver or kidney disease is predisposed to digitalis toxicity since the liver inactivates the drug and the kidney excretes it. In addition to hypokalemia, increased tendency toward toxicity may occur with alkalosis, hypercalcemia, hypomagnesemia, and hypothyroidism.

Specific nursing actions include observing the client's pulse before administration of digitalis. Bradycardia, increased rate, and arrhythmia are warning signs. The toxicity may be mild and persist for long periods as gait disturbances and confusional states. Serum digitalis levels help determine the milder cases.

Outcome criteria of successful nursing intervention against digitalis toxicity

1. The client no longer shows signs and symptoms of digitalis intoxication.
2. The client or the caregiver understands the early signs of digitalis toxicity and the need for pulse observation.
3. If the elderly client is responsible for administering his own drugs, a plan is set up to ensure correct dosage.
4. The client or caregiver can give the rationale for daily potassium intake (dietary or prescribed if he is on diuretics).

After restoration of cardiac function, the nurse should review with the caregiver or client the events that led to the toxicity. For many elderly, whose problem is remembering whether the one daily dose has been taken, cooperative problem-solving is needed. A pill taken with the first cup of coffee may solve the problem of remembering. Little calendar boxes can be constructed with a compartment for each day of the week. On Sunday a pill is placed in each compartment; when empty, the dose has been taken. Discharge planning will include caution to report loss of appetite (no ingestion of potassium), or nausea, or use of purgatives. Pulse counting is an important skill.

Drug misuse and abuse

The first question the nurse should ask about the elderly person who exhibits confusion is: what drugs is this person taking? In many instances the nurse is responsible for administering the drugs. Drug administration is not difficult, and the present controversy over whether the drug should be administered by pharmacists or nurses, or by what level of nursing preparation, is academic to the real questions concerning the need for knowledge of drug effects; the observation of its effect on the client; and finally, the judgment of when to withhold the medication and report its effects or lack of effect on the client. Unfortunately, these questions have been ignored, and the elderly person has been the victim of drug abuse and drug misuse.

Drug abuse is intentional excessive use of a drug to alter the way one feels (Olson and Johnson, 1978). On the other hand, misuse is unintentional, as in medication errors. For the elderly, both have grave and frequent consequences. One of the most abused drugs is alcohol. Today, alcoholics are living to old age, and an increasing number of elderly are turning to alcohol as an easily accessible drug in old age to ease the pain of grief, depression, loneliness, or boredom and even for physical pain itself (Butler and Lewis, 1977). Fig. 9-4 shows the solitary drinking at high noon of a old man in a park where there are many others like himself. Some are lonely because their families could not tolerate their frequent drunkenness, while others have no family. Socialization and food programs can help combat such escapes from loneliness (Fig. 9-5).

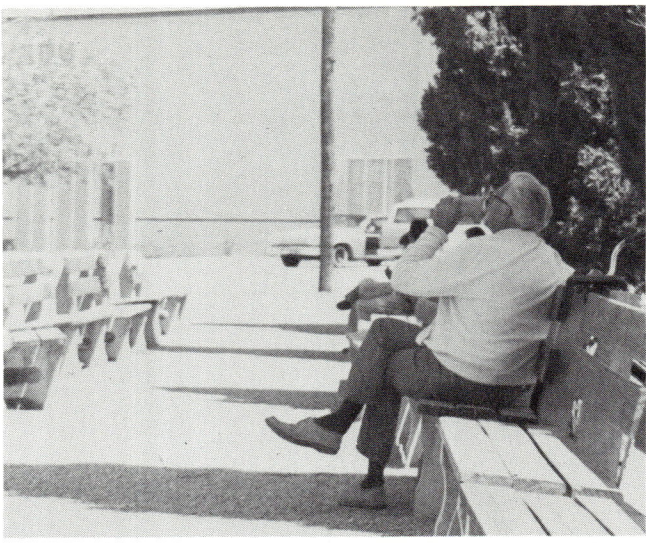

Fig. 9-4. Solitary drinker at high noon. A wine bottle is hidden in the brown paper bag. The need alcohol is meeting is not so easily disguised. (Photograph by C. D. Falk.)

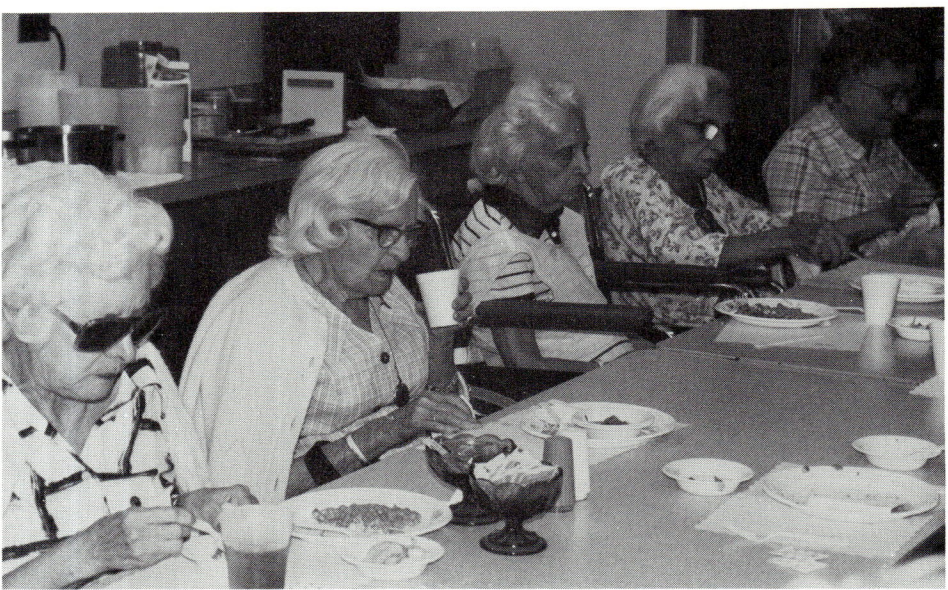

Fig. 9-5. The socialization and nutrition programs offer an opportunity to be with other people and to enjoy a hot meal in a family atmosphere. Federal funds have made such programs available in almost every community. (Photograph by C. D. Falk.)

Alcoholism is not confined to the lonely old men on park benches, however. It is a grave problem in retirement communities where the middle class have left their lifetime identity with work and community to move to "fun in the sun." Happy hour becomes a day-long rite. The Veterans' Administration hospitals particularly have a high rate of alcoholism among the older men in the domiciliaries. Ebersole and Hess (1981) describe the community efforts to help the elderly alcoholic. For example, nearly every town has its Alcoholics Anonymous unit, which usually includes many women alcoholics.

Christopherson, Bainton, and Escher have a grant to study alcoholism among the rural elderly in Arizona. Sixteen percent of their sample described themselves as heavy drinkers, with men consistently outdrinking women (Knetzger, 1979). Christopherson found the Mexican-American man especially had a problem, which was concealed by his spouse and family. Ethnic groups were particularly aggravated by a sense of isolation, limited recreational activities, frustration, and feelings of discrimination from society outside the barrios.

The physical and behavioral effects of drugs and alcohol in combination are important whether the client is an occasional, moderate, or chronic drinker. The Federal Drug Administration (FDA) bulletin (1979) on alchohol-drug interactions estimates that of the 100 most frequently prescribed drugs, at least half have an ingredient that reacts adversely with alcohol. The statistical estimate of alcohol-drug interactions is 2,500 deaths and 47,000 emergency room admissions per year. Chronic alcoholics may have liver damage that alters drug effects. Even abstaining alcoholics need drug doses that differ from those required by the nondrinker to obtain a therapeutic drug level.

Drugs that react with alcohol to compromise brain support include:

1. Antianginal and antihypertensive agents (see hypotension in this chapter)
2. Antidepressants and stimulants—may cause hypotension
3. Antihistamines—drowsiness and inability to think
4. Antidiabetic agents (hypoglycemics)—potentiate hypoglycemia (see hypoglycemia)
5. Barbiturates—respiratory depression with hypoxia may lead to coma and death
6. Benzodiazepines (Librium, Valium, and Dalmane) and meprobamate (Equanil)—reduce attention span and alertness
7. Major tranquilizers (phenothiazines) (see hypotension)
8. Narcotics—depressant for the central nervous system; respiratory depressant—hypoxia

Sedative hypnotics

The widespread insomnia problem of the elderly is often a manifestation of depression that can be attributed to the life situation (Butler and Lewis, 1977). The solution is often a social one—the restoration of ability to love and be loved. Frequently, there is no one to make the effort. *The problem becomes a medical one, for the physician is the legal gatekeeper to the sleeping pill.* From 1971 to 1977 there was a 39% decrease in hypnotic prescriptions (Institute of Medicine study, 1978). Barbiturates had dropped from 47% of hypnotic prescriptions in 1971 to 17% in 1977, and flurazepam (Dalmane) had increased from a newly discovered drug to 53% of the prescriptions in 1977. The IOM report challenges the impression that the benzodiazepine hypnotics are safer and more effective than the barbiturates and says that neither drug is ideal. The committee making the report commented on the increased likelihood of adverse reaction with patients of advancing age and patients with diminished kidney function.

The report emphasized that treatment for insomnia be restricted to short-term use. Sleep laboratories had shown loss of sleep-promoting properties within 3 to 14 days of continuous use. The buildup of flurazepam

Table 9-4. Plasma half-life values for barbiturates and flurazepam in adults*

Drug	Half-life in hours in adults
Flurazepam (Dalmane)	50-100
Amobarbital (Amytal)	16-24
Butabarbital (Butisol Sodium)	62-138
Pentobarbital (Nembutal)	21-48
Phenobarbital	72-96
Secobarbital (Seconal)	20-28

*Adapted from FDA Bulletin, Vol. 9, No. 3, p. 17.

in the body led to an unwanted carry-over effect in the daytime with drowsiness, poor coordination, and poor mentation. The plasma half-life of sedative hypnotic drugs is shown in Table 9-4, indicating that for some drugs it may be 4 days.

Unexpected toxic reactions with alcohol can occur when the client taking nighttime sedatives drinks alcohol on the following day or even the second following day.

The IOM report (1978) advises physicians to look for and treat the underlying disorders that cause insomnia and to restrict the ordering of hypnotics. The nurse is often the person who makes the contact with the physician for the institutionalized client. Her description of the problem, professional anxiety to treat, and the easy answer found in hypnotics have led to the routine passing of "sleepers" at night. A hypnotic ordered "p.r.n." is given regularly without assessing its need. The nursing assessment of the client should include an estimation of the insomnia and its probable cause. Many older people do not sleep all night but are up and down. There is no harm in this, except to the anxious caregiver. A sociable hot drink and time in a rocking chair with company will often result in drowsiness and spontaneous sleep. The number of hypnotics given on the evening shift probably reflects the philosophy and need of the nurses more than the need of the client. Night is traditionally the time for quiet. But the elderly may have a quiet day during which their naps cared for sleep needs. There should be a nightroom for those who do not sleep and are not harmed by it, just as there is a dayroom. The nightroom would have hot milk, hot tea, Postum, or coffee. There should be rocking chairs and music by earphones to listen to all-night radio programs. The elderly want to be part of the action rather than lying sleepless in bed staring at the dark and worrying about some personal problem. There would be little confusion from hypnotics in such an environment, and clients would be alert at breakfast.

The physician may be the gatekeeper for hypnotics, but nurses hold the key to the gate.

Tardive dyskinesia

In the past 10 years the effects of using neuroleptics, or tranquilizers, to treat the mentally ill or the elderly who were confused, agitated, and depressed has brought a drug-induced problem called "tardive dyskinesia." Tardive refers to tardy or late-appearing, and dyskinesia derives from the Greek root "kinesia," meaning movement. It is assumed to be the result of long exposure to neuroleptics, and Crane (1973) estimates that the "percentage may rise to 50 among the patients over 60 who have been exposed to neuroleptics for three years or longer" (p.127). A study of outpatients at Mount Sinai Medical Center reported 40% of the patients had tardive dyskinesia, although some were presenting subtle, barely detectable symptoms (Horowitz, 1978). Horowitz also found it in patients who had been taking phenothiazines for as little time as 3 weeks. Weiss and Santelli (1978) have reported that intermittent administration of haloperidol (Haldol) produced movement disorders in nonhuman primates when given continuously for several months, then discontinued for 508 days. Drug sensitivity persisted, and dyskinetic episodes occurred.

The dyskinesia resembles Huntington's

chorea or parkinsonism. The symptoms may be mild and not interfere with activity, or they may be so severe that breathing, swallowing, and speaking are problems. The facial symptoms interfere with social interaction (Chapter 7). Other signs and symptoms include:
1. Rhythmic and involuntary movements of face and limbs
2. Cheek puffing
3. Lip smacking or pursing
4. Chewing movements of mouth and lips
5. Undulation of the tongue and repeated tongue thrusts in a flycatcher movement
6. Stiffness of neck and arms
7. Difficulty in swallowing and speaking
8. Rotation of ankles and constant movement of hands

The client who is receiving any of the neuroleptics should be watched for early detection of the tremor and movements of the mouth. The treatment should be to discontinue the drug. Often this is not done, and the client will be given some antispasmodic, such as those given for Parkinson's syndrome, in addition to his neuroleptic. The issue concerning discontinuing the drug has become a medicolegal one. An editorial written by the 1973 FDA-American College of Neuropsychopharmacology Task Force states: "Because of lack of adequate substitutes for the neuroleptic drugs in the treatment of psychosis, tardive dyskinesia has been accepted as an occasionally unavoidable price to be paid for the benefits of prolonged neuroleptic therapy" (Horowitz, 1978).

The legal aspects of neuroleptic therapy have resulted in a few suits against the physician and drug manufacturer with a verdict for the client. Since the symptoms may come much later, the client may not be able to trace back to the specific drug. Physicians have not accepted responsibility for drug reaction.

Tardive dyskinesia holds many implications for nurses. The nurse who administers neuroleptics to the elderly or who supervises their care should be aware of the potential hazard. No drug should be used past its point of usefulness. Clients admitted to institutions are often given neuroleptics to cover the "relocation shock." There are other methods available that require human interaction and do not result in dyskinesia. Relocation is described in this book as a stressful event requiring excellent nursing care. That care cannot be exchanged for tiny colored pills with the same effect. Long-term care institutions should have special personnel trained in dealing with the agitated or depressed person. Ritualization in treating the elderly confused and agitated client has resulted in viewing drug therapy as indispensable. In some centers all clients are placed on Mellaril until they are docile and adjusted. The treatment is called the Mellaril routine and includes increased doses until the client misses a breakfast because he is too drowsy to eat. The nurse who participates in such ritualized therapy without trying other alternatives is party to the development of the tardive dyskinesia. Administrative, economic, and political pressures have led to senseless ritualization of drug therapy that may lead to continuation of the drugs for persons who are unimproved or even asymptomatic for many months and years (Horowitz, 1978).

Prognosis of tardive dyskinesia is poor on the basis of present knowledge of treatment. Research is being done on the use of choline (found in eggs, fish, liver, and soybeans) to relieve the condition, with reports of mixed results.

Neuroleptics implicated in tardive dyskinesia

Phenothiazines: chlorpromazine (Thorazine); thioridazine (Mellaril); trifluoperazine (Stelazine)
Butyrophenones: haloperidol (Haldol)
Thiothixenes: (Navane)

Is tardive dyskinesia a political affair? Is the government involved? The success of the neuroleptics have led to large profits by the pharmaceutical companies that produce the drugs. There is pressure on Congress to leave the situation as it is. It is an economic problem as well as a medical and legal one.

The situation is so recent that the nurse should keep herself informed of developments on all fronts. In the meantime, she does her client a service by being fully aware of the newest findings in tardive dyskinesia.

CHAPTER 9 SUMMARY
Confusional states secondary to compromised brain support

Cause	Signs and symptoms	Prevention	Nursing intervention
Hypoxia	Confused behavior, restlessness, impaired memory, dyspnea, and abnormal blood gas values		Immediate: care of confusion (Chapter 8)
Anemic hypoxia (hypoxia caused by reduction in amount of hemoglobin or blood available for oxygen transport)			
Gradual blood loss Gastrointestinal tract bleeding	Gradual blood loss compensated until large amount lost, pallor, weakness, and hemorrhage	Monitor aspirin ingestion	Assist in restoration of hemoglobin or blood cells Teach dietary intervention and medical self-help
Pernicious anemia Lack of intrinsic factor Lack of vitamin B_{12}	Weakness to loss of use of extremities, confusion, and soreness and burning of tongue	None known	Provide replacement of vitamin B_{12} Assist in neurologic restoration and adaptation to disease
Folic-acid deficiency Lack of folic acid in diet	Same as for pernicious anemia	Diet that includes fresh fruit and vegetables	Teach dietary need Assess life-style and assist in modification
Hemolytic anemias (destruction of blood-forming organs) Drugs and infection	Loss of red blood cells Acute: chills, fever, irritability, pain, and oliguria		Support client's physiologic status Assist with the medical regime
Histotoxic anemia Conditions that threaten the narrow range within which the neurons function			
Fluid and electrolyte imbalance Dehydration	Apathy and confusion, thick, ropy saliva, anorexia, oliguria, weak pulse, arrhythmias, shock level with hypovolemia, decreased blood pressure, deeper respiration, dehydration, muscle weakness, abdominal distention (K^+ deficiency)	Monitor fluid intake and drugs ingested	Provide fluids and replacement safely Teach preventive measures

Continued.

CHAPTER 9 SUMMARY
Confusional states secondary to compromised brain support—cont'd

Cause	Signs and symptoms	Prevention	Nursing intervention
Hypocalcemia Decrease of Ca^{++} in blood serum	Tetany, irritability, change in mental status, acidosis, and positive Chvostek's sign. Increase in nerve activity	Dietary intake of calcium	Facilitate Ca^{++} replacement. Provide safety and supportive care for client with demineralization. Teach about calcium replacement and plan for discharge
Hypercalcemia Serum calcium level above 5.7 mEq/liter	Depression of nerve activity, apathy, lethargy, depression, decreased gastrointestinal activity, anorexia, skeletal and cardiac muscle weakness, thirst, and polyuria	Promote mobilization. Avoid excessive vitamin D, antacids, and total milk diet	Restore fluid volume. Prevent fracture. Teach specific prevention and specific treatment for cause
Temperature imbalances Hyperthermia — core temperature above 100° F (37.7°C)	Apathy, weakness, increased body temperature, change in mental status, and fast pulse and respiration	Avoid infection and high ambient temperature	Relieve hyperthermia. Observe for source. Support client and share his experiences of hallucinations and illusions
Hypothermia — core temperature below 95° F (35° C)	Decreased body temperature, mental status sluggish, and confused to comatose	Note high-risk persons. Avoid low ambient temperature. Obtain drug profile. Check on those who live alone for warm housing and beds	Restore body temperature safely. Teach to prevent recurrence. Refer to community agencies
Azotemia Kidney failure	Behavioral changes, gastrointestinal signs of anorexia, cardiorenal signs of pitting edema, dyspnea, decreased urinary output, bleeding, laboratory tests and results, anemia	Can be controlled, but prevention impossible at this time for the elderly	Restore fluid and electrolyte balance as part of delegated medical regime. Monitor and observe. Give supportive care. Teach and plan with family for discharge or for peaceful death

Care of the client with confusion secondary to compromised brain support

Hypoxemic hypoxia			
Ventilatory problems	Confusion, dyspnea, use of accessory muscles, cough, and poor chest expansion	Reduce stress	Prevent accumulation of secretions
Poor gas exchange		Prevent accumulation of secretions	Assess observations
Aging changes in chest and lungs			Teach cough, deep breathing, positioning, and pain relief
Environmental insults to lungs			Teach to live within limitations
Hypoxia from poor perfusion of blood to brain			
Cardiac failure	Confusion, dyspnea, edema, orthopnea, basal pulmonary rales, and liver engorgement	Minimize cardiac stress, both physiologic and emotional	Conserve cardiac strength by reducing energy demands
Aging changes			Reduce fluid volume
Disease that reduces cardiac output			Plan discharge for life-style compatible with cardiac limitations
Hypotension			
Vasodilatation from drugs or poor circulatory reaction to change in position	Dizziness, confusion, and syncope	Treat cause	Relieve emergency and provide blood to brain
		Teach client how to change from horizontal to vertical position	Help determine cause and institute preventive regimen
		Arrange for observation	Plan for discharge
Increased intracranial pressure			
Subdural hematoma	Change in behavior, headache, increased blood pressure, decreased pulse and respiratory rate, and motor signs of weakness and loss of reflexes	Prevent falls and jolts to head	Give postsurgical care
			Restore premorbid personality by maintaining link with life history and reality
Normal pressure hydrocephalus (NPH)	Recent onset of confusion, gait disturbance, and later incontinence	None known	Give postsurgical care
Dilatation of ventricles of brain with fluid and crowding of cortex and other brain tissue		Early detection	Restore orientation
			Assist family to accept condition
Hyperglycemia			
Adult-onset diabetes with added stressors	Thirst, polyuria, dehydration, confusion, hypotension, coma, and abnormally high blood glucose level	Predict stressors: burns, hypothermia, drugs, and dehydration	Rehydrate and restore electrolytes in intensive care setting

Continued.

CHAPTER 9 SUMMARY
Confusional states secondary to compromised brain support—cont'd

Cause	Signs and symptoms	Prevention	Nursing intervention
Hypoglycemia Sudden reduction or gradual reduction of blood glucose below functional level	Confusion, nocturnal headache, diplopia, nightmares, apprehension, coma, seizures, and abnormally low blood glucose level	Adequate diet; if prevented by inability to take food, hypoglycemic drugs withheld	Restore blood glucose Teach prevention at discharge
Drug toxicity Polypharmacy Altered physiology of the aged Interaction of drugs	Confusion, other signs dependent on nature of drug: digitalis, phenothiazines, or sedatives	Prediction of likelihood in face of polypharmacy, age, and physiologic status	Prevent toxicity Withhold drug Plan at discharge for a new life-style requiring fewer or no drugs

REFERENCES

Abbey, J.: Personal communication, 1974.

Adams, R.D., and others: Symptomatic occult hydrocephalus with normal cerebrospinal fluid pressure, N. Eng. J. Med. **273**:117-126, 1965.

Agate, J.: Common symptoms and complaints. In Rossman, I., editor: Clinical geriatrics, Philadelphia, 1971, J.B. Lippincott Co.

Allen, E.T.: Prolonged immersion in cold water, Nurs. Times **70**:1928, 1974.

Alpers, B.J., and Mancall, E.L.: Clinical neurology, Philadelphia, 1971, F.A. Davis Co.

Barber, J.M., Stokes, L.G., and Billings, D.M.: Adult and child care, St. Louis, 1977, The C.V. Mosby Co.

Besdine, R.W.: Treatable dementia in the elderly—task force draft, May 1978, National Institute of Aging.

Brocklehurst, J.C.: The urinary tract. In Rossman, I., editor: Clinical geriatrics, Philadelphia, 1971, J.B. Lippincott Co.

Brown, F.R.: Problems of the heart and major blood vessels. In Phipps, W.J., Long, B.C., and Woods, N.F., editors: Medical-surgical nursing: concepts and clinical practice, St. Louis, 1979, The C.V. Mosby Co.

Brown, M.M.: Drug-drug interactions among residents in homes for the elderly, Nurs. Res. **26**(1):50, 1977.

Butler, R.N., and Lewis, M.I.: Aging and mental health, ed. 2, St. Louis, 1977, The C.V. Mosby Co.

Caird, F.I., and Dall, J.L.C.: The cardiovascular system. In Brocklehurst, J.C., editor: Textbook of geriatric medicine and gerontology, Edinburgh, 1973, Churchill-Livingstone Co.

Caranasos, G.J., and others: Drug-induced illness leading to hospitalization, J.A.M.A. **228**:713-717, 1974.

Carter, A.B.: The neurologic aspects of aging. In Rossman, I., editor: Clinical geriatrics, Philadelphia, 1971, J.B. Lippincott Co.

Cassmeyer, V.: Management of persons with impaired regulatory mechanisms. In Phipps, W.J., Long, B.C., and Woods, N.F., editors: Medical-surgical nursing: concepts and clinical practice, St. Louis, 1979, The C.V. Mosby Co.

Coleman, J.H., and Evans, W.E.: Drug interaction with alcohol, Alcohol Health Res. World, Winter 1979.

Crane, G.E.: Clinical psychopharmacology in its 20th year, Science **181**:124-128, 1973.

Daly, B., and Norman, A.: Respiratory assessment. In Phipps, W.J., Long, B.C., and Woods, N.F., editors: Medical-surgical nursing: concepts and clinical practice, St. Louis, 1979, The C.V. Mosby Co.

Daly, B., Phipps, W., and Brown, F.: Management of the person with impaired oxygen-carbon dioxide exchange. In Phipps, W.J., Long, B.C., and Woods, N.F., editors: Medical-surgical nursing:

concepts and clinical practice, St. Louis, 1979, The C.V. Mosby Co.

Duncalf, D., and Kepes, E.R.: Geriatric anaesthesia. In Rossman, I., editor: Clinical geriatrics, Philadelphia, 1971, J.B Lippincott Co.

Ebersole, P., and Hess, P.: Care of the aged: nursing roles and functions, St. Louis, 1981, The C.V. Mosby Co., Chapter 8.

Epstein, L.J., and Simon, A.: Organic brain syndrome in the elderly, Geriatrics 22:145-150, 1967.

Exton-Smith, A.N., and Windsor, A.C.M.: Principles of drug treatment in the aged. In Rossman, I., editor: Clinical geriatrics, Philadelphia, 1971, J.B. Lippincott Co.

Federal Drug Administration bulletin: Alcohol-drug interactions, 9(2), Rockville, Md., 1979, Department of HEW Food and Drug Administration.

Federal Drug Administration bulletin: Update on sedative hypnotics, 9(3), Rockville, Md., 1979, Department of HEW Food and Drug Administration.

Feist, R.R.: A survey of accidental falls in a small home for the aged, J. Gerontological Nurs. 4(6):15-17, 1978.

Goldfarb, A.I.: Aging in humans. In Goldman, R., and Rockstein, M., editors: The physiology and pathology of human aging, New York, 1975, Academic Press, Inc.

Green, M.F.: Hypothermia and the elderly, Queen's Nurs. J., November 1975, pp. 214-216.

Groer, M.E., and Shekleton, M.E.: Basic pathophysiology, a conceptual approach, St. Louis, 1979, The C.V. Mosby Co.

Harris, R.: The management of geriatric cardiovascular disease, Philadelphia, 1970, J.B. Lippincott Co.

Horowitz, J.: The hidden cost of mind-medicines, Hum. Behav. 7(5): 53-55, 1978.

Hurwitz, N.: Predisposing factors in adverse reactions to drugs, Br. Med. J. 1:536-539, 1969.

Institute of Medicine report: Sleeping pills: insomnia and medical practice, Office of Publications, National Academy of Science, Washington, D.C., 1978.

Irvine, R.F.: Hypothermia in old age, Practitioner 213(1278):795-800, 1974.

Jaffe, J.: Common lower urinary tract problems in older people. In working with older people, vol. 4, 1971, Department of Health, Education and Welfare, pp. 141, 143-145.

Johnson, M.: Outcome criteria to evaluate postoperative respiratory status, Am. J. Nurs. 75(9):1474-1475, 1975.

Katzman, R.: Cerebrospinal fluid physiology and normal pressure hydrocephalus. In Gerson, S., and Terry, R., editors: Aging, vol. 3, New York, 1976, Raven Press.

Kayne, R.C.: Drugs and the aged. In Burnside, I., editor: Nursing and the aged, New York, 1976, McGraw-Hill Book Co.

Kinney, M.: Management of the person with neurological manifestations. In Phipps, W. J., Long, B.C., and Woods, N.F., editors: Medical-surgical nursing: concepts and clinical practice, St. Louis, 1979, The C.V. Mosby Co.

Klocke, R.A.: Influences of aging on the lung. In Finch, C.E., and Hayflick, L.E., editors: Handbook of the biology of aging, New York, 1977, Van Nostrand Reinhold Co.

Knetzger, J.: Drinking: a problem for many older Americans, *Arizona Daily Wildcat*, Tucson, University of Arizona Press, Feb. 16, 1979, p. 3.

Kolata, G.B.: Blood sugar and the complications of diabetes, Science 203:1098-1099, 1979.

Lancet editorial: Normal pressure hydrocephalus, Lancet 2(8046):1011-1012, 1977.

MacLean, D., and others: Metabolic aspects of spontaneous rewarming in accidental hypothermia and hypothermic myxdema, Q. J. Med. 43:471-487, 1974.

Miller, P.L.: Problems of the urinary system. In Phipps, W.J., Long, B.C., and Woods, N.F., editors: Medical-surgical nursing: concepts and clinical practice, St. Louis, 1979, The C.V. Mosby Co.

Mitten, C.J., and Phipps, W J.: Endocrine dysfunction. In Phipps, W.J., Long, B.C., and Woods, N.F., editors: Medical-surgical nursing: concepts and clinical practice, St. Louis, 1979, The C.V. Mosby Co.

Myers, R.D., and Veale, W.L.: Body temperature: possible ionic mechanism in the hypothalamus controlling the set point, Science 70:95-97, 1970.

National Institutes on Aging: A winter hazard for the old: accidental hypothermia, DHEW publication no. (NH)78-1464. Washington, D.C., 1978, U.S. Government Printing Office.

Nicolas, F., and others: Circulatory and metabolic disturbances in accidental hypothermia, Bull. Physiopathol. Respir. 11:757-785, 1975.

Olson, J., and Johnson, J.: Drug misuse among the elderly, J. Gerontological Nurs. 4(6):11-14, 1978.

Ozuma, J.M., and Foster, C.: Hypothermia and the surgical patient, Am. J. Nurs. 79(4):646-648, 1979.

Phipps, W.J., Long, B.C., and Woods, N.F., editors: Medical-surgical nursing: concepts and clinical practice, St. Louis, 1979, The C.V. Mosby Co.

Pinel, C.: Accidental hypothermia in the elderly, Nurs. Times 71:1848, 1975.

Ritchey, D.P.: Effects of human aging on drug absorption and metabolism. In Goldman, R., and Rockstein, M., editors: The physiology and pathology of human aging, New York, 1975, Academic Press, Inc.

Rifkin, H., and Ross, H.: Diabetes in the elderly. In Rossman, I., editor: Clinical geriatrics, Philadelphia, 1971, J.B. Lippincott Co.

Roberts, S.L.: Renal abnormalities in aging. In Burnside, I.M., editor: Nursing and the aged, New York, 1976, McGraw-Hill Book Co.

Rockstein, M.: The biology of aging in humans, an

overview. In Rockstein, M., and Goldman, R., editors: The physiology and pathology of human aging, New York, 1975, Academic Press, Inc.

Rockstein, M., and Sussman, M.: Biology of aging, Belmont, Calif., 1979, Wadsworth Publishing Co.

Rodstein, M.: Heart disease in the aged. In Rossman, I., editor: Clinical geriatrics, Philadelphia, 1971, J.B. Lippincott Co.

Rosen, S.: Weathering, New York, 1979, M. Evans Co., Inc.

Sadikali, F., and Owor, R.: Hypothermia in the tropics, Trop. Geogr. Med. **26**:265-270, 1974.

Scribner, B.H., editor: A teaching syllabus for the course on fluid and electrolyte balance, ed. 7, School of Medicine, University of Washington, Seattle, 1969.

Seymour, G., and others: Confusional states in the elderly. Paper presented at the International Congress of Gerontology, Tokyo, Japan, Aug. 24, 1979.

Shields, E.M.: Introduction to drug therapy for older adults, J. Gerontological Nurs. **1**(1):8, 1975.

Shirrifs, C.G., and Bresher, P.D.: Hypothermia, abdominal pain, and lactic acid in phenoformin-treated diabetes, J. Br. Med. **3**:506, 1970.

Soltis, B.: Fluid and electrolyte imbalance. In Phipps, W.J., Long, B.C., and Woods, N.F., editors: Medical-surgical nursing: concepts and clinical practice, St. Louis, 1979, The C.V. Mosby Co.

Spencer, H., Baladad, J., and Lewin, I.: The skeletal system, osteoporosis. In Rossman, I., editor: Clinical geriatrics, Philadelphia, 1971, J.B. Lippincott Co.

Steinman, M.: The Catch-22 of antipsychotic drugs, *New York Times Magazine,* March 18, 1979.

Stone, M.H.: Normal pressure hydrocephalus, Nurs. Clin. North Am. **9**(4):667-676, 1974.

Timiras, P.: Developmental physiology and aging, New York, 1972, The Macmillan Co.

Tripp, A.: Hyper- and hypocalcemia, Am. J. Nurs. **76**:1142-1145, 1976.

Wachman, A., and Bernstein, D.S.: Diet and osteoporosis, Lancet **1**:958, 1968.

Weiss, B., and Santelli, S.: Dyskinesias evoked in monkeys by weekly administration of haloperidol, Science **200**:799-801, 1978.

Wilson, S.F.: Neuronursing, New York, 1979, Springer Publishing Co., Inc.

10

CARE OF THE CLIENT WITH SENSORIPERCEPTUAL PROBLEMS

Linda Ree Fraelich Phillips

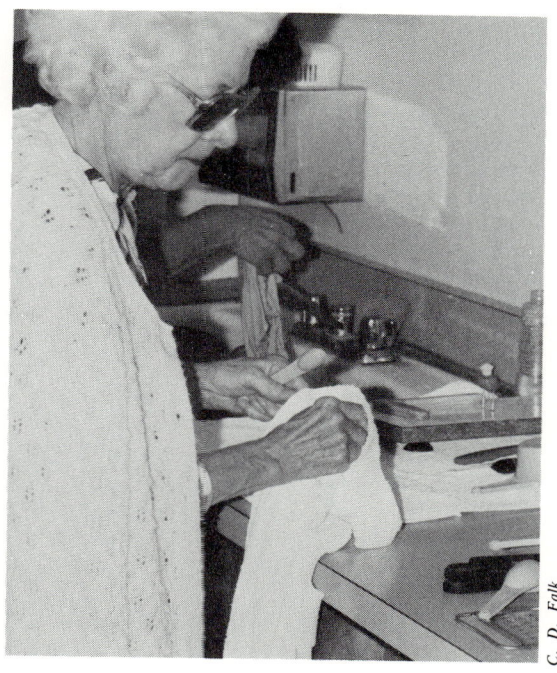

Anna Black is 72 years of age. She resides on a unit in a nursing home that is specially designed for people who need careful supervision. She was placed on that unit because she is confused and she wanders. In addition to being confused, she is blind, her hearing is impaired, and English is not her primary language.

Ms. Black is one of 20 similar patients who were observed in an informal study of confused people on the special unit (Phillips, 1979). All of the residents in the study were over the age of 65, with an average age of 78. Thirteen of the residents had a diagnosis of organic brain syndrome or related diagnosis. Although the remaining seven residents had diagnoses unrelated to their mental states, they were all placed on the unit because of their confusion. For the most part, all residents on the unit, like Ms. Black, were described by the nursing staff as "confused and disoriented to time and place." In addition, three of the residents were described as having hallucinations and one as having compulsive behavior.

Other characteristics were common in the group. Three residents were limited in their ability to speak by aphasia. Four were limited in their ability to communicate because their primary language was not English. Five had visual impairments that were not helped by glasses or they did not wear their glasses; one was totally blind. Of 20 residents, only four had good vision, with or without glasses. Seven residents had a documented hearing impairment, with two of these suffering a bilateral hearing loss. None of the hearing impaired elderly was significantly helped by the use of a hearing aid.

What implications do these findings have for a discussion of confusion? Some evidence indicates that the way in which elderly people perceive and interact with the environment is related to confusional states. Decreased vision has been related to decreased mental competency by Weinberg (1975) and Snyder, Pyrek, and Smith (1976). Eisdorfer (1960), Weiss (1965), and O'Neil and Calhoun (1975), have demonstrated a relationship between lower scores on mental status tests and compromised sensory functioning. The aging process is characterized by many changes in the sensory apparatus. Virtually every sensory modality is affected by these primary changes and accompanying pathologic changes. Therefore, sensory alteration as a possible cause of confusion among elderly people cannot be ignored.

SENSORY ALTERATION: THE ISOLATING EXPERIENCE

Sensory alteration is defined as the state produced by "a situation in which reception or perception of stimuli is blocked or altered, or in which the environmental stimuli themselves are blocked or altered" (Chodil and Williams, 1970, p. 455). Subsumed in the concept of sensory alteration are (1) sensory deprivation, or the limitation of sensory input, from whatever source, below the level to which the person is accustomed; (2) sensory overload, or the increase of sensory input over the level to which the person is accustomed; and (3) sensory distortion, or the alteration of sensory input to a degree that the person can no longer ascertain the relationships between stimuli or perceive identifying cues in the input. It has been shown that when a normal, healthy young person is placed is an isolating situation where any one of these is induced, profound behavioral changes result (Heron, Bexton, and Hebb, 1953; Bexton, Heron, and Scott, 1954; Doane and others, 1959; Scott and others, 1959; Jackson and Ellis, 1971; Brownfield, 1972; Bolin, 1974). Although not adequately investigated, the effects of illness and aging appear to facilitate the sensory alteration experience (Greenwood, 1928; Mendelson and Foley, 1956; Ziskind, 1960; Jackson and others, 1962; Kornfield, Zimberg, and Malm, 1965; Leiderman and associates, 1968; Ellis, 1972; Bolin, 1974; Oster, 1976).

Common to all of the experiments conducted and all of the anecdotal reports given to date is a set of environmental conditions that promote sensory alteration. Brownfield (1972) calls these "characteristics of isolation situations." They are (1) confinement to a limited space; (2) separation from people, place, or things to which the person is attached or dependent; (3) removal from a total environment of usual sensations; and (4) imposition of invariable or monotonous stimulation. Confinement can be accomplished by actual physical restraint, such as wrist, leg, or body straps and barriers, such as doors or walls; by potential physical restraint, such as threats or commands; and by psychologic restraints, such as time restrictions, curfews, or deadlines. The chemical restraint of sedative and tranquilizers can be considered in this category. Separation can be accomplished by actual loss, through death or destruction, or by potential loss, through disrupted, censored or delayed communication, distance, and conflicting duties or responsibilities. Removal from the usual sensations can be accomplished by decreased social interaction or confinement; the key issue is a reduction in or relative absence of normal levels of sensory stimulation. Imposition of monotonous stimulation can be accomplished by making the stimulation so invariable that it is no longer perceived. It is important to note that monotony of stimulation is independent of intensity of stimulation. An intense visual, auditory, or tactile experience can become as monotonous as a muffled one. For example, a soldier can sleep during an artillery barrage but probably will awaken when the noise stops (Brownfield, 1972). For the elderly person whose life resources are already limited, institutionalization may produce an isolating situation that meets these characteristics quite closely.

Various theories have been proposed to explain the reactions of individuals to sensory alteration. The most widely accepted are the optimal level of stimulation theory and sensoriatasis, or the drive for sensory variation. Basically, these theories state that an individual must maintain an optimal range, level, and variety of external stimulation to maintain awareness. The individual will act so that optimal levels of stimulation are maintained. Therefore, at times, there will be motivation to increase stimulation and at other times to decrease stimulation. Brownfield (1972) suggests that each individual has a personal optimal level that may stem from early postnatal levels of stimulation. Zuckerman (1969) suggests that evidence for individual differences in lifelong optimal levels of sensory stimulation is found in everyday life.

Contrast the individual who needs absolute quiet for cognitive activity and the person who can work only with the din of music and voices around him. Consider persons who manage their lives so that every event is repeated, regular and predictable and those whose lives are in continual uproar because of their need to vary their stimulation and maintain a high level of excitement (p. 529).

This is the contrast between the habitual "sensation seekers" and those who are "sensation reducers."

In addition, the uniquely personal optimal range of stimulation can shift based on (1) the task in which the individual is engaged, (2) the previous level of stimulation, and (3) the present overall state of the individual (Brownfield, 1972). Some of the individual variation seen in different desires for stimulation can be attributed to the reinforcing qualities of sensory variation.

Schultz (1965) argues that learning and behavior can occur in situations in which the organism is reinforced *only* by variation in sensory input. Exploration, manipulation, curiosity, and play are probably examples of this. Some experimenters suggest that even pain can be a reinforcing experience if it serves to increase the stimulation level from minimal to optimal (Leuba, 1955). *The concept of individual differences in the optimal level of stimulation and variation is crucial in a conceptualization of sensory alteration.*

Cerebral mechanisms have been used to explain sensory alteration. It is thought that the anterior two thirds of the reticular activating system (RAS) of the brain serves a major function in monitoring stimulation, altering attention, and maintaining arousal. The template-matching model is used to explain the function and activity of the RAS under normal circumstances (Bruce, 1977). The template-matching model states that the RAS is "programmed" with predictable expectations about acceptable inputs. Changes in the intensity and characteristics of input to the RAS result in a mismatch with the existing template. Stimuli are then projected onto the cerebral cortex for fine analysis and perception. For awareness and arousal, it is necessary that a certain number of stimuli "mismatch" with the template.

Diffuse nerve pathways converge in the RAS. Sources of stimulation for the RAS are (1) external, or from the peripheral and visceral sensory receptions; and (2) internal, or from the cerebral cortex itself. From either of these sources, the activation is nonspecific and interchangeable. Either can result in arousal of the individual. Duffy (1962) states that, under normal conditions, the interchange of internal and external stimulation is primarily facilitative. If stimulation from either source becomes excessive, the results are impairment or blocking of the RAS and disturbances of awareness and attention. Sensory overload seems to interfere with the neural "directing" of

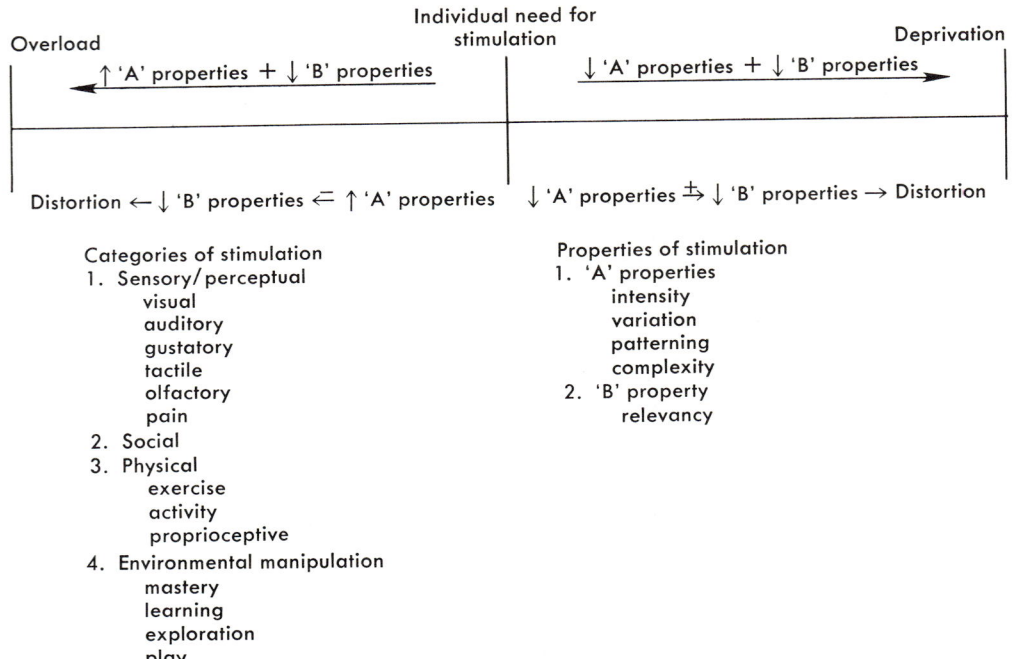

Fig. 10-1. Model of sensory alteration.

stimuli. In sensory deprivation, it is thought that low levels of environmental stimulation in combination with uncontrolled internal stimulation produce inappropriate imagery and cognitive disorganization.

The information processing theory of perception helps explain sensory alteration. All of the stimuli entering the central nervous system (CNS) at any time are potentially overwhelming. The role of the CNS is to screen, organize, and structure the input in such a way that the individual can make sense of the internal and external environment. Certain stimuli are perceived and others are undetected because some are simply not strong enough to exceed the threshold for perception. The sensory threshold is not, however, an all-or-none concept. A great deal of individual variation exists in signal detection among healthy people.

"The proportion of correct detections of a stimulus (especially a weak one) depends on not only the observer's discriminative capacity but on . . . the criteria set of deciding whether a stimulus was present or not" (Schiffman, 1977, p. 9). This introduces the idea of relevance in relation to sensory alteration. Not only must stimuli be within the bounds of variability and intensity, but they must also be perceived by the individual as meaningful or relevant. The meaning ascribed to a particular stimulus, therefore, determines, to a certain extent, whether or not it will be perceived. This helps to explain why sensory distortion has a deleterious effect. The individual must be able to make sense of the various stimuli to behave competently (Freedman and Greenblatt, 1959; Davis, McCourt, and Solomon, 1960; Brownfield, 1972).

Fig. 10-1 is a model devised to help explain sensory alteration. Following the model, the reception and perception of sensory stimuli can be viewed on a continuum ranging from overload to deprivation, with the individual need for stimulation at the midpoint. The sources or categories of stimulation arise from at least four areas: (1) sensoriperceptual, including visual, auditory, tactile, gustatory, olfactory, and pain; (2) social, including all forms of relationships, ranging from intense and significant to casual; (3) physical, including exercise and activity; and (4) evironmental manipulation, including mastery, learning, exploration, and play. Each of these categories of stimulation possesses certain properties that are divided into two groups. The 'A' group of properties consists of (1) intensity, or the strength of stimulation; and (2) variation, or the amount of change in the stimulation. Subsets of variation are patterning, or the degree to which the sensory input is predictably organized, and complexity, or the degree of intricacy in the variation. The 'B' property consists of relevancy, or the degree to which the stimulation makes sense to the individual. When there is an increase, above the individual need in either of the 'A' properties, the result is sensory overload. Conversely, when there is a decrease in either of the 'A' properties, below the individual need, the result is sensory underload or sensory deprivation. As the 'A' properties increase or decrease, there is a decrease in the 'B' property of relevance. This decrease is related to sensory distortion, overload, and deprivation.

Reaction to the alteration in sensory input results in the constellation of behavioral manifestations that are characteristics of sensory alteration. These can be roughly categorized as:
1. Effects on sensory function
2. Cognitive and intellectual effects
3. Hallucinations
4. Emotional effects

Any of these, singly or in combination, can be interpreted as or can produce confusion.

Effects on sensory function

The most common sensory effects reported by subjects during and after sensory alteration experiences of isolation are: (1) apparent movement of the room that is independent of movement by the subject, (2) changes in the size and shape of people and objects, (3) expansion and contraction of objects in the room, (4) distortions of shape, (5) the tendency of straight lines to appear curved or wavy, and (6) colors becoming intensified or luminescent (Freedman, 1961). Subjects report perceptual changes similar to those reported by people ingesting hallucinogenics or by Alice after eating the famous mushroom in Wonderland. The effects usually disappear after 20 minutes of normal stimulation, but some have persisted as long as 24 hours after termination of isolation.

Freedman (1961) attributes these changes to a partial breakdown in those processes that are used to organize and stabilize the world. It is thought that spatial and body orientation is a learned phenomenon that requires constant verification by the person. New learning can result in a reorganization of the subject's perspective of the world, but new learning requires environmental cues that are consistent and predictable.

In the normal relationship of an adult human to his environment, "up" is always "up" and "down" is always "down." If he should wear inverting prisms, "up" becomes "down" and "down" becomes "up." This reversal continues becoming the basis for learning a whole new spatial order. . . Whether "up" is always "down" is relatively unimportant provided that the relationship is *continuous* and *predictable* (Freedman, 1961, p. 19).

Sensory alteration presents a situation in which the environment provides no continuous or predictable cues about organization. The relationships between objects and self that were previously ordered are no longer perceptible because the pattern is missing from the environmental cues.

Cognitive and intellectual effects

The most common cognitive effects that have been reported are (1) the inability to concentrate, (2) the inability to control the direction of thoughts, (3) difficulty recalling information and problem solving in some areas, and (4) regression into fantasy. The duration of these effects ranges to several days after the experiment, depending on the total time spent in isolation (Scott and others, 1959; Zubek and associates, 1961). Some subjects report a "sharpening" of intellectual powers during isolation. However, as noted by Scott and associates (1959), Shurley (1960), and Zubek and others (1961), this "increase" in intellectual powers may be more an increase in the ability to visualize or to recall visual images. The subjects who note these changes also report that they cannot work with their thoughts, even though they are quite clear. Kracke (1967) believes that isolation affects reasoning and higher level organizing abilities but may have little influence on the more automatic functions, such as language and simple arithmetic.

Freedman (1961) suggests that cognitive function is related closely to the social isolation involved in sensory alteration. Social isolation may lead to an impairment of the person's ability to test and verify usually shared realities. Kracke, (1967) on the other hand, believes cognitive functioning is affected by sensory alteration because the individual's attention is drawn inward toward fantasy rather than outward toward testing the external environment.

Hallucinations

The most common hallucinations reported have ranged from simple, including (1) seeing dots, colors, and geometric shapes; (2) hearing water running, the sound of wind, the mechanical sounds; and (3) feeling bodily changes such as itching and numbness of the fingers and toes; to complex, including (4) seeing meaningful objects, such as people, animals, and landscapes; (5) hearing voices or music; and (6) feeling the body as light and floating. Some people report tasting and smelling odors that are not present in the environment (Jackson and Ellis, 1971). Hallucinations have been associated with both the amount of light and the amount of tactile stimulation present in the setting. They are more likely to occur in diffuse lighting than in total darkness (Kracke, 1967). The relative absence of tactile sensation speeds the appearance of hallucinations (Lilly, 1956). Kracke (1967) believes hallucinatory activity is caused by the subject's need for external stimulation and the unbalanced presence of internal stimulation. It is thought that the hallucinatory material is directly related to the internal need states of the subject.

Emotional effects

These effects include (1) emotional lability, (2) irritability, (3) brooding and dwelling on imaginary injuries, and (4) moods that are inappropriate, such as amusement or elation (Kracke, 1967). Depression, anxiety, and fear that ranges to panic have been reported by some subjects (Jackson and Ellis, 1971). Ziskind (1960) reports noncompliance and belligerence may result from being deprived of sight.

Kracke (1967) states that emotional disturbances can be explained by a gradual regression of attention and energy toward the self, which results in an impairment of behavioral control mechanisms. The emotional effects may also be precipitated by the isolation experience. Stress arises from boredom and loneliness, enforced regression and dependency, and the frustration of individual drives.

In addition to these subjective manifestations of sensory alteration, objective changes have also been noted. Experimenters and observers report that early in an isolation experience the subject sleeps for a prolonged period. As isolation continues, sleep decreases, with long periods of fitful wakefulness taking its place. Subjects usually try to increase their attempts at self-stimulation during extended isolation with such activities as singing, tapping the fingers, and restless random movement. Masturbation is another form of self-stimulating behavior observed among some individuals in isolation.

In summary, sensory alteration produces a wide range of subjective and objective manifestations. Some of the effects noted are remarkably similar to characteristics associated with confusion among elderly people. However, most of the observational and experimental reports concern normal, healthy people. In addition, most experimental work has been confined to the investigation of sensory deprivation. Specific investigations of sensory distortion and overload are few. It is not empirically or practically clear how all these concepts relate to adult, hospitalized individuals in general, or to elderly clients in particular. More work needs to be done to identify the relationships among sensory alteration, illness, and aging. It would, however, be beneficial to consider some of the literature dealing directly with this subject before discussing the implications of sensory alteration for the nursing care of the aged in the prevention of confusion.

SENSORY ALTERATION, ILLNESS, AND AGING

The literature indicates that sensory alteration has been studied most among three groups of hospitalized people. The first of these are those individuals who are immobilized because of treatment method. In 1956, Mendelson and Foley reported psychotic-like states among patients with bulbar poliomyelitis who were being treated with tank-type respirators. These patients seemed to be adversely affected by the physical restrictions of the respirator and the constant auditory input associated with respirator operation. Leiderman and others (1968) reported similar effects among polio patients and stated that the hallucinations of these patients centered on the sounds of machines and other mechanical sounds. They hallucinated about moving in machines as well. Jackson and associates (1962) reported disorientation, confusion, and anxiety among orthopedic patients shortly after immobilization. Bolin (1974) interviewed orthopedic patients who had been immobilized for long periods and found that many reported disturbed sleep and dreams that were quite different from those they had at home. During the course of dreams two patients in the sample tried to remove the traction apparatus and get out of bed. Leiderman and others (1968) reported that the reactions to immobilization were most dramatic for patients with body casts, orthopedic tongs, and complex traction. Casual observations of orthopedic nurses indicate that patients on CircOlectric beds and Stryker frames may have profound reactions similar to those reported in the literature.

A second group of observed patients are those who have had eye surgery, eye patches, or who are suddenly and temporarily blind. These patients comprise mainly those with cataracts and detached retinas. Mental and behavioral disturbances have been noticed among this group since as early as 1928 (Greenwood). Jackson and O'Neil (1966) report that of 78 patients studied after eye surgery, approximately half displayed perceptual and sensory disturbances that were not related to their age, use of drugs, or physical status. The most profound disturbances occurred on the second postoperative day. Ziskind (1960) reported noncompliant behavior among eye-patched patients, such as trying to pull off the eye patches and trying to get out of bed.

A third group is patients who have had cardiac surgery or who have been in intensive care units. Kornfield, Zimberg, and Maim (1965) report emotional and behavioral changes among postoperative cardiac patients, which they relate to the monotony of respirator and monitor sounds and the lights and presence of unfamiliar sights. These changes are related to sensory distortion. DeMeyer (1967) reports that patients had subjective feelings of sensory overload related to the number of staff present in the intensive care unit, the loss of a sense of time, the presence of continual lights, and the amount of equipment in the intensive care unit. Sixty-seven percent of patients in the Ellis study (1972) reported unusual sensory experiences while in the intensive care unit.

Experimental research relating aging and sensory alteration is minimal. Conceptually, however, Oster (1976) has postulated the effect of sensory alteration or restriction on the elderly client. According to Oster, primary effects on cognition arise from immobilization and the recumbent position, both common "treatments" for previously active elderly people who are institutionalized. He suggests that the recumbent position causes the central nervous system to "disengage," predisposing the elderly to sensory alteration and confusion. "In terms of comparison with the functioning of an engine it might be said that the brain is 'in neutral' when the patient is physically inactive, and becomes 'engaged' when the patient is in the standing position— 'the cephalopedal reflex.' The brain starts to function when the feet touch the floor"

(p. 462). Oster's observations about the effect of immobilization and recumbency are supported by investigations with healthy adults. Zubek and MacNeil (1967) report that the combined effects of isolation and recumbency are most profound, but that prolonged periods in the recumbent position alone is enough to precipitate complex and vivid dreams, worry, fright, hunger, and subjective restlessness.

The physiologic and psychophysiologic changes associated with sensory restriction among elderly people are represented in Fig. 10-2. For Oster, the end result of decreased sensory input is brain cellular atrophy, the ultimate cause of confusion. As stated earlier, this assertion has not been satisfactorily confirmed.

In summary, the constellation of behaviors that nurses call confusion is characterized by disruptive and noncompliant behavior, inattention and memory deficits,

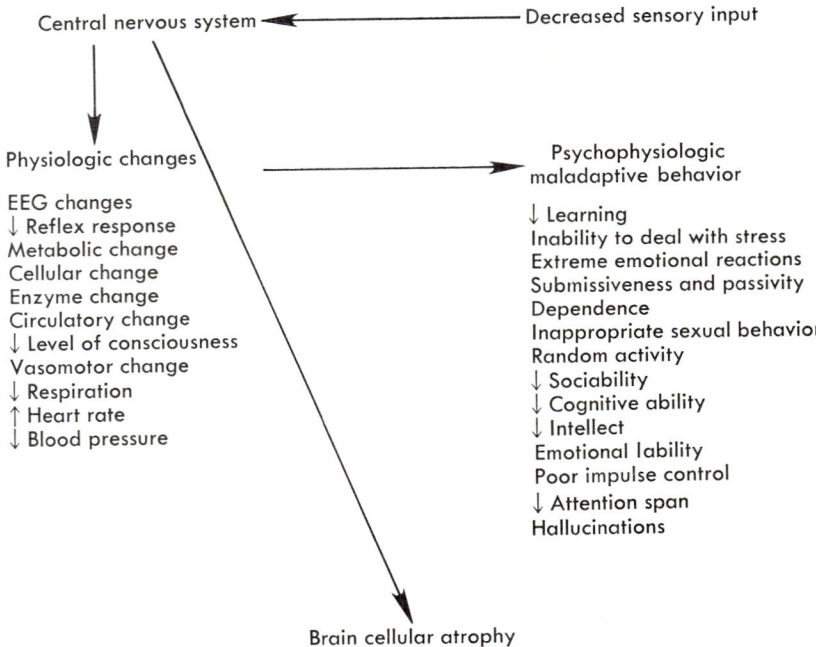

Fig. 10-2. Changes associated with sensory restriction. (From Oster, C.: Sensory deprivation in geriatric patients, J. Am. Geriatr. Soc. **5:**462-463, 1976.)

and inappropriate verbalizations indicative of hallucinations. These same behaviors can be produced by altering the sensory input, by imposing immobility, and by isolation. The implications of this for the elderly are important. Older clients who come to the attention of the health professionals are functioning at a certain level. Some have compromised sensory apparatus as a result of aging, but they have adapted. Some have moderate chronic sensory alteration that could be relieved in the home setting if it were recognized as such. Often confusion is not evident at all prior to institutionalization. Under the care provided in the institutional setting, elderly people may become extremely and sometimes permanently confused. Probably the key to this is change that is imposed on them by caregivers—changes in usual routine, their usual environment, and their usual levels of sensory input. It should be remembered that although changes are sometimes necessary, there are means by which the environment and interactions with the client can be structured to minimize the impact of change.

In addition, sensory alteration does not occur in a vacuum. When an elderly person is admitted to the hospital, complex social and cultural events occur that often lead to states of confusion. For an elderly person, every hospitalization and every contact with a health care worker means the potential limitation of independence. Many older people are deemed unable to care for themselves during a hospitalization or during a visit with their health care worker. If one cannot care for one's self, someone else must provide care. This means major life-style changes. Older people, with or without their consent, are sent to the homes of their children or to nursing homes. Nursing homes are often perceived as terminal and, in reality, often are. Even the placement in the home of an adult son or daughter may mean an end to independent life as the elderly person knew it. Therefore, hospitalization and illness may result in depression, anxiety, and panic for older people, which jeopardize cognitive functioning and interfere with the ability to not be confused.

IMPLICATIONS OF SENSORY ALTERATION FOR THE NURSING CARE OF THE AGED

Elderly people may be particularly prone to the confusion associated with sensory alteration because of physiologic changes within their sensory apparatus. Some of these changes are related directly to the normal aging process, whereas others are related to pathologic changes that are commonly found in the older age groups. Both of these are discussed in this chapter.

In general, the sensory changes of aging result in a diminished receptive ability, making the older person prone to sensory deprivation. Since they are less sensitive to "normal" levels of stimulation, they need quantitatively more intense stimulation to exceed the perceptual threshold. Sensory alteration among the aged, however, is simply not a matter of sensory deprivation. The sensory changes of aging produce a complex reception situation. Many changes of aging are "spotty," meaning that parts of one sensory modality may be entirely intact, whereas other parts are impaired. For example, with impaired hearing, usually only the reception of certain ranges of tone are affected. When the television is loud enough for the elderly client to hear the midrange tones, he is bombarded with sounds in the low ranges where his hearing is relatively normal. This predisposes to sensory overload for some ranges of tone and deprivation for others. The spotty nature of aging changes also causes the elderly to clearly receive only bits and pieces of stimulation rather than the stimulation in its entirety. The result of this situation is sensory distortion. Deprivation, distortion, and overload may therefore coexist for the elderly client. To further complicate the matter, there is some research evidence suggesting that with increasing age, there is a decrease in sensation-seeking behavior and in the optimum range of sensory stimulation (Zuckerman and others, 1964). This suggests that older people may tolerate isolation better than younger people and that older people are more prone to sensory overload than would be expected. As a result, it is difficult to judge what are the acceptable and normal levels of sensory stimulation for the individual older person.

The four sections that follow discuss clinical nursing considerations for the client who is experiencing sensory alterations that result from age-related changes, situational factors, or caregiver factors. First, sensory alteration itself is considered; then the three sensory modalities of vision, hearing, and touch are discussed. In each of these four sections, four separate areas are studied. These are (1) high-risk factors, (2) fourth-level or functional assessment, (3) prevention, and (4) intervention.

The following definitions are used throughout this chapter:

1. High-risk factors—those factors that cause an individual to be particularly vulnerable to the effects of sensory alteration. These factors arise from three sources: the client, the setting, and the caregivers.

The client himself may be at high risk for sensory alteration by virtue of physiologic changes associated with aging or illness that interfere with his perception or reception of stimuli or by virtue of certain psychologic factors that predispose him to the effects of sensory alteration.

The setting may be a high-risk factor because of the prescribed treatment forms or the structural characteristics affecting the stimuli available to the client. Either of these can distort, disrupt, monotonize, mute, intensify, or disorganize stimuli in such a way that variation, intensity, or relevance of the stimuli is affected. Examples of prescribed forms of treatment are bed rest, eye patches, and hearing aids. Structural characteristics of the environment include the level of lighting, the use of wall intercommunication systems, and the physical environment of the institution.

The caregivers may contribute to the high-risk situation because of their personal attributes, their role definitions, or their expectations for the behavior of elderly clients. For example, efficiency and organization tend to be highly valued attributes among nurses. Frequently, elderly people are expected to behave in such a way that neither the institutional routines nor the nurse's routines are disrupted. These expectations often result in a situation wherein the very behaviors that would facilitate the client's interpretation of stimuli, such as wandering, exploring, and verbally communicating, are viewed as disruptive. Thus, older people may be discouraged or prohibited from meeting these needs by nursing behaviors aimed at organizing the environment for the nurse's own purposes.

Although one of the three factors can predominate, in most cases the three interact to produce the high-risk situation. However, defining high-risk factors according to these three categories helps identify specific problems to address for nursing treatment and program planning. The nurse primarily has control over only two of these three areas: the setting and caregivers. Client factors may not be amenable to direct nursing treatment because they often reflect irreversible physiologic changes. This puts the emphasis for nursing in the areas in which nurses have the most control.

2. Fourth-level or functional assessment—those actions or maneuvers that aid in identifying the extent of a client's problems. The fourth level of nursing assessment (see Chapter 5) is the basis for planning the treatment measures for the client. The assessment actions proposed are extensive, but none is particularly complicated. Assessment activities should be selectively performed over time to obtain an accurate data base from which to plan action.

3. Prevention—those actions that help to relieve sensory alteration that, if neglected,

may produce confusional states. These are instituted prior to the onset of confusion. The common theme of the prevention section is the concept of the prosthetic environment. This concept means, literally, that the environment is structured so the client can achieve maximum function, just as other types of prostheses, such as canes, eyeglasses, and artificial limbs, maximize function. To create the prosthetic environment, the client is actively involved in identifying, planning, and implementing the changes necessary to facilitate his understanding to prevent confusion.

4. Intervention—those actions that help relieve the sensory problems that appear to be contributing to the confusion. The common theme of intervention is organized, structured enrichment of the environment and the care situation.

SENSORY ALTERATION
High-risk client factors

Sensory alteration among the elderly is often characterized by multiple moderate deficits that compound each other, with no single, severe or acute deficit.

From the research to date, it can be inferred that certain attributes and characteristics make a person particularly susceptible to the effects of sensory alteration. Unfortunately, these attributes and characteristics have been studied only in relation to young, healthy subjects. As a result, generalization to older individuals can only be inferred. In addition, the assumption is often made that increasing age alone makes a person more susceptible to the effects of sensory deprivation. According to Brownfield (1972), this has yet to be verified among those elderly people with normal sight, hearing, and touch. Most experimental work has not controlled for the age variable. Of the few studies that have, the results have contradicted the assumption that increasing age and increasing susceptibility to sensory deprivation are related. Zuckerman and others (1964) demonstrated that the optimal level of stimulation and sensation-seeking behavior decreases with increased age. This may indicate, as stated earlier, that older individuals tolerate the isolation experience better than younger ones. Clinical research with eye-surgery patients is often used to substantiate the assumption that older individuals tolerate sensory deprivation better than younger ones, since bizarre experiences are more common among patients with detached retinas than among cataract patients at a rate of about two to one (Ziskind, 1960; Jackson and O'Neil, 1966). On the whole, patients with detached retinas are a younger group of people. However, many other variables other than age make these two groups different. These are rarely accounted for and include the rapidity of onset, the length of confinement and immobilization, and bilateral versus unilateral eye patches. The results of the age-related experiments in sensory alteration are therefore inconclusive.

Although there is evidence that age alone is probably not related to an increased susceptibility to sensory deprivation, there is reason to suspect that age in combination with other variables does increase susceptibility. As has been demonstrated, age in combination with sensory deficits makes the person more prone to sensory alteration. This relationship is supported by many researchers (Birren and others 1963; Schaie and associates, 1964; O'Neil and Calhoun 1975). Relocation and age can produce bizarre behavioral manifestations (Butler and Lewis, 1977). The behavioral manifestations demonstrated with relocation are much like those that people demonstrate during sensory alteration situations. These manifestations are most severe among the very old, those with concurrent sensory deficits, and in situations where the environment is strikingly different from the client's previous one. Other research helps to explain why relocation and increased age contribute to sensory alteration. McCaffery (1968) suggests that the less able the person is to perceive pattern and meaning in the environment and the less opportunity the person has to explore the environment, either because of physical immobility or fear, the more likely sensory alteration experiences are. Both of these situations probably occur more frequently among the aged. Maxwell, Bader, and Watson (1972)) support the latter view, stating that behavioral manifestations are most bizarre, or at least as perceived by caregivers, whenever the person has a limited opportunity to learn and practice the territorial rules in a new enviroment. In addition, Oster (1976) states that age and immobilization are related to the appearance of sensory alteration behaviors.

Certain other characteristics and attributes related to the incidence of sensory alteration among the young may have implications for the aged. The most successful subjects in the sensory alteration experiments have been those who report the ability to entertain themselves and to enjoy solitude. These include individuals who have a history of enjoying books rather than television and who do not rely on outside sources of stimulation, such as nonsmokers. People who consider themselves to be introspective seem to tolerate deprivation quite well (McCaffery, 1968). There is no indication of how well these "loner" types of people tolerate sensory overload or distortion experiences.

Much research has been devoted to the investigation of the effects of field dependence and body orientation on sensory deprivation. According to McCaffery (1968), field-dependent people rely on external stimulation for the validation of self and reality. These people tend to be rigid and to depend heavily on the concrete quality of stimulation. The body-oriented people, on the other hand, are flexible and use internal and abstract stimuli as well as external stimuli in their perceptions. Field-dependent people tolerate isolation less well than body-oriented people. There is, however, some controversy about this point. Women are usually thought to be more field-dependent than men and should logically be less tolerant of isolation. However, findings do not support this position. No clear sex differences have been demonstrated from the sensory deprivation experiments (Brownfield, 1972), although some research indicates that women tolerate isolation slightly better than men. Therefore, the variable of field dependence may not be the significant one, but rather some other variable that is associated with rigidity and reliance on external stimulation other than field dependence, which is yet to be identified.

According to McCaffery (1968), there is evidence that individuals with average or below average intelligence tolerate isolation better than highly intelligent people, particularly if they also tend to have a calm and placid personality. Individuals who are basically dependent seem to tolerate sensory restriction better, as do people who are low in impulsiveness and high in conformity. Those who are comfortable producing their own stimulation in the form of singing or reciting also seem to be better able to tolerate deprivation. Those who habitually react promptly to discharge tension in stressful situations tolerate the experience better than those whose response is delayed. Tension discharge is accomplished by this first group through verbalization, motor activity, or somatization.

The level of motivation of the subjects to participate in a deprivation experiment has been found to be significant to their reaction (Brownfield, 1972). Therefore, if the hospitalized patient perceives the reason for his confinement as important to his future health and well-being, the experience is tolerated better. If however, the reason for confinement is perceived as threatening, particularly if it jeopardizes some significant aspect of the person's life, the experience is tolerated less well (McCaffery, 1968).

A previous history of isolation experiences has proved helpful to many subjects in the sensory deprivation experiments. Subjects are helped significantly if they know the duration of their confinement (McCaffery, 1968; Brownfield, 1972). It has been suggested that the predeprivation life circumstance and physiologic state have a major effect on the individual difference displayed by subjects in isolation. In addition, the preexperiment instructions and information have been shown to be significant (Brownfield, 1972).

McCaffery (1968) suggests that individuals who are prone to hypnagogic states are more prone to sensory alteration experiences. "Patients who are taking certain drugs, who sleep or doze intermittently, or who ordinarily have difficulty waking up will probably have many mental symptoms" (p. 81). Leiderman and others (1968) confirm that hypnotics and sedatives can reduce the level of awareness and impair sensory discrimination. They state that these kinds of drugs produce a synergistic effect that precipitates the appearance of sensory alteration symptoms among some patients.

High-risk setting factors

The environment of the incapacitated elderly person is often characterized by lack of variety, lack of personal contacts, and lack of meaning. These factors have been implicated as significant in the research into acute and chronic sensory alteration. Although only about 5% of the elderly population are institutionalized in long-term care settings at any given time, the effect of institutional living can be profound for those individuals. In the acute care setting there are multiple people and things that impinge on the client and jeopardize his functioning, yet he can still be lonely and deprived of significant personal contact, variety, and meaning. In the nursing home setting, the problem is further compounded by days that are invariable and personnel who are only more or less interested in the individual residents. Even in the home environment, these three variables may be present. Thus, for the elderly person, the potential for sensory alteration is present in any setting. In addition, certain other setting factors have been found to be important experimentally.

The type of confinement has also been found to be significant. Individuals tolerate chair confinement much better than confinement to a bed, and the bed is better tolerated in a large area than in a small space. Confinement to a very small place, such as a tank respirator or water immersion tank, rarely fails to produce symptoms of sensory alteration experimentally (Brownfield, 1972). Lying on one's back in bed seems to produce more symptoms than lying on one's side (Shurley, 1972).

Brownfield (1972) suggests that assurance that basic needs will be met is probably significant in the experimental setting. If the person is relatively sure that eating, toileting, and sleeping needs will be met, reactions will be less severe. There has been some conjecture that this is the reason that the tank immersion experiments have produced such bizarre results. The person has little assurance that needs will be met. If these have been shown to be important with healthy subjects, how much more important they must be for individuals who are ill, uncomfortable, and totally dependent.

The degree of social restriction has been implicated as an important variable in sensory alteration. Even when the subject is severely restricted and exposed to all manner of input manipulations, the experience is better tolerated when some social contact is provided. This is true even if the social contact is on an intermittent basis. Isolated groups of people show less reaction to sensory monotony than individuals isolated alone. Even when sensory input is "normal," social isolation alone may be enough to produce a disruption in perceptual, cognitive, and behavioral functioning (Brownfield, 1972). It has been suggested that social isolation is one of the most devastating things about the sensory alteration experiments.

Along with the degree of social restriction, the amount of communication with the experimenters and the assurance that the experimenters will promptly answer the subject's requests for release have been shown to be significant. Healthy subjects tolerate isolation much better if they are provided with some means of at least occasionally communicating with the people on the "outside." When the subject feels trapped, with no possible escape and no means of communication, the results are likely to be rapid and profound (Brownfield, 1972).

The number and type of modalities involved in the deprivation experience are important for the strength of the subject's response. Schultz (1965) reports that light deprivation is more stressful than deprivation of sounds. The strength of response seems also to be related to how significant that particular modality is for the particular individual (McCaffery, 1968). In addition, the deprivation of more than one modality is more significant than one alone. McCaffery reports that deprivation of both sight and hearing, for example, produces a more profound reaction than deprivation of either of these alone.

The "closeness" of the barrier that is producing sensory alteration also seems to affect the outcome of the experiment. For example, when sight is deprived by eye patches, the reaction is different than when it is altered by darkness. When hearing is altered by a soundproof environment, the reaction is different than when hearing is altered by a lack of a hearing prosthesis or by earplugs (McCaffery, 1968). It is also thought that if the individual feels a responsibility toward the deprivation experience, the response will be more profound.

The amount of physical activity permitted to a subject during an isolation experience is the last setting factor to be discussed. The more physical activity permitted, the less reaction occurs as a result of sensory alteration. Even when subjects are totally deprived of sight or hearing, if they are permitted to move around or exercise, the reaction seems less profound than when they are input-deprived and restricted in their movements as well. It may be that sensory input from the bones and muscles helps ameliorate the effects of deprivation in other sensory systems (McCaffery, 1968; Brownfield, 1972).

High-risk caregiver factors

Basically, the experimenter variable has not been investigated or controlled in any of the experiments on sensory alteration. "In spite of his effect on the research design, his observation and interpretation of data, his biases and predispositions, the conclusions of research rarely take this into consideration" (Brownfield, 1972, p. 139). This problem not only has implications for the validity of the research reported about sensory alteration but has marked implications in the clinical setting as well, where the caregiver is roughly analogous to the experimenter. Many older individuals are devoid of personal social support systems. In the home, often the caregiver is the only person with whom the elderly individual has contact on a regular basis. In the institutional setting, the professional caregivers are usually the most consistent sources of social interaction, with the individuals from the outside being only occasional visitors. If, as Brownfield suggests, lack of control for experimenters has implications for research, the totally unpredictable effect of caregiver input in the clinical setting has an even more significant effect on the outcome of care for the elderly.

Brownfield identifies four experimenter variables that are probably important from a research perspective. These can be used to specify clinically the caregiver effect on sensory alteration. First, the experimenter's expectations for the results of the experiment probably have an unmeasured effect. Subjects in an experiment will react to a certain extent as the experimenter expects they will. There is reason to believe that this is also true in the clinical setting. During one clinical study of the elderly, it was observed that elderly individuals could be shaped into behaving in aberrant ways simply by the reinforcement pattern of the nursing staff (Phillips, 1976). Since many caregivers expect that older individuals will be confused and will not behave as younger individuals would in the same circumstance, they reinforce the client for inappropriate behavior and ignore his appropriate behavior. In the course of another study (Phillips, 1979), it was observed over and over that the client got the nurse's attention most often when he was doing something strange, such as lying on the floor, crying or screaming, or hitting another resident. During times when the residents were quiet and behaving in a "normal" manner, the nurses tended to take their breaks, talk among themselves, or do their charting. These behaviors of the nurse ignore appropriate client behavior. There is every reason to believe that this same phenomenon occurs when the problem includes sensory alteration. Caregivers may shape clients into certain behavioral responses in relation to sensory alteration that are quite different from those they would display if shaping were not occurring.

The second variable is the experimenter's role in the subject's life.

Depending upon the subject's perception of the experimenter as an authority figure, or of the particular stereotype, he may be guided in any expression of behavior that could affect his relationship with the perceived experimenter. This may lead to a suppression of response, or an effort to please, or any form of behavior designed to insure the continuance or abolition of the subject-experimenter dyad (Brownfield, 1972, p. 140).

This problem is particularly important when one considers that many older individuals are dependent on the caregivers for every aspect of their daily existence. Caregivers have tremendous power as authority figures over the lives of vulnerable older individuals. This power can affect the client basically in two ways. First, the client's response to sensory alteration may be hastened by the anxiety he feels in the situation. He may hesitate to share his early experiences, which is important to his well-being, for fear he will be considered crazy by the caregivers. Second, the client may be afraid that any attempt to increase his stimulation level, such as through verbalization, wandering, or exploring, may break the rules and will be viewed negatively by the caregivers, resulting in punishment. Thus, he loses the opportunities to alter his sensory experience using familiar means and to ameliorate his confusion.

The third variable is "experimenter ignorance." By this Brownfield means the assumptions that experimenters make about behavioral responses that are independent of what the subject is actually feeling or experiencing. For example, in the clinical setting, the caregiver may assume that the behaviors seen are related to senility. As a result, no attempt may be made to ascertain the underlying reason for the behaviors. Often, the only step taken is to limit the offending behaviors by some form of restraint. This usually intensifies rather than corrects the situation. Many caregivers are not even aware that sensory alterations can result in strange behaviors and that the situation is actually correctable.

The last variable identified by Brownfield is the experimenter's sex.

Sex, particularly that of the experimenter who places the subject in an isolation chamber, invariably leads to the arousal of feelings, attitudes, ideas and fantasies which are related to the normal psychological interaction between sexes, but may become more pronounced under the peculiar experimental conditions of isolation (Brownfield 1972, p. 140).

Little is known about the influence of the caregiver's gender and the response of an elderly person. One study did show that older females are more anxious about the touch of men than women (DeWever,

1977). But generally, the effect of gender on the client is simply unknown. Phillips (1976, 1979) has observed that in the nursing home setting, elderly women react very positively to interaction with young men. This interaction is often characterized by joking, flirtation, and affection. Older women, however, tend not to discuss personal problems and concerns with young men. Male residents seem to relate more comfortably about personal problems to young men than women, often seeking the advice of male administrators about these matters, rather than the help of the predominantly female nursing staff. It is possible that the anxiety caused by the interaction of gender, the caregiving role, and the nature of the problem has an effect on the appearance of sensory alteration experience, but this needs yet to be explored.

Other caregiver factors not identified by Brownfield possibly have a role in the appearance of sensory alteration experiences. These include the age of the caregiver, the type of setting, the role of the caregiver (whether a nurse, social worker, nursing assistant, or volunteer), and the personal attributes of the caregiver.

Fourth-level assessment for sensory alteration

Nursing history
Observation of the client's behavior
Observation of the client's environment
Observation of the client's situation
Eliciting subjective data relative to sensory alteration experiences

---

Consideration of the patient's history and personal characteristics, careful observation, and the eliciting of subjective data from the patient are key elements to assessing for sensory alteration. The following questions need to be answered during the history-taking process (adapted from McCaffery, 1968; Jackson and Ellis, 1971):

1. What experiences has the client previously had with isolation or overstimulation? How did he react to them?
2. What have his prior sick experiences been like?
3. Does he have the capacity for self-stimulation and self-entertainment? Does he enjoy solitude or consider himself to be a loner?
4. Does he have ways to release tension that he uses comfortably and successfully, such as verbalizing? Can he perform physical exercise? If so, what type? Level of endurance?
5. What sources does his usual stimulation arise form? Are these sources outside of himself or sources that he creates himself? How much does he interact with others? How much does he verbalize?
6. Is he prone to hypnagogic states? Nightmares?
7. What opportunities for problem solving and control does he have?
8. What does he know about what is happening to him? In what areas would teaching information be helpful?
9. How effective are the physical comfort measures that are being provided?
10. What purpose does he feel his present situation serves? For example, what does he feel he is in the hospital (institution) for? Does he see an end to the confinement? Does he feel himself to be confined?

The answers to these questions will help to identify those who are at high risk for sensory alteration and to make some predictions about the experiences the client may have.

Observations need to include consideration of the client's behavior, environment, and situation. The client behaviors that can be anticipated during sensory alteration experiences can only be inferred from the literature. Only the most common will be discussed here, but, depending on the client and his situation, any unusual behavior should be considered as a part of the assessment. In the laboratory setting, it has been observed that individuals who are experiencing sensory deprivation begin the experience with prolonged sleep. As the experience continues, sleeping time is reduced and long periods of wakefulness can be observed. During these times, subjects attempt to relieve deprivation by self-stimulating activities, including singing, restlessness, masturbation, and random movements. In the hospital studies, noncompliant behaviors such as pulling out tubes, taking off traction, and pulling off eye patches often accompany sensory deprivation, as does wandering and seemingly purposeless activity.

Although not explored in the literature, it may be that individuals who are experiencing sensory overload or distortion attempt to decrease these experiences by various forms of withdrawal, such as sleep or attempts to move away from the stimulation. Overload and distortion that continue may create agitation, irritability, and anxiety states. Prolonged sensory alteration of any type may be accompanied by a general stress reaction, with symptoms of tachycardia, hypertension, alterations in breathing, perspiration, paleness, cool skin, tremulousness, increased blood sugar, increased blood sodium and chlorides, and decreased blood potassium (Jasmin and Trygstad, 1979). Any of these symptoms accompanied by irritability, withdrawal, agitation, and restlessness should alert the nurse to the possibility of sensory alteration, depending on the situation and the environment.

The environment of the client should be observed critically. It needs to be determined what the client can see, hear, smell, and taste from his perspective and position. The types of restraints present need to be determined, including physical, chemical, potential or threatened, and psychologic restraints, as defined on p. 172. It also must be determined what types of restrictions are present in the environment. Restrictions can arise as a result of rules, physical disabilities, or impositions by the treatment plan.

The client's situation must also be assessed carefully. What types of sensory input are available to him? What sensory restrictions are present by virtue of the aging process, a pathologic process, or a treatment method? If sensory restrictions are present, the type, extent, and duration need to be determined. The client's sensory deficits need to be considered to determine if correction is effective or even possible. In addition, the people in the client's environment need to be observed. What are they like? What are their personal characteristics that could contribute to either overload, or distortion? How many people are usually in contact with the patient and how consistent are they? How much interaction occurs between the client and the individuals who surround him? These considerations should help the nurse determine whether or not sensory alteration is present or is likely to be a problem for the client.

Last, subjective data needs to be elicited from the client. Eliciting such information, unless the client is very frightened by what is happening to him and brings up the subject himself, can be very difficult. Many clients fear their experiences will make others think that they are "crazy" or "going crazy." It is helpful to preface your questions with statements such as, "Many people have unusual thoughts when they are in the hospital. Have you been experiencing any of this?" Another nonthreatening approach is to call the experiences "bad dreams." For example, "Some people tell me that they have bad dreams while they are here. Have you been having any problems with this?" (Jackson and Ellis, 1972). Sensory alteration experiences can be quite bizarre and frightening to the client, and it is important that the person who questions him is accepting and reassuring and, above all, nonjudgmental. Subjective data should be elicited in areas of dream content; sensory disturbances; cognitive disturbances; sense of time; sense of place, person, and purpose; daydreams and fantasies; and illusions and hallucinations.

Prevention

The approach to preventing confusion among clients who are at high risk for sensory alteration is multifaceted. The following suggestions have been found to be helpful.

1. *Structure and enrich the environment but be sure that the client has control over inputs, sanctioned privacy, and means of escape from activity.* Very little is known about the optimal levels of stimulation that are most therapeutic to elderly clients. As a result, it is very important that a variety of activities and inputs be provided. Much like a smorgasbord, the activities should be available, but the choice of activities should be individually determined by the clients. Control over inputs also includes self-regulated, self-stimulation activities. Such activities may include the use of radios, television, large-print magazines, and newspapers. When radios or televisions are available, it is essential that the client have ultimate control over whether the device is on or off. Background entertainment can turn into background noise and disturbance if the device is turned on and allowed to run continually. When used intermittently, such media can increase the total amount of stimulation. Stimulation devices, however, are in no way a substitute for human interaction. The client still needs to have the opportunity to share with other people what he has heard or read. Stimulation devices are best used as the basis for focused interaction through which the client can be helped to resocialize and foster relationships.

Sanctioned privacy and time to be alone are essential for the elderly client. We provide few opportunities in the institutional setting for privacy. Clients are usually required to share their bedrooms, their eating facilities, their kitchens, and virtually every waking moment in the company of others who are more or less strangers. Very few caregivers could tolerate a similar situation in their own lives. Small rooms need to be provided in the institutional setting where clients can be alone or where they can entertain a few of their friends. These rooms need to be simply furnished for easy navigation by clients in wheelchairs. Space needs to be provided outside the facility where the client can go safely to be alone and enjoy the outdoors. Negotiations between roommates need to be facilitated so that each is assured periods of inviolate privacy. Caregivers need to make a special effort to respect the closed door or the drawn drape by announcing their presence and requesting permission to enter. Structured "do-not-disturb" time is essential in the institutional setting where communal living is the norm.

The client needs to have a sanctioned, easy means of escape from stimulation. Whether in a group setting or in a relatively solitary endeavor, a means of escape enhances the sense of control. This has been verified in the sensory deprivation studies as well. The client needs to know how to move in and out of situations. Those with mobility problems must be carefully arranged so they can move out of a situation with as little effort as possible. Escape methods and routes need to be arranged with the client prior to his beginning an activity.

2. *Reduce the total number of barriers present.* Barriers can include physical, sensory, or psychologic restrictions. Some of the barriers in institutions are necessary because of the restrictions imposed by group living. If the barriers that are problematic to the client are absolutely necessary, describe the rationale to him. Although he may not accept the reason, knowing the reason is helpful. Negotiate as much as possible for mutually agreeable rules. Be prepared to bend the rules and restrictions to allow the client to retain control of some areas. For example, one woman in a nursing home was unsafe when she smoked unsupervised, as demonstrated by her setting some of the shrubbery on fire. The nursing staff restricted her smoking for safety purposes, but these restrictions were quite un-

acceptable to the resident and caused much distress. In negotiation, it was mutually agreed that the client could smoke as much as she chose, as long as she was in the nursing home lobby. In the lobby, she could use a disposable butane lighter, which would extinguish if dropped, but she was not permitted to use either a conventional lighter or matches. Through negotiation the restrictions that the client found so disturbing were bent to be mutually agreeable to all parties.

3. *Attend to the individual client's problems related to sensory deficits.* (More specific information is provided in the remaining sections of this chapter.) Sensory deficits may be one of the major reasons that elderly people experience sensory alterations. As much as possible, the sensory deficits of the client should be evaluated and corrected. The environment should be individually constructed so that the person with sensory deficits can function as independently and successfully as possible. The creation of such a prosthetic environment requires creativity and the participation of the client, the nursing staff, and the administrative personnel. Carefully analyze the environment and the way the client functions in it to determine what obstructs and facilitates function. Analyze the client's activities so that only those portions of the acitvities that the client cannot perform are assisted and the client's overall independence is not jeopardized.

4. *Provide consistency in staffing, routines, and activities that is mutually agreeable to both the staff and the client.* Consistency is a difficult problem in the institutional setting. First, the elderly person may be faced by more interactions with people in one day in an institution than he has encountered in one day in his entire life. Reducing the total number of people with whom the elderly person must interact is desirable. The caregiver's assignments should *not* be rotated on a frequent basis. Rather, a system needs to be devised that carefully matches the skills and talents of the staff members to the needs and interests of the clients. Client and caregiver need to be assigned together for periods long enough to build relationships and establish trust in each other. One of the most positive aspects of group living situations for the elderly is that such living arrangements afford the potential for relationship building among a group of people whose past relationships are essentially gone.

Often, the staff response to this suggestion is something like: "This is fine for the 'good patient.' But what about the patient who is difficult? Won't that drive the caregiver who is assigned to that person crazy?" Perhaps it will; however, consider the following points. First, a great deal of selectivity and sensitivity needs to be put into the assignment process so that caregivers and clients are fairly compatible and no caregiver is overburdened with all "difficult" clients. Second, perhaps the reason the client appears to be difficult is because he is so frustrated with the way his needs are currently being met. Third, dealing with difficult patients, with the support of coworkers and supervisors, can be one of the most rewarding and valuable learning experiences a nurse can have. Agreed, there may be pain in the process, but perhaps it is most painful because the experience is permitted to occur without support. There need to be mechanisms by which the caregivers can share their experiences, both good and bad, and offer mutual support and assistance. This creates a situation in which the nurse grows, everyone on the unit grows, and the patient is provided with consistent, quality care that is as nonconfusing as possible.

There needs to be consistency in routines on the unit. Nursing units probably appear chaotic to clients who reside on them. The caregiver needs to communicate how the unit is organized and who does what and to identify for the client consistent routines and time frames. The client's personal routines need to be structured in ways that are agreeable to him and consistent from day to day. In addition, ways must be devised to manage the unexpected events that contribute to feelings of disorganization. A frequent question caregivers ask in regard to handling the unexpected with clients is: "When something unusual happens, what should we tell the clients?" For example, Mr. Jones, a long-term resident of the facility who consistently participates in unit activities, dies. Should the other residents be told? Or Ms. Brown, a nursing assistant who has a positive relationship with many residents, has a family emergency and must suddenly take a leave of absence. How is this handled best? Or there is a delay in the breakfast trays, and at nine o'clock there is still no meal. The clients should be told what amounts in the long run to the least confusing, threatening, and upsetting answer: the truth. Adequate explanations are essential for creating an environment where there is mutual trust and support. This kind of an environment helps lend order to chaos.

Another area where consistency is difficult is in hospital activities. Institutions are characterized by sporadic bursts of activity that can be distressing and disorienting. Clients need to have these flurries of activity explained to them. A characteristic of an acute-care setting is that during the diagnostic and recovery phases, the patient is taken from place to place for one upleasant experience after another. For example, the patient is repeatedly taken to x-ray and other laboratories for diagnosis, often while he is sick, in pain, and hungry. During the recovery phase, a single day may mean a trip to physical therapy, occupational therapy, inhalation therapy, and the x-ray department. Although some of these trips are unavoidable, steps should be taken to reduce the stress as much as possible. Nurses should use sensitivity and consultation with the patient to determine the sequence of tests and the number of tests that are scheduled in one day. If possible, someone who can explain to him what is happening should accompany the elderly patient and can act as an advocate during the procedure. Even if the trip is unavoidable, overload can be decreased if someone is with the patient to facilitate the process and help make it as painless as possible.

5. *Increase the total amount of knowledge the client has about procedures and treatments*. The chance of sensory alteration experiences are increased when the client cannot perceive pattern and organization in his situation or his surroundings. Teaching, support, and information are more than "frills" for elderly people in the institutional setting. These activities are essential so that the elderly client can understand what is happening to him physiologically, physically, and emotionally. Increased knowledge can lead to a decreased incidence of confusion.

6. *Reduce the incidence of relocation, and when relocation is unavoidable, involve the client in the planning*. Relocation has been extensively studied among the elderly. There are certain facets of relocation that are particularly detrimental. When the relocation is sudden, unplanned, and done without the awareness or participation of the client, the results can be disastrous. When, for example, an elderly patient is relocated from his home following a fall resulting in a hip fracture, confusion is almost inevitable. Not only is there amnesia surrounding the trauma of the accident, but there is usually pain, disorganization, and exhaustion accompanying such an accident, which contribute to confusion. Although the relocation is unavoidable under these circumstances, the impact on the elderly person is very detrimental. The same is true when an elderly person is perpetually relocated within a facility for the convenience of the care staff. Such practices should be minimized as much as possible. However, not every relocation is as traumatic as these. For example, when a new facility is opened and clients must be transferred to a new permanent location, relocation can be comfort-

ably managed if the client is involved in the decision-making and planning processes. If the client is given the opportunity to anticipate the move, understands the reason for the move, the plans for his new residence (makes plans to decorate or place the furniture as he chooses), the trauma of relocation is reduced. Therefore, sudden, unexpected, and unplanned relocations of elderly people for the convenience of the caregivers should be avoided.

7. *Exploration, manipulation, and play are necessary for all people but should be particularly encouraged as a prevention for sensory alteration among the elderly.* Knowledge of the environment requires more than merely being told about it. Acquisition of knowledge involves the experience that the client gains as he explores and manipulates the environment. Within the bounds of safety, there should be no curtailment of the client's needs to wander, explore, handle and touch, ask questions, or just simply verbalize. For those individuals who are dependent on others for ambulation, provisions need to be made so they can meet these needs as well. Although these activities may "feel" disruptive to the nursing staff and may contribute to the staff's overload, they are essential to the prevention of sensory alteration that leads to confusion.

8. *Increase the total opportunities for successful problem solving, planning, and control on the part of the clients.* Provide the support the client needs to be successful in these attempts.

In the institutional setting, we systematically strip our clients of opportunities to conduct their affairs and their lives. We strip the responsibilities of living from the client, leaving only the sick role as the basis for their behavior model. Within their physical and emotional capabilities, elderly people need to have responsibilities for self and responsibilities for the group. On admission or shortly thereafter, a contract should be devised with the client that specifies those activities the client is responsible for and those the staff is responsible for. This assigns some of the responsibility for self-care activities to the client himself and increases his opportunities for independent decision making and problem solving. During negotiation, the client's level of function needs to be carefully determined so that the contract is realistic and fair. As the client's level of function increases or decreases, the contract should be renegotiated. Under such a system, the staff has the responsibility to fulfill every part of their bargain and to provide the materials and supports needed for the client's successful fulfillment of his part of the contract.

Responsibilities for the other residents, the group, or family members should be negotiated on an individual basis within the social, physical, and sensory limitations of the people involved. A contract should be negotiated with nearly every client that involves some group responsibility, no matter how small. Even the most withdrawn or physically limited people can be helped to see that even small contributions help the group as a whole. For some clients, the contract may be as simple as consistently using the ashtray rather than throwing cigarette butts on the floor. For other clients, responsibilities can be more complex, involving wiping the tables after meals, helping another resident to the table, feeding another resident, or passing out desserts.

Sensory alteration experiences are more likely to occur when the client sees no purpose to his existence and lacks opportunities for control of independent decision making and problem solving. As one nursing assistant observed in a long-term care setting, "Normal people have times when they work, relax, and play. Here no one works. They only have things to entertain them. Most of these people have worked all of their lives, and now they just sit. I wonder if that is why some of them come to me and ask me how they are going to get to work?" Prevention of confusion arising from sensory alteration, then, involves helping the client to perceive purpose and responsibility for his existence.

9. *Increase the amount of predictability in the environment.* Set goals with the client that are time-oriented and help him to see that he is moving in the direction of the goal, with things happening as expected.

Some individuals have defined aging as the process of becoming a spectator. When one is a spectator, there is neither predictability nor control over the things that are happening. Rather, everything is planned and carried out by someone else; the spectator merely looks on. This situation, which predisposes to sensory alteration, can be alleviated through goal setting. While some things happen in the institutional setting over which there is little control, they are certainly the exception. Through the mutual identification of goals and recognition of progress toward the goals, the incidence of confusion related to sensory alteration can be decreased.

10. *Discuss with the client what he is thinking and feeling.* Many staff members fear discussing emotionally charged subjects with elderly individuals because "it might upset the client." In addition, clients hesitate to express their thoughts or feelings for fear that the caregivers will reject them or see them as emotional, senile, or "crazy." Clients need the opportunity to discuss what is "happening inside their heads" with people who are nonjudgmental, accepting, and supportive. If the subject under discussion leads to an emotional outburst, the expression of these feelings helps the client to vent these emotions and to gain a perspective about the problem. The support given the client during a discussion is important. The client and staff must realize that many people who are restricted experience delusions, hallucinations, sensory aberrations, and cognitive disorders, but this kind of experience does not mean they are "going crazy." Let the client know that these kinds of thoughts and feelings are better expressed than suppressed and that there are means by which the unpleasant experiences can be decreased.

11. *Help the client develop means of self-stimulation, particularly if the means he has always used are now compromised.* If the client has always relied on reading or needlework and now has poor eyesight, find an alternate means of self-stimulation. He might appreciate being read to, having talking books, or learning poetry by sound. Encourage him to recite memorized passages to himself and others. Many older individuals can be heard reciting nursery rhymes, since often this is the only poetry remembered. This is a very acceptable self-stimulation activity, along with singing and humming and exercising while counting the number of movements aloud. Any form of self-initiated and self-regulated activity can serve the purpose of increasing the stimulation level from minimal to acceptable.

12. *Facilitate interaction between the client and the others in his environment and provide opportunities for group activities and group interaction.* Any form of interaction acceptable to the client is important to consider. Equally important is that the person has success in the experience. Group interactions are most successful when they are semistructured and focused on sharing between group members. Group work with elderly people has been the topic of many publications. For more specific ideas please refer to the works of Burnside (1973, 1976, 1978) and Ebersole (1976, 1978).

13. *Help the client identify his strengths and construct his environment to minimize his weaknesses.* When a person is faced with multiple losses, including the loss of function, it is sometimes difficult to see what strengths are left that enhance self-worth. It is helpful if the client can identify with you how he has successfully managed in the past and what have been his lifelong assets. Help the client to identify which deficits are particularly problematic to him and the alternatives he has in his environment. It is particularly important that the

individual see himself as a successful, capable person who has resources and controls to prevent confusion.

14. *Provide all the necessary cues for the client to be successful in the environment.* A great deal of time may be spent turning the world of elderly clients into a guessing game in the name of assessing orientation. Assessment time needs to be separated from intervention time. When assessment is not occurring, we need to be conscious of providing the elderly person with all the information he needs to be successful in his world. This includes reinforcing environmental cues, cues about orientation to time and place, and cues about the individuals who interact with the client. Do not expect the elderly client to remember everything told him. Each of us, young and old, remembers selectively, repeats the same subject to the same people, and forgets things that other people consider to be overwhelmingly important. The client may have fewer potential stimuli to help him remember. Do not hesitate to repeat, reexplain, and reinforce. Do not be tempted to say, "I told you that a moment ago" or "You told me that story yesterday." As we provide information consistently and repeatedly and positively reinforce remembering and appropriate responses, the elderly client will begin to remember more and more as his stress levels decrease.

Intervention

The organizing objectives for the nursing care given to a client who is experiencing sensory alteration are:
1. To provide a sense of control for the client
2. To provide a sense of organization for the client
3. To help the client focus his thoughts and to determine purpose for his activities
4. To help the client achieve his optimal level of stimulation

Each of these overall objectives will be considered more specifically in six separate areas related to the sensory alteration experience:
1. Boredom and inactivity
2. Overload or distortion
3. Slowness of thought and excessive daydreaming
4. Thought disorganization
5. Anxiety and panic
6. Emotional lability

The content presented in these areas has been adapted, in part, from the suggestions of Chodil and Williams (1970).

For simple problems such as boredom or inactivity

1. *Provide a variety of activities over which the client has control.* The client needs to feel that he is in control of the amount and types of input he is receiving and has ways of increasing his general stimulation level. He should be given several activities to choose from and helped to make a comfortable choice. The activities identified may include diversional activities, socialization activities, or self-care activities. All should have a component of human companionship and should be self-limiting. The client needs to be able to see an end to the activity identified and to be given permission to discontinue it when he wishes. The client should be helped to see that by engaging in activities, he is providing himself a means of escape from his boredom.

2. *Regular exercise, within the physical limitations of the client and treatment restrictions, needs to be provided.* Even if the client is in traction or is on complete bed rest, it is possible to provide a certain amount of physical activity in the form of passive movement. For those with no restrictions, physical activity should be as vigorous as possible. Wheelchair bowling, throwing pillows, and hammering nails can all be used by the person in an institution. Reinforce with the client that one of the best ways to relieve the boredom experienced in the institutional setting is to engage in physical activity.

3. *Provide the client with opportunities to explore and manipulate the environment.* If the client feels like wandering, let him wander and explore safely. If he feels like handling the objects in the environment, provide ways for him to do so. Help the person rediscover the environment as if it is totally new.

For overload or distortion

1. *Provide a sense of control over the sensory input and the stressors in the environment.* First, help the client to identify what elements of the environment are causing him distress. If he is experiencing diffuse discomfort from multiple stimuli, it may be difficult for him to determine exactly what is bothering him. In this case, the nurse needs to use her own assessment skills to help the client focus on the noxious stressors. Is it the number of people, the noise level, or the speed at which activities are performed and circumstances change? Are there elements in the environment that the client is misinterpreting or that cause his perceptions to be distorted? Next, assure the client that his feelings of agitation and distress are not unusual and that many people experience the same types of feelings under the circumstances. Then, help the client identify ways to control the input; a sense of control is essential. Provide the client with permission and ways to seek privacy.

2. *Act to reduce the client's anxiety.*

a. Teach the client relaxation and "centering" techniques similar to those in Appendix D. Encourage him to use these at least twice daily and whenever he feels his anxiety level is building.

b. Explore how the client is perceiving the environment so that misperception can be corrected. Provide an explanation for the sensory events in the environment that could be misinterpreted. Sounds, sights, odors, and tastes need to be explained. Where do they come from? What do they mean? What are they? If, for example, noises are causing difficulty to the client, take the client to see what is causing the noise and explain to him why the noise is occurring. Or, if there is a flashing light in the setting, explain the purpose of the light and try to eliminate it from the client's field of vision.

c. Encourage the client to participate in structured activities. Help him to retain control over activities. Help the client establish schedules and routines and then communicate these to others in the environment. Give the client permission to maintain control over as many activities as possible. Even if the client does not have ultimate control over an activity, he can participate in deciding how and when the activity will occur. For example, if a spinal tap is to be performed, inform the patient and help him negotiate with the physician for a mutually agreeable time. During the procedure, encourage him to turn himself on his side and to say when the procedure may begin. Regular exercise is another activity the client can control. Help the client decide how and when he will exercise within his physical limitations. Making appointments with the client for care activities and helping him to have a sense of control over time help a great deal in this process.

d. Give descriptions and anticipatory information about forthcoming procedures or events. For example, if a catheterization is needed, the client needs to know why, who will do it, what he is expected to do, what kind of equipment will be used, and how it will feel. If he is being taken to a group activity program, the client should know who will be there, what will happen, what he is expected to do, how he can leave, and where the event will occur.

e. Teach an appropriate means of summoning help. Teach the client what communication devices are present and how they work. Make sure the call light is within his reach and he knows exactly how to use it. Then, respond to his calls. Nurses register disgust about the client who bangs on the side rails and yells to get attention. However, often this client does not understand the more acceptable communication system or has been reinforced for yelling because the call light does not get results. Yelling always does. Reliability and consistency help build trust.

For slowness of thought and excessive daydreaming

1. *Provide consistent interaction with other people.* Provide goal-directed, focused converstion on topics of meaning to the client. Conversation can be initially focused on pictures, the newspaper, food, or other immediate sensory input. Having the client describe to you a familiar activity may be helpful. For example, if the client is a retired steel worker, you might have him focus on the steel-making process by describing it or what he did in his job. The important thing is that the client participates and helps direct a conversation with a person who is willing to listen and spend time with him.

2. *Help the client focus on his thoughts.* Depending on the client's cognitive abilities and past interests, the following suggestions may be helpful:

   a. Have the client help you solve some of the problems encountered in his living environment, such as how to arrange his cupboard or his furniture or how to perform some of his care activities.

   b. Have the client help you solve a problem, such as giving you advice on things familiar to him, such as plumbing or auto problems.

   c. Have the client teach you something, such as how to plant a garden, how to can peaches, or whatever is a part of his knowledge repertoire.

   d. Involve the client's family in helping the client participate in their problem-solving, such as managing money or balancing the check book.

   e. Give the client puzzles or games that require problem solving or logic. Depending on the degree of cognitive involvement, many of these suggestions may be at a level higher than the client's ability at that point in time. When necessary, give the client cues so that he can solve the problem successfully or scale down the problem so that he can manage it. Make every attempt to make his problem-solving attempts successful and meaningful, and reinforce the client for his successes.

For thought disorganization

1. *Help the client impose structure and organization on his world.* It may be that the client needs to be helped to find structure through consistency and schedules. The institutional environment that looks so structured to the workers can appear chaotic to individuals who are suddenly relocated and unable to determine the reason for certain organizational features. Explain how the organization works and what features you, the nurse, use to impose structure.

2. *Provide benchmarks for time and activity so the client can predict what will happen and can impose order on the events around him.* Orient the client to time through the use of clocks and environmental cues. Help the client to see the passage of time by establishing one-step goals that are reinforced when obtained. For example, say to the client that breakfast will be over by eight o'clock and then reinforce that it is over. Then tell the client that his bath will be completed by ten o'clock and reinforce this as well.

3. *Introduce activities and people one at a time.* Allow the client plenty of time to assimilate each new thing occurring in the environment or happening to him personally. Do not put the client in a position that requires dealing with multiple stimuli and inputs without support and explanation. Remind the client what is going on, and who you and those around him are. Do not expect that he is going to remember, and do not turn his life into a guessing game by constantly asking him. During periods of thought disorganization is not the time to be assessing for orientation. Rather, it is the time to be:

4. *Providing all the cues the client*

196 Confusion: prevention and care

needs to maintain his orientation and sense of reality.

For anxiety and panic

1. *Provide reference points so the environment can be perceived as predictable and consistent.* Take the responsibility for the client's orientation into your own hands. Calmly, simply, and reassuringly tell him exactly what is happening around him and to him.

2. *Assure the client that you are in control of the situation and that you will help him regain his own sense of control.* If you can identify it, explain the sensory source for his experience. Let him know that his feelings and experiences are not uncommon among people in institutional settings, and reinforce that he is not "losing his mind" or "going crazy." Assure him that you will help him deal with his experiences and that you will not leave him alone without telling him where you are going, when you will be back, and how he can find you if he needs you.

3. *Help the client set one-step goals that will move him toward feeling more secure.* For example, if the client is experiencing panic because it is the middle of the night, tell him what time it is. Tell him when sunrise will be and assure him that he will be less fearful in the daylight. Then help the client assess his own movement toward meeting his goal. Place a clock where he can see it. Reinforce with him the passage of time and the approach of daylight. By seeing progress toward the established goals, the clients helps relieve his sense of anxiety and panic.

For emotional lability

1. *Accept that the client will be emotionally labile during periods of restriction and stress.*

2. *Help the client to see the appropriateness of his feelings and emotions and help him to identify their source.* Often there are sound reasons for the client's anger, unhappiness, depression, or anxiety. Accept the client's right to these feelings and help him express them.

3. *Help the client to find ways of expressing his emotions that are harmful neither to himself nor to others.* Appropriate expressions of these feelings might include increased physical activity, increased touching, screaming, or crying. Giving permission to the expression of feelings is the most therapeutic approach to helping the client deal with them.

Outcome criteria of successful nursing intervention against sensory alteration

1. The client reports and demonstrates that his anxiety level has decreased
2. The client's activities appear purposeful to both him and his caregiver
3. The client perceives pattern and organization in his environment and responds appropriately
4. The client is able to discuss those sensory experiences that are disturbing and to share his perceptions
5. The client's problem solving is logical and organized to both him and those around him
6. The client is no longer confused

The suggestions found in the assessment, prevention, and intervention portions of this section are summarized at the end of this chapter.

SENSORY ALTERATION IN RELATION TO TOUCH
High-risk client factors

Only a limited amount of information regarding the physiologic effects of aging on the sense of touch is available. This may be related to the complexity of the topic. The sense of touch is associated with the following separate processes: temperature sensation, vibratory sense, pressure sense, pain, proprioception or position sense, crude touch sense, fine touch sense, and two-point discrimination or localization sense (Guyton, 1971; Geldard, 1972). To further complicate the situation, individuals do not use these processes separately to gather information about the world. Rather, they use these processes in combinations called "touch blends" (Geldard, 1972). Through touch blends, individuals can make absolutely reliable and valid interpretations of the world around them. A correct judgment can be made about an object's qualities on the basis of touch alone. For example:

"Oiliness" reduces to weak pressure accompanied by warmth, with movement enhancing its reality. "Hardness" is uneven, cold pressure with a good boundary while "softness" requires an uneven, warm pressure of poor boundary. "Stickiness" takes a variable and moving pressure, while "clamminess" is essentially "a cold softness perceived with movement and supplemented by unpleasant imagery" (Geldard, 1972, p. 314).

Therefore, it is the interaction of touch processes that produces the "feel" of an object, not the presence of one isolated characteristic.

To even further complicate the discussion of touch, two distinct neurologic pathways exist for the conveyance of touch information: the spinothalamic system and the lemniscal system (Guyton, 1971). At least three distinct areas of the brain are involved in the reception and interpretation of touch information: the thalamus, the sensory cortex I, and the sensory cortex II. Interpretation of the results of touch experiments is thus an extremely complex matter, whether the subject is young or old.

Nevertheless, certain facts are known about the tactile senses of aging people. First, there seems to be a general decrease in somesthetic sensitivity across all sensory modalities among the elderly. It is incorrect, however, to assume that these deficits occur to *all* elderly people. Rather, every study conducted reports a less than 50% incidence of somesthetic loss among the subjects examined. In addition, there is great diversity in the types and degrees of the losses of sensation reported. The degree of loss varies from mild to severe, with most losses reported in the mild to moderate range. There is no uniformity in either the parts of the body affected by loss or the modalities involved (Kenshalo, 1977). It does, however, appear that losses of sensation tend to be caudocephalad, appearing earliest and most severely in the feet, legs, and "tail." To illustrate this point, Howell (1949) reported that among his sample of 200 elderly men, vibratory sense loss was most marked after the eighth decade of life with 10% of the over 80 sample reporting a deficit involving the ankle, 28% reporting a deficit involving the shin, 28% reporting a deficit involving the knee, and 90% reporting a deficit involving the sacrum.

Second, on exploring vibratory sense further, there seems to be a decrease in this sense among some people over 60 years of age who are considered to be normal and neuropathologically free. According to many researchers, the loss of vibratory sense begins around age 50, is more severe in the lower extremities, is fairly uniform for all frequencies of vibration for men, and affects women mostly in the higher frequencies and not the low (Keighley, 1946; Rosenberg, 1958; Goff and others, 1965; Perret and Regli, 1970). Pearson (1928) first reported the occurrence of this loss and noted that of his 150 subjects, 48% had a decreased vibratory sense that could be attributed to aging alone. Although the incidence of this impairment seems high, the degree of impairment for normal people is slight to moderate. A severe impairment of vibratory sense seems to be associated with organic brain syndrome (Bender, 1975).

Third, there is a decrease in localization sense among older people. The incidence of this impairment increases in direct proportion to increasing age. In a study of 64 normal subjects between the ages of 40 and

64, Bender, Fink, and Green (1953) found a 36% error rate on the face-hand test (p. 207) during the first trial; all subjects correctly perceived being touched in two places on the second trial, after the experimenter corrected their misperception. In the same study, 287 elderly subjects between the ages of 65 and 95 were tested in a similar manner. Ninety-six percent of these subjects were able to discriminate being touched in two places on the second trial after being corrected. Failing at the face-hand test with eyes open is considered diagnostic of organic brain syndrome (Bender, 1975). Again, in these experiments, the pattern of error among the older subjects was caudocephalad with the face being dominant over the hand and the thigh being dominant over the foot.

Fourth, the studies involving both temperature sense and pain sense have been very inconclusive in establishing a relationship between either of these and aging. In regard to temperature, Clark and Mehl (1971) report that older subjects detect warmth almost as well as young subjects, but their "old" subjects ranged only to 67 years of age. In a study of three elderly subjects, Kenshalo (1970) reports a sensitivity to warmth and cold similar to that found in college students. However, his sample was too small for generalization. It is known that older subjects seem to have difficulty coping with extreme environmental temperatures (Krag and Kountz, 1950). Therefore, although their perception of heat and cold may be intact, their thermal regulating system may be impaired (Kenshalo, 1970).

The sensitivity to pain as a function of aging has been studied extensively. Results have varied widely, probably based on the inability of most investigators to separate the affective-emotional components of pain and the effects of subject expectation and instructions from the pain experience itself (Kenshalo, 1977). The animal model has been used in an attempt to make this separation, and it appears that older mice are tolerant of greater amounts of pain than younger mice (Nicak, 1971). However, as always, the transfer between the animal subject and the human subject is neither easy nor direct. The Clark and Mehl (1971) study with human subjects did, however, support the idea that older people of both sexes do experience less pain for the same amount of intensity than younger subjects. Kenshalo (1977) suggests that older people may use different criteria for reporting pain, tending to be more certain than younger subjects that pain is present before reporting it. Studies with pain relief seem to indicate that older subjects both react more strongly and more frequently to the placebo effect than younger subjects, as well as receiving more relief from active pain agents than do younger subjects (Bellville and others, 1971; Lasagna 1971).

Fifth, touch sensitivity has not been studied extensively among the older population. However, it appears that some aging people have a decrease in touch sensitivity in the skin of the palms and soles, with touch being fairly well preserved on the hairy surfaces of the body (Kenshalo, 1977). Kenshalo (1977) reports that Ronge (1943) showed a decrease in the number of touch spots over the body surface until the sixth decade of life. After the sixth decade, the total number of touch spots and touch sensitivity increased, perhaps from structural skin changes that make the skin easier to deform. The samples of these studies have, however, not been representative enough of the total population of elderly people to infer the incidence in changes of sensitivity to touch.

There has been some attempt to investigate the changes of kinesthetic sense among the aged. Generally, it is thought that there is a decrease in position sense for the lower extremities, with older subjects making more errors in judging the direction of lower extremity movement. However, the threshold at which movement is detected does not seem to be affected by aging (Kenshalo, 1977). The incidence of active movement deficiencies for such activities as the finger-to-nose, heel-to-knee, and finger-to-heel tests among the aged has not been satisfactorily determined, but in the few studies done with "normal" elderly people, the incidence seems to be low (Kenshalo, 1977).

In addition to these points, certain disease processes common among the aged affect tactile perception. These include diabetic and other peripheral neuropathies, strokes, herpes zoster, and nutritional polyneuropathies (Alpers and Mancall, 1971; Rossman, 1972). Some of the decrease in tactile sense found among aged people may be attributed to concurrent spinal arthritis and arteriosclerotic myelopathy (Bender, 1975).

The relationship between simple aging and changes in tactile sense has not been investigated to any extent. In addition, there has been no documentation that all, or even most older people have changes in their perception of touch. Based on these sparse findings, it would be difficult to build a case that older people are at high risk for sensory alteration as a result of tactile deficits alone. There is, however, a growing body of literature that indicates that elderly individuals have a need for tactile stimulation as a means of relieving the sensory deprivation that arises from other sources and as as a means of establishing rapport. These references are *not* based on physiologically decreased tactile sensitivity as the cause of sensory deprivation. Rather, they are based on the following four assumptions about the nature of touch, aging, and illness.

1. Touch is a means of communication established early in life through which most human feelings can be conveyed (Barnett, 1972; Huss, 1977). Touch is a primary nonverbal means of communication. As such, it conveys certain basic meanings, often more effectively than words. Mintz (1969) states that the meanings of touch include direct libidinal gratification, symbolic mothering, a sense of being accepted, and a sense of reality. It should be noted that in Western culture, direct libidinal gratification is often exclusively associated with touching, as if touch held no other meaning (Jourard and Rubin, 1968; Egan, 1970; Huss, 1977). Dominian (1971) also stresses that touch conveys reassurance. The language of touch frames and enriches the words used during an interaction. Touch conveys the quality and intent of words that are used (Frank, 1957). Touch conveys primary emotion, often without the need for words.

As a means of communication, touch conforms to the codified rules for appropriate usage determined by the culture (Hall, 1968), just as other cultural language forms do. These rules are learned during childhood and determine how a member of a given culture will perceive being touched (Frank, 1957).

2. The need for touch does not diminish with increasing age and may even increase markedly during times of stress and illness (Burnside, 1973; McCorkle, 1974; Huss, 1977). The typical pattern of touching in Western society is that a child first learns about his world of people and things through tactile communication and stimulation. Around the age of 3 (often earlier for boys), the frequency of touching by the mother and significant others decreases. At about age 5 or 6 the child has almost completely replaced tactile communication with verbal means. The cultural expectation is that the "adult" way to communicate is verbal rather than tactile except under certain circumscribed conditions.

Most adults equate touch with sexual contact. Thus touching between people of the same sex, between parents and their adult children, and between health care workers and their clients tends to be perfunctory for fear of misinterpretation of more intimacy than is desired. As a result, children, adolescents, and adults in Western culture suffer from "skin hunger" (Huss, 1977). In addition, until recently, it was fairly commonly considered that adults who acknowledged a need for touch were displaying infantile behavior. In an investigation of "the need to be held" among adult women, Hollender (1970) reports that even though many women express this need, those who do often equate it with "childishness." As Hollender presents it, the need to be held is quite different from the need for sexual activity, although sexual activities are often bartered or used as a substitute for the need to be held. Being held provides a sense of protection, security, comfort, contentment, and love among healthy women. Hollender indicates that the need to be held may also be experienced by healthy men, but his studies involved female subjects only.

In addition to being a need of healthy people, the need for touch may be intensified during stress and illness. Barnett (1972), for example, notes that inherent in the sick role in Western society is the mandate that the patient relinquish temporarily his adult responsibilities and delegate responsibility for self-care and decision making to someone else. This sets the stage of regression and a kind of "therapeutic childishness." Augmenting this, Dominian (1971) notes that this regressive state creates an intense need for human contact in the form of touch.

3. Touch is therapeutic and the use of touch can increase the well-being of a sick person (Aguilera, 1967; Mintz, 1969; Burnside, 1973; Kreiger, 1974a; McCorkle, 1974; Zefrom, 1975). Using a sample of 60 seriously ill people, McCorkle (1974) demonstrated the positive effects of touching on the quality of the nurse-patient interaction, the speed of establishing rapport, and the way in which the patient evaluated the nurse's care. In a study with psychiatric patients, Aguilera (1967) showed touch to be effective in increasing verbal interaction, rapport, and approach behaviors by the patients, as well as producing positive changes in the attitudes of the nurse toward the patients. Using a single case study, DeThomaso (1971) discussed the use of touch as a means of ameliorating the effects of loneliness and anguish among psychiatric patients.

In addition to increasing the sense of well-being, some researchers advocate touch as a means of healing. Krieger's work (1972, 1974, 1975, 1979) has dealt with therapeutic touch by the "laying on of hands." The act consists of "the simple placing of the hand for about 10 to 15 minutes on or close to the body of an ill person by someone who intends to help or to heal that person" (Krieger, 1975, p. 784). Under controlled laboratory conditions, Krieger has repeatedly demonstrated an increase in the hemoglobin levels of ill subjects, which she attributes to the therapeutic laying on of hands. Krieger, Zefrom (1975), and others argue that touch is more than "a nice thing to do." It is an untapped resource that nurses possess to effect wellness among their clients.

4. For many elderly people who are devoid of stimulation from other sources (because of pathology or deficits in other sensory modalities), touch is one sensory pathway that remains relatively intact with aging. Therefore, touch can be used to increase the overall sensory input to "normal levels," as well as to communicate (Burnside, 1973; Preston, 1973; Huss 1977). Very little can be done to improve seriously altered sight or hearing of elderly people. The tactile sense, on the other hand, remains fairly intact for most normal elderly people and touch can be easily manipulated by the caregivers.

This assumption has been used extensively in the group work with elderly people of Burnside (1973, 1976, 1978) and Ebersole (1976, 1978). For example, using touch as an intervention technique with a group of six regressed elderly individuals with an average age of 79, Burnside (1973) reported that the clients learned to use affective touch with each other, began to display interest in their surroundings, and increased the level of their interactions in general. The amount of spontaneous behavior such as laughing, clapping, and smiling also increased. Using the case study approach, Preston (1973) also advocated the use of touch for regressed elderly clients.

Chronic brain syndrome can indeed be "a misery" to live with. But the distress can be ameliorated to a degree by non-verbal communication—an outstretched hand to invite participation, a gentle pat or wave to convey recognition, a warm, friendly smile, and other gestures to soothe, to hold attention, and above all to make contact (p. 206).

It should be acknowledged that in group work with the elderly, the use of touch has not been the only variable manipulated and therefore may not be the actual "cause" of the behavior changes that have been noted. Invariably, the subjects have also been exposed to other forms of intervention, including reality therapy, music therapy, and exposure to social and other types of rewards. However, when touch has been combined with other specialized treatments of the patients as people, the outcomes have been noteworthy.

Tactile deprivation

There is a growing body of literature demonstrating that people in Western society experience "touch or skin hunger" for most of their adult lives. In addition, if it is shown that touch can make a difference in the sense of well-being and the state of health among elderly people, why is it that the elderly are often deprived of touching experiences? The answer probably lies in the nature of aging and touching in this society. Touching in Western culture is reserved for close friends and significant others. As a person ages, more and more of the people who have provided touch input are lost through death. Older people tend not to replace the lost people in their lives. As a result, fewer people provide touch stimulation, and the very old person may be virtually untouched. As stated by Huss:

Perhaps the elderly in our society are deprived the most because of impersonal care in nursing homes and the loss of loved ones. Their distance receptors of vision and hearing decrease in functional capacity; thus limiting experiential capability. These disabilities, compounded by the lack of meaningful touch with others, make their isolation even more acute. The elderly cling to those possessions that can be handled or that evoke memories of lost contact (p. 13).

It is not the sense of touch or the meaning of touch that decreases, but the external sources of touch that decrease and make elderly people high risk for touch deprivation. As one elderly widow lamented, "No one has hugged me since Ed died."

Tactile overload and distortion

Sensory overload and distortion related to the sense of touch arise from basically two sources: physiologic and psychologic. McCaffery (1968) identifies pain as the most significant source of physiologic overload for the sense of touch. Pain, from whatever source, is distracting and disturbing and can produce behavioral changes much akin to other types of sensory overload. Pain among the elderly may not be taken seriously; many assume aging is a painful process, and certain aches and pains are normal. This is not necessarily true. As with the young, pain among the elderly is always a warning signal requiring investigation and therapeutic or palliative intervention.

Discomforts such as pressure are another source of physiologic overload. The pressure of lying in one spot, from not being able to move a limb or a part, or the pressure of an external device on the skin such as a cast or traction can produce tactile overload. Excesses of temperature, either hot or cold, are another discomfort. In the presence of circulatory changes, many older people do not experience the intensity of temperature extremes as they once did. It might be difficult for them to identify that their source of restlessness arises from excesses of temperature. The unpleasantness of rough handling can be a source of overload. Many older people, for example, must be coaxed to bathe in nursing homes. Some of this is undoubtedly related to the discomfort and unpleasantness of the bathing experience. The lack of privacy, the cold shower room, and being held in a forceful shower may be a part of the experience related to sensory overload and discomfort.

Psychologic sources of overload for older people may arise from the nature of touch itself. The experience of being touched conveys certain messages. Some of these messages are culturally determined. "Rules concerning affective touching are consistent within a culture because culture determines how the member's sensoriums are programmed and, consequently, how the members perceive sensory experience" (DeWever, 1977, p. 164). On the whole, North American adults are greatly affected by the Anglo-Saxon heritage that dictates that touching is not usually acceptable (Graves, 1966; Jourard, 1966; Hall, 1968; Watson, 1969). Violation of the touch taboo can result in higher anxiety levels for some people (DeAugustinis and others, 1963). The elderly are, of course, not immune to this kind of cultural training.

Some researchers have found that aversion to touching is related to social status. Henley (1973) states people of higher status are permitted to touch people of lower status without evoking anxiety. The reverse is not true. Gender is an important variable in the response to touch. For young people, there is a high degree of anxiety associated with two members of the same sex touching (Egan, 1970). Among the elderly, the reverse of this is true, particularly for females (DeWever, 1977). It is, therefore, socially determined to a certain extent whether or not the touching experience will be pleasant and comforting or overloading and misinterpreted. DeAugustinis and others (1963) projected that among patients, affective touching is misinterpreted about 50% of the time. No such figures are available that are specific to the elderly.

In addition to cultural and social determination, certain personal factors seem to influence whether the touching experience will be well received or overloading and anxiety producing. This is analogous to the meaning of language for certain individuals. It is well known that certain words hold a "loaded" meaning for certain individuals, based on their backgrounds and experiences. This loading may have little to do with culture or the society. So it is with touching. Touch conveys personal meanings that can be ascribed to only one individual. Certain people are, for example, simply "nontouchers." This was demonstrated in the DeWever study by quoted client comments. All of these people reported being comfortable with touching but added: "I see no point to touching;" "Touching is unnecessary;" "I don't like to be felt;" and, in reference to touching, "I don't like informality" (pp. 168-169). This same aversion to touching was reported by some of the subjects in the Hollender study (1970).

Aside from personal variation, some overloading and distortion are related to who is doing the touching, the setting, where on the body the touch occurs, and when it occurs. Touching by a relative stranger is probably not well received under the best of circumstances. Even if the stranger is a professional person, any touching other than that related to business may not be well received. All of the studies on touching have involved touching of the upper extremities only. The place on the body being touched may be an important, unstudied variable. The DeWever study, for example, showed that older people found having their hand touched more acceptable than having an arm placed around their shoulders. At what point during the illness or relationship the touch occurs seems to be important in whether or not it will produce anxiety. DeThomaso (1971) reports that touching is more appropriate at different stages in a relationship. These stages seem to be related to different levels of permission given by the patient and the patient's ability to reach out to be touched at that time. Touching that violates the person's privacy and need for aloneness is very anxiety producing for most individuals. The duration of the touch is a relatively unexplored variable in relation to anxiety. Some people may tolerate a short pat quite well but may become very restless and anxious if someone holds their hand for 15 minutes. An elderly woman discharged from the hospital after treatment for sciatica commented: "That massage the physiotherapist gave me was wonderful. When I am terminally ill, I intend to take my last $200 to spend on having my back massaged."

In summary, the touching experience may be related to both a sense of well-being and comfort and a sense of discomfort and anxiety. The precise factors that relate to each of these have been fairly unexplored in the research, but it seems clear that the reception of the reaction to touch is individual. The way to render a client less high risk for sensory alteration related to touch is to help him to determine the amount of touching that he needs and that makes him comfortable.

High-risk setting factors
Tactile deprivation

Certain methods of treatment predispose to the deprivation of touch. For example, people who are isolated because of infectious disease, particularly a wound infection, are usually not touched any more than is absolutely necessary to provide care. It is often felt among the nursing staff members that they will become vulnerable to the client's disease by touching him. This fear seems to be particularly acute among nonprofessionals, the group that delivers the bulk of the care to elderly individuals. Treatments for burns and skin diseases often prevent or inhibit touching. Orthopedic devices, such as casts and traction and other complicated setups, inhibit both the nursing staff and family and friends from touching the patient for fear of disturbing the equipment.

The institutional environment can lead to regression among elderly individuals. Often, the most intensely affected are the elderly whom the caregivers expect to have regressive behavior anyway, for example, the person who is admitted with a diagnosis of senility. Regression increases the need for touching, but within the institutional environment there is no guarantee that this increased need will be met. Abram (1969) identifies that regression is often displayed by demanding behavior that irritates both physicians and nurses. The result is that these regressed people are the most likely to be ignored and untouched.

Generally, just being in an institutional setting decreases the likelihood of being touched. Institutionalization means being separated from the few people who have previously provided touch. It is not unusual to find the person who has slept beside a loved one for 50 years crawling into bed with a total stranger in the middle of the night in an institution. As disturbing as this is to the nursing staff and to the stranger, this is a display of the deprivation of touch by someone now separated from a loved one. In addition, being in an institution means being among individuals who do not necessarily have the warm feelings that result in affective touch. The deprivation of touch is probably more severe in the acute care setting, where the focus is on curing, short-term stays, and youth. It may be that the elderly in acute care settings receive less touching by the staff. It is also possible that they receive the same amount of touching as the younger, more desirable patients, but their deprivation is more acute because they have fewer people on the outside able to supplement their needs for affective touching on a consistent basis. Touch deprivation is probably less severe in long-term care facilities as the client becomes a long-term resident. The longer he resides in the institution, the more likely he is to have established caring relationships with others. As demonstrated in Fig. 10-3, spontaneous touching between residents in long-term care facilities is not at all unusual, and it serves as a source of comfort and support to both parties.

Lack of variation in the institutional setting is implicated in all forms of deprivation, and touch deprivation is no exception. The

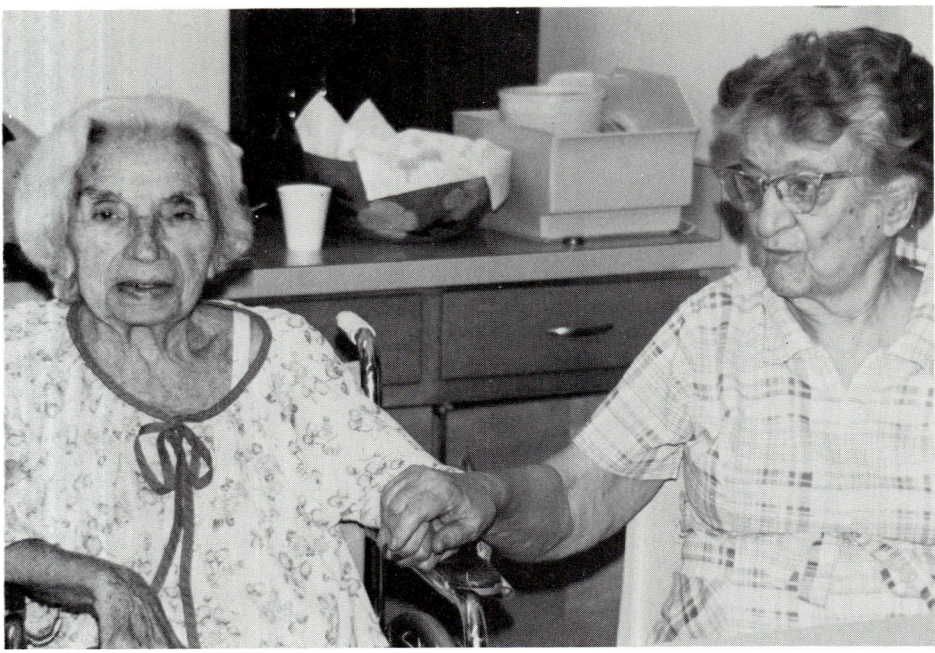

Fig. 10-3. Touching. (Photograph by C. D. Falk.)

tactile apparatus of clients who do not dress in street clothes is stimulated by few different stimuli. Institutional sheets and gowns are all smooth and lack variation in texture. Many older individuals respond well to soft blankets or fur pieces directly against their skin as a source of tactile variation. Therefore, in addition to less affective touching, many older people experience a total deprivation experience that includes lack of variation.

Tactile overload and distortion

Painful manipulation as a result of treatment methods can contribute to sensory overload and distortion. At particularly high risk are those individuals who are seen in teaching hospitals and have an "unusual condition." One older woman related having a total of seven interns, residents, and staff physicians examine her prolapsed rectum during one examination period. She found this exposure upsetting and anxiety producing. This kind of experience is not limited to physicians' examinations. In settings where multiple individuals share the responsibility for client care, baths and intrusive procedures may be done by many different caregivers every day. An elderly client may have one nurse's aide give the bath, another get him out of bed, one nurse start an IV, and another perform a catheterization—all in the space of 3 hours. The greater the number of instrusive procedures requiring the laying on of hands, the greater is the risk of tactile overload. The more painful the procedures or the longer the pain experienced by the client, the greater is the overall risk involved.

Restraints may be a form of stimulation producing overload. As the person is snugly affixed to a chair, wheelchair, or bed and struggles against the restraint, the more overload is produced. Sudden position changes, such as standing or being turned in a CircOlectric bed or Stryker frame, may produce overload to the proprioceptive apparatus. Strange devices such as wires and tubes coming from the body may distort the sense of body integrity and overload the sensory apparatus.

High-risk caregiver factors

The prohibition of touch as a helping technique used by caregivers dates to the Victorian era. Not only was there a general emphasis on sexual prudery and a clear association on the exclusive relationship of sexuality and touching, but freudian psychology also had a major effect on the delivery of health care. Four attitudes emerged during that period that still influence what is considered appropriate behavior for a caregiver in relation to clients. First, Freud emphasized the divorcing of magic and religion from the practice of medicine. Both of these had used touching extensively as therapeutic techniques. Second, the practice of psychiatry had to be kept apart from any hints of depravity. The content of freudian analysis often relates to sexuality. It was thought that permitting therapists to touch their clients would jeopardize the reputation of the new field. Third, Freud emphasized the need for the client to learn to meet his own needs rather than to depend on an outside person for gratification. He felt that physical contact between the helper and the client would hinder this process and prolong the therapy experience. Fourth, Freud emphasized that the focus of the situation was on the client's needs and feelings; the therapist was to be a "blank wall" on which feelings and needs could be projected. Early therapists thought that touching would complicate the care situation as the feelings and needs of the therapist became superimposed on those of the client (Mintz, 1969). Although these attitudes were originally directed at the psychotherapeutic community, their influence on other health care professionals is clear. A general mandate to psychotherapists to remain noninvolved with the client contributed to the current touch taboo in the health care setting.

Recently, therapists have recommended more and more involvement between the helper and the client (Mintz, 1969). Interestingly enough, the emphasis on more involvement has not been accompanied by a concurrent emphasis on more touching in traditional circles (Fromm-Reichman, 1950). The touch taboo remains a viable part of the health care workers' behavioral repertoire.

Huss (1977) states that nurses are the most likely of the health professionals to use touch with comfort. Still, as Johnson (1965) notes, the use of touch by nurses is complicated by many factors. Among these are the types of touch used and the ways in which touch is used in combination with verbal communication. The degree to which a nurse will use touch and the results of the use of touch depends, in part, "on how the patient and the nurse interpret touch, on their own personal background, on how their culture regards touch, and on their current level of social maturity" (Johnson, 1965, p. 60).

Fourth-level assessment for tactile alteration

Nursing and medical history
Eliciting subjective data relative to the tactile sense
Temperature sense
Pain sensation
Position sense
Light touch
Deep touch
Localization sense by the face-hand technique
Ability to determine the nature of objects
Ability to distinguish and respond to texture
Response to affective touching

In summary, nurses may deprive elderly clients of affective touch for many reasons.

Many nurses are inhibited from touching by their perception of what constitutes appropriate behavior between clients and nurses. These perceptions are usually learned from professional role models and in the academic setting. Some nurses are inhibited by the fear that clients will misinterpret their use of touch and the situation will be uncontrollable (the "dirty old man" problem). Many nurses are inhibited by their own cultural backgrounds and experiences, which affect their personal perception of the meaning of touch. Johnson (1965) also believes that the lower the level of social maturity and the younger the nurse, the less she will tend to use affective touch with clients, unless she is taught and supported in her attempts.

Since the incidence of tactile sensory deficits among elderly people has not been documented in the literature, it is essential that each elderly client be considered individually, with no assumptions made about his ability or lack of ability to use the touch sense. In addition, the elements of the assessment should be given priorities, moving from those abilities immediately involving safety and sensory alterations, such as temperature sense, proprioception, and affective touch, to those abilities less important to the client's ability to function in the environment, such as vibratory sense. The testing of vibratory sense is probably more important diagnostically than functionally and therefore will not be considered at all in this assessment.

For some clients, particularly those who have recently been hospitalized in an acute care setting, it is possible that a complete neurologic examination has been done, including evaluation of the touch sense. This information can be helpful to the nurse if it provides enough factual material on the functional level of the client. Unfortunately, as with many of the assessment measures commonly used by physicians and nurses, the language of one group may interfere with that of the other. Since the physician's focus is on diagnosis and the nurse's is on functional abilities, the nurse will often need to repeat major parts of the assessment using the nursing focus. This is particularly critical for those clients who have histories of diseases that affect touch perception, such as diabetes or stroke.

As before, the logical place to start with the assessment is with a nursing history. Unfortunately, changes in the tactile sense are often insidious and are frequently not recognized by the client. However, the following questions may be helpful in permitting the client to identify the changes he is experiencing:

1. Do you notice any change in your ability to feel warmth, cold, or pain?
2. Do you have tingling or numbness of any body part?
3. Do you feel awkward when you are walking or do you fall frequently?
4. Does this awkwardness seem to be associated with dizziness? (With proprioceptive problems, dizziness is not involved.)

Even if the answers to these questions are negative, it is still necessary for the nurse to investigate for possible tactile deficits that make the client's functioning difficult.

Among the elderly population, temperature sense is most frequently and severely affected in the lower extremities. This, however, does not preclude testing of other parts of the body. As outlined in the short assessment form in Chapter 6, temperature sense is tested in the following manner.

Fill one test tube with 115° to 120° F (46° to 49° C) water and a second with 40° F (4.4°C) water. A cold metal object can be substituted for the tube of cold water, but this may "feel" different to the client and give a clue as to which is cold other than by temperature alone. The client closes his eyes and is then touched on various parts of his body alternately with the tubes of water. Ask him to report which is hot and which is cold. Begin by applying the tubes to the solar and plantar surfaces of the feet and the inner and outer aspects of the legs. Then test the hands and arms. Anticipate a decreased sensation on both the palmar surface of the hand and the plantar surface of the foot. Test the face and covered portions of the body last. Remember that as you handle the tubes, the water inside will change temperature and it may be necessary to change the water during the test. Also, as you handle the tubes, you will begin to accommodate to the temperature of the tubes; they will not "feel" as hot or cold as they did in the beginning. For this reason, measure the temperature of the water as you change it rather than relying simply on touch. Areas of the body where it is particularly difficult for the client to determine temperature should be noted carefully. If you detect a serious deficit in the client's ability to sense either hot or cold, teaching should begin immediately. Caution the client to use the most sensitive portions of his body to "test" water before bathing and other potentially harmful substances before taking hold of them.

Cutaneous pain sensation is carried in the same afferent fibers of the nervous system as temperature sense. Many people, therefore, recommend the testing of either one or the other. If, however, time permits, both can be tested. Conventionally, cutaneous pain sensation is tested using a safety pin and alternately touching the client with the "sharp" and "dull" parts of the pin. The test is conducted in a manner similar to the temperature assessment, beginning with the feet and legs, moving to the hands and arms, and finishing with the face and covered body parts. The areas where deficits are found are noted in the record, and teaching begins during the assessment process.

Proprioceptive sense is comprised of active and passive elements. The passive elements are tested by asking the client to close his eyes. Various appendages of the body are then lightly touched on the sides and moved either upward or downward. Ask the client to describe to you where in space the appendage is located. The most usual appendages tested are the great toe, the foot, the fingers, the thumb, and the hand. It is essential that the body part be touched only on the sides since the gentle pressure exerted against either the top or bottom of it would give the client a clue as to movement associated with pressure and not proprioception. Again, the most common places for proprioceptive losses to occur are in the feet and legs.

Active proprioceptive abilities are tested by using the finger-to-nose, heel-to-knee, and finger-to-heel tests. With eyes closed, the client is asked to touch one body part to another. The "normal" person is able to touch his nose, for example, with his finger with eyes closed and has no difficulty. The client is observed closely as he performs these activities and deficits are noted. (Although these tests are usually considered to be indicative of coordination and not proprioceptive abilities, Kenshalo [1977] stresses that the proprioceptive elements of these movements cannot be overlooked.)

A wisp of cotton is used to test the client's ability to "feel" sensations in the light touch range. Begin with the lower extremities, move to the upper extremities, and then test the face and covered body parts. Lightly apply the cotton to the skin, being careful to not depress the skin, and ask the client to tell you when he detects feeling. This test is usually performed first with eyes closed, then with eyes open if the client has had difficulty. Most deficits are found on the palmar surfaces of the hand and fingertips and plantar surfaces of the feet and toes. Light touch is usually well preserved among the elderly on the body parts with light hair growth, such as the backs of the hands, arms and legs.

Deep touch is assessed by touching the client on various parts of his body with your fingertip after he has closed his eyes. Be certain to depress the skin with your touch. Because of aging skin changes, deep or crude touch sense is usually well preserved or hypersentitive. Again, note the client's reaction and record the areas with deficits or hypersensitivities.

The face-hand technique is a test for localization sense. Using the full palm of your hand, lightly touch the client in two places simultaneously. After the client closes his eyes, begin with his right cheek and touch the ipsilateral hand. Ask the client where he is being touched. If he reports he is being touched only on his face (the most common error), correct the misperception and tell the client you will try again. Touch the client lightly on the right cheek and the contralateral hand and ask him where he is being touched. Many older individuals have difficulty perceiving being touched in two places without anticipatory information, and some continue to make mistakes even after correction. After several trials during which the left and right sides of the face and the contralateral and ipsilateral hands are touched, the pattern of client responses and the types of errors are recorded. This technique is repeated with the client's eyes open if he has had difficulty with eyes closed.

Astereognosis is the inability to identify an object by touch. Most individuals can identify an object placed in their hands by touch alone. A deficit in this area can lead to misperception of the environment, particularly for those people who are temporarily sightless, without eyeglasses, or blind. The materials used in testing can include a coin, a key, a bar of soap, and a toothbrush. Actually, any object can be used that has a fairly distinctive "feel." The client is asked to close his eyes and extend his hands. Various objects to be identified are placed in his hands, which he can manipulate in any way. Any problems or deficits are carefully recorded.

The identification of textures can be tested by having the client close his eyes and identify the nature of what is touching him. Testing materials can include a terry cloth towel, a smooth sheet, a piece of fur, and a blanket. Equally important to assessing the ability to identify textures is the assessment of the types or variety of textures that usually touch the client and his favorable or unfavorable responses to them. Texture variety is limited for most individuals in institutions and for those who are bedfast at home. Attempts made to increase this variety can be stimulating to the client.

The most effective means of assessing the response to affective touch is by observation. The following kinds of questions should be answered as you observe the client and his interactions with others:
1. Does the client touch other people?
2. Do they touch him?
3. How do they touch?
4. Under what circumstances is the client touched and under what circumstances does he touch others?
5. Who usually initiates the touching?
6. How does the client respond to being touched? Does he move back from touching or does he accept being touched?
7. Does he seek touching? Does he reach out to touch or be touched?

It is also beneficial to ask the client how he regards touching, under what circumstances touching is used in his family, and if he considers himself to be a person who enjoys touching.

Since the client's response to touch is often dependent on the toucher's attitude and manner, it is also essential that the nurse and the nursing staff assess their own attitudes toward touching. Many nursing personnel fear that their use of touch will be misinterpreted or that touching will lead to a situation they will be unable to control. Female staff have reported to us that "touching women is all right, but touching men is not." These attitudes need to be brought into the open and the attitudes and expectations of the staff members matched to the attitudes and needs of the clients under their care.

Prevention

1. *Anticipate that the need for touch will increase during periods of stress, illness, loneliness or depression.* It is well documented in the literature that when a person is encountering personal difficulties, the need for affective touch increases. As human beings, we respond to the increased needs of those around us. Instinctively, when our friends are ill or needy, we

reach out to them. We touch them, hold their hands, kiss them, and use touch freely. As health care workers, we do not usually share the same level of intimacy with our clients. We often do not respond in the same way to the people for whom we care when they are ill or needy. We assume our "nurse" or "therapist" role, shed our "human" role, and fail to respond to the humanness of the situation. To prevent confusion among our elderly clients, it is essential that our "nurse" or "therapist" role not interfere with our humanness. For the elderly, often the caregiving staff constitutes the only group of individuals who display consistency and caring. Literally, as age advances and the client's outside sources of caring decrease, we become, in every sense, family members, friends, and significant others. As elderly clients face the pains and losses that may accompany aging, we may be the only human beings left with whom they can share their deepest and most intimate moments. As a result, a key to preventing confusion among elderly individuals involves learning to respond to our clients as other human beings who are experiencing difficulties that only the caring and support of another person can ameliorate. Affective touch is a large part of this intimate sharing experience.

2. *Attend to the physical comfort of the client to remove sources of overload and to increase his general stimulation level within comfort ranges.* Sick individuals confront many forms of discomfort directly under our control. For example, every effort should be taken to remove sources of pressures. Bedridden patients should be turned frequently and massaged at regular intervals, not only to decrease the chances of decubiti formation, but to decrease the chances of confusion arising from unrelieved discomfort. The wheelchair-bound client who is able should be taught ways to relieve pressure and discomfort, either by wheelchair push-ups, limb rearrangement, or independent transfers. In addition, we frequently hear reports and see evidence of elderly clients in nursing homes and hospitals being left to sit in wheelchairs far beyond their tolerance for sitting. This practice is supposedly aimed at increasing the client's stamina for sitting. However, prolonged sitting can instead increase the client's total discomfort input to intolerable levels. Every effort should be taken to carefully plan such "sitting" experiences. The client needs to be carefully observed for his tolerance level, which may be as short as 5 minutes. He should be transferred back to bed for rest shortly after his tolerance level is reached, with a gradual increase in the amount of time he remains sitting. Such a program may mean the client is transferred from bed more frequently during the day, with short periods of sitting time, but the net result will probably be increased sitting tolerance and increased strength, with a decreased chance of confusion arising from discomfort and fatigue.

Complaints of pain from a client should be investigated for source and relief measures. Pain medications are by no means the only tools available to help elderly clients in pain. Massage and repositioning are helpful, as is the judicious application of warm or cool compresses. Relaxation techniques may be used, whereby the nurse literally "talks" the client into a relaxed posture, helps him to "center," and directs his imagery to pleasantness and well-being and away from pain. Later, as the client responds to these techniques, he can be taught to use them independently. Appendix D contains examples of relaxation programs found to be useful with anxious and uncomfortable people. In addition, Jasmin and Trygstad (1979, pp. 70-76) present an excellent discussion of various centering techniques. Self-hypnosis has also been used successfully for pain control by many clients. A self-hypnosis program is best instituted by enlisting the help of a person trained in hypnosis. When the program is underway and the client is comfortable with the technique, the nursing staff can support and reinforce the client in his use of hypnosis.

The environmental temperature is often a source of discomfort for elderly people. Procedures that require body exposure should be undertaken in the warmest possible environment. Baths, for example, should be given in a warm room, with bath blankets and warm clothing available afterward for the client. If showers must be given, the room and water should be warm and the force of the water gentle. A general atmosphere of relaxation and comfort should surround the bath experience, rather than the production-line hustle and bustle that often accompanies bathing. Other procedures requiring exposure should be similarly considered. Whenever possible, such procedures should be conducted in a slow, relaxed manner, giving every attention to the client's warmth and the relief of his tension. Privacy is of utmost importance.

3. *Plan carefully for manipulative or exposing procedures so that a minimum of people are involved and the amount of manipulation is minimized.* In the acute care setting, it is often difficult to control the number of procedures that an elderly person is exposed to in one day. However, it should be possible to some extent to control the number of caregivers and the speed of the procedures. Sometimes, by increasing the time between intrusive procedures, rest periods can be provided. In the extended care and long-term care setting, it is much easier to control both the number of procedures performed daily and the number of caregivers who perform such procedures. Staff consistency and attempts to decrease manipulation and exposure can help prevent sensory overload that leads to confusion. The amount of privacy the client has during these procedures is also helpful.

4. *Provide ways for the client to explore and manipulate his environment, the objects in it, and the treatment apparatus that will be used with him.* A primary way that people become familiar with their environment is by tactile exploration. The tactile sense can be used to demystify many of the experiences that elderly people have in the health care setting. For example, many nurses keep unsterile equipment available, such as catheter equipment and hypodermic syringes, for the client to manipulate and explore prior to the procedure. Knowing that a catheter is soft rubber, how the balloon works, and where in the body the catheter is placed helps to decrease some of the fear. Having the client explore his body after a catheterization, with your guidance, may decrease the likelihood that he will attempt to pull the tube out. Let him feel how the catheter is attached to his body, where it enters, and what distortions in his body integrity the tube creates. Get a mirror and let the client see how the placement of the tube looks. This kind of exploration, along with verbal explanations, can be done with virtually every object the client is exposed to in the institutional setting, with the exception of those items that would cause him harm, such as radiation materials. Manipulation of the equipment and thorough explanations help the client to become an active participant.

One way older people remain in contact with their life histories is through the personal objects around them. An elderly person admitted to the hospital should be encouraged to bring personal items from home, such as pictures, pillows, and clothing. In the long-term care setting, personal furniture is quite comforting and should be within the reach of the elderly client. He should be encouraged to handle them and share their significance with others. Contact with personal items provides links to the past that may prevent confusion among those who are relocated and separated from their past lives.

5. *Educate staff members, significant others, and the client about skin lesions, radiation therapy, infections, burns, and treatment apparatus so the client may receive as much affective touch as possible.* Certain disease conditions seem to isolate the client and predispose him to a decreased

amount of affective touching. Included in this group of conditions are those considered to be disfiguring, communicable, or dangerous to either the client or the person interacting with him. Many individuals react adversely to skin lesions, from whatever cause, for fear of "catching" them. Communicable diseases are associated with stigma regardless of the actual mode of transmission. Radiation therapy creates among staff members a fear of too much radiation exposure and of associated illnesses. Complicated pieces of equipment create the fear that the client will dislodge the equipment and harm himself. These reactions can be alleviated, to some extent, by education and support. If the fear involves "catching" the disease, the individuals involved should know the disease's communicability, the mode of transmission, the amount of contact necessary to contract the disease, and the precautions needed to prevent transmission. If only "enteric precautions" are necessary to prevent transmission, for example, the staff and others should understand the disease is not transmitted in other ways and other types of contact with the client are safe. If the disease state or equipment actually does limit the amount of movement or contact the client can have, the degree to which contact can be provided should be determined. Nursing care needs to be planned so the client receives the maximum amount of interpersonal contact and tactile stimulation within the limitations of the situation. Many times the nursing actions planned to protect the nursing staff are not really needed and end up creating more harm to the patient.

6. *Provide opportunities for mutually consenting clients to touch each other.* If the nursing personnel does not interfere with touching between clients, many elderly people who are independently ambulatory can meet their own needs for affective touch with those around them. Prohibitions about touching between clients are, in some institutions, explicit. Such institutions have rules that prohibit contact between clients of opposite sexes, and some even limit the amount of body contact "permitted" between married couples. Most frequently, however, rules that prohibit touching are implicit. The staff may raise their eyebrows when couples are found kissing or holding hands, may walk indiscreetly through closed doors or curtains, or may openly ridicule any touching seen between clients. Most of the touching that occurs between clients is not explicitly sexual in nature. Rather, the need to be touched or held is more a reflection of the need for security and comfort. This need is often expressed in the form of body contact with another human being. Even if the contact is explicitly sexual, that really should be of no concern to the nursing staff, unless one of the individuals is expressing discomfort or the desire to not be involved. The primary way to *not* prohibit touching between clients is to provide privacy. Within institutions, closed doors and drawn curtains should be inviolate. Nurses can take the responsibility to educate other staff members about the clients' rights to touch each other. Providing avenues for open discussion of this topic between staff members prevents the frequent covert ridicule. It is thought that tactile contact is a primary way for individuals to stay in "touch" with reality. Permitting such contact may be an important way to prevent confusion that arises when contact with reality is lost.

7. *Provide routine rituals involving touch as time benchmarks to induce relaxation and provide tactile stimulation and variety.* Rituals and routines are one means of signifying the passage of time. For example, a nightly ritual might include warm foot and hand soaks, massage, and "tucking in" the client. The morning ritual of washing the face and hands and applying makeup can signify the day is beginning. Rituals that include the "laying on of hands" can be very significant to the client and can provide reinforcement of the passage of time. Carefully planned and consistently executed, these rituals can be used as a

means of helping the client to remain time-oriented.

Intervention

The nursing objectives for intervention against tactile alteration are:
1. To determine the types of touch to which the client responds best
2. To use affective touch to a degree comfortable to the client
3. To use touch to punctuate verbal communication and to hold the client's attention
4. To manipulate the tactile experience to provide external stimulation and variation
5. To use verbal and visual communication to explain tactile experiences
6. To plan position changes and ambulation around proprioceptive deficits
7. To use warmth as a means of reducing agitation and restlessness
8. To use deep massage to induce relaxation and to create a sense of comfort

1. *Carefully determine the types of touch to which the client responds best*. Use these forms, such as warmth or cold, texture, massage, and affective touch, to provide meaningful touch input. Evaluate the response continually.

The touch experience is individually received and perceived by the people involved. As has been demonstrated, being touched and touching are loaded with cultural, social, and individual meanings that make it most difficult to predict the response. Therefore, interventions that will decrease a sensory alteration experience but not contribute to overload, anxiety, and confusion must be individually tailored for the people involved. Any measure instituted to alter the touch experience for the client must be carefully evaluated at every step to determine its acceptability and effect. Although the touch experience is easily manipulated, interventions that alter touching must be carefully and thoughtfully manipulated to produce the desired effects. Clients will find the following interventions to be selectively acceptable, depending on their response set. A certain amount of care must be taken with their use.

2. *Use affective touch to a degree comfortable to the client.* Comfort is usually related to the amount of familiarity between the client and the caregiver, as well as their social and cultural backgrounds. Often, it is not the amount of touching the elderly person is exposed to, but the quality of these experiences that makes the difference in response. The gentle affective touch of a caring individual is far more appropriate than the indiscriminate use of touch by multiple noncaring people. In this latter situation, the touching experience can lead to discomfort, anxiety, and overload rather than comfort.

An affective touch can be warm and comfortable, empathic and supportive, or surprising and delightful. For example, in one nursing home, the elderly men in wheelchairs passed their days sitting in front of the glass-enclosed nursing station. The head nurse, who was busy inside the nursing station, would quite unpredictably come out of the station, give one of the men a big hug, and plant a kiss on his cheek. None of the old men ever knew who would be next, and the day passed quickly in anticipation. Before the day had passed, everyone sitting outside had been given one or two kisses. Life was not nearly so exciting when that particular nurse was off duty. Affective touching can include anything from a pat to hand holding, hugs, and kisses. Underlying all affective touching there must be warmth, acceptance, and a genuine liking for the other individual as a person.

For many people, affective touching can also be used as a response to primary emotions such as crying, screaming, or pacing. Anyone with a small child knows that one of the most effective ways to quiet uncontrollable outbursts of emotion is to gather the child in your arms and hold him close. Although some people are further agitated by touch and a strong elderly person who is agitated and violent may be more than a nurse can handle, neither situation is usual. Often, the nurse is dealing with a frail elderly person with an incomprehensibly strong emotion who would welcome external control from a source other than the conventional cloth or leather restraints. Often, warm, caring body contact that is strong and reassuring is enough to quiet an outburst.

When the client reaches out for affective touch, it is important that the caregiver not withdraw. Since our culture is so focused on the idea of a direct connection between affective touching and sexual advances, it is sometimes difficult for caregivers not to withdraw from a client's touch. In a workshop recently conducted on this topic, many of the participants expressed the fear that if they did not withdraw from the touch of an elderly person (a man in particular), they were giving tacit approval for a sexual advance. They feared the situation would end up being embarrassing and uncomfortable for both people. After this fear was openly discussed, the group decided on the following. First, in the actual experience of the participants, such a situation was incredibly rare. Only one person out of a group of twenty had experienced the seductive advances of an elderly person in the last 5 years. Therefore, although the fear was expressed by many of the participants, the realization of that fear was very infrequent. The myth of the "dirty old man" is, in reality, a myth. Second, the group agreed with Whiteley (1978), who demonstrates that seduction is a process involving a group of behavioral cues and a certain intimate context, not an isolated behavior. If the caregiver uses affective touch in a caring way that omits all other courtship cues and the client reaches out to be touched, also omitting the other courtship cues, the action is likely not to be misinterpreted. Third, the group decided that by virtue of health, strength, and the caregiver role, the caregiver is *always* in control of the situation. It is basically the caregiver's behavior and not the client's that determines what will occur within the context of a situation. Therefore, withdrawing from a client's touch for fear of creating an uncontrollable situation is unwarranted. Without belaboring the point, elderly individuals reach out to be touched because they are afraid, lonely, or in need of honest, warm, human contact. Although caregivers have the personal right not to be touched if touching makes them uncomfortable, this is the caregiver's, not the client's problem, and should be handled as such. Those caring for the elderly should work with their own feelings about touching so this powerful tool can be offered without fear or misgivings.

3. *Use touch to punctuate verbal communication and to hold the client's attention as you communicate with him.* When an elderly client is confused, one of the best ways to get and hold his attention is through a gentle touch on his arm or hand. Touching as you talk can help the client concentrate on what you are saying and can help keep him from being distracted by the multiple stimuli around him. It is ineffective to try to interact with a confused client who is babbling, talking incessantly, or restlessly moving around until you have gotten his attention. Touch can be used to quiet these activities so more appropriate social behaviors can emerge. One frequent observation made of well-meaning caregivers is that they will approach a client and try to wait patiently until the person has stopped rambling before interacting. They will ask a question or start the conversation and then patiently wait through more rambling, with the expectation of eliciting understandable communication. After many attempts to communicate, they will leave the situation saying, "You just can't get through to him." By providing undivided attention to rambling and babbling, the caregiver is providing positive reinforcement for aberrant behavior. Touch can be used to break this cycle. The client usually quiets if you place your finger over his lips or yours in a "shushing" motion when he begins to ramble. Touch provides the caregiver with a tool to control incoherent responses and to

positively reinforce responses of a more desirable nature.

4. *Manipulate the tactile experience to provide external stimulation and variety for the client.* Many types of sensory input can be provided through the media of touch. Using a terry cloth towel to "vigorously" rub the client after a bath increases stimulation, as does the use of lotions and skin oils. A cool astringent to the face after washing is soothing to some people. Even the most withdrawn clients seem to respond positively to the stimulation that tactile input provides. Observations of the client will tell you which kinds of tactile stimulation are best received and produce the most positive responses.

5. *If the client has difficulty localizing tactile stimulation or has difficulty determining the nature of objects by touch, use verbal and visual communication to explain what is happening.* For example, it is quite common for older individuals to be frightened when they are turned because they fear that the person is not going to hold them and keep them from falling. It may be that these older individuals do not perceive being touched in two places and perceive that only their shoulders are being supported. Show the client where you are placing your hands, tell him what you are doing, and reinforce your concern for his safety during the turning procedure. If you are going to touch the confused client with an object, show him the object, tell him what it is for, and describe to him what the object might "feel" like. During the procedure check with the client to determine what he is perceiving of the tactile experience.

6. *Plan position changes and ambulation around proprioceptive deficits.* Individuals with proprioceptive problems may have difficulty with sudden position changes and with "finding" and protecting their limbs during transfers and ambulation. Such a client needs to be taught to "look" for his limbs, to be visually aware of their placement, since he may not be able to feel where his limbs are in space. Occasionally, a client with propriceptive problems will see his limb and not recognize it as a part of himself, and such a statement is usually interpreted as confusion by the observers (Ullman, 1962). Visual and verbal communication concerning their limb placement is essential for these individuals. During ambulation, the client must consciously check that his knee is locked, and to not step forward until he is reasonably sure that his lower limb is in a position that will support his weight. Usually, ambulation programs stress that the client not look down at his feet, because this is likely to alter balance. However, with proprioceptive problems, looking down may be the only way to assure safe ambulation; in this case, balance should be addressed as a separate problem.

7. *Use warmth as a means of reducing agitation and restlessness.* Many elderly individuals have difficulty adjusting to ambient air temperatures. When everyone else in the room is comfortable, the elderly individual may feel cold or uncomfortable and be unable to determine the source of the discomfort. Some of the restlessness and agitation observed in a confused client may be the result of his attempt to increase muscle movement in order to "feel" warm; the behavior may be motivated by discomfort at a subconscious level. Layers of clothing and the liberal use of blankets are helpful to these clients. Tucking the person in bed may create a sense of safety and security that will be the difference between restlessness and agitation and comfort and sleep.

8. *Use deep massage to induce relaxation and to create a sense of comfort and well-being.* Massage provides tactile input, especially for those people who do not respond well to spontaneous affective touch. In addition, the calming effect of massage is well known. Many nurses use only one form of massage, such as a back rub, forgetting that elderly people respond positively to massage of other body parts. Leg massage may not be possible because of problems with thrombus formation in the

lower extremities, but foot rubs after a foot soak are extremely relaxing. Massage of the hands, arms, face, and head will often induce sleep, eliminating the need for other soporifics.

Outcome criteria of successful nursing intervention against tactile alteration

1. The client reports and demonstrates that his anxiety level has decreased
2. The client and caregiver report comfort and appear comfortable with the amount of affective touching used
3. The client's level of awareness, not his anxiety, is increased by the use of tactile input
4. The client is no longer confused

The suggestions found in the assessment, prevention, and intervention portions of this section are summarized at the end of this chapter.

SENSORY ALTERATION IN RELATION TO VISION
High-risk client factors

Visual acuity is compromised with normal aging. Snyder, Pyrek, and Smith (1976) found that among 295 extended care residents over 65, 24% were legally blind and 35% had low visual acuity (20/70 to 20/200) even with corrective lenses. Visual changes of the aging eye involve multiple structures. The first change involves the cornea, which becomes less translucent and takes on a smoky appearance with progressive aging. As the corneal cells become hypertrophic and the endothelial cells flatten, astigmatism is produced. Light transmission of the cornea decreases and refractive surfaces increase (Hatton, 1977). The results of corneal changes are sight distortion and the need for more external light to produce a satisfactory image on the retina. The second change involves the sclera. Its decreased opacity permits stray light to enter the eye; as a result, images tend to wash out, necessitating more striking color contrasts for satisfactory visual perception. Third, the "floaters" found within the vitreous increase in the aging eye. These floaters are often described by the person as black spots floating within the field of vision that are worrisome and distracting. Although this is usually a benign condition, the presence of increasing numbers of floaters may also be an early symptom of a detached retina (Leighton, 1973).

Fourth, there are profound changes in the lens with aging. Because of a loss of lens elasticity by age 45 and a subsequent decrease in the capacity to accommodate to near vision, most people have a reduction in visual clarity for near objects that makes focusing nearly impossible. This condition is known as presbyopia (Leighton, 1973). The lens also becomes rigid and thicker. "Yellowing of the lens" refers to protein pigments that accumulate in the lens that alter color vision, particularly for shades of brown, beige, and blue. Reds and yellows are usually perceived best (Hatton, 1977). Senile cataracts—a clouding of the lens that makes vision progressively difficult—are so common among elderly people that some authors suggest they are simply an exaggeration of the normal aging of the human lens (Nordmann, 1965).

A fifth senile change in the aging eye occurs in the retina. Both arterial and venous occlusions occur in the retinal blood vessels. Pathologic changes associated with hypertension and diabetes are superimposed on normal aging changes (Duke-Elder, 1967). In the area of the macula, senile macular degeneration results in progressively poor vision, the only treatment for which is increased magnification (Fig. 10-4).

Sixth, the pupil of the eye may be affected by senile miosis. With this problem, the size of the pupil decreases, and the diameter narrows. As a result, a decreased amount of light is able to reach the retina of the eye and more time is required for light-to-dark accommodation (Buseck, 1975).

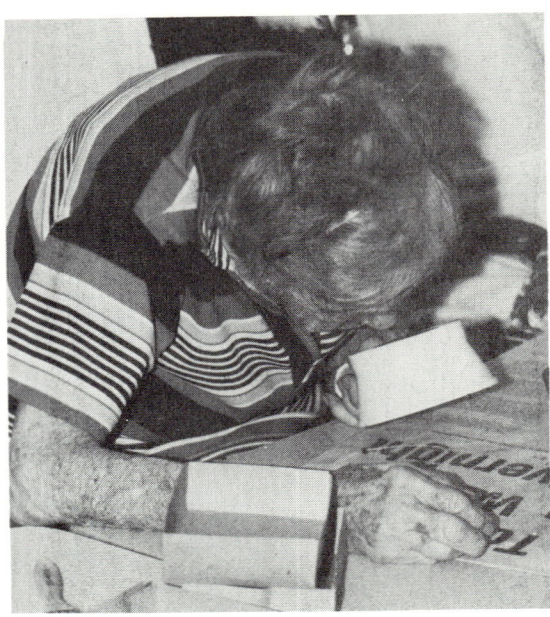

Fig. 10-4. This client has severe macular degeneration and reads headlines only by using magnification. (Photograph by C. D. Falk.)

Last, some rather uncomfortable changes involve the exterior apparatus of the eye. Changes in the upper and lower eyelids can result in irritation of the cornea and conjunctiva. An outward deviation of the eyeball as a result of muscle weakness, known as exotropia, is not uncommon (Buseck, 1975). The field of vision can be altered simply by the mechanical displacement of the eyeball from a loss of orbital fat and ptosis. An obstruction of the nasolacrimal apparatus is fairly common among the elderly. It results in excessive watering of the eye, which distorts vision and causes discomfort. Some people experience a reduction in tear formation that causes dryness and irritation and predisposes to inflammation of the external surface of the eyeball (Leighton, 1973; Buseck, 1975).

The pathologic changes that result in altered vision for elderly people are many. The incidence of glaucoma increases with age, with a major pathologic effect of damage to the optic disk, which can produce blindness or severe alterations in the visual field such as tunnel vision (Leighton, 1973). The microaneurysms of diabetic retinopathy cause rather peculiar and unpredictable changes in the field of vision. People who have had a cerebral vascular accident may have a severe visual field impairment in the form of homonymous hemianopia, which literally causes half of the world to disappear. Diplopia, another neurologic problem, frequently occurs among the aged. In fact, transient visual changes such as brief visual losses, diplopia, and ptosis may be premonitory signs of carotid insufficiency and impending stroke (Buseck, 1975). Some of the changes in visual acuity associated with aging are portrayed in the picture series in Fig. 10-5. The implications of these for safety and ambulation are clear from the photographs.

Trauma, infectious diseases, tumors, and toxic problems of the eye are not uncom-

Text continued on p. 221.

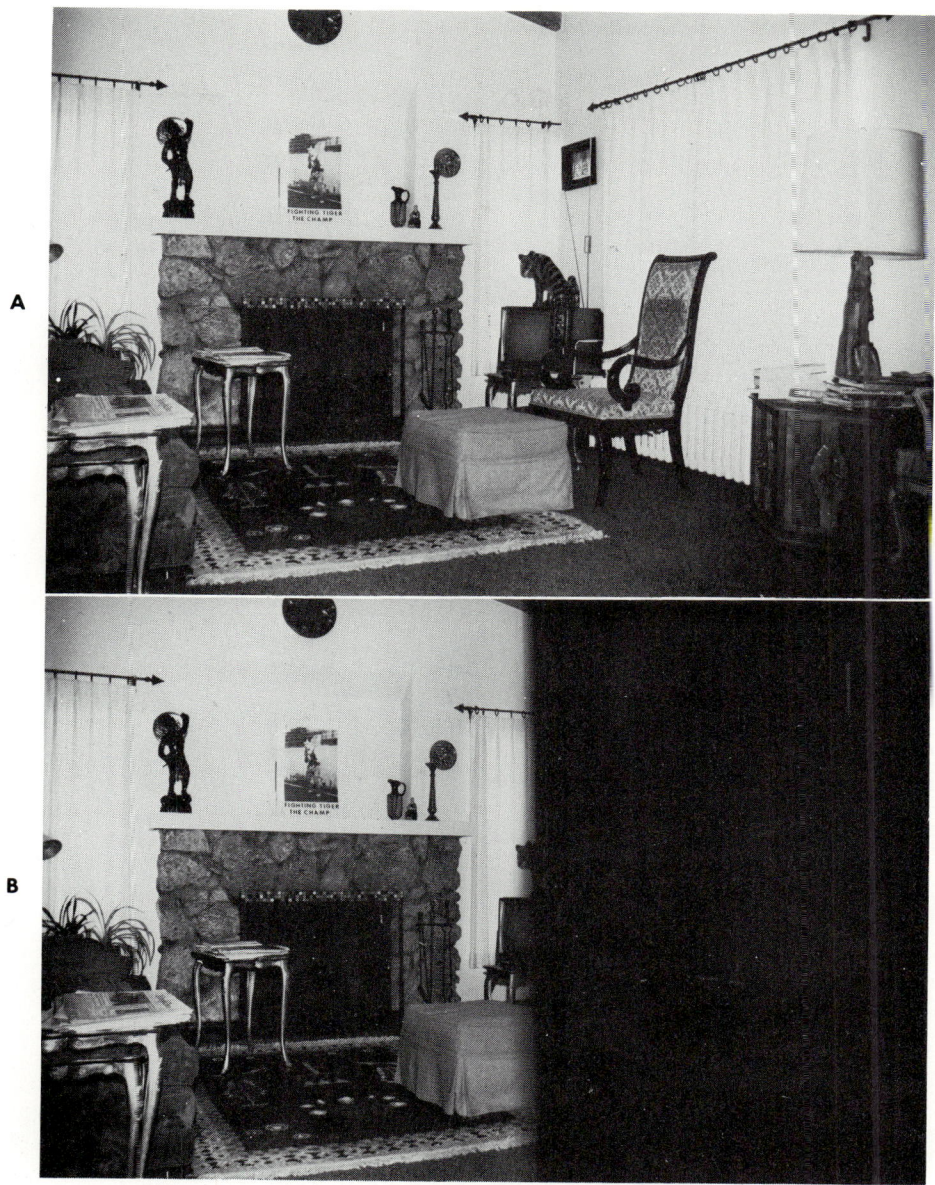

Fig. 10-5. Photo series depicting common visual problems of the aged. (Notice the potential obstacles and how these are affected by visual changes.) Living room seen by: **A**, Client with visual correction of 20/20. **B**, Client with homonymous hemianopia following a cerebral vascular accident. (Photographs by C. D. Falk.)

Continued.

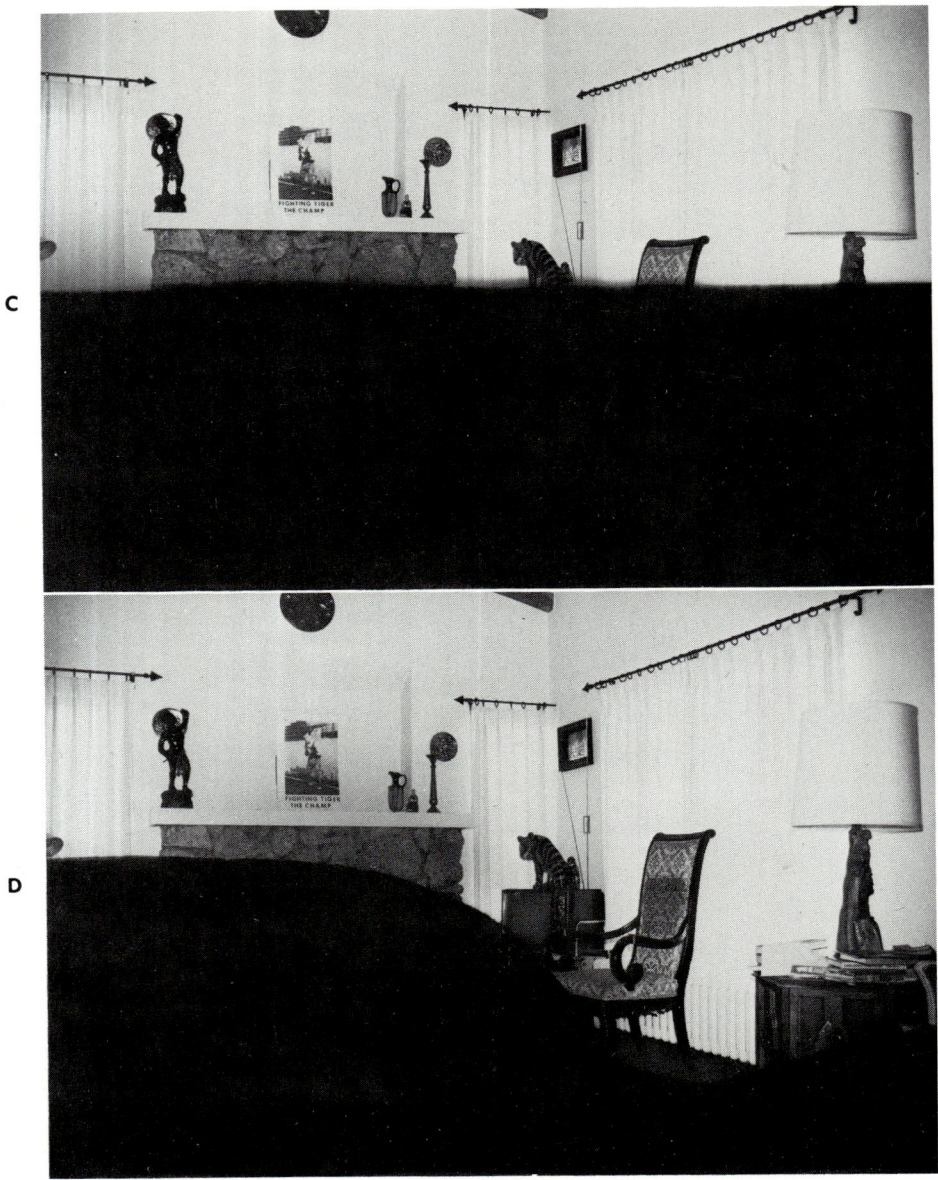

Fig. 10-5, cont'd. C, Client with inferior hemianopia following a cerebral vascular accident; **D**, Client with a detached retina.

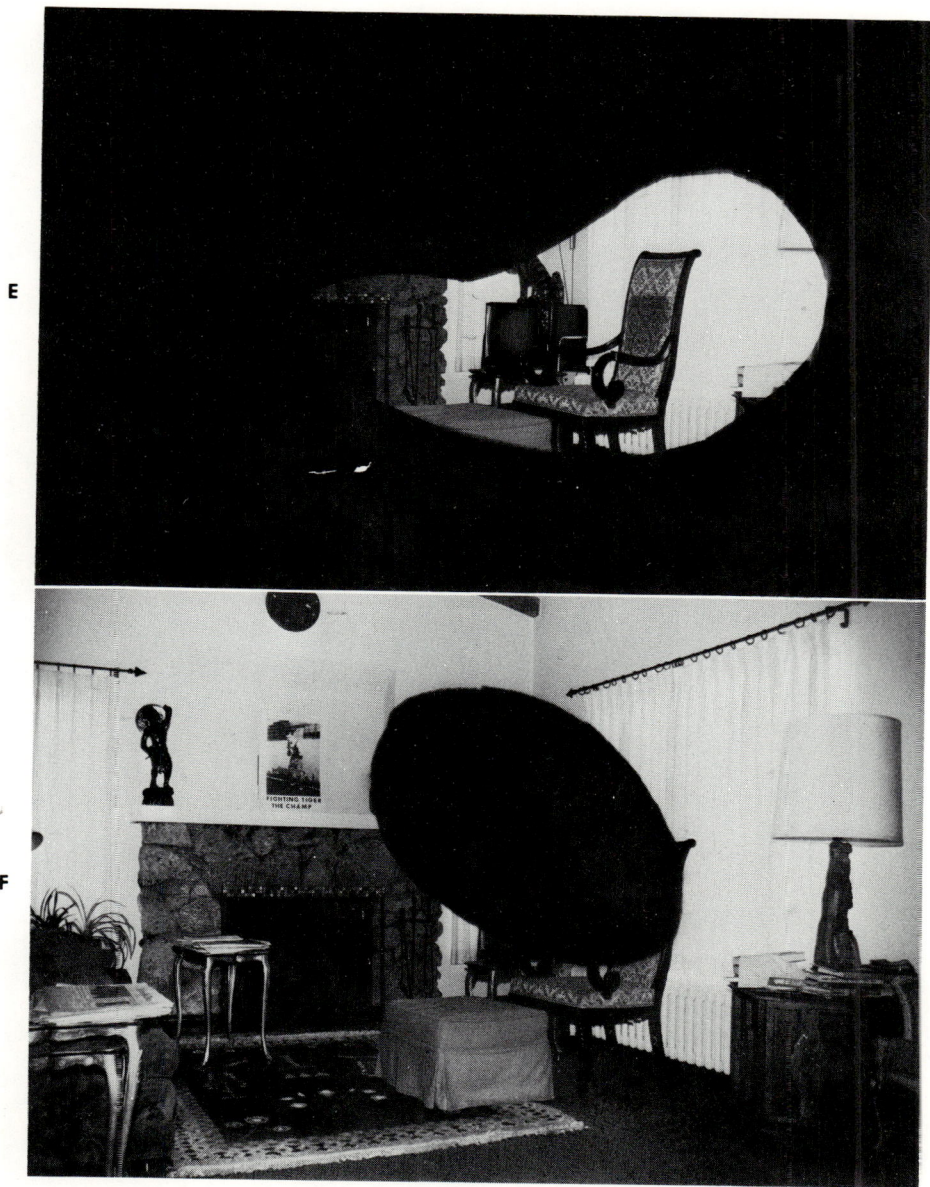

Fig. 10-5, cont'd. E, Client with advanced glaucoma; **F**, Client with macular degeneration.
Continued.

220 *Confusion: prevention and care*

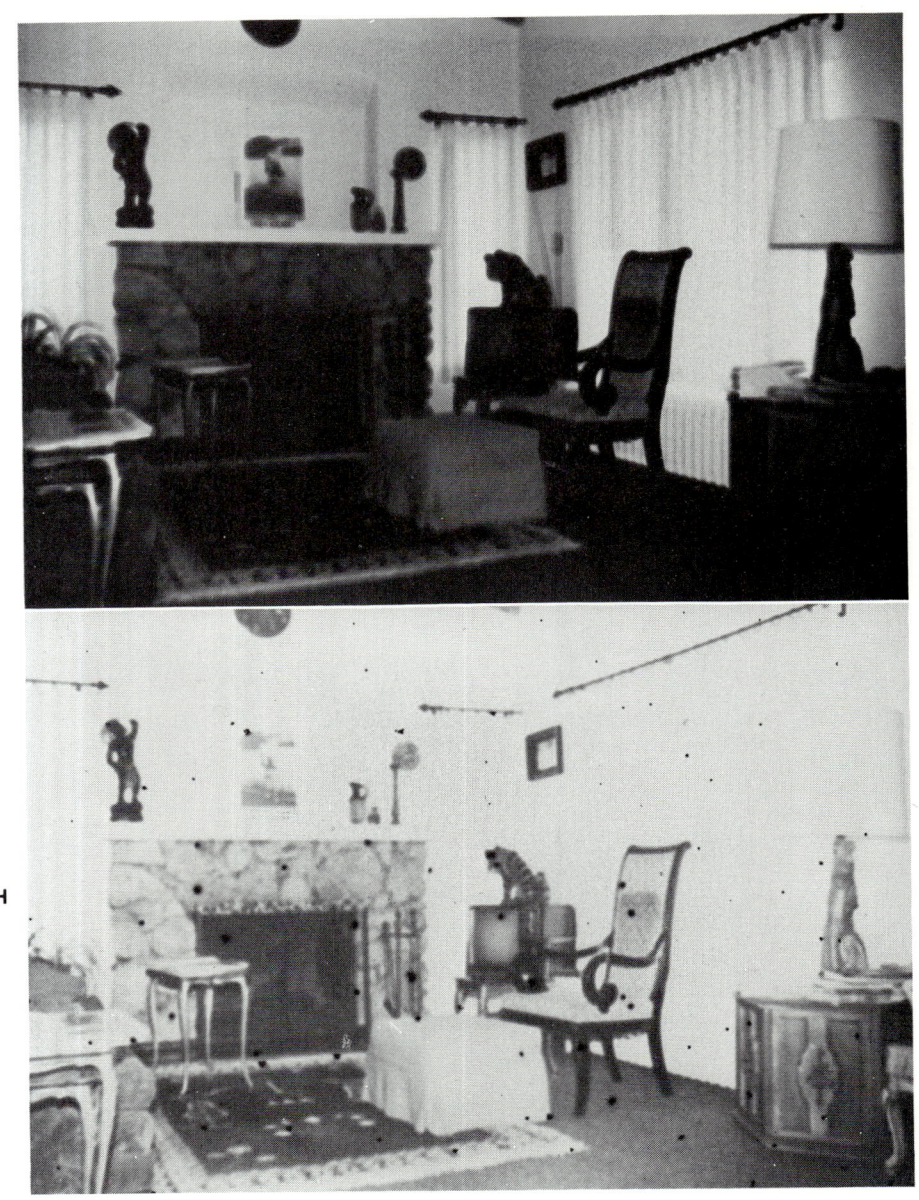

Fig. 10-5, cont'd. G, Client with cataracts; **H**, Client with corneal damage.

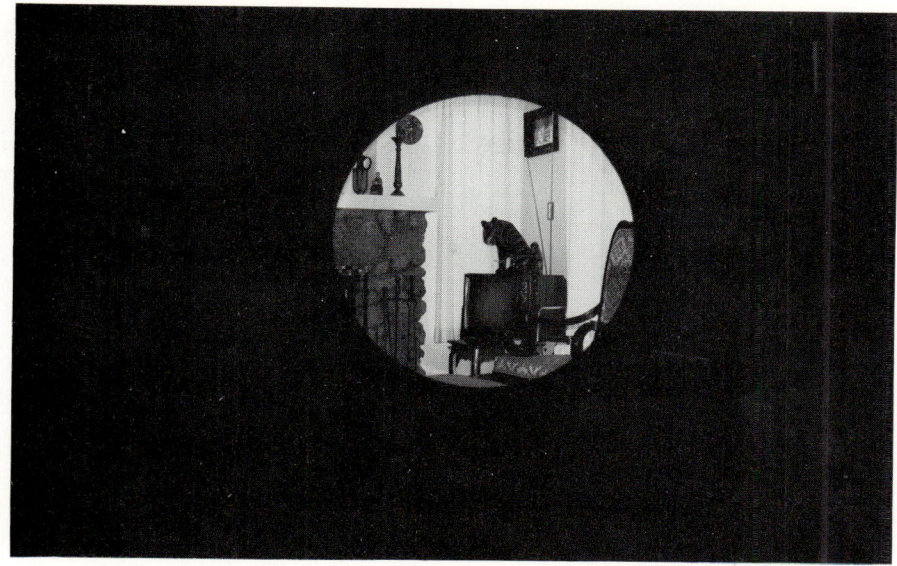

Fig. 10-5, cont'd. I, Client with tunnel vision (retinitis pigmentosa).

mon among the aged. Often, the trauma is self-inflicted as the older person rubs and scratches irritated eyes (Buseck, 1975). Eye irritations not only arise from physical changes in the exterior of the eye, but from chronic exposure to cold, wind, dust, and air pollution. Buseck (1975) reports that herpes zoster, a viral infection, often affects the eyes of older people. After the acute phase of the disease, during which there is pain in the forehead, upper eyelid, and eyeball, there may be a persisting residual anesthesia. This loss of sensation may predispose the individual to abrasions and scarring of the cornea if proper precautions are not taken. Tumors of the eyelid may also occur among the elderly. These usually are basal cell carcinomas characterized by persistent ulcerations and crusts. Finally, the sight of an elderly person may be affected by the toxicity of hypervitaminosis, particularly involving vitamins A and D (Buseck, 1975).

Most of the visual changes of elderly people have an insidious onset and are progressive. The implication for sensory deprivation is chronicity. Many individuals do not realize the extent of their visual limitations because the onset has been so slow. Snyder, Pyrek, and Smith (1976) demonstrated that visual acuity and the caregiver's assessment of mental function are intimately related. Since most of our mental competency tests are based primarily on the appropriateness of response to environmental stimuli, it is not difficult to see that limitations in visual acuity may interfere with the ability to interact and interpret the environment accurately and may lead to inappropriate behavior. Weinberg (1975) suggests the mental status influences visual status. The result is circular. The less an older client sees, the less clear his mental functioning; the more compensated his mental function, the more difficulty he has perceiving what he sees in the environment.

In addition to chronic sensory deprivation, a number of older individuals develop acute sensory deprivation as a result of a sudden loss of sight. Conditions such as glaucoma, detached retina, retinal vascular disease, and hemianopia can all produce a sudden loss of sight.

Although not as numerous, certain physiologic changes of aging can contribute to sensory distortion and overload. An uncorrected astigmatism, for example, can produce an insidious distortion of the world as seen by the elderly person. This can affect depth perception and the perception of the relationships between objects. Certain changes associated with the exterior of the eye, such as tearing and burning, cause distortions of vision and light perception. Lights may seem to be intensified or glaring because of irritation and pain in the exterior eye. Glaucoma can produce halos and alterations of color perception that contribute to sensory overload and distortion. Overdoses of certain drugs, for example, digitalis, can affect the perception of colors and lights. Narcotics may affect the perception of relationships, sizes, and shapes of objects.

High-risk setting factors
Visual deprivation

Sight may be altered or lost completely because of the method of treatment or the characteristics of the environment. For example, sudden blindness, the ultimate deprivation experience, can be simulated through the application of eye patches or by subjecting an individual to a totally dark environment. Sight may be altered by insufficient light or the lack of a previously used prosthesis, such as eyeglasses or a magnifying glass. Many institutionalized individuals are unable to clean their own glasses. The buildup of sticky fingerprints can render the glasses virtually useless, resulting in visual alteration.

An unexpected visual alteration results from bed rest. Consider for a moment the types of sights available to a bedfast person. In the institutional setting, if the person is seated in bed, a wall or wall cabinet is straight ahead. When lying down, the ceiling is straight ahead. On one side of the bed is usually a blank wall framed by bed rails. On the other side of the bed are usually unfamiliar objects, such as an over-the-bed table, suction machines, or bottles of fluid, all framed by bed rails. From most bed positions, it is very difficult to see the faces of individuals who are standing. When the client is lying on his side, for example, the most available view of a person standing beside the bed is the person's chest and upper arms. This problem is even more pronounced if the client has a spinal deviation that limits the range of motion of his neck. Windows are usually accessible to only half of the clients in health care facilities, and then on only one side of the bed. These effects are shown in the pictures series in Fig. 10-6.

Colors in institutions also contribute to the deprivation experience. Pastel colors such as blues, beiges, and pinks are often impossible for the elderly person to distinguish. These may not even be perceived by the client as distinct colors. Dark shades of blue, brown, black, and charcoal are probably not distinguishable except under the most intense lighting conditions (Hatton, 1977). Since beige, pastel yellow, and green are frequently used on walls and for bedspreads, between-the-bed curtains, and draperies in institutional settings and are poorly perceived by elderly clients, texture is probably the only distinctive characteristic among them. Elderly individuals have difficulty distinguishing white china on a white tablecloth, white towels and white soap against the background of white or beige bathroom tiles, and pastel or white uniforms against the faces of caregivers. Thus, depending on colors and object-to-background contrasts, the environment may appear sparsely furnished and very unstimulating, and people become faceless and unidentifiable.

Visual overload and distortion

Contrast glare is a painful problem experienced by most elderly clients that contributes to sensory overload and distortion. Sunlight shining into a darker room can be almost intolerable. Light is intensified as it is reflected off shining wheelchairs, walkers, plastic-covered furniture, and waxed floors. Even china and silverware reflect more light than is comfortable.

Lighting is a tremendous problem in

Care of the client with sensoriperceptual problems 223

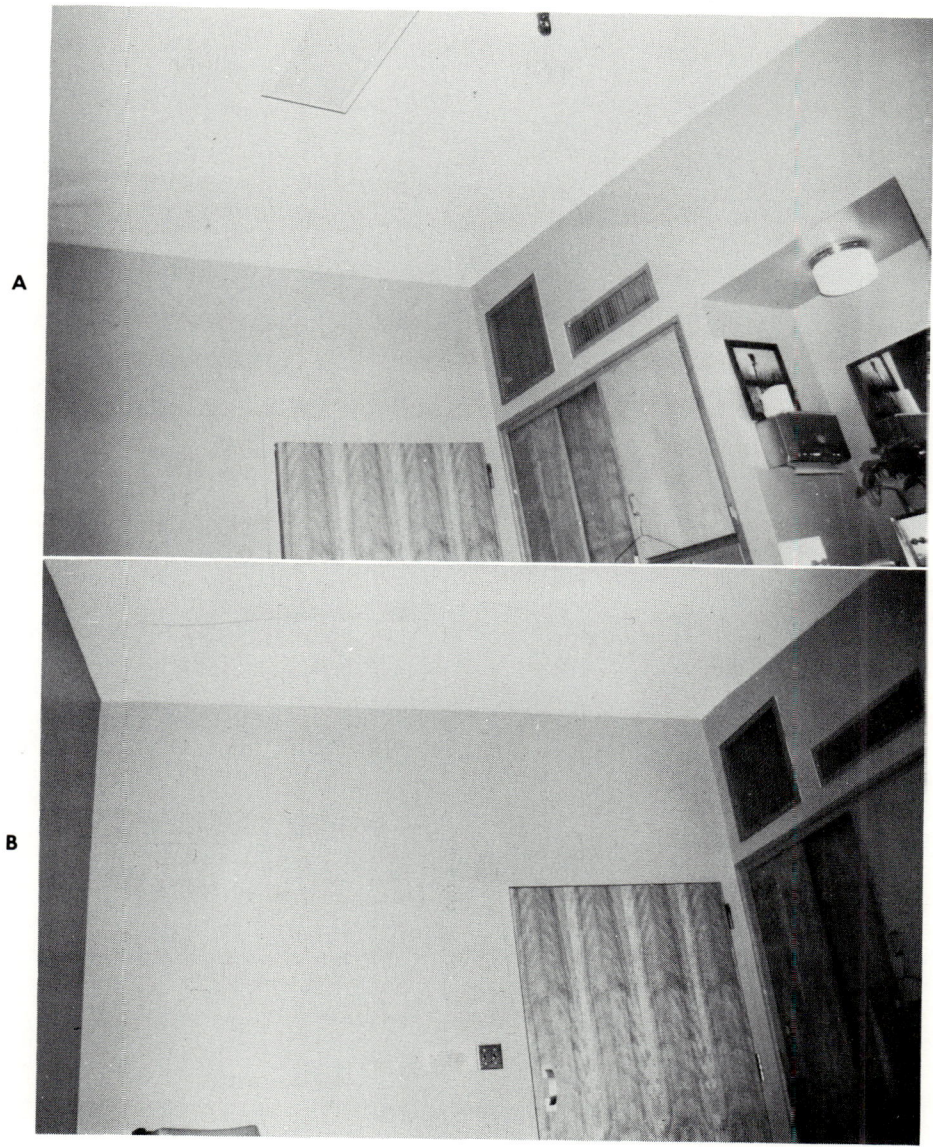

Fig. 10-6. Views from the client's bed. **A,** Lying flat; **B,** Semi-Fowler's position. (Photographs by C. D. Falk.)

Continued.

224 *Confusion: prevention and care*

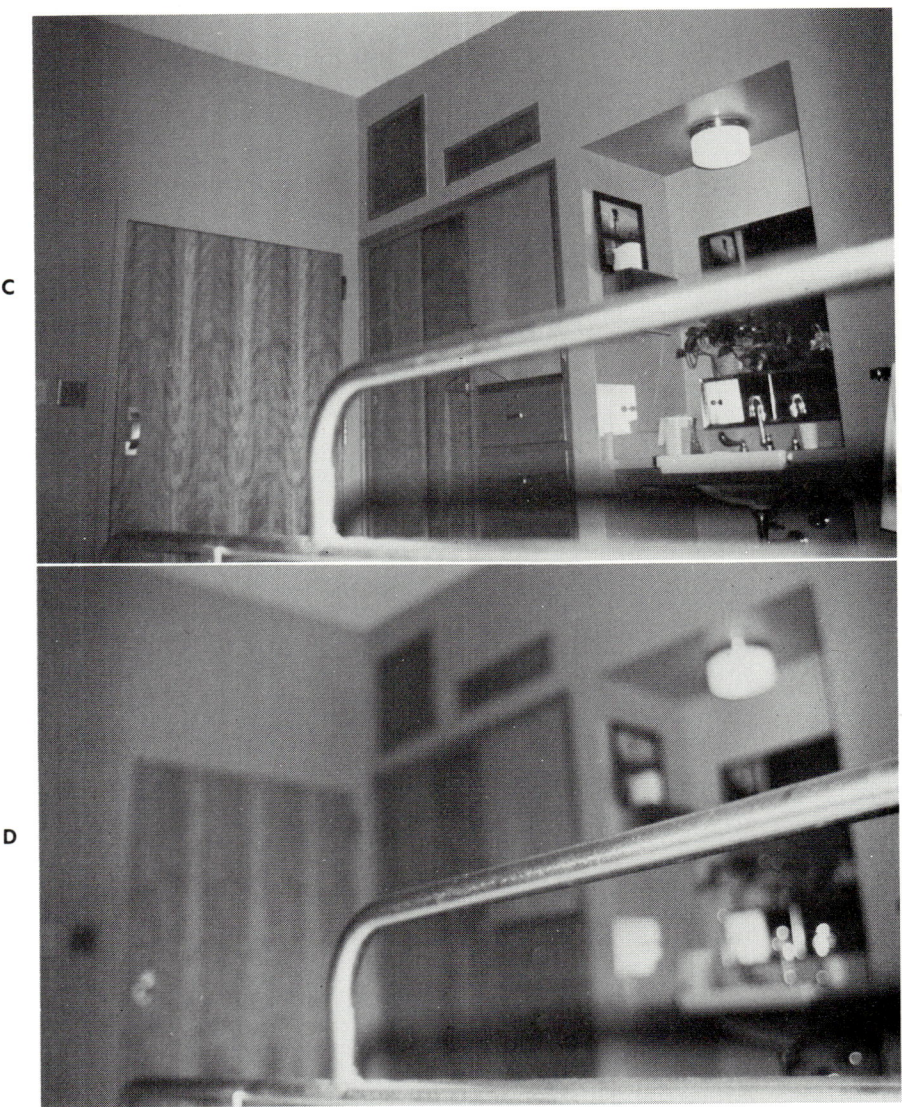

Fig. 10-6, cont'd. C, High Fowler's position looking to the door; **D**, High Fowler's position looking to the door without corrective lens.

Care of the client with sensoriperceptual problems   225

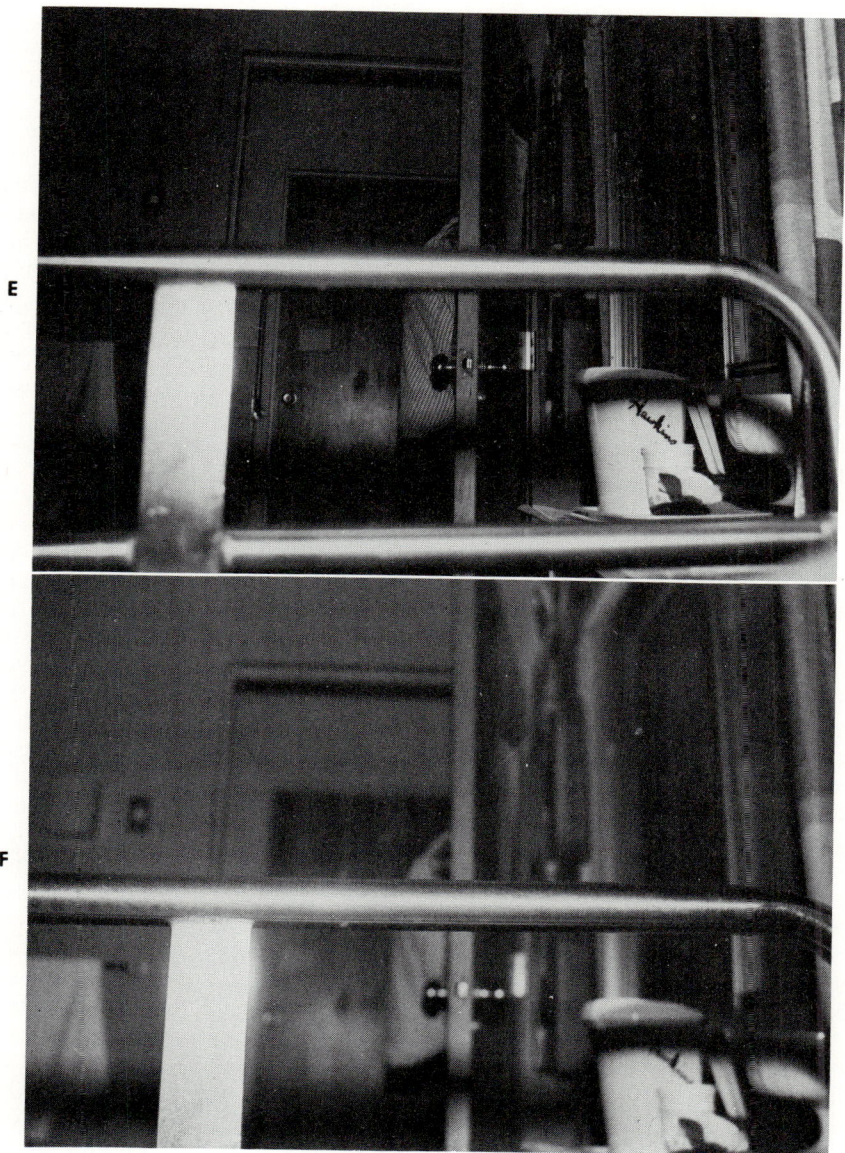

Fig. 10-6, cont'd. E, Lying on side; **F,** Lying on side without corrective lens.

health care facilities and in homes for the elderly. The elderly client needs quantitatively more light to perform detailed tasks. However, the more intense the lighting, the more glare is produced. Elderly people usually cannot accommodate quickly to changes in lighting. Walking from the sunlight into a darker room produces blindness for a prolonged period. Turning on a light in a dark room can produce the same effect as looking directly at a flashbulb (Hatton, 1977). Even moving into a shadowed area can produce the illusion of unequal ground. Many elderly people have fallen after perceiving a ground shadow as a step.

Other sources of distortion and overload arise from treatment methods. Consider, for example, the client who has had his eye patches removed and is faced with the problem of again becoming accustomed to lights and sights. New glasses can produce temporary distortion, particularly when an elderly client is fitted for the first time with bifocals. Bifocals are designed so the lowest level offers comfortable reading sight. This means the client must adapt to the insecurity of not seeing his feet or the ground when he is walking. Prism glasses, given to individuals who must remain flat in bed to facilitate reading and daily activities, can create special problems. Switching back and forth between unaided vision and vision assisted by prism glasses can be extremely disorienting. For example, one elderly client who had been using prism glasses for several days suddenly had an attack of panic. She reported she could no longer distinguish between up and down and was perceiving herself to be on end and falling to the floor.

Equipment in the client's environment can contribute to distortion and overload. Unless the sensory input is ordered, explained, and understood, many elderly clients experience the acute effects of sensory overload.

High-risk caregiver factors

With senile eye changes, the client's visual field and visual acuity determine what he is actually perceiving of the people in his environment. Clients with presbyopia may see rather well at a distance and may be able to see facial features of a caregiver who is standing at arm's length. However, without glasses, these clients usually cannot clearly see objects or people who are closer than arm's length. Clients with senile macular degeneration usually have difficulty distinguishing fine details at any distance. Such clients may, however, at least recognize the person who moves to the distance of a handshake or closer. Retinal vascular changes can result in "spotty" fields of vision, with portions of people or objects absent or indistinct, depending on whether the image falls on one of the "blind spots" of the retina.

Overload and distortion related to the caregivers arise from several areas. Elderly individuals need quantitatively more time to assimilate and respond to new experiences and people. Often, the elderly person who feels physically vulnerable perceives running, fast movements, and rushing with alarm, frustration, and feelings of impending danger. Crowds of people may be frightening for the same reason. Frustration is associated with rushing. The caregivers do not seem to care enough or are too busy to give the elderly client time to gather his thoughts and respond for himself.

Particularly in the institutional setting, the number of people the individual comes in contact with has implications for distortion and overload. With staff changing by shift and with task fragmentation, one client may be in contact with as *few* as ten people during any one day. That number can then be multiplied by the number of staff days off and the number of times staff are rotated from client to client to give an estimate of the extent of the problem. Often, because the client must relate to so many people to meet his needs, he is unable to determine exactly who is responsible for what. This in itself predisposes to overloading and confusion. As one client said, "I feel like a parcel post package. Shuffled from place to place and no one will take me in."

Large numbers of visitors and volunteers further compound the problem. Many untrained "outsiders" are uncomfortable and ignorant about dealing with older people who have visual problems. Often, they approach the client, speak to him, and then awkwardly try to make conversation, all the while making no attempt to identify themselves. One client with severe macular degeneration stated, "They come in here and they stare at me. I'm not sure if I know them or if they know me. If I could see them, it might be different. I am not a freak to be stared at." This type of exchange can be frustrating as well as disorienting to the client.

To a great extent, what we know about other people comes from what they look like within the context of the situation and from their verbal communications. Facial expressions, body movements, and eye contact often reveal more about what a person is saying than the words used. Thus, sensory alterations can arise from not having the caregivers stand, sit, or position the environment in such a way that the client can perceive all the subtle cues necessary for successful interaction.

Fourth-level assessment for visual alteration

Nursing and medical history
Opthalmologic findings
Test for functional visual acuity
Visual field assessment
Inspection of the eyes
Test extraocular muscle strength
Test color vision
Environmental assessment

Assessment of sensory alteration related to sight consists of a series of data-gathering procedures ranging from performing actual visual examinations to critically surveying the environment to identify problem areas. The assessment procedures in this section are more specific for fourth-level diagnosis than the screening procedures introduced in Chapter 6.

Obtaining baseline data about the client's visual status during initial contacts is desirable, particularly if problems were identified during the screening assessment. This information can be used to prevent confusion and to help the nurse detect subtle changes in vision that may occur later. In the Snyder, Pyrek, and Smith (1976) study, of the 295 long-term care residents who received visual screening, 81% had no record of eye care since coming to the facility. This does not necessarily mean that they had not received care. However, there was no record or indication of the care, and the client could not provide the information. This may or may not be indicative of the eye care of the general elderly population, but these findings should raise the nurse's index of suspicion relative to the need for vision assessment. Therefore, she should approach the visual assessment with the assumption that even though the client is wearing glasses, his sight may not be adequately corrected. The client's visual problem may not be correctable with glasses, or his glasses may have been purchased in a dime store.

Assessment may begin with the nursing and medical history. Ascertain the duration of visual problems, the nature of these problems, the types of medical care the client has received for visual problems, the type of prostheses that has been prescribed, and when the last eye examination was performed. Discuss with the elderly client or his caregiver how the client has accommodated for visual problems in the past and how the prosthesis has been used. Suggesting and arranging for an ophthalmologic examination may be one of the most important results of the nursing assessment of visual status. The nurse should have access to the ophthalmologic findings for a complete understanding of the client's visual problems.

Functional visual acuity can be tested using lettered charts constructed from white cardboard and black ink pens or premade letters such as those pictured in Fig. 10-7. For those clients who can read, dark letters on a white background can be used. Begin

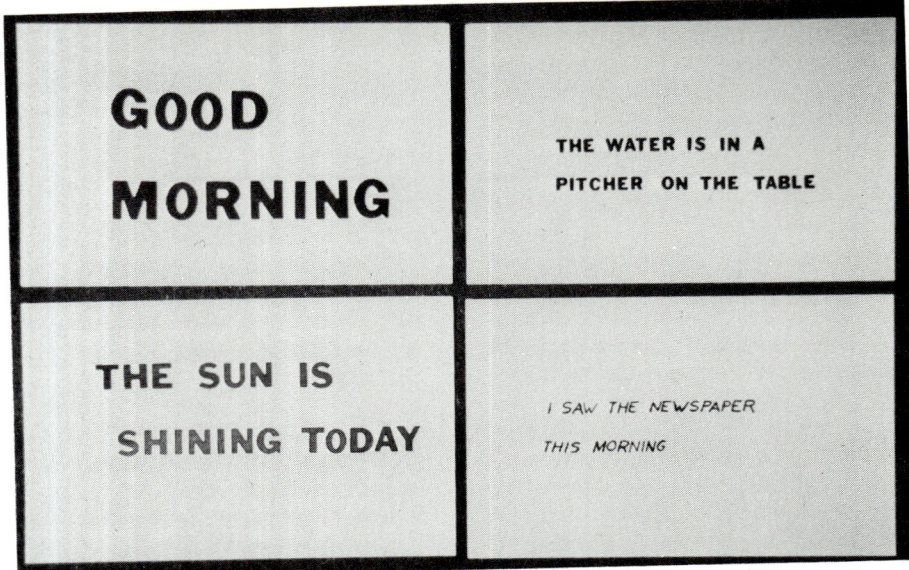

Fig. 10-7. Cards for testing visual acuity: *Upper left,* ¾-inch letters; *lower left,* ⅝-inch; *upper right,* ½-inch; *lower right,* 3/16-inch.

the testing with the largest letters (¾ inch). Have the client hold the card at arm's length and read the words aloud. The distance at which the card is held is then increased and decreased to determine the client's visual acuity at various distances. Progress to smaller print (⅝ inch, ½ inch, 3/16 inch, and book print). Do not use newspapers to test visual acuity. The print of newspapers is not black enough, nor is the paper white enough. In addition, newspaper is thin; light and colors leak through from one page to the next.

Functional visual acuity can also be tested using objects or pictures in the client's room. If you use pictures of objects, make sure the color contrasts are striking. Multicolored or complex pictures are not as useful as pictures of one or two objects. If the client has limited vision, he may have difficulty responding when many objects or colors are present in one picture. Be sure that you use a picture familiar to the client. If the client does not know the name of the object, he may not respond for that reason alone. Visual acuity should be tested with and without glasses, since clients do not usually wear their glasses in bed. After you have tested the client's functional visual status, make detailed notes on his chart or the nursing care plan so others may be aware of the findings.

The client's visual fields should be assessed to ascertain where people should stand, where needed objects should be placed, and generally, how much of the environment is being perceived. There are several ways to assess visual fields. The peripheral fields can be tested by facing the client at a distance of about 1½ feet. Instruct him to look at your nose or mouth and to cover one eye with a piece of cardboard. Cover your own eye on that side. Your visual field will serve as the "normal" and will be compared to the client's. Slowly bring your fingers into the client's peripheral vision. Ask him to tell you when he first sees your fingers. The examination is then repeated with the other eye. Some nurses prefer to use paper and pencil tests

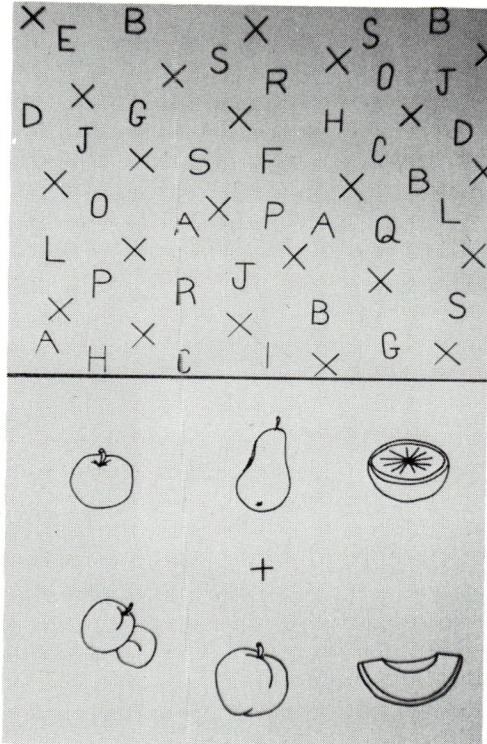

Fig. 10-8. Tests for hemianopia. *Top,* Client circles all X's. *Bottom,* Client looks at center cross and identifies the surrounding objects.

to assess visual fields. Fig. 10-8 shows an example of two such tests. In the top test, the client is asked to circle all of the X's on the page. Watch the client closely as he performs this task. People who have accommodated on their own to a visual field problem will move their eyes, head, or the paper to view the entire page. In the bottom test of Fig. 10-8, the client is asked to look directly at the cross in the middle of the paper and identify the objects on the paper. If time prohibits the use of either of these tests, careful observation of a client as he performs such activities as eating or bathing often reveals a visual field problem. For example, a client with an uncompensated visual field defect will neglect to eat everything on his plate because he cannot see the food placed in his blind spots. When the plate is turned, he will finish the meal. Often, he will request soap or toilet articles, even though these articles are directly in front of him. Certain items that are outside of his altered field of vision simply do not exist for him.

Inspection of the eyes is an essential part of a visual assessment. Tearing and irritation should be noted. Crusts around the eyelids and lesions around the eyes should be examined. Unusual discharges from the eye may be indicative of infections or irritations that could be relieved with medical treatment. Looking into the pupil of an aging eye may reveal the beginnings of an undetected cataract. Redness of the conjunctiva may be the first sign of untreated glaucoma.*

Since exotropia or deviation of the eyeball is not unusual with increasing age, the eyes should be inspected for placement of the eyeball in the socket as the person looks straight ahead. In addition, the muscle strength of the extraoccular muscle can be tested with finger following, using the six cardinal directions of eye movement. Observe the movement of both eyes as they converge on your fingers. As the client follows your finger with his eyes, observe for deviations in movement and nystagmus or fine tremors of the eyeball. Ask the client if he experiences unusual sensations or sights as he follows your finger. Diplopia, or double vision, can cause severe perceptual problems. It stems from weakness or paralysis of the extraoccular muscles and can be detected with finger following (Prior and Silberstein, 1973). In mild forms of diplopia, where only slight muscle weakness is present, the double vision is experienced only when the client attempts to look in the same direction as the weakened muscle. Severe diplopia, on the other hand, usually persists continuously and is most severe when the

---

*For more information, please refer to Mehner, F.: Patient assessment: examination of the eye, Am. J. Nurs. **74**(11):1-16, 1974, a programed instruction.

client attempts to look in the same direction as the paralyzed muscles.

Testing the client's color vision helps the caregiver determine ways to enrich the visual world. For example, if the individual has difficulty discriminating colors such as blues or browns, the environment can be constructed using those colors to which the person is more sensitive. Shades of colors can be applied to white cardboard sheets to assess the person's ability to distinguish primary colors, secondary colors, and various shades of colors. Expect that the perception of bright primary colors will be fairly intact among most elderly individuals and that they will have more difficulty distinguishing pastels and muted shades.

The last phase of the visual assessment involves a careful survey of the environment as the client sees it. Be particularly sensitive to color contrasts, lighting arrangements, sources of glare, and shadows (Fig. 10-9). Critically survey the environment at different times of the day and from

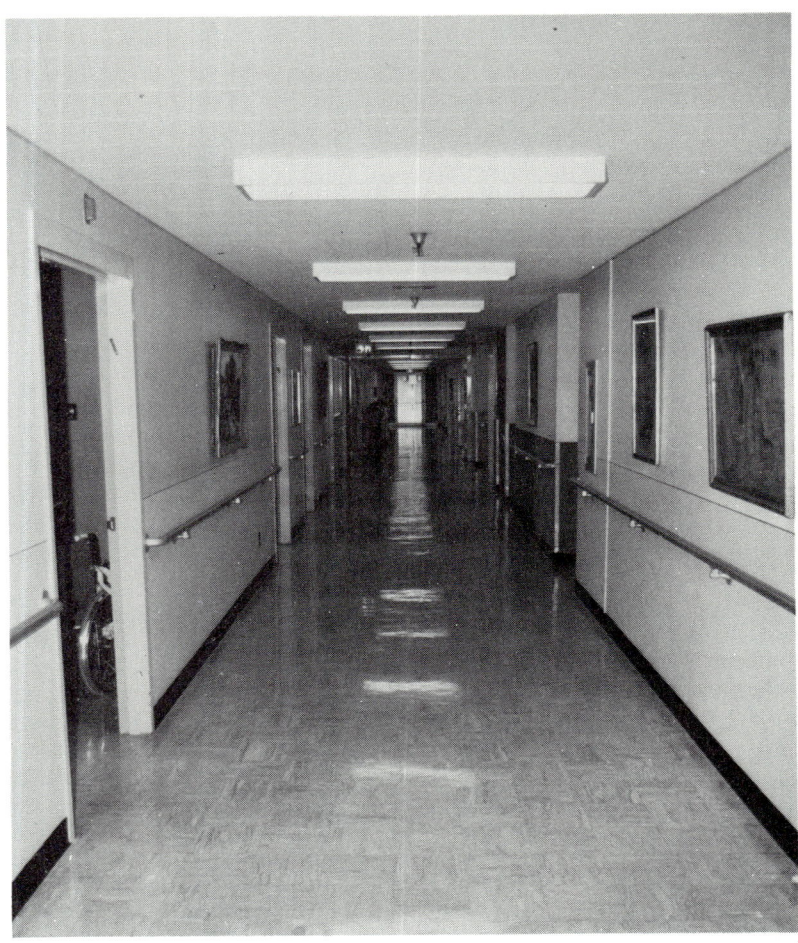

Fig. 10-9. View of a nursing home hall early in the morning. Notice the tunnel effect from the glare, which can cause difficulty for the older person. (Photograph by C. D. Falk.)

different angles. Compare the changes you see with the times when the individual displays wandering, agitation, or confusion. Is it possible that various types of confusion (for example, the "sundown syndrome") are directly related to different visual perceptions as the natural and artificial lighting effects change?

Communicating the results of the assessment is an essential step. The staff, client, and his caregiver should be aware of the visual problems you detect. Plan with them for ways to offset visual problems and to intervene for the confusion that may arise from visual impairments.

Prevention

Prevention of confusion among those clients experiencing visual problems is focused on making the environment predictable and structured, as well as visually richer. When planning enrichment of the environment, remember the client is the only judge of what constitutes enrichment and what constitutes deprivation and overload. The enriched environment can be provided, but the degree of involvement by any client is highly individual.

This section also explores the concept of the prosthetic environment as a means of maximizing function. The realization of such an environment requires a creative staff and the active involvement of the individual clients to make it as meaningful to each as possible. This section is divided into preventive measures for the person who is totally blind and additional preventive measures helpful for the person with altered sight. Some of these measures have been adapted from Burnside (1976).

For clients with severe visual handicaps

1. *Help the client organize his experiences and his environment.*
   a. Introduce yourself to the client initially and announce who you are each time you come in contact with him. Introduce the other people in his environment, whether they are visitors, other caregivers, or other clients. The client who is blind should know who is approaching and why they are there. We often assume sight-deprived individuals become quite sensitive by using other sensory modalities. This may be true for the person who has been blind for a long time but is probably not true for the person who is suddenly blinded, ill, or otherwise preoccupied.
   b. Help the blind client explore the environment through smell, touch, hearing, and locomotion. The blind individual must be given vivid descriptions of the environment. When he is ambulated or pushed in a wheelchair he should be oriented to the destination and given directions to reach the destination. Look for environmental cues that will help the client maintain his orientation to place. Point out the odors as you pass the kitchen and the breeze as you pass an open door. Give opportunities for the client to manipulate the objects in the environment. Point out the different textures as he touches objects, describing the object, its color, and its purpose.
   c. Provide explanations for the sensory events in the environment. Tell the client that the sound of heavy carts in the hall means that it is mealtime, for example. If a person in the client's environment is smoking, let the client know. The odor of a match or a cigarette smoldering in an ashtray smells like anything else burning. Panic reactions can be averted by careful and thoughtful explanations.
   d. Arrange the environment so that the person is comfortable and aware of an object's location. Involve the client in this process so that he has control over his environment as much as possible. Explain to the paraprofessional, staff, family members, and cleaning staff that nothing in the room should be moved without the client's permission. If necessary, place adhesive tape on the furniture and on the floors and write on the tape what goes there so everyone knows the position of articles in the room. If it is necessary to make changes, discuss

them with the client. If a new piece of equipment is needed in the room, give him as many options as possible and let him decide on the object's location.

2. *Teach the client a means of remaining or becoming oriented to time by using environmental cues.*

For example, take the face off of a clock and teach the person how to tell time with it. If the blindness is permanent, suggest the crystal be taken off the client's watch so he can tell time. Chiming clocks are also helpful to the blind. Be sensitive to changes in the environment and use these as points of orientation. If you make rounds every 2 hours, tell the client the approximate times so he can gauge his personal time. If the mailman comes around 10 AM or if meal trays come at 7:30 AM, 11:30 AM, and 5:30 PM, tell the client so these can serve as benchmarks. Noises occurring at the change of shifts may serve as a point of orientation. The warmth of the sun on the window or on the bedsheet may be a way of determining time. When you have established a daily routine with the client, do not deviate from it.

Every institution has distinctive characteristics that denote different days. For example, music therapy may be offered Monday, Wednesday, and Friday. These can be identified and used for orientation to day.

Orientation to month is more difficult. You may be able to obtain a calendar with raised letters, but if not, devise one. Use a peg board that has the number of pegs equal to the number of a month, for example. Explain to the client what month it is and how he can interpret the pegs. Reinforce differences in the changes of the seasons. Whatever system you devise, teach it to the client so that orientation to time is not merely a guessing game.

3. *Devise a means by which the client can ambulate independently.*

For the person who is eye-patched temporarily, independent ambulation probably is not indicated. But if blindness is permanent, independent ambulation is an important goal. Many long-term care institutions have handrails on the walls that can serve as guides and safety devices. Even individuals in wheelchairs can learn to use these to pull themselves along and to become independent. Do not assume that blindness by itself prohibits independent ambulation. Lack of physical strength, lack of coordination, and medical prohibitions *may* limit independent ambulation, but blindness, by itself, does not.

4. *Provide liberal sensory input via other sensory modalities, along with verbal descriptions.*

Blind individuals respond well to experiences where they can use their other senses. Many socialization groups reported in the literature have used kittens, dogs, and various textures of cloth for tactile stimulation; perfumes, cooking odors, and flowers for olfactory stimulation; music, rhythm bands, and talking for auditory stimulation; and different tasting foods for gustatory stimulation. With these cited exceptions, we use few of the potential enjoyable sensations to stimulate our clients. For example, gardening provides the opportunity for all of the pleasurable stimulations derived from being outside: the warm sun, the cool breeze, and the fresh odors of the outdoors. Working the soil provides the warmth and the smell of the earth. When the client is growing and cultivating flowers and herbs, he can learn about his different plants by their odors and their feel, and at the same time, he has the satisfaction of helping living things thrive. We organize clubs for bird-watching, but what about clubs for bird-listening? Learning to identify birds by their various songs and teaching others about them can be exciting and also promotes our self-esteem. In home environments, we keep houseplants and pets of all kinds, we encounter children, and we create an environment of warmth and comfort. We do little of this for the homebound or institutionalized elderly, and the blind are particularly devoid of pleasurable stimulants. This is a largely untapped area, limited only by our imagination.

5. *Explore each area of the activities of daily living for each client to ascertain what environmental manipulation would support independent functioning.*

Each activity of daily living needs to be considered separately and each activity broken into its component parts to determine how to facilitate independence. For example, independent bathing requires that the client (1) know where the bathroom is; (2) have a means of getting to the bathroom; (3) know where his toilet articles are kept; (4) can gather the articles and get them to the bathroom; (5) can undress and dress; (6) can safely get in and out of the tub or shower; (7) can safely remain in the tub or shower without being harmed; (8) can turn the water on and off easily and safely; and (9) have such personal items as soap, towel and shampoo arranged in accessible positions. Any one of these areas may need to be supplemented by the nursing staff.

The next step is to determine the client's current abilities in each area, his potential abilities, and those areas that are restricted because of safety factors. The environment itself should be considered to determine which facets obstruct independence and which facilitate it. Obstructive facets should be altered in whatever way possible. For example, the person may need help getting in and out of the tub and turning the water on and off without being burned. On the other hand, he is able to collect his own toilet articles and get to the bathroom if he uses a wheelchair with a cloth carrier attached to the side. He can wash himself except for his back and legs. If the client has any functional sight, his personal toilet articles should stand out against the white tile background, for example, a dark blue towel, green soap, and green shampoo in a clear, shatterproof bottle. Making these distinctions, following through with the necessary environmental alterations, and helping in only those areas where the client needs help is the essence of creating the facilitative environment for the person with visual alterations.

The following suggestions may be helpful for various activities of daily living. This list is by no means exhaustive or complete. The interested reader may want to consider further study on this subject through the use of an occupational therapy textbook.

a. Dressing. If the client has difficulty choosing and reaching his own clothing, help him select the clothing. Lay it out on the bed in the same accessible way each day. It is helpful to many visually impaired individuals to use a button sewed into the back of the neck and waist of each garment as a dressing cue. Small buttons, snaps, and zippers replaced by large buttons or Velcro fasteners are helpful to many individuals who are both sight-deprived and arthritic or who have difficulty manipulating small objects. For individuals who have difficulty reaching or seeing their feet, sometimes "starting" their socks or stocking is enough to enable them to complete the task. Some people are quite successful at using a cardboard "sock guide" that opens the sock and has a string tie for pulling the sock on. Elastic shoelaces help the client slip on tied shoes without having to see. Arranging his clothes closet according to colors and outfits may be helpful in allowing the sight-deprived client to choose color-coordinated outfits without help.

Occasionally, the person's problem is compounded by hemiplegia. There is no reason why sight-altered people cannot be taught the same one-handed techniques for dressing taught to other hemiplegic patients.*

b. Toileting. The obvious problems with independent toileting for elderly individuals with visual problems include navigating to the bathroom and safely transferring to the toilet. A visual disturbance by itself does

---

*These techniques are presented simply in the publications entitled *Strike back at stroke* (U.S. Department of Health, Education and Welfare. Public Health Service, Washington D.C., 1964, U.S. Government Printing Office) and in other similar publications.

not prohibit these activities. Barring other problems that must be dealt with separately, such as poor balance, poor coordination, and orthostatic hypotension, navigating and transferring can be easily taught and consistently reinforced with good results. A not-so-obvious problem associated with toileting concerns the client who is dressed in his unaltered clothing and then requires undressing assistance as well. The unassisted client may not be able to remove his clothing quickly enough to prevent an accident. It is helpful to replace the zippers and buttons in his slacks with Velcro strips, which require a slight tug to open rather than the ability to see and find a zipper pull. Men and women alike have found that creating a U-shaped opening in the front of their slacks (similar to the openings found on the U.S. Navy bellbottom trousers) to replace the traditional fly facilitates manipulation of clothing. It is helpful for women to wear slacks that are one size too large, with elastic waists for easy manipulation. Men are often more satisfied with slacks one size too large as well. Many women prefer loose skirts rather than slacks because of their easier manipulation.

Undergarments can be a real problem especially for the sight deprived woman. Tight girdles often prohibit getting to the toilet on time. Wearing a girdle that has no crotch and not wearing underpants helps in these circumstances as does splitting the undergarment at the side seams and sewing a "Velcro" strip in. It is best to convince the woman to wear a tight girdle only for special occasions.

c. Eating. Most nurses know to teach the person with visual disturbances to find his plate and place setting by using the clock face as a guide. However, other things are equally as helpful. For instance, the plates used for elderly people with visual disturbances should be plain white; figures or designs on the plates can be easily confused with food. These white plates should stand out on a background tablecloth of a dark brown, black, or deep red. This will help individuals with even minimal visual acuity. Brightly colored food is then placed on the white plates, also standing out. A menu that included fish, rice and cauliflower on the same white plate would be difficult to see. Tell the client what he is eating to help him more directly identify the food on the plate. The use of plate guards is helpful for people with visual disturbances since they can push the food against it and be relatively assured they will end up with food on their fork. "Training cups" rather than regular cups and glasses are helpful for some individuals who spill their drinks frequently. However, in cases where they are not well accepted, nonbreakable glasses and cups only half filled may prevent spilling. Glasses with stems can be easily tipped and are not desirable for the person with a visual disturbance.

If the client has difficulty eating independently because he spills food on himself, several alternatives may help him. Plastic bibs can be used, but these are not well received by older individuals. Washable smocks used for mealtime and then removed and washed are far more acceptable to the older person. Many older individuals feed themselves much better when they know they are wearing old clothes rather than their very best. The better clothing can be donned when the meal is finished. Having the sight-impaired elderly person use the same place setting for every meal also facilitates independent eating.

d. General comments. Older people with visual problems, both in and out of institutions, can be taught to cook, clean, make their beds, use the telephone, and ambulate with safety and independence. In addition, they can be helped to perform a wide variety of recreational and business activities independently. The important components of the plan consists of assessing their capabilities, capitalizing on their strengths, and manipulating the environment to be as facilitative and helpful as possible.

For clients with specific alterations of sight

In addition to previous suggestions:

1. *Assess the precise nature of the sight problem and plan accordingly.*

Adequate intervention for sight-deprived clients is impossible unless the exact nature of the sight problem is known. For example, measures effect against visual field defects are quite different from those effective against decreased visual acuity. Therefore, assessment of the sight problem is the first step.

2. *For defects in functional and reading sight:*

a. Obtain and use appropriate prosthesis. Arrange with the staff and client for the glasses to be placed consistently in a convenient place so that the client has access to them at all times. Everyone who has contact with the client should know that he wears glasses, and where they are kept, and should encourage their use. If necessary, this information can be posted on the client's bed or wheelchair. Cleaning glasses should be a part of the daily activities of living for each elderly client in a health care facility.

b. Wean client to independent ambulation, if at all possible. Learning the territory is essential for the client, as is gaining strength and endurance. As time progresses, control and mastery of the environment are enhanced if the client can get up and go when he wants to. Concentration on socialization and group activities is the usual approach taken with older clients. While social interaction in groups is desirable, the client still needs to have control over his group participation and to be able to seek privacy. As he becomes proficient at independent locomotion, he can move in and *out* of groups as he desires and can ultimately control the amount and intensity of his overall sensory input.

c. Promote focused communication and social interaction. After observing and interacting with many elderly individuals with visual problems, it is strikingly apparent that they often have difficulty maintaining perfunctory social interaction. After the topics of health and the institutional food are exhausted, the client is left with little to say. Think for a moment about how most of us start and maintain interaction when we are building a relationship. We focus our interaction on things we see in the immediate environment, such as some activity or the weather, or we discuss what we have seen on television or read in the newspaper. The person with altered vision is at a real disadvantage in social interaction unless he has learned the social skill of focusing conversation on other than visual experiences. Therefore, the nurse needs to teach the client, other staff members, visitors and family members how to foster and maintain social interactions. For example, communication can be focused on shared sensory experiences other than visual ones, such as things that are heard, felt, or smelled in the immediate environment. Interaction may be focused on the remembered past, using the techniques of reminiscing therapy. Newscasts can be used to help the client initiate and maintain communication. Reading passages from books or poetry and then stopping for discussion can be used as a socialization technique, as can audiotapes on various topics. The process of communication need not be difficult or awkward, if the client and untrained people who come in contact with him receive support and guidance during the initial contacts. The nurse can provide this and enable the visually limited client to retain his sense of competence and pleasure about social interaction.

d. Provide adequate lighting. Elderly people generally need quantitatively more light to perform detailed tasks than the young. This becomes increasingly important as a visual alteration becomes worse. When an elderly person is reading or doing hand work, the work area should be brightly lighted, with care to avoid glare. It is recommended that most lighting in institutions for the aged be indirect, with direct lighting provided for tasks requiring fine discrimination. There should be adequately shaded lights in the environment that the elderly client can pull down to directly illuminate his work. The lighting inside a room should be of the same intensity as the lighting coming in from the window. Older people can experience a great deal of discomfort if they look out on bright daylight from a darker room. Sunscreens can be used to filter the intensity of the outside light without significantly darkening the room, or the lights inside can be left on when intense sunlight streams into the room. Rheostats on the inside lights make it possible to change the intensity of inside lighting without a "flashbulb" effect.

e. Use a color coding system to enrich the visual stimulation aid orientation. Bright colors enrich the environment. The surfaces in nursing homes should have matte finishes rather than glossy ones. A color coding system that uses bright colors may be used to help the client recognize special places he uses routinely. For example, if all the women's bathrooms have bright red doors, and all of the men's bathrooms have bright green doors, the chances of the client finding the appropriate bathroom are increased. In most institutions, all halls look the same. Therefore, if the walls in one hall are painted with a broad bright pink band, and the walls in another hall are painted with a broad bright blue band, the chances of the client finding the hall with his room are also increased. Color coding can also be used to help a client distinguish his own space and belongings. His door may be painted bright yellow, along with the furniture in his room, the back of his wheelchair, and the tags in the back of his clothing. Since all beds look alike, use of bright bedspreads may overcome the problem of one client crawling onto another's bed.

f. Use the client's name, printed on belongings in large black letters, or identifying pictures to help him identify his personal things. In most institutions names are printed on the doors for the convenience of the staff. Large print must be used for the client's sake.

g. Use variety in colors and types of objects, with descriptions to enrich visual perception. Clients respond to flowers, foods of various colors, animals, soft, bright clothing, gaudy jewelry, and bright pictures. Their response to a hand mirror held close to their faces is often remarkable. Many people have spent 5 years in nursing homes, never clearly seeing their own face because the mirrors in the bathrooms are too far away and not at the right angle for a wheelchair. When individuals are largely confined to one room, the potential for variation in visual experiences is limited. The setting needs to be changed as often as possible. For example, a semicomatose patient who requires tube feedings and oxygen has been in her room for more than 18 months. Periodically, the staff moves her bed so she can have different views. When the bed is turned toward the windows, there is a spectacular view of the mountains. When the bed is turned toward the door, there is a view of the activity in the hall. Occasionally, they move her bed, with all the equipment, into the hall and remain with her, explaining and describing the events around her. She is presented with flowers and pictures in close-up. She is shown a mirror, and the staff describes her appearance to her. Even though the staff is only occasionally rewarded by a response from the patient, they believe that this variety increases the quality of her existence, and it probably does.

h. Relieve eye irritations. Some people have altered sight that arises from the irritations associated with the aging eye. For these individuals, "artificial tears" can relieve the irritation and tearing that gives rise to blurred vision. Some clients report that cool, moist compresses placed over the eyes are helpful. Some elderly clients are prone to the collection of debris in the canthus of the eye, which can predispose it to infection and further alter sight. Gently clean the area around the eyes at frequent intervals and remember that anything put directly into the eye must be sterile. Some physicians prescribe antibiotic ointments or drops that help relieve blurred vision if they effectively control the infection.

3. *For defects in the visual field*:

a. Construct the environment as individually as possible so the client can compensate for the defect. Staff and visitors need to be instructed where to stand for maximum visualization. Food and personal articles should be placed in precisely the right position to be seen. Clients should be approached from a visible position. Having people "pop" into the visual field at close quarters can be very startling and disturbing. Every attempt must be made to maximize whatever good vision the client has.

b. Attend to safety. Elderly clients with visual defects may become progressively less willing to ambulate independently and to explore the environment if they feel they may be endangered by their lack of vision. One way to help the client achieve maximum function is to teach him to scan the environment. Clients with visual field defects often do not realize that if they move their heads from side to side as they walk, they are more likely to see all of their environment. "Spotting exercises" sometimes help the client learn how to scan. These involve using a flashlight in a darkened room and teaching the person to follow the light as it is projected on the wall. As the client becomes proficient following the light, the light is flashed on different areas of the wall for the client to find. Scanning can also be taught by having the person view a picture or look out a window and describe the scene. The client should learn to pay particular attention to those areas not in his field of vision but that he may see by moving his head.

4. *For defects in extraocular muscle movement*, attend to diplopia. When a client has a weakened eye muscle, diplopia occurs when he tries to look in the direction of the weakened muscle. If weakness is the only problem, diplopia can be averted by having him move his head to visualize those things on the weakened side. However, if the extraocular muscle is totally paralyzed and the eye is constantly everted in the opposite direction, the only measure that provides comfort and reduces visual distortion is patching the involved eye.

5. *For defects in the environment*:

a. Decrease visual monotony. The environments that clients encounter in institutions are often quite different from those they have at home. The visual environment, particularly in the long-term care facilities, should be as visually pleasing and stimulating as possible. A great amount of effort must go into planning the living environment for the elderly.

b. Increase the identifiability of people. People are just as much a part of the client's environment as the rooms or the furniture. For that reason, staff members must make a special effort to distinguish themselves individually to the patient. Conventional name tags are of use only to the visitors; tags should be at least 4 inches high to be visible to elderly people experiencing normal visual changes. Caregivers should wear bright colors easily differentiated from skin tones and bright lipstick that allows the clients to see their faces and mouths. Well-manicured and brightly colored nails add depth to the nurse's hands and help define her personal boundaries. Even perfumes and after-shaves worn by the staff help to distinguish one individual from the next. Since clients may have difficulty telling each other apart, these special efforts should be made with the clients as well.

c. Attend to the effects presented by nighttime. As artificial lighting predominates at night, special visual problems are created. Shadows are extremely difficult to interpret for the client with a vision problem. Illusions can be created by shadow-to-light contrasts or as the bedfast individual looks out on a bright corridor from a darkened room. A night-light burning in the room of an elderly client can prevent nighttime accidents. However, in the sensory deprivation experiments cited previously, hallucinations were present more often under partial light conditions than under no-light conditions. Therefore, although night-lights need to be used for safety, they should be shaded and diffused, with just enough light to illuminate the walking area. Leaving a light on in the bathroom with the door slightly ajar is not a suitable substitute for a well-designed night-light.

Intervention

The key to intervention for those who are experiencing confusion resulting from visual problems is a structured and organized enrichment of the environment. This kind of intervention requires sensitivity to the environment and to the client himself. For the client with a visual problem, the caregiver serves as a resource. Through interaction with the caregiver, the client can validate and interpret his visual experiences. Through the staff, the client can organize and structure his perceptions and begin to rely on consistency and predictability in a setting that he cannot see well.

The nursing objectives for this section are:

1. To provide an unchanging structure and organization to which the client is oriented
2. To act to reduce anxiety

In addition, the reader is referred to Chapter 8, the previous prevention section, and the section on sensory alteration for other suggested interventions.

1. *Provide an unchanging structure and organization to which the client is oriented.* Elderly blind people need to have the opportunity to find consistency and predictability in at least some parts of their life. The parts that need to be structured should be determined by the individual. Some clients enjoy moving from event to event during the day, but require an inviolate bedtime routine. Others like consistency throughout the day, with infrequent surprises for variety. If he is able, the client should decide. Once the decision has been made, schedules, routines, and rituals should be communicated to everyone in contact with the client. For blind individuals, the most needed routines are consistent placement of objects in the environment and consistent rituals around such daily activities as bathing and eating. However, only the client himself can decide what will make him most comfortable.

2. *Act to reduce anxiety.*

a. Speak to the client before touching him so as not to startle him. If he is hearing impaired as well, use very gentle touch to get his attention before performing any task. Every time you come into the room, the client should know you are there and who you are. Use his name, introduce yourself, and give an explanation of why you are in the room.

b. Explore how he is perceiving the environment and discuss misperceptions.

c. Teach an appropriate means of summoning help.

Outcome criteria of successful nursing intervention against visual alteration

1. The client reports and demonstrates that he can interact comfortably with an environment that he cannot see
2. The client reports and demonstrates that his anxiety level is reduced
3. The client is successful in his environment most of the time
4. The client can comfortably discuss his visual perceptions of the environment
5. The client is no longer confused

These measures in the assessment, prevention, and intervention portions of this section are summarized at the end of this chapter.

SENSORY ALTERATION IN RELATION TO HEARING
High-risk client factors
Physiologic manifestations

It is estimated that by the age of 65, 50% of the male population and 30% of the female population suffer a hearing loss that interferes with social interaction (National Center for Health Statistics, 1971). The term presbycusis is applied to an auditory decline associated with simple aging. It should be noted that there is a great deal of controversy about the idea of hearing loss being a "normal" consequence of aging. Some audiologists state that loss of auditory functions is a symptom rather than a disease. Whether the loss occurs at age 6 or 65, these audiologists state that there are always underlying identifiable pathologic causes, some of which are preventable or treatable (Rupp, 1970; Myerhoff and Paparella, 1978). Hinchcliffe (1962) and Fisch (1973), on the other hand, state that deterioration of sensory perception in the aged occurs in all sensory modalities. Therefore, it is reasonable to assume that declining auditory function occurs as a result of aging. Perhaps, they state, it is the expected degree of loss, not the loss itself, that spells the difference between normal aging and pathologic processes. To date, the relationship between increasing age and decreasing auditory function is a simple correlation rather than a causal relationship. Thus, the practitioner's index of suspicion for active pathology should be high no matter at what age hearing loss is reported.

Presbycusis is a progressive, bilateral, symmetric hearing loss that is sensorineural in nature. The major manifestations are (1) a progressive loss of hearing in the higher frequencies that can usually be detected audiometrically but may not have a significant effect on functional hearing; and (2) a primary loss of discrimination that may not be detectable by audiometric examination for pure tones but significantly affects sound discrimination (phonemic regression) (Yarrington, 1976). The functional abnormalities found with presbycusis include impaired sound localization, impaired auditory sensitivity, increased response time to verbal stimuli, and sometimes tinnitus (Fisch, 1973). According to Pastalozza and Shore (1955), "pure" presbycusis can be differentiated from hearing deficits that arise from auditory pathology by certain criteria. The characteristics of "pure" presbycusis include no history of ear disease, negative otoscopic and rhinoscopic findings, patient's age of 60 years or over, no history of a severe generalized disease, audiometric indications of sensorineural hearing loss, bone conduction almost equal to air conduction, right and left ear air conduction almost equal, and a gradual and progressive onset of the impairment.

Schnuknecht (1955, 1964) identifies four basic types of presbycusis that can be differentiated histologically. The first is epithelial atrophy or sensory presbycusis. This is associated with degeneration at the basal end of the cochlear duct of the organ of Corti. It is manifested by an abrupt high-tone hearing loss and appears in middle age. The second type is neural atrophy or neural presbycusis. It is associated with degeneration of the spiral ganglion cells of the cochlea. The onset of this type occurs later in life and is characterized by the loss of auditory discrimination or phonemic regression. This type is affected by a decreasing number of neurons to decode and transmit the auditory message. The problem with this presbycusis is not necessarily that the person cannot hear but that he cannot understand what he hears. Often, audiometrically, his hearing remains essentially normal (Rupp, 1970). This finding is present whether or not a hearing aid is in use. Metabolic presbycusis is the third type identified by Schuknecht. This seems to result from problems with the physical and chemical processes by which energy is made available to the sensory organs. It is associated with a decrease in the production of endolymph. The last type is mechanical presbycusis. It is associated with a stiffening of the basilar membrane and an interference with the motion mechanics of the cochlear duct.

Since presbycusis is not the only condition that results in adult-onset deafness, it is of benefit to briefly review other types of hearing loss among the elderly. According to Meyerhoff and Paparella (1978), hearing loss may be congenital or delayed. Congenital hearing loss is present at birth and rarely presents a diagnostic problem among the elderly. Congenital deafness may, however, present a management problem in old age. Delayed deafness, which develops later in life, is the type most commonly associated with the hearing loss of aging. In addition, hearing loss may be progressive or stable. It may have a genetic basis or may be nongenetic and result from environmental influences. All of these have implications for the elderly.

Using the Meyerhoff and Paparella classification system, the following are types of delayed deafness found among elderly people.

1. *Genetic deafness alone*. Otosclerosis is a primary example of this type, involving is a disease of the labyrinthine capsule of the middle ear. It is often responsive to surgical intervention. Otosclerosis usually appears during the third or fourth decade of life and is characterized by a progressive conductive or mixed hearing loss. A second example of this type is familial progressive sensorineural hearing loss. This may occur at any time and is characterized by a specific audiometric configuration and fairly good speech discrimination. Presbycusis can also be classified under this heading, but Myerhoff and Paparella emphasize that many nongenetic factors effect the onset of presbycusis.

2. *Genetic deafness with other abnormalities (syndromes)*. A prime example of this group is Paget's disease, the incidence of which is increasing among elderly men. The hearing loss associated with Paget's disease is either sensorineural or mixed. A second example is the hearing loss found among people with rheumatoid arthritis. This hearing loss is usually of the conductive or mixed type and may respond to steriod therapy. It may also be associated with Friedreich's ataxia, Alport's dominant syndrome, and van der Hoeve's syndrome (osteogenesis imperfecta tarda).

3. *Nongenetic deafness*.

a. Inflammatory disease. Infections and allergic inflammations may be responsible for conductive as well as sensorineural hearing loss. For example, the aged population is as susceptible to otitis media as the younger population. Chronic otitis media may be bacterial and may be the manifestion of more serious diseases, such as diabetes or tumors of the nasopharynx. Elderly individuals with chronic debilitating diseases are prone to middle ear infections, or such infections may be a result of the late-appearing damage from childhood infections (Ruben, 1971). Primary tuberculosis of the middle ear is appearing with increasing frequency. Congenital, secondary, or tertiary syphilis may cause middle ear damage. Even upper respiratory tract infections, influenza, measles, and mumps may be the cause of bilateral, sensorineural hearing loss among the elderly.

b. Chronic ototoxicity. The list of substances that cause reversible or irreversible damage to the auditory system is increasing daily. Antibiotics, including neomycin, kanamycin, bacitracin, streptomycin, and dihydrostreptomycin, are implicated, as well as diuretics (ethacrynic acid and furosemide). Aspirin may cause reversible sensorineural hearing loss. Lead and mercury have been shown to be toxic to the inner ear.

c. Traumatic injury. The most recently implicated of the traumatic agents affecting hearing loss is noise. Hearing loss can result from either continuous exposure to moderately loud noise or a brief exposure to a large noise impulse. Butler and Lewis (1977) discuss that in societies where background noise remains under 40 decibels, the hearing loss associated with aging is minimal. In the world that most of us experience, normal speech occurs at 60 decibels, and busy traffic registers 70 decibels. Even the noise level in a quiet restaurant is at a level of 50 decibels (Butler and Lewis, 1977). Of course, at particular high risk are those clients whose living arrangements or occupations have caused them to be chronically exposed to high levels of noise. The sensorineural loss of hearing associated with high noise levels is irreversible.

d. Metabolic disorders, vascular insufficiency, Meniere's disease, and central nervous system disease. Each of these can produce a hearing loss among the elderly. The types of metabolic disease that can affect hearing include hypothyroidism, adrenopituitary disorders, hyperparathyroidism, renal disease, and abnormal glucose tolerance. Vascular insufficiency is usually associated with a sudden hearing loss. Not to be overlooked in this category are receptive aphasias, where there may be essentially nothing wrong with the hearing apparatus, but the ability of the individual to understand speech is compromised. Meniere's disease is associated with a fluctuating hearing loss, vertigo, and tinnitus. It may be caused by allergic, inflammatory, or metabolic phenomenon or may be idiopathic. Diseases such as multiple sclerosis may cause a hearing loss that is associated with disease of the central nervous system.

The manifestations of hearing loss among the elderly are multiple. Older people may hear speech but not be able to understand it. They may have lost the ability to hear high frequencies or distant sounds. As the hearing loss progresses, the elderly person may have more difficulty understanding women's voices than men's. The raised or shouting voice, particularly in unfamiliar surroundings, begins to cause frustration and confusion rather than understanding.

Psychologic manifestations

To appreciate the sensory deprivation effects of hearing loss, it is beneficial to consider the psychologic levels of hearing and their effect on the normal person. Normal hearing is composed of a mixture of hearing on the symbolic level, the warning level, and the primitive level. The first of these, the symbolic level, is closely associated with the process of social interaction. Words are symbolic substitutions for events, objects, feelings, and processes. People who share a common language can share these things through a common cultural definition. By the use of words, communication is almost as complex and flexible as the nature of experiences themselves. Language helps to clarify and organize thoughts and permits moral values to be shared and reinforced. Language permits conceptualization at a high level of abstraction. The inability to hear at the symbolic level produces social isolation and interferes with the enjoyment of the esthetic qualities of human existence (Ramsdell, 1970).

Campanelli (1968) suggests that the interference with social interaction resulting from hearing impaired at the symbolic level may not even be perceived by the individual involved. Rather, the father of a family, for example, slowly isolates himself, denying hearing loss. Often he complains that people on the outside speak too softly and, after all, he has no difficulty understanding his own family. The family members themselves may not be aware of the degree to which they help the hearing-impaired individual compensate for his loss. They escalate the intensity of their voices, turn up the television, and do all manner of unconscious things to facilitate communication. Often family members become tired and frustrated with the situation and seek help. Even at that point, the hearing-impaired person still denies the presence of a problem.

The second level of auditory function is known as the warning level. By using this level of hearing, people are able to make the necessary adjustments to a potentially hostile environment. Although sight can provide a certain amount of information about the environment, sound waves are not limited by walls or corners. Although we can see only in one direction at a time, we can simultaneously receive sounds from multiple sources and from multiple directions. The localization of sound is an important ability of those with normal hearing, as is the ability to determine the approximate source and distance of warning sounds. It is believed that the loss of hearing at this level, however, is the easiest to compensate for. Although the inability to distinguish warning sounds produces a sense of insecurity, it does not necessarily produce a profound emotional upset (Ramsdell, 1970).

The third level of hearing is primitive hearing. A loss of hearing at this level profoundly affects the psychologic state of the affected individual. Primitive hearing permits the individual to sense the variety of background noises that provide a sense of being part of a living, active world. Hearing at the primitive level creates the background of feeling and the affective tone of the world.

It relates us to the world at a very primitive level, somewhere below the level of clear consciousness and perception. The loss of this feeling of relationship with the world is a major cause of the well-recognized feeling of "deadness" and also of the depression that permeates the suddenly deafened and, to a less degree, those in whom deafness develops gradually (Ramsdell, 1970, p. 437).

For those with normal hearing, it is difficult to imagine a world in which the sounds of birds, the wind, and the breathing of a sleeping loved one are absent. This is an acute loss of essential sensory input.

There are many behavioral manifestations related directly to hearing loss. How any given individual reacts to hearing loss is determined by the extent and degree of the loss, the rapidity of onset, the degree to which the client acknowledges the loss, his general physical condition, and whether he is in familiar surroundings with familiar people or is in a new place, being forced to communicate with strangers. Feelings of loss and depression are dominant themes that underlie the behaviors of hearing-impaired clients. These may be manifested by apathy, sleep disturbance, anxiety, insecurity, and physical complaints (Ramsdell, 1970). Since hearing confirms our integration into a living world and helps us define our individual boundaries (Conover and Cober, 1970), the loss of hearing can produce disorganization of behavior and thought. Often, seemingly unreasonable anger, erratic behavior, and acting out may be present if the client feels no one in his environment is making an adequate effort to communicate or if he views what is asked of him as meaningless (Perron, 1974).

In one study that examined the relationship between hearing loss, not speaking English, and a history of alcoholism to the appearance of "mental symptoms" following eye patching, Ziskind (1960) found the following. Forty-two percent of the clients with mental symptoms who had a cataract extraction were hearing impaired, whereas only 29% of that same group who displayed no mental symptoms were hearing impaired. Those who displayed mental symptoms clearly had a higher frequency of hearing impairment. Examining the combination of hearing loss and not speaking English, Ziskind found that 57% of those displaying mental symptoms had both problems, whereas only 31% of those displaying no mental symptoms had this combination of problems.

Feelings of suspicion found among the hearing impaired are often given a psychiatric label. However, Ramsdell (1970) indicates that most individuals have underlying suspicions and feelings of insecurity that are simply aggravated and stimulated to the surface by a hearing loss.

The tendency toward paranoid reactions exists to some degree in nearly all of us, but it is generally kept under control. Since control is lessened when a person is depressed, sensitiveness and suspicion are more easily aroused. *Deafness seems to be a powerful stimulus to any latent paranoid trend in the personality*, possibly because of the invariable association of depression and deafness (p. 444).

It is, in addition, very easy to translate what seem to be interrupted conversations and half-heard remarks into critical unfriendly comments when one simply does not understand what is going on.

In summary, hearing loss itself can produce behavioral manifestations such as anger, acting out, paranoia, and depression, which may be interpreted by an onlooker as confusion. Furthermore, since hearing is the basis and the means by which much of the world is shared and organized, deprivation of hearing can result in thought disorganization and difficulties in the definition of self.

High-risk setting factors

As defined in the section on visual alterations, setting factors that produce sensory alteration in relation to hearing include those imposed on the client through the environmental and social setting or through some treatment method. The lack of a hearing prosthesis is one of the most common factors that leads to deprivation of sound for elderly individuals. There are, of course, pathologic conditions for which hearing aids are of minimal benefit. However, only a skilled audiologist can make the determination of whether a prosthesis would be of benefit or not. In answering the question, "Who needs a hearing aid?", one audiologist states the current position on the subject.

Professional opinion is so varied that it is impossible to establish any true authoritarian set of figures as to when a hearing aid is indicated. In recent years, the pendulum has swung back and forth until it has reached a point where each clinician relies on his own experience to determine his own criteria. In general terms, hearing aids should be fitted *any time* a patient is having difficulty utilizing his hearing socially or occupationally . . . A hearing aid should be fitted whenever it will help the individual using it to hear better (Teter, 1976, p. 231).

In order to avoid the fraud that has been perpetrated against many elderly people by unscrupulous peddlers, McNamee (1978) suggests that the best policy is to have the device prescribed and fitted by the audiologist rather than a person who is simply in the business of selling hearing aids.

In addition, there are many reasons why an elderly person either does not have a hearing aid, refuses to be fitted with one, or has one but does not use it.

First, hearing loss tends to be a hidden disability in our society. Often, clients do not want to acknowledge their deficits and feel that the presence of a hearing appliance produces a social stigma. This attitude is further perpetuated by hearing aid advertisements that have the "no one will know you wear one" approach. Even the current search for smaller and more hidden hearing devices is an indication of the hidden nature of the disability and the amount of social disapproval that surrounds it.

Second, a hearing aid in no way substitutes for normal hearing. As Campanelli (1968) cautions:

He (the client) should be counseled that a hearing aid is just that—an aid—not a new hearing mechanism. Furthermore, the aid is a mechanical creation that, because of its size and component parts, has rather critical limitations which are inherent in the design of the hearing aid. These aspects affect tonal quality particularly (p. 85).

Often, there is a certain amount of disillusionment after the purchase of a hearing device. Sounds do not have the quality they are remembered to have, mechanical squealing may be introduced, and such sounds as the turning on and off of the refrigerator are suddenly new and disturbing. Every sound, not just important ones, is magnified. Some of this disillusionment can be avoided if the client has been properly counseled, taught, and helped to cope with the limitations of hearing aids. If not, many clients who have finally accepted the idea of a hearing aid will abandon its use.

Rupp (1970) identifies a third set of problems with hearing aids specific to elderly people. Poor memory can result in failure to turn off the aid at night, to change the batteries, and to remember which batteries are new and which are used. Poor vision and limited dexterity result in difficulty inserting the ear mold, manipulating the small controls, and keeping the instrument clean and functioning properly. Slowed learning coupled with instruction given too rapidly result in inability to use the unit properly and to its best advantage. Thus, the hearing device becomes more trouble than it is worth.

Lack of money and transportation can be reasons for not obtaining a hearing aid, and lack of social and occupational rewards can be reasons for not using it. The use of a hearing prosthesis requires the client to learn an entire new set of responses and a new way of hearing. The teaching approach must be supportive, encouraging, and tailor-made to the needs of an older learner.

An important reason clients in institutional settings do not use their hearing aids is that they do not have access to them. Many times, the people around the client do not offer him the hearing aid, or the caregivers do not provide the social rewards that make using it pleasant. Often, caregivers themselves do not know how to operate the hearing device and cannot help with it. Caregivers place such a low priority on hearing aids that batteries are permitted to wear out long before replacements are obtained. Burnside (1972) states that nurses simply do not know enough about hearing aids. "Batteries get lost and wear out and nurses state that in non-metropolitan areas batteries are difficult to obtain" (p. 297).

From our experiences in dealing with nurses and their clients with hearing difficulties, one other observation can be made. When a client cannot communicate—when he cannot hear—nursing care is much easier. The nurse is not called on to talk during care, the client cannot and does not have to be answered, and many emotionally charged subjects can be avoided. For example, one elderly client is routinely without batteries for her aid. "She is a 'fiddler'," the nurses report, and as a result, her batteries wear out faster than they can be replaced. She *is* a fiddler, but communication with her is intense, difficult, and exhausting. It is just easier for everyone when she cannot hear. Thus, the caregivers' feelings about individual clients influence whether or not the hearing aid will be offered or maintained.

For the elderly person in an institutional setting, other sources contribute to sound deprivation and monotonous input. Cut off from the usual sources of social interaction, these people must often rely on the telephone to maintain contact with their significant others. Few hospitals are equipped with amplification devices on the bedside telephones. Even the ringing of the phone can be missed if the person's hearing is compromised. The intercommunication systems in institutions were designed to save the nursing staff a few steps. However, for a person with a hearing impairment, these are almost useless. First, without seeing the person who is speaking, it is very difficult for hard-of-hearing people to understand what is being said to them. Second, intercoms are rather modern and sophisticated forms of communication. Many elderly people become quite confused by voices "coming from the wall" and are unable to determine the source of the sounds. How much better it is for a caregiver to appear in response to a call light, fulfill the request, communicate in an understandable manner, and serve as a source of social stimulation and caring as well.

For the person with impaired hearing, major sources of sound overload and distortion arise from the environment. Background noises, loud and soft, are a constant problem on the nursing unit. A great deal of noise is generated from simply meeting the client's needs. Noise arises from food carts, cleaning equipment, and each of the people who operates them. This is the loud and sporadic noise usually associated with rushing and activity. During the change of shifts, a great deal of noise is created by the staff greeting each other and describing their day. Snyder and others (1978) demonstrate that wandering and confusion increase during these periods of high noise levels.

Interesting problems are created by the devices that we ordinarily associate with relaxation and entertainment. Radios, television, and music of all types can cause overload problems for people with compromised hearing. Overload results from increasing the volume levels the person can supposedly hear, but by doing this, the treble tones are increased in relation to bass tones, and the person is exposed to overload in the lower tones. Music in the high keys serves to frustrate and distract rather than relax, as these tones are distorted for the person with presbycusis (Hatton, 1977).

Any device or treatment that suddenly increases the quality of speech discrimination or the ability of the person to hear can potentially produce overload. The problems associated with new hearing aids have been discussed. However, even the person who has had plugs of earwax for many years and is suddenly relieved must learn to adjust to louder noise levels. Surgery can correct some hearing deficits. Postoperatively, the patient needs to be protected from excessive noises until he determines the levels of sound that are most comfortable for him.

High-risk caregiver factors

Communication with the hard-of-hearing person can be exhausting and time consuming and requires effort and creatively. In many care settings, the caregivers simply are unable or unwilling to expend the time and energy required to communicate effectively. Many caregivers do not have the physical, intellectual, or emotional resources to help the client combat the problem of sound and communication deprivation. Administrative supports are usually not built into the care delivery system to help caregivers communicate effectively. In settings where the staff to client ratio is low, the caregiver gets little opportunity to communicate in a meaningful way and less opportunity to mobilize resources between communication sessions. In addition, professional caregivers are not usually monetarily or socially reinforced for their communication skills. Only their organizational abilities and efficiency displays are rewarded by the administrative structure. With other types of clients, the caregivers can safely rely on other people, including residents and visitors, to fulfill some of the individual's stimulation needs. With the hearing-impaired individual, for whom no communication system has been devised, participation with other people is tedious, frustrating, and difficult. As a result, it is the primary caregivers who must supply most of the stimulation required by the client. This further complicates the role of the professional caregiver.

Caregivers can have certain personal qualities that make communication with the hearing-impaired client problematic. For example, many people do not articulate well and mumble their native language. Many people have distracting body and hand movements that draw attention away from the interaction. Resting the head or chin on the hand while talking can interfere with lip movement, as can smoking or chewing gum. Caregivers may use slang expressions that are consistent with their own cohort group. However, most caregivers do not share a common language of slang with their clients, who may be 25 years older or more. Special problems are created whenever the client and the caregiver speak a different primary language. Under the best of circumstances this can interfere with communication, but it is lethal to communication with the elderly individual who has impaired hearing.

Often, it is assumed that hard-of-hearing people can be helped to hear if the caregivers shout. This is not true. Increasing loudness usually serves only to increase the voice pitch and not the bass tones, resulting in language confusion and anxiety. In addition, opportunities for privacy and intimacy are lost. The client's business becomes everyone's business. Intimate one-to-one relationships simply cannot be established through shouting.

The rate of speech and the number of people talking at one time can produce overload and distortion. When sentences and words run together rapidly, speech discrimination becomes particularly difficult. When a large group of people are talking together, speech discrimination for the person with a hearing loss can be impossible. Several elderly clients have reported that the number of words used to convey the message can contribute to overload. "Tell me just what I need to know, don't tell me a story" is the type of instruction received from the hearing-impaired elderly person.

Caregivers can contribute to the total sensory alteration experience of elderly people by adding to deprivation, overload, and distortion. Taken together, the results may ultimately be confusion.

Fourth-level assessment for auditory alteration

Nursing and medical history
Drug and occupational history
Elicitation of subjective data about hearing loss
  Symbolic-level hearing assessment
  Warning-level hearing assessment
  Primitive-level hearing assessment
Environmental assessment
Observation of social interation patterns
Assessment of client's ability to use a hearing prosthesis

Under most circumstances, the client comes into contact with the care providers with very little actual information related to his hearing status. It may be obvious to all that he wears a hearing aid or that he has a hearing difficulty, but the exact nature of the problem may not even be known to the client. The fourth-level assessment is designed to elicit information that will help the caregiver accurately identify the client's hearing problem. It includes early detection of hearing loss; assessment of the symbolic, warning, and primitive levels of hearing; and assessment of the physical and social environment to detect external sources of sensory alteration. Although lacking the precision of an audiometric examination, this assessment should be useful in helping the caregiver structure the environment and hearing inputs to facilitate hearing and communication to the greatest possible extent.

It is important to note that the three levels of hearing (primitive, warning, and symbolic) are assessed separately. They are considered as three distinct abilities, any one of which can be compromised or not compromised independent of each other. We often hear nursing personnel state that "the client can hear what he wants to" or "that he can hear more than he lets on," based on their observation that he "seems" unable to communicate but turns his head when he hears a door slam. These impressions of clients' hearing abilities are unfair based on the concept that warning-level hearing is distinct from symbolic-level hearing. A client can retain abilities in one area and still have tremendous problems with speech discrimination and communication.

A nursing, medical, drug, and occupational history can help with early detection of a hearing loss. Early detection affords the affected individual the opportunity to be audiometrically examined and properly treated or trained to cope with the problem. Remember, not all hearing losses encountered among elderly people are the *result* of aging. Many may respond to medical or surgical treatment, many are helped with amplification, and if neither of these is possible, teaching a client to read signs and speech early may significantly increase the quality of his life.

The nurse conducting the assessment should be particularly attuned to investigating the possibility of a hearing loss, even if the client *seems* to be able to hear, when he reports having worked for many years at an occupation related to high, unprotected noise levels or having taken ototoxic drugs for many years. In addition, as stated before, many systemic illnesses, such as tertiary syphilis, tuberculosis, influenza, Paget's disease, and rheumatoid arthritis, are associated with a hearing loss. When encountering such clients, the nurse should be particularly careful to investigate the client's current hearing status. The following questions help the client or family members identify the presence of a hearing loss early.

Questions for the client include:
1. Do you find yourself shouting to get your point across?
2. Do you frequently fiddle with the volume controls on the television or radio?
3. Do you find yourself asking people to repeat fairly often?
4. Do you go out socially? Do you go out less now than you did? Do you know why you go out less?
5. Do people sometimes mumble?
6. Do you find that talking to another person while in a group of people is particularly difficult?

Questions for significant others include:
1. Do you find yourself shouting at the client to get your point across?
2. Is the television or radio at the client's house sometimes so loud that you are uncomfortable?
3. Does the client ask you to repeat frequently?
4. Does the client sometimes seem to be ignoring you?
5. When many people are present, is communicating with the client worse?
6. Is the client going out socially less frequently? Do you know why? Does the client tell you that other people are unfriendly? Does he tell you that his acquaintances mumble?

This cursory assessment of hearing status should be conducted at regular intervals. Many times, the loss has progressed substantially before the client or his family is overtly aware of it. These kinds of questions help them to identify the loss earlier than might otherwise be possible. Referral to a source of audiometric testing is essential if a hearing loss is suspected.

The symbolic level of hearing is the level used in everyday communication (Ramsdell, 1970). The following is a list of words that can be used to crudely determine the extent of a symbolic hearing loss and to identify those areas where the client's hearing is fairly intact. For many people, hearing loss involves only certain letters or combinations of letters, such as f, th, s, and sh. Many individuals have difficulty when certain letters fall in a particular place in the word, such as at the beginning or the end. For example, many older clients with hearing problems will have difficulty distinguishing th from f at the beginning of the word and cannot tell the difference between *fat* and *that*. This word list helps to crudely diagnose these problems.

smart, off, with, that, thin, will, cat, room, all, jaw, does (Shore, 1978)

To perform this test, stand behind the client about 3 feet away. Using a normal speaking tone, pronounce the words for the client to repeat. Note words that are difficult for the client. If he has any difficulty repeating words in the list, repeat the test. This time, face the client with your face and mouth well lighted. Again pronounce the words using a normal speaking tone. Note problem words. When performing this test, pronounce the words clearly and leave enough space between words to allow for adequate response time.

The warning level of hearing permits the client to identify potential threats in the environment, such as the ringing of a fire alarm or the sound of someone approaching (Ramsdell, 1970). Since the warning level often occurs at a level that is not quite conscious, the patient must be instructed to listen for the sound used in testing. However, using these instructions makes the testing situation quite artificial. Remember, the *best* the client is able to hear warning sounds under these artificial conditions, where it is quiet and he is listening for the sound, is probably the very *best* he can do under any circumstances. Thus, his best performance should not be considered his usual performance. In order to have hearing intact at the warning level, the client should be able to both identify and localize distant sounds.

Sound identification is tested by using a sharp sound in the distant environment, such as a ringing telephone, a slamming door, or a bell or buzzer. Ask the client to listen for the sound and identify what he considers to be its source. Use your own hearing as a gauge of how compromised the client is in the ability to identify distant sounds.

Sound localization is tested by using a distinct sound that moves around, such as a bell, buzzer, or doors slamming in different directions. Ask the client to listen for the sound and identify its direction. Again, your hearing can be used as the gauge of whether or not the client is having problems. If the client has difficulty localizing distant sounds, his ability to localize sound within his own room can be tested using a loudly ticking clock. Ask the client to close his eyes and identify the direction of the ticking as you move around the room holding the clock.

Primitive-level hearing is used to identify indistinct background noise and the sounds of living things, such as the singing of birds, the rustle of the wind in the trees, and the breathing of someone who is sleeping (Ramsdell, 1970). To test this, ask the client if he can hear birds that are singing nearby or other indistinct environmental noises. In addition, you can test primitive-level hearing using whispers. Ask the client to repeat two-syllable words such as "cowboy" or "toy boat" that you whisper standing behind him. A softly ticking watch can be used to determine the distance at which he can hear the sound. Sometimes, simply asking the client if he sometimes perceives that the environment is "dead" is enough to help him identify a problem with primitive-level hearing.

Environmental sources of overload, distortion, and deprivation can best be identified by caregivers who increase their sensitivity to the total hearing environment of the client. The nurse should identify sounds in the environment that increase her own sense of agitation. The environment must also be surveyed for those sounds the nurse understands but which are alien to someone who is new to the environment, such as food carts, other clients crying out, and air conditioners. The quality and quantity of client interactions should be observed to determine the difficulties that interfere with satisfaction or success. Individuals who care for the client should be observed to see if there are any personal peculiarities that interfere with communication, such as distracting body language, chewing gum, or mumbling. The client's use of his hearing prosthesis also must be assessed, and consultation should be sought with experts to determine if the hearing aid could be enhanced. Noises that produce overload and distortion for clients are often not recognized unless the caregivers display a great deal of awareness.

Prevention

1. *Act to detect hearing losses as early as possible*. Among elderly people, the first step in preventing confusion related to hearing impairments is the early detection of a hearing loss. Hearing needs to be assessed at least at every physical examination for people over 50 years of age. Nursing clinics that serve the "drop-in" clientele and public health nurses who visit the elderly in their homes should know how to screen elderly people for hearing loss and where to refer them for audiometric examinations. When hearing losses are detected early, measures can be instituted and taught that will prevent confusion in the future. For example, many authors (Heffler, 1960; Hoople, 1960; Alpiner, 1963; Campanelli,

1968; Rupp, 1970), recommend people at all ages who are experiencing a hearing loss should be offered the opportunity to learn speech or lipreading. This is a difficult skill to master and requires a functional level of sight, but the earlier such training is started, the more likely the client will become proficient in its use. In addition, signing or sign language is a helpful skill that is rarely taught to elderly people as an alternate means of communication. Signing as a communication and expressive art form can be taught to elderly people to enhance contact with the outside world, enhance the expression of thoughts and feelings, and prevent the confusion that arises when either of these are inhibited.

2. *Use and teach the "Principles of Sensitive Communication" with hearing-impaired people.* McNamee (1978) has developed the "Principles of Sensitive Communication," which should be used by and taught to all people who encounter clients with hearing difficulties. These principles help create a therapeutic milieu that enhances communication and prevents confusion:

   a. The responsibility for understanding does not rest entirely with the hard-of-hearing client. Understanding is a responsibility shared by all people who communicate with the hearing-impaired person.

   b. Reassurance is important since many people with hearing impairments misunderstand or misinterpret the sounds they receive. Caregivers have the responsibility to ascertain the client's level of understanding, as well as to help validate correct interpretations from distorted ones.

   c. Medications affect the client's ability to hear and pay attention. If a hearing problem exists that varies in intensity with time of day or from day to day, caregivers should investigate the medications the person is receiving to determine if they are interfering with the communication process.

   d. Caregivers have the responsibility to speak clearly, slowly, and articulate well.

   e. If the client does not understand the message being conveyed after it is repeated twice, the caregiver has the responsibility to find an alternate means of conveying the message. Under these circumstances, the nature of the words themselves probably is making the reception of the message difficult. There is nothing more frustrating to all concerned than trying over and over again to say the same thing.

   f. A hearing impairment should never be used as an excuse to talk over the client or to make no attempt to communicate. There are very few people with whom communication is absolutely impossible, and there is no better way to reinforce feelings of insecurity and mistrust than to talk to a third person in the presence of a client when the client does not understand what is being said.

   g. It is the responsibility of the speaker to assess the use of gestures to determine if they enhance or detract from communication. Useless and distracting gestures should be eliminated as much as possible.

   h. Accusations that hearing-impaired people hear only what they want to hear are unjust. People's ability to hear and their energy to communicate varies with their physical and emotional states and with other stimuli in the environment. In addition, people may retain their ability to hear warning-level sounds, for example, but lose their ability to discriminate functional speech from background noise.

   i. Impatience does not help anyone.

3. *Use the word list to diagnose sound problems and structure communication to avoid difficult sounds.* It is helpful for many elderly individuals with hearing problems if verbal communication is structured, as much as possible, around the word list (see p. 247) used for assessment (Shore, 1978).

By carefully analyzing the client's mistakes during the assessment of symbolic hearing, those who communicate with the client can be alerted to those combinations of sounds that present special problems. By careful and thoughtful consideration, it might be possible to avoid words with such combinations of letters or to devise certain hand signs that indicate which of the problem combinations are being used in the word.

4. *Help the client and his family establish two-way communication.* Confusion may be prevented by helping the client establish a two-way communication system that is useful with nursing personnel as well as with his family and friends. Often, this requires the nurse to be an instructor for all parties involved, helping them to find the most effective ways of communicating, reinforcing their efforts, supporting them through the frustrations and discouragements, and helping them establish realistic expectations for communication and interaction. One of the most difficult parts of communicating with hearing-impaired clients is the limitations they perceive for the topics of communication. Often, they confine their conversations to the concrete, here-and-now facets of life, such as food, sleeping, and bowel movements. To convey feelings and dreams seems fairly impossible to them. If the nurse can help the client and his friends establish a level of communication that is flexible and intimate, using signs, pantomime, and carefully chosen words, she has indeed performed a valuable service.

5. *Act as an interpreter for the client during interaction.* Another valuable service that a consistent nursing staff can perform for a hearing-impaired client is to serve as interpreter, much in the same way they would for a person who speaks a foreign language. For example, telephone contacts with significant others may be extremely difficult when the person has impaired hearing. The staff may need to convey messages over the telephone so that the client can remain in close contact with his family and friends. When people visit who are not aware of the communication system, a member of the nursing staff may need to sit by the client and interpret the conversation. This will help to reduce the amount of misunderstanding and misinterpretation that can take place, as well as to increase the likelihood of a successful social interaction. For the client who also has a sight impairment, it may be necessary to help him understand the contents of his cards and letters by summarizing their content and writing who they are from on large pieces of paper with large, dark letters. In addition, many individuals with hearing impairments need to be helped to interpret their own behavior toward others in terms of what attracts and what repels people. For example, when the client shouts or speaks inappropriately, people tend to move away. Having someone he trusts point out these behaviors helps the client learn to communicate more effectively.

6. *Facilitate the learning process when the client receives a new hearing aid.* Individuals with new hearing devices need to have special measures applied to prevent confusion. The successful wearing of a hearing aid depends on early fitting and extensive counseling regarding its use. "The presbycusic patient, wearing a hearing aid for the first time, must learn to listen rather much like a newborn infant" (Campanelli, 1968, p. 85). It takes practice and patience on both the part of the client and the caregiver to effect mastery of a hearing aid. By planned practice with word lists that emphasize various vocal sounds, the client can be helped to increase his acuity for the sounds that present him with specific difficulties. Careful attention to selective listening can increase the client's auditory acuity, and he can be helped to increase his sensitivity to both auditory and visual cues. The earlier the client is helped to use a hearing aid to listen selectively, the more likely his success and the less his overall discomfort (Campanelli, 1968). Also, early counseling about fitting and patient, reinforcing

instruction about the device will result in the less disillusionment and a greater likelihood that the client will continue to use it.

7. *Use environmental devices that augment hearing to facilitate independence.* In the institutional setting and in the home environment, many amplification devices can be used to facilitate hearing and enhance communication, keeping the person independent and in touch with the world. A hearing aid, of course, is one of these. Others include amplification devices for the telephone and television earphones that intensify and concentrate sounds for only the person who is having difficulties. Doorbells and telephones can be adapted to flash a light instead of ringing, permitting the client with a hearing problem to "see" when someone wants to talk to him. Alarm clocks can be fitted to vibrating pillows to facilitate independence and self-reliance. Some regions of the country have found "hearing ear" dogs to be helpful to some hearing-impaired individuals. The various telephone companies and medical supply houses have other devices also helpful in creating the prosthetic environment.

8. *Provide forms of recreation that do not require hearing.* The quality of life for a hard-of-hearing client can be enhanced by the use of visual rather than auditory entertainment. Such clients should be offered the opportunity to attend silent films or plays performed in pantomime. People with hearing difficulties can be helped to enjoy the outdoors and share these experiences with those around them. As the client's enjoyment of his current life situation increases, the less likely he is to withdraw into a confusional state.

9. *Facilitate group participation and interaction.* Participation in groups and focused socialization is as important for the hearing-impaired client as it is for the visually impaired one. With a hearing impairment it is easy for the client to become so inwardly drawn that he is unable to socialize and even forgets how to. Teaching such a client to focus on the other individuals in the group and give them his full attention may be the first step in facilitating socialization. He may have lost the ability to listen sensitively, which interferes with socialization. Listening skills, in addition to hearing, include focused attention on facial expression, body language, and feeling tone. Touch can be used to increase these skills and is often helpful with groups of hearing-impaired individuals. Helping clients develop the abilities needed for satisfactory interaction requires a high degree of skill on the part of the caregivers, but it is by no means an impossible task.

10. *Provide consistent staffing patterns and adequate support to the caregivers.* Staffing for the elderly person with a hearing impairment should be consistent. Time should be given to the caregivers to recoup after intensive interactions. Communicating with the hard-of-hearing client is one of the most exhausting and time-consuming requirements of nurses in geriatric settings. The people who perform these tasks must be rewarded and supported in their efforts. Staff who deal with the hard-of-hearing client need to have time to help the client organize his experiences in order to prevent confusion. They must be alert to the environment so as to explain sounds and events that the individual perceives but does not understand. The most important feature of such a staff must be the desire to build relationships, establish trust, and to provide consistency and dependability.

Intervention

The nursing objectives are as follows:
1. To establish a two-way communication system with the client
2. To increase understanding of the client through active listening
3. To facilitate verbal communication
4. To facilitate verbal communication for the client using a hearing aid
5. To help the client organize and validate his experiences by interpreting the "sound" environment to him

Some of the interventions suggested here

are adapted from the work of Burnside (1976).

1. *Establish a two-way communication system with the client.* First and foremost, interventions against confusion for clients experiencing sensory alterations because of hearing problems must be based on the establishment of a two-way communication system between the client and the others in his environment. Communication is more than simply imparting information to the client and telling him what to do. Communication with clients involves both parties imparting, receiving, and understanding information, as well as sharing thoughts, feelings, and experiences. Most of us think of communication as the spoken word, but this is not the only form. Reading and writing can be used to communicate with the client whose sight is adequate. Reading is often facilitated if the caregiver uses dark marking pencils on white paper. It is often necessary to make the letters as high as 3 inches to be recognized. Bright pictures or drawings to communicate some ideas, and careful gestures, demonstrations, and pantomime can also be used. Touch is an excellent form of communication. The client needs to be given every possible facility to understand the message, including adequate lighting, careful choice of an appropriate mode of communication for the message, and the necessary repetitions and reinforcements until understanding is achieved. The mode of communication is unimportant as long as it is mutually understood and consistently used by those in contact with the client.

2. *Listen to the client actively and intently to increase your understanding of him.* In addition to conveying the message, the caregiver must be prepared to use every possible means to understand the message the client is trying to get across. Many people with hearing problems have difficulty articulating. Some speak too loudly or too softly. They often watch the receiver's face closely to see the kind of reception their message is having. Many clients will stop in midsentence to ask for nodded reinforcement that their message is being received. This type of reinforcement is essential. Be very aware of your body language and facial expressions as you listen. Individuals with hearing impairments may be quite sensitive to your facial expressions, and these should be appropriate to the conversation. Often, when listening, your body language and facial expressions convey more understanding, caring, and confidence than words ever could. Listening to and communicating with an elderly client with hearing problems helps him validate his reality and decrease the confusion that surrounds many of the experiences he has within his setting.

3. *Use every means to facilitate verbal communication.* There are various ways in which speech communication can be facilitated.

   a. Face the client at the distance of a handshake.
   b. Make sure that your face is well lighted.
   c. Before speaking to the client, get his full attention. Gently touch his arm and make sure that you have direct eye contact before trying to speak.
   d. Direct communication at the more functional ear.
   e. Your speech should be slowly and distinctly spaced, with pauses between words and sentences. For those with presbycusis, lower the pitch of your voice.
   f. A slight increase in your speech intensity with a lowered pitch might be helpful to convey the message, but if shouting seems necessary, find another way of communicating what you have to say. Sometimes a stethoscope can be used to amplify sound for the client by placing the earpieces in his ears and speaking into the bell.
   g. Watch the client closely for feedback cues. His face will tell you if the message is being received. Give him plenty of time to respond.
   h. Be succinct. Long stories only frus-

trate and exhaust the listener who is having difficulty hearing. Often in the process, the intent of the message is lost.
  i. If your primary language is different from the client's, be prepared to use an alternate form of communication.
  j. Make an attempt to decrease the competition from background noise as much as possible.

4. *Facilitate verbal communication for the client using a hearing aid.* For the clients with a hearing aid, special steps must be taken to assure the reception of verbal communication:
  a. It is important that every caregiver knows how the client's aid is operated and adjusted.
  b. Every day, the caregiver should check that the hearing aid is operational. The hearing aid should be in place in the client's ear every time he is trying to communicate, day or night. Some clients, although not usually those with presbycusis, have two hearing aids, one for each ear. Each of these needs to be checked daily.
  c. Know how the batteries are to be placed in the hearing aid. Each client should have a supply of batteries on hand, and these should be given to him as soon as he requests them. Most clients know when the batteries in their hearing aid are losing power; they should not have to wait until the battery is dead before being given a replacement.
  d. Know how to clean and insert the ear mold for the client. Many problems arise simply because the ear mold has not been properly positioned.
  e. Check with the client so that he remembers to turn his aid off at night. It may help to mark the on-off switch with nail polish to remind the client which switch is which. A hearing aid left on and laid on a hard surface will squeal loudly. Listen for and turn off squealing aids that are not being used.
  f. When you are speaking to a person with a hearing aid, be sure the microphone is facing you. With severe impairments and for people who use a "body aid," it may be helpful if you hold the microphone in your hand as you speak.
  g. It is never necessary to shout into the microphone. Speak slowly and clearly into the microphone as if you were speaking into a telephone, and lower the pitch of your voice slightly.

5. *Interpret the "sound" environment, helping the client organize and validate his experiences.* Intervening for confusion also involves interpreting sounds not understandable to the client, validating his experiences, and organizing the environment to make it understandable by using his intact senses. One of the most valuable services nursing personnel can perform is to help the client separate correct interpretations of situations from distorted ones. Often, not only must alien sounds be interpreted, but also the conversations the client has had with others. With speech discrimination problems, it is not unusual for the client to misinterpret what has been said to him and use the distorted perceptions to anticipate imaginary problems or events. Many hearing-impaired clients have only half-heard a staff discussion about the diagnosis of cancer of the patient down the hall, interpreted it as having to do with him, and then worried for days about his supposed diagnosis. Often, anticipatory information and teaching opportunities that would decrease confusion are lost to individuals who cannot hear. The nurse can intervene in these cases to provide the information the client needs to prevent confusion through an alternate means of communication. Sensory input from other sources is important for maintaining orientation among hearing-impaired clients, as long as this input is structured, organized, and understandable. Often, reading materials such as magazines with pictures and large print can be used to help the client keep in touch with the world. Being out-

doors often helps orientation. Massage, warm baths, and the use of perfumes and oils bring pleasurable sensations and esthetic enjoyment into the client's life, as well as sensory input. In addition, these facilitate the building of trusting relationships between the client and those who minister to him. Individuals with hearing impairments need to be able to share and reflect on their experiences, whether the topic is a book they have read, something they have heard, an object they are seeing outside, or the catheterization performed that morning. Sharing helps clients organize their own experiences and validate their own perceptions and helps treat the confusion they may already be experiencing.

Outcome criteria of successful nursing intervention against auditory alteration

1. The client and those around him communicate in a successful and comfortable manner
2. The client is able to use his hearing prosthesis to its best advantage
3. The client reports and demonstrates that his anxiety level is reduced
4. The client is no longer confused

The suggestions found in the assessment, prevention, and intervention sections are summarized at the end of this chapter.

SUMMARY

As described by McCaffery (1968), sensory alteration is the result of a problem with the man-environment interaction phenomenon. We believe that confusion is also, to a great extent, the result of a problem with the man-environment interaction phenomenon and that confusion and sensory alteration are intimately related. In this chapter, we explored the phenomenon of sensory alteration and the high-risk factors common among elderly people that predispose to sensory alteration. These included the factors that arise from the client himself, such as the physiologic changes in the sensory apparatus of aging individuals; from the setting, such as the methods of treatment and the structural features of the environment; and from the caregivers, such as their personal characteristics, attitudes, and values. In addition, we presented fourth-level assessment procedures, preventive measures, and interventions in four areas: sensory alteration in general, touch, vision, and hearing. The suggestions provided in this chapter are meant as stimuli to help readers look critically at their own situations, their own clients, and themselves. These suggestions should serve as guides to thought, investigation, and experimentation. As we learn more about the aging process, the future should hold exciting possibilities for the treatment and prevention of the confusional states we encounter that are related to sensoriperceptual problems.

CHAPTER 10 SUMMARY
Sensory alteration among the elderly
Sensory alteration in general

Fourth-level assessment	Prevention	Intervention

Nursing history
Observation of the client's behavior
Observation of the client's situation
Observation of the client's environment
Elicitation of subjective data relative to sensory alteration experiences
	1. Structure and enrich the environment, but be sure that the client has control over inputs, sanctioned privacy, and a means of escape.
	2. Reduce the total number of barriers present. Negotiate so rules are mutually satisfactory and agreeable.
	3. Attend to client's problems related to sensory deficits.
	4. Provide consistency in staffing, routines, and activities mutually agreeable to the staff and client.
	5. Increase total amount of knowledge the client has about procedures and treatments.
	6. Reduce the incidence of relocation, and when relocation is unavoidable, involve the client in planning.
	7. Encourage exploration, manipulation, and play.
	8. Increase the total opportunities for successful problem solving, planning, and control on the part of the client.
	9. Increase amount of predictability in environment.
	10. Help the client discuss what he is thinking and feeling. Be nonjudgmental, accepting, and supportive.
	11. Help the client develop means of self-stimulation, particularly if the means he has always used are now compromised.
	12. Facilitate interaction between the client and the others in his environment and provide opportunities for group activities and group interaction.
		A. For simple problems with deprivation, such as boredom or inactivity:
		  1. Provide a variety of activities over which the client has control.
		  2. Provide for regular exercise within the client's physical limitations.
		  3. Provide the client with opportunities to explore and manipulate the environment.
		B. For simple problems with overload or distortion:
		  1. Provide sense of control over sensory input and stressors in environment.
		  2. Act to reduce the client's anxiety.
		    a. Teach the client relaxation and "centering" techniques similar to those in Appendix D.
		    b. Explore how the client is perceiving the environment so misperceptions can be corrected. Provide an explanation for sensory events in the environment.
		    c. Encourage the client to participate in structured activities. Help him to retain control over activities.
		    d. Give anticipatory information to the client.
		    e. Teach an appropriate means of getting help.
		  3. Provide regular exercises within the client's physical limitations.
		C. For slowness of thought and excessive day dreaming:
		  1. Provide consistent interaction with other people.

Continued.

CHAPTER 10 SUMMARY
Sensory alteration in general—cont'd

Fourth-level assessment	Prevention	Intervention

	13. Help the client identify his strength and construct his environment to minimize his weaknesses.
	14. Provide all the necessary cues for the client to be successful in the environment.
		2. Help the client focus his thoughts.
		  a. Have the client help you solve some problem encountered in his daily living.
		  b. Have the client help you solve your problem.
		  c. Have the client teach you something.
		  d. Involve the client's family in helping the client participate in their problem solving.
		  e. Give the client puzzles or games requiring problem solving or logic.
		D. For thought disorganization:
		  1. Help the client impose structure and organization on his world.
		  2. Provide benchmarks for the passage of time.
		  3. Introduce activities and people one at a time.
		  4. Provide the client with the information he needs to cope successfully.

CHAPTER 10 SUMMARY
Sensory alteration in general—cont'd

Fourth-level assessment	Prevention	Intervention
		E. For anxiety and panic: 1. Provide reference points so that the environment can be perceived as predictable and consistent. 2. Assure the client that you are in control and that you will assist him to regain his sense of control. 3. Help the client set one-step goals that will move him toward security. Reinforce with him that time is passing and that he is moving toward his goals. F. For emotional lability: 1. Accept that the client will be emotionally labile during periods of restriction and stress. 2. Help the client to see the appropriateness of his feeling and emotions. Help him to accept his right to these feelings. 3. Help the client to find appropriate ways to express his emotions that are neither harmful to himself nor to others.

Continued.

CHAPTER 10 SUMMARY
Sensory alteration related to tactile problems

Fourth-level assessment	Prevention	Intervention

Nursing and medical history
Elicitation of subjective data relative to tactile sense, with assessment of:
  Temperature sense
  Pain sensation
  Position sense
  Light touch
  Deep touch
  Localization sense by the face-hand technique
  Ability to determine the nature of objects
  Ability to distinguish and respond to textures
  Response to affective touching
	1. Anticipate that the need for touch will increase during periods of stress, illness, loneliness, or depression. Act to meet this need.
	2. Attend to the physical comfort of the client to remove sources of overload and to increase his general stimulation level within comfort ranges.
	3. Plan carefully for manipulative or exposing procedures so that a minimum of people are involved and the amount of manipulation is minimized.
	4. Provide ways for the client to explore and manipulate his environment, the objects in it, and the treatment apparatus that will be used with him.
	5. Educate staff members, significant others, and the client about skin lesions, radiation therapy, infections, burns, and treatment apparatuses so that the client may receive affective touch.
	6. Provide opportunities for mutually consenting clients to touch each other.
	7. Provide routine rituals involving touch as time benchmarks to induce relaxation and provide tactile stimulation and variety.
		1. Carefully assess the types of touch to which the client responds best.
		2. Use affective touch to a degree comfortable to the client.
		3. Use touch to punctuate verbal communication and to hold the client's attention as you communicate with him.
		4. Manipulate the tactile experience to provide external stimulation and variety for the client.
		5. If the client has difficulty localizing tactile stimulation or has difficulty determining the nature of objects by touch, use verbal and visual communication to explain what is happening.
		6. Plan position changes and ambulation around proprioceptive deficits..
		7. Use warmth as a means of reducing agitation and restlessness.
		8. Use deep massage to induce relaxation and to create a sense of comfort and well-being.

CHAPTER 10 SUMMARY
Sensory alteration related to visual problems

Fourth-level assessment	Prevention	Intervention

Nursing and medical history
Ophthalmologic findings
Test for functional visual acuity
Assessment of visual field
Inspection of eyes for abnormalities or lesions
Test for color vision
Assessment of environment
Test for extraocular muscle strength by finger following
	A. For clients with severe visual handicaps:
	  1. Help the client organize his experiences and his environment.
	    a. Introduce yourself and others in the client's environment every time you come in contact with him.
	    b. Help client explore environment through smell, touch, hearing, and locomotion.
	    c. Explain sensory events in the environment; introduce and explain new experiences.
	    d. Arrange environment as client directs and do not move anything without his participation in decision.
	  2. Teach the client a means remaining or becoming oriented to time by using environmental cues such as adapted clocks or calendars.
	  3. Devise a means by which the client can ambulate independently.
	  4. Provide liberal sensory input via other sensory modalities, along with verbal descriptions.
	  5. Explore each area of the activities of daily living for each client to ascertain what environmental manipulation would support independent functioning.
	    a. Dressing.
	    b. Toileting.
	    c. Eating.
		1. Provide an unchanging structure and organization to which the client is oriented.
		2. Act to reduce anxiety.
		  a. Speak to the client before touching him so as not to startle; use his name.
		  b. Explore how the client is perceiving the environment and discuss misperceptions.
		  c. Teach an appropriate means of summoning help.

Continued.

CHAPTER 10 SUMMARY
Sensory alteration related to visual problems—cont'd

Fourth-level assessment	Prevention	Intervention

	B. For clients with specific alterations of sight (in addition to previous measures):
	1. Assess the precise nature of the sight problem and plan accordingly.
	2. For defects in functional and reading sight:
	  a. Obtain and use appropriate prostheses.
	  b. Wean client to independent ambulation, if possible.
	  c. Promote focused communication and socialization.
	  d. Provide adequate lighting.
	  e. Use a color coding system to enrich the visual environment and aid orientation.
	  f. Use client's name or identifying pictures to help him identify his personal things.
	  g. Use variety in colors and types of objects, with descriptions to enrich visual perception.
	  h. Relieve eye irritations.	

CHAPTER 10 SUMMARY
Sensory alteration related to visual problems—cont'd

Fourth-level assessment	Prevention	Intervention

	3. For defects in visual field:
	  a. Construct the environment as individually as possible so the client can compensate for the defect.
	  b. Attend to safety; teach scanning of the environment as a means of dealing with permanent defects, including "spotting exercises."
	4. For defects in extraocular muscle movement:
	  a. Teach client to move his head to avert diplopia.
	  b. When diplopia is severe, provide an eye patch.
	5. For defects in the environment:
	  a. Decrease visual monotony.
	  b. Increase the identifiability of people.
	  c. Attend to the defects presented by nighttime.	

Continued.

CHAPTER 10 SUMMARY
Sensory alteration related to hearing problems

Fourth-level assessment	Prevention	Intervention

Nursing and medical history
Occupational and drug history
Elicitation of subjective data relative to hearing loss
   Symbolic-level hearing assessment
   Warning-level hearing assessment
   Primitive-level hearing assessment
Environmental assessment
Observation of social interaction patterns
Assessment of client's ability to use hearing prosthesis
	1. Act to detect hearing losses as early as possible.
	2. Use and teach the "Principles of Sensitive Communication" with hearing-impaired people.
	   a. The responsibility for understanding is shared between the client and the caregivers.
	   b. Reassurance is important since the client may misunderstand or misinterpret sounds.
	   c. Medications affect the client's ability to hear and pay attention.
	   d. Speak clearly, slowly, and articulate well.
	   e. If you must repeat something more than twice, find a different way of conveying the message.
	   f. Never use a hearing impairment as an excuse to talk over or around a client.
	   g. Use gestures only if they enhance communication.
	   h. Accusations that the hearing-impaired client hears only what he wants to hear are unjust.
	   i. Impatience does not help.
		1. Establish a two-way communication system with the client.
		2. Listen to the client actively and intently to increase your understanding of him.
		3. Use every means to facilitate verbal communication.
		   a. Face the client at the distance of a handshake.
		   b. Make sure your face is well lighted.
		   c. Get the client's attention by gently touching him before speaking.
		   d. Know which side is most affected by the hearing loss.
		   e. Use slowly spaced speech, leaving pauses between words and sentences.
		   f. Lower the pitch of your voice; use a normal tone or speak slightly louder. Do not shout.
		   g. Watch for feedback cues. Give plenty of time for the client to respond.
		   h. Be succinct.
		   i. If your primary language is different from the client's, be prepared to use an alternate means of communication.
		   j. Make an attempt to decrease background noise competition.

CHAPTER 10 SUMMARY
Sensory alteration related to hearing problems—cont'd

Fourth-level assessment	Prevention	Intervention

	3. Use the word list (p. 247) to diagnose sound problems and structure communication to avoid difficult sounds.
	4. Help the client and his family establish two-way communication.
	5. Act as an interpreter for the client during social interaction.
	6. Facilitate the hearing process when the client receives a new hearing aid.
	7. Use environmental devices that augment hearing to facilitate independence.
	8. Provide forms of recreation that do not require hearing.
	9. Facilitate group participation and interaction.
	10. Provide consistent staffing patterns and adequate support to the caregivers.
		4. Facilitate verbal communication for the client with a hearing aid.
		  a. Know how the hearing aid operates.
		  b. Make sure the aid is in operation.
		  c. Know how the batteries are placed.
		  d. Know how to clean and insert the ear mold.
		  e. Check to see that the client remembers to remove and turn the device off at night.
		  f. Make sure the microphone is facing you as you speak. It may help to hold it in your hand as you speak.
		  g. Do not shout. Speak slowly and clearly as if you were speaking into a telephone. Use a slightly lower voice pitch.
		5. Interpret the "sound" environment, helping the client organize and validate his experiences.

REFERENCES

Abram, H. S.: Psychological responses to illness and hospitalization, Psychosomatics **10**:218:223, 1969.

Aguilera, D. C.: Relationship between physical contact and verbal interaction between nurses and patients, Psychiatr. Nurs. **5**:5-21, 1967.

Alpers, B. J., and Mancall, E. L.: Clinical neurology, Philadelphia, 1971, F. A. Davis Co.

Alpiner, J. G.: Audiological problems of the aged, Geriatrics **18**:19-26, 1963.

Barnett, K.: A theoretical construct of the concepts of touch as they relate to nursing, Nurs. Res. **21**:102-109, 1972.

Bellville, J. W., and others: Influence of age on pain relief from analgesics: a study of postoperative patients, J.A.M.A. **217**:1835-1841, 1971.

Bender, M. B.: The incidence and type of perceptual deficiencies in the aged. In Fields, W. S., editor: Neurological and sensory disorders in the elderly, New York, 1975, Stratton Intercontinental Medical Book Corporation, pp. 15-32.

Bender, M. B., Fink, M., and Green, M.: Patterns in perception on simultaneous tests of face and hand, Arch. Neurol. Psychiatry **66**:355-362, 1953.

Bexton, W. H., Heron, W., and Scott, R. H.: Effect of decreased variation in the sensory environment, Can. J. Psychol. **8**:70-76, 1954.

Birren, J. E., and others, editors: Human aging: a biological and behavioral study, U.S. Public Health Publication No. 986, Washington, D.C., 1963, National Institute of Mental Health.

Bolin, R. H.: Sensory deprivation: an overview, Nurs. Forum **13**:240-258, 1974.

Brownfield, C. A.: The brain benders, New York, 1972, Exposition Press.

Bruce, R. L.: Fundamentals of physiological psychology, New York, 1977, Holt, Rinehart & Winston.

Burnside, I. M.: Accoutrements of aging, Nurs. Clin. North Am. **7**:291-301, 1972.

Burnside, I. M.: Touching is talking, Am. J. Nurs. **73**:2060-2063, 1973.

Burnside, I. M., editor: Nursing and the aged, New York, 1976, McGraw-Hill Book Co.

Burnside, I. M.: Working with the elderly: group processes and techniques, North Scituate, Mass., 1978, Duxbury Press.

Buseck, S. A.: Visual status of the elderly, J. Gerontological Nurs. **2**:34-39, 1975.

Butler, R. A., and Lewis, M. I.: Aging and mental health: positive psychosocial approaches, St. Louis, 1977, The C. V. Mosby Co.

Campanelli, P.: Audiological perspectives in presbycusis (Part I), Eye Ear Nose Throat Mon. **47**:3-9, 1968.

Campanelli, P.: Audiological perspectives in presbycusis Part II), Eye Ear Nose Throat Mon. **47**:76-82, 1968.

Carter, A. B.: The neurological aspects of aging. In Rossman, I., editor: Clinical geriatrics, Philadelphia, 1971, J. B. Lippincott Co., pp. 123-140.

Clark, W. C., and Mehl, L.: Thermal pain: a sensory decision theory analysis of the effect of age and sex on 'D', various response criteria, and fifty percent pain threshold, J. Abnorm. Psychol. **78**:202-212, 1971.

Chodil, J., and Williams, B.: The concept of sensory deprivation, Nurs. Clin. North Am. **5**:453-463, 1970.

Conover, M., and Cober, J.: Understanding and caring for the hearing impaired, Nurs. Clin. North Am. **5**:497-506, 1970.

Davis, J. M., McCourt, W. F., and Solomon, P.: The effects of visual stimulation on hallucinations and other mental experiences during sensory deprivation, Am. J. Psychiatry **116**:889-892, 1960.

DeAugustinis, J. R., and others: Ward study: the meanings of touch in interpersonal communication. In Fard, S., and Marshal, M., editors: Some clinical approaches to psychiatric nursing, New York, 1963, Macmillan Publishing Co., Inc.

DeMeyer, J.: The environment of the intensive care unit, Nurs. Forum **96**:163-171, 1967.

DeThomaso, M. T.: Touch power and the screen of loneliness, Perspect. Psychiatr. Care **9**:112-118, 1971.

DeWever, M. K.: Nursing home patients' perception of nurses' affective touching, J. Psychol. **96**:163-171, 1977.

Doane, B. K., and others: Changes in perceptual function after isolation, Can. J. Psychol. **13**:210-219, 1959.

Dominian, J.: The psychological significance of touch, Nurs. Times **67**:896-898, 1971.

Duffy, E.: Activation and behavior, New York, 1962, John Wiley & Sons, Inc.

Duke-Elder, S.: Systems of ophthamology, vol. IX: disease of the retina, London, 1967, Kimpton.

Ebersole, P. P.: Reminiscing and group psychotherapy with the aged. In Burnside, I. M., editor: Nursing and the aged, New York, 1976, McGraw-Hill Book Co., pp. 182-196.

Ebersole, P. P.: Group work with the aged: a survey of the literature. In Burnside, I. M., editor: Nursing and the aged, New York, 1976, McGraw-Hill Book Co., pp. 182-196.

Ebersole, P. P.: A theoretical approach to the use of reminiscence. In Burnside, I. M., editor: Working with the elderly: group processes and techniques, North Scituate, Mass., 1978, Duxbury Press, pp. 139-154.

Ebersole, P. P.: Establishing reminiscing groups. In Burnside, I. M., editor: Working with the elderly: group processes and techniques, North Scituate, Mass., 1978, Duxbury Press, pp. 237-254.

Egan, C.: Encounter: group processes for interpersonal growth, Belmont, Calif., 1970, Brooks/Cole Publishing Co.

Eisdorfer, C.: Developmental level and sensory impairments in the aged, J. Projective Techniques **24**:129-132, 1960.

Ellis, R.: Unusual sensory and thought disturbances after cardiac surgery, Am. J. Nurs. 72:2021-2025, 1972.

Fisch, L.: Special senses: the aging auditory system. In Brocklehurst, J. C., editor: Textbook of geriatric medicine and gerontology, Edinburgh, 1973, Churchill-Livingston Co., pp. 265-279.

Fowler, E. P.: Presbycusis: the aging ear, Ann. Otol. 68:764, 1959.

Frank, L. K.: Tactile communication, Genet. Psychol. Monogr. 56:209-255, 1957.

Freedman, S. J.: Perceptual changes in sensory deprivation, suggestions for a cognitive theory, J. Nerv. Ment. Dis. 132:17-21, 1961.

Freedman, S. S., and Greenblatt, M.: Studies in human isolation, WADC, Technical Report 39-226, U.S. Air Force, Wright-Patterson AFB, Ohio, 1959.

Fromm-Reichmann, R.: Principles of intensive psychotherapy, Chicago, 1950, University of Chicago Press.

Gardner, W. R.: Attention: the processing of multiple sources of information. In Friedman, E., and Friedman, M. P., editors: Handbook of perception, vol. II, New York, 1974, Academic Press, Inc., pp. 23-56.

Geldard, F. A.: The human senses, New York, 1972, John Wiley & Sons, Inc.

Goff, C. B., and others: Vibration perception in normal man and medical patients, J. Neurol. Neurosurg. Psychiatry 28:503, 1965.

Graves, T. D., and Watson, O. M.: Quantitative research in prosemic behavior, Am. Anthropologist 68:971-985, 1966.

Greenwood, A.: Mental disturbances following operation for cataract, J.A.M.A. 91:1713, 1928.

Guyton, A. C.: Textbook of medical physiology, Philadelphia, 1971, W. B. Saunders Co.

Hall, E. T.: Proxemics, Curr. Anthropology 9:83-95, 1968.

Hatton, J.: Aging and the glare problem, J. Gerontological Nurs. 3:38-44, 1977.

Heffler, A. J.: The Montifiore home hearing conservation program, Geriatrics 15:106, 1960.

Henley, N. M.: The politics of touch. In Brown, P., editor: Radical psychology, New York, 1973, Harper & Row Publishers, Inc.

Heron, W.: The pathology of boredom, Sci. Am. 196:52-56, 1957.

Heron, W., Bexton, W. H., and Hebb, D. O.: Cognitive effects of deceased variation to sensory environment, Am. Psychol. 10:13-18, 1953.

Hinchcliffe, R.: Aging and sensory thresholds, J. Gerontol. 17:45-50, 1962.

Hollender, M. H.: The need or wish to be held, Arch. Gen. Psychiatry 22:445-453, 1970.

Hoople, G. P.: Care of the hearing in the elderly, Geriatrics 15:180, 1960.

Howell, T. H.: Senile deterioration of the central nervous system: clinical study, Br. Med. J. 1:56-58, 1949.

Huss, A. J.: Touch with care or a caring touch?, J. Occup. Ther. 31:11-18, 1977.

Jackson, C. W., and Ellis, R.: Sensory deprivation as a field of study, Nurs. Res. 20:46-54, 1971.

Jackson, C. W., and O'Neill, M.: Experiences associated with sensory deprivation reported by patients having eye surgery. In Ross Roundtable on Maternal and Child Nursing: Patients with sensory disturbances: implications for nursing practice and research, Columbus, 1966, Ross Laboratories, pp. 54-69.

Jackson, C. W., and others: The application of findings for experimental sensory deprivation to cases of clinical sensory deprivation, Am. J. Sci. 243:558-562, 1962.

Jasmin, S., and Trygstad, L. N.: Behavioral concepts and the nursing process, St. Louis, 1979, The C. V. Mosby Co.

Johnson, B. S.: The meaning of touch in nursing, Nurs. Outlook 13:59-60, 1965.

Jourard, S. M.: An exploratory study of body-accessibility, Br. J. Soc. Clin. Psychol. 5:221-225, 1966.

Jourard, S. M., and Rubin, J. E.: Self-disclosure and touching: a study of two modes of interpersonal encounters and their interrelationship, J. Hum. Psychol. 8:39-48, 1968.

Keighley, R.: An instrument for measurement of vibration sensation in man, Milbank Mem. Fund Q. Bull. 24:36-48, 1946.

Kenshalo, D. R.: Psychophysical studies of temperature sensitivity. In Neff, W. D., editor: Contributions to sensory physiology, New York, 1970, Academic Press, Inc., pp. 19-74.

Kenshalo, D. R.: Aging changes in touch vibration, temperature, kinesthesis and pain sensitivity. In Birren, J. E., and Schaie, K. W., editors: Handbook of the psychology of aging, New York, 1977, Van Nostrand Reinhold Co., pp. 562-579.

Kornfield, D. S., Zimberg, S., and Malm, J. P.: Psychiatric complications of open-heart surgery, N. Engl. J. Med. 273:287-292, 1965.

Kracke, W. H.: The maintenance of the ego: implications of sensory deprivation research for psychoanalytic ego psychology, Br. J. Med. 40:17-27, 1967.

Krag, C. L., and Kountz, W. B: Stability of body functions in the aged: effects of exposure to the body to cold, J. Gerontol. 5:227-235, 1950.

Krieger, D.: The response of in-vivo human hemoglobin to an active healing therapy by direct laying-on of hands, Hum. Dimension 1:12-15, 1972.

Krieger, D.: The relationship of touch with intent to help or to heal to subjects' in-vivo hemoglobin values: a study in personalized interaction. In American Nurses Association Ninth Nursing Research Conference, San Antonio, Tex., March 21-23, 1973, Kansas City, 1974a, American Nurses Association, pp. 39-58.

Krieger, D.: Healing by the laying-on of hands as a facilitative of bioenergetic change: the response of in-vivo human hemoglobin, Psychoenergetic Systems 3 (1), 1974b.

Krieger, D.: Therapeutic touch: the imprimature of nursing, Am. J. Nurs. **75**:784-787, 1975.

Krieger, D.: Therapeutic touch, Nurs. Times **72**:572-574, 1976.

Krieger, D.: Searching for evidence of physiological change, Am. J. Nurs. **4**:660-661, 1979.

Lasagna, L.: Influence of age on analgesic pain relief, J.A.M.A. **218**:1831, 1971.

Leiderman, H., and others: Sensory deprivation, clinical aspects, Arch. Intern. Med. **101**:389-396, 1968.

Leighton, D. A.: Special senses: aging of the eye. In Brocklehurst, J. C., editor: Textbook of geriatric medicine and gerontology, Edinburgh, 1973, Churchill-Livingston Co., pp. 254-263.

Leuba, D.: Toward some integration of learning theories: the concept of optimal stimulation, Psychol. Rev. **1**:27-33, 1955.

Lilly, J. C.: Mental effects of reduction of ordinary levels of physical stimuli on intact healthy persons, American Psychiatric Association Reports, no. 5, 1956.

Maxwell, R. J., Bader, J. E., and Watson, W. H.: Territory and self in a geriatric setting, Gerontologist **12**:413-417, 1972.

McCaffery, M.: Nursing practice theories related to cognition, bodily pain, and man-environment interactions, Los Angeles, 1968, UCLA Students' Store.

McCorkle, R.: Effects of touch on seriously ill patients, Nurs. Res. **23**:125-132, 1974.

McNamee, C.: Communicating, Can. Nurse **74**:28-29, 1978.

Mendelson, J. H., and Foley, J. M.: An abnormality of mental function affecting patients in tank-type respirators, Trans. Am. Neurol. Assoc., Richmond, Va., 1956, William Bird Press, p. 136.

Meyerhoff, W. L., and Paparella, M. M.: Diagnosing the causes of hearing loss, Geriatrics **32**:95-99, 1978.

Mintz, E. E.: Touch and the psychoanalytic tradition, Psychoanal. Rev. **45**:365-376, 1969.

National Center for Health Statistics, Department of Health, Education, and Welfare: Health in later life, Washington D.C., 1971, U.S. Government Printing Office.

Nicak, A.: Changes of sensitivity to pain in relation to postnatal development in rats, Exp. Gerontol. **6**:111-114, 1971.

Nordmann, J.: Present state and perspectives in research of the lens, Invest. Ophthalmol. **4**:384-397, 1965.

O'Neil, P. M., and Calhoun, K. S.: Sensory deficits and behavioral deterioration in senescence, J. Abnorm. Psychol. **5**:579-582, 1975.

Oster, C.: Sensory deprivation in geriatric patients, J. Geriatr. Soc. **24**:461-464, 1976.

Pastalozza, G., and Shore, I.: Clinical evaluation of presbycusis on the basis of different test of auditory function, Laryngologist **65**:1135-1163, 1955.

Pearson, G. H. J.: Effect of age on vibratory sensibility, Arch. Neurol. Psychiatry **20**:482, 1928.

Perret, E., and Regli, F.: Age and the perceptual threshold for vibratory stimuli, Eur. Neurol. **4**:65-76, 1970.

Perron, D.: Deprived of sound, Am. J. Nurs. **74**:1057-1059, 1974.

Phillips, L. R.: The imprisonment model. Unpublished manuscript, 1976.

Phillips, L. R.: Sensory changes of aging, sensory alteration experiences, and confusion among the elderly. Unpublished manuscript, Preliminary examination, Tucson, University of Arizona, 1979.

Preston, T.: When words fail, Am. J. Nurs. **73**:2064-2066, 1973.

Prior, J. A., and Silberstein, J. S.: Physical diagnosis: the history and examination of the patient, St. Louis, 1973, The C. V. Mosby Co.

Ramsdell, D. A.: The psychology of the hard-of-hearing and deafened adult. In Davis, H., and Silverman, S. R., editors: Hearing and deafness, New York, 1970, Holt, Rinehart & Winston, pp. 453-461.

Rosenberg, G.: Effect of age on peripheral vibratory perception, J. Am. Geriatr. Soc. **6**:471-481, 1958.

Ruben, R.: Aging and hearing. In Rossman, I., editor: Clinical geriatrics, Philadelphia, 1971, J. B. Lippincott Co., pp. 247-252.

Rupp, R. R.: Understanding the problems of presbycusis, Geriatrics **25**:100-107, 1970.

Schaie, K. W., and others: A study of auditory sensitivity in advanced age, J. Gerontol. **19**:453-457, 1964.

Schiffman, H. R.: Sensation and perception: an integrated approach, New York, 1977, John Wiley & Sons, Inc.

Schnuknecht, H. F.: Presbycusis, Laryngologist **65**:402-419, 1955.

Schnuknecht, H. F.: Further observations on the pathology of presbycusis, Arch. Otolaryngol. **80**:369, 1964.

Schultz, D. P.: Sensory restriction: effects on behavior, New York, 1965, Academic Press, Inc.

Scott, T. H., and others: Cognitive effects of perceptual isolation, Can. J. Psychol. **13**:200-209, 1959.

Shelby, J. P.: Sensory deprivation, Image **10**:49-55, 1978.

Shore, H.: Sensory deprivation. Mainstreaming the elderly, Conference, University of Kansas, Overland Park, Kan., 1978.

Shurley, J. T.: Profound experimental sensory isolation, Am. J. Psychiatry **117**:539-545, 1960.

Shurley, J. T.: The hydro-hypodynamic environment. In Cleghorn, R. A., editor: Proceedings of the Third World Congress of Psychiatry, Montreal, June 4-10, 1961, Toronto, 1972, University of Toronto Press, pp. 232-236.

Snyder, L. H., Pyrek, J., and Smith, K. C.: Vision and mental function of the elderly, Gerontologist **16**:491-495, 1976.

Snyder, L. H., and others: Wandering, Gerontologist **18**:272-280, 1978.

Snyder, L. H., and others: Environmental changes for socialization, J. Nurs. Administration **8**:44-50, 1978.

Teter, D.: Clinical considerations of hearing aids. In Northern, J. L., editor: Hearing disorders, Boston, 1976, Little, Brown & Co., pp. 228-240.

Ullman, M.: Behavioral changes in patients following strokes, Springfield, Ill., 1962, Charles C Thomas Publishers.

Watson, O. M.: On proxemic research, Curr. Anthropology **10**:222-224, 1969.

Weinberg, H.: On adding insult to injury, Gerontologist **16**:4-10, 1975.

Weiss, A. D.: Role and importance of sensory functions in aging. In Jeffers, F. D., editor: Duke University Council on Gerontology: Proceedings 1961-1965, Durham, N.C., 1965, Duke University Regional Center for the Study of Aging.

Whiteley, M. P.: Seduction and the hospitalized patient, J. Nurs. Educ. **17**:34-39, 1978.

Yarrington, C. T.: Presbycusis. In Northern, J. L., editor: Hearing disorders, Boston, 1976, Little, Brown & Co., pp. 178-184.

Zefrom, L. J.: The history of the laying-on of hands in nursing, Nurs. Forum **14**:350-363, 1975.

Ziskind, E.: Observations of mental symptoms in eye-patched patients: hypnagagic symptoms in sensory deprivation, Am. J. Psychiatry **66**:895, 1960.

Zubek, J. P., and others: Perceptual changes after prolonged perceptual isolation, Can. J. Psychol. **16**:83-100, 1961.

Zubek, J. P., and MacNeil, M.: Perceptual deprivation phenomenon: role of the recumbent position, J. Abnorm. Psychol. **72**:147-150, 1967.

Zubek, J. P., editor: Sensory deprivation: fifteen years of research, New York, 1969, Appleton-Century-Crofts.

Zuckerman, M.: Theoretical formulations: I. In Zubek, J. P., editor: Sensory deprivation: fifteen years of research, New York, 1969, Appleton-Century-Crofts, pp. 407-432.

Zuckerman, M., and others: Stress response in total and partial perceptual isolation, Psychosom. Med. **26**:250-260, 1964.

11

CARE OF THE CLIENT WHOSE CONFUSION RESULTS FROM DISRUPTION OF PATTERN AND MEANING

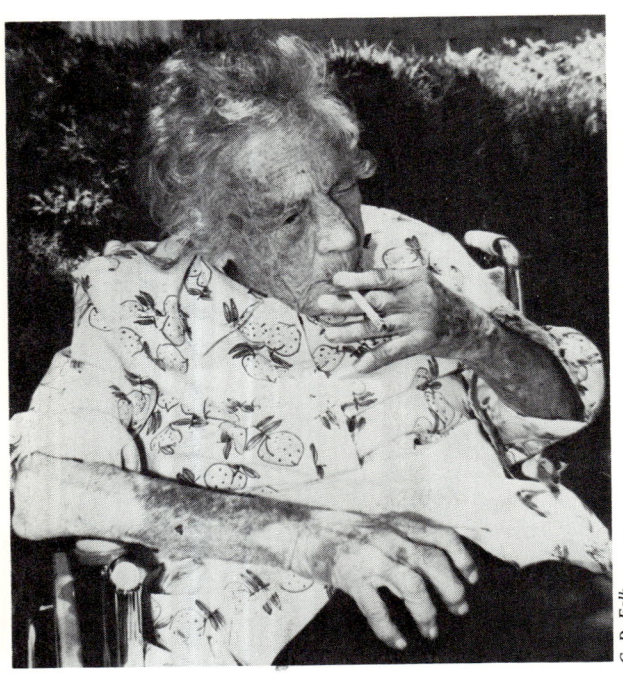

In Chapter 2, we introduced the idea that confusional states can arise from problems with interaction. Using the concept of interaction in its broadest sense, we presented in Chapter 9 interaction problems in the physiologic realm that can result in confusion among elderly people. In Chapter 10 we discussed interaction problems involving the sensoriperceptual apparatus that can result in confusion. The unifying principle throughout this presentation has been that, ordinarily, people interact continually with internal and external stimuli that are characterized by or at least perceived as having stability, predictability, and meaning. When the pattern and meaning of stimuli are disrupted or no longer perceived, for whatever reason, acute confusion results. In this chapter, another component of interactional problems will be presented—the confusion that arises from interactions with an external environment in which either the pattern or the meaning is disrupted.

This chapter will be organized into two sections. First, the confusion that arises when stressors disrupt the pattern and meaning perceived by the client in his personal milieu is discussed. The concepts that unify this section are crisis and stress. Second, the confusion that arises when the social context interferes with the client's perception of pattern and meaning is explored. The concepts unifying this section are imprisonment and social breakdown. Both sections identify the conceptual perspective, the clients who are in the high-risk category, the fourth-level assessment procedures that specify the problems, and the measures that prevent and intervene against the appearance of confusion.

STRESSORS AND THE CLIENT'S PERSONAL MILIEU

For those readers previously oriented to the idea that confusion among the elderly arises solely from physiologic difficulties or problems with drugs, it may be difficult to conceive that serious, long-standing, and even permanent confusion can arise from a disruption in the pattern and meaning of life experience that is unrelated to physiology. However, consider the following quotation: "Helen Hayes, the actress, confessed, 'For two years (after her husband's death) I was crazy as you can be and still be at large. I didn't have any really normal minutes during those two years. It wasn't just grief. *It was total confusion*' " (Caine, 1974, p. 98) (italics added). Using this quotation, plus many of her own experiences, Caine describes the feelings and thoughts that surround the death of a spouse. Most of us, at least intellectually, can identify quite closely with Caine's moving account and can acknowledge that widowhood produces devastating grief, depression, anxiety, emptiness, and loneliness. But two additional things can be learned from this quotation and from Caine's experiences. First, acute confusion accompanies this "normal," but major stressor, and second, the confusional state may persist over months or even years.

Many of us have experienced the feeling of acute, total confusion that accompanies a major stressor, although we may have never thought of it in those terms or called it "confusion." We can ask the question, then, Is the acute confusion that accompanies a major stressor for a person of any age the same acute confusion that is displayed by many elderly people? Many times it is. If so, why is it that the confusion each of us has experienced is momentary and intermittent, and the confusion displayed by many elderly people persists? Part of the answer to this, of course, is that many elderly people have fewer physical and social resources. They may have compromised brain supports to the point that combating and recovering from the confusion is difficult. However, another part of the answer is frequently overlooked by all of us. In our culture, we all have certain expectations concerning the appropriate magnitude and duration of the reaction to a major stressor. Using the death of a spouse as an example, we expect that the widow will show a great magnitude of grief behaviors immediately following the death and that the magnitude of grief behaviors will diminish over time. Time for the grieving person in our culture is measured in months, not years. We are programmed to believe the grief process will be fairly well resolved by the first anniversary of the death, and if confusion accompanies the death experience, it, like grief, will be resolved within that first year. However, using Helen Hayes' words, "It wasn't just grief." The death of a spouse is no simple matter, and it becomes increasingly complicated with increasing age. As Caine indicates, radical life changes accompany this one major stres-

Table 11-1. Life change events that may occur with the death of a spouse

Personal injury or illness
Change to different line of work
Change in financial state
Mortgage over $10,000
Foreclosure of mortgage or loan
Change in living conditions
Revision of personal habits
Son or daughter leaving home
Trouble with in-laws
Change in residence
Change in work hours or conditions
Change in social activities
Change in sleeping habits
Change in eating habits
Vacation
Christmas

sor that complicate the grieving process and may account for why confusion persists. Table 11-1 uses items from Holmes and Rahe (1967) Social Readjustment Rating Scale, as does Caine (1974), to illustrate the events that may accompany the death of a spouse. This table demonstrates that one major stressor, the death of a spouse, may precipitate other major and minor stressors in a ripple effect. Confusion may arise when the individual has neither the time nor the resources to resolve the first stressor before the next one occurs. Set within this framework, elements of both crisis theory and stress theory can be used to explain the confusion that arises because of a disruption of the client's perception of pattern and meaning.

Stressors as the source of confusion

Fig. 11-1 shows a model in which various types of stressors are seen as the precipitating factors that may eventually lead to confusion as a form of individual decompensation. This model, used to organize this section, is adapted from the concepts presented by Selye (1976). The general form of the model is as follows (the numbers presented in the text correspond with the numbers that appear on the model):

1. Personal, social, and cultural stimuli are perceived by the individual as stressors.
2. Stressors set off the alarm phase of reaction, in which both cognitive and experiential components components are present.
3. In the cognitive component of the alarm phase, the individual engages in a balancing process through which he, consciously or unconsciously, identifies the personal resources and the personal liabilities that constitute his coping (or noncoping) abilities in relation to his particular stressor and to his perception of the aging condition. The experiential component of the alarm phase involves the experiences perceived by the individual in relation to the particular stressor, such as loneliness, helplessness, hopelessness, and ambivalence, and in relation to his total situation. The relationship between the experiential component and the cognitive component is reciprocal. Even if, for example, the person has adequate resources to outweigh his personal liabilities, the experiences associated with the stressor may be so overwhelmingly negative, so filled with loneliness and hopelessness, that his personal resources are rendered neutral. In this case the experiences themselves become liabilities. In addition, for the elderly, it may be that the experiential component is "preset" by multiple and continuing stressors or by his perception of the aging condition, rendering his resources neutral.
4. There are three possible outcomes for the alarm phase: adaptation, resolution, and growth; crisis; and chronic tension or stress.
5. Two possible outcomes exist for both crisis and chronic tension or stress: adaptation, resolution, and growth; and decompensation. Confusion is one example of decompensation; death, psychosis, depression, and suicide are others.
6. The relationship between crisis and chronic tension or stress is reciprocal. One possible resolution of crisis, for example, is chronic tension or stress, with the individual failing to grow and adapt but continuing to function at his precrisis level, a state not as detrimental as crisis but not as healthy as adaptation. Conversely, chronic tension or stress may lead to crisis to the point that other stressors compound the problem or the individual's frustration level is exceeded and exhaustion intervenes. Crisis, in this view, can be considered an outcome of chronic stress, much in the way decompensation and growth may be outcomes of chronic stress.
7. As long as the individual has not terminated his existence with passive or active suicide, or he has not been overwhelmed by physiologic exhaustion, he may experience one end result of decompensation—adaptation, resolution, and growth—provided positive energies intervene during

Care of the client whose confusion results from disruption of pattern and meaning

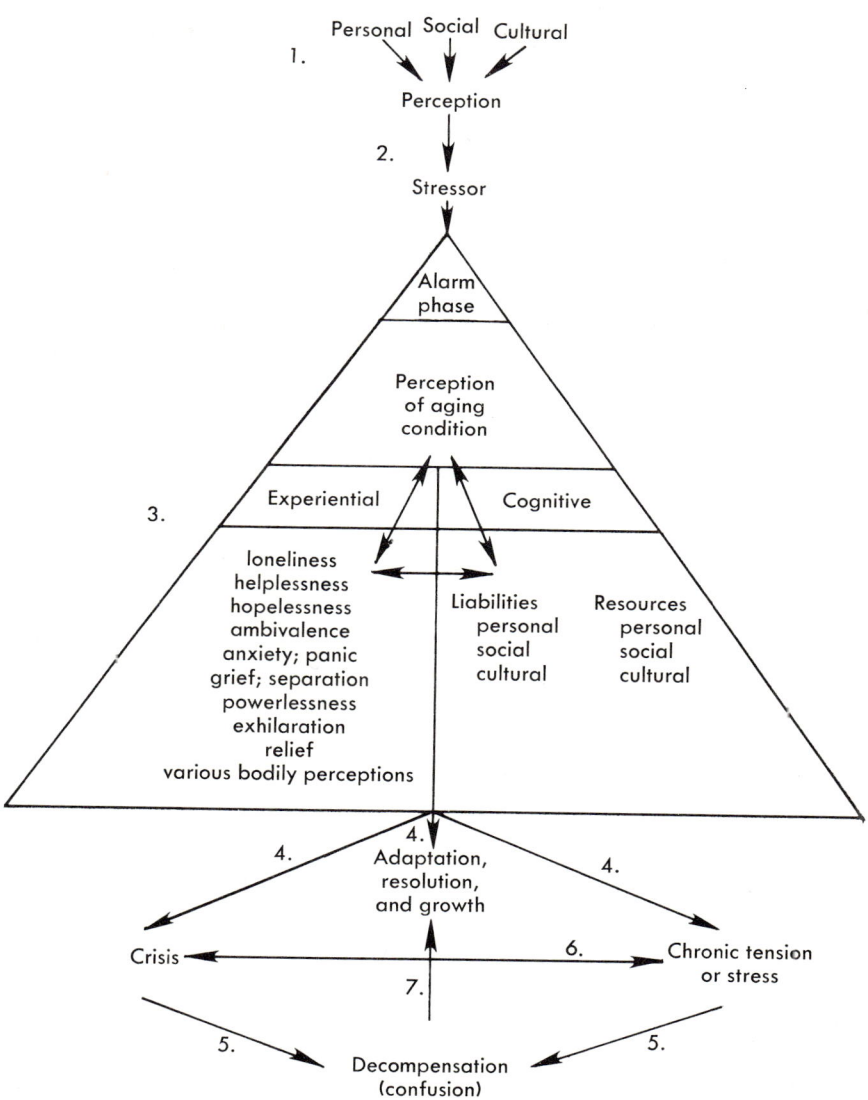

Fig. 11-1. Relationship of stressors to confusion.

decompensation. It must therefore be emphasized that confusion, psychosis, and depression are not necessarily terminal outcomes.

Each of the major components of this model will be specifically discussed in relation to elderly people.

Stressors

A stressor is a stimulus that differs from the routine multiple stimuli encountered in our day-to-day interactions by its crucial nature and magnitude.

A routine stimulus is one to which the organism can respond more or less automatically, one that poses no problem in adjustment.... A *stressor*, however, can be defined as a demand made by the internal or external environment of an organism that upsets its homeostasis, restoration of which depends on a nonautomatic and not readily available energy expending action (Antonovsky, 1979, p. 72).

The individual reaction determines whether an event constitutes a routine stimulus or a stressor.

Stressors may arise out of the personal/interpersonal, social, or cultural milieu of the individual. Table 11-2 demonstrates some of the common stressors that arise from the personal/interpersonal milieu of the elderly individual. This table was developed from taped autobiographies of noninstitutionalized, elderly adults (Phillips, 1976).

Three dominant themes or categories are presented in this table: losses, rejection, and powerlessness. Each of these can be considered to be a constant characteristic of the aging condition for many people, as well as potential, individual stressors. In addition, elderly people are exposed to other personal/interpersonal stressors at a fairly high rate. These include illness, accidents, malnutrition, intrapsychic fear related to past experiences, intrapsychic fears related to physical vulnerability and the fear of victimization and aggression, and certain maturational conflicts, such as the immediacy

Table 11-2. Common stressors that arise from the elderly individual's personal/interpersonal milieu

I. Losses
   A. Loss of relationships with people
      1. Loss of significant others and confidants
      2. Loss of peer group and collegial relationships
   B. Financial losses
   C. Loss of possessions
   D. Awareness of declining health
      1. Deterioration of own health
         a. Discomforts and pain
         b. Confinement and immobility
         c. Physical changes
         d. Monotony of daily encounters
         e. Absence of personal privacy
         f. Enforced idleness
         g. Awareness of death
      2. Deterioration of significant others' health
         a. Confinement
         b. Burden of caring for others
II. Rejection
   A. Feeling forgotten
   B. Being forgotten
   C. Feeling unworthy or unacceptable
III. Powerlessness
   A. Powerlessness against others and the world
      1. Vulnerability and being a spectator
      2. Unreliability of others
      3. Unpredictability of others and the fates
      4. Indignities and dependence
      5. Being exposed to propaganda
         a. Being talked into what is not wanted
         b. Having information withheld
         c. Not having accurate information
   B. Powerlessness against time
      1. Not knowing the duration of confinement
      2. Sensing a meaningless existence
   C. Sensing threats to life and health

Table 11-3. Stressors in both long-term and short-term care settings

1. **Threats to life and health**—the client's apprehension about his fate, whether in the form of the fear of death following acute trauma or surgery, the fear of permanent disability, or the fear of the dying process
2. **Discomforts**—the physical complaints of the client in regard to pain, cold, fatigue, poor food, lack of care, etc.; the client's apprehension regarding his ability to regulate discomforts and being assured discomforts will be attended to
3. **Loss of a means of subsistence**—the client's concern about economic conditions in general, economic conditions of significant others, his own economic conditions, and economic concerns about illness
4. **Deprivation of intimacy**—the loss of physical closeness, sexual satisfaction, close affiliations, and friendships
5. **Enforced idleness**—the client's concern about his inability to perform usual tasks, engage in necessary tasks for survival, such as cooking and shopping, and engage in recreational activities
6. **Restriction of movement**—physical immobility, monotony of daily encounters, and the absence of personal privacy
7. **Isolation**—the client being apart from his usual environment, apart from his usual acquaintances or old friends, and perceiving that the caregivers are uncaring
8. **Threats to family structure**—the fear of a loss of family status or family role and the realization of failing health and loss of resources of close family members
9. **Capricious behavior of those in charge**—the client's perception that his caregivers are unpredictable
10. **Propaganda**—the client not having accurate information about his status, feeling that information is being withheld, and being talked into something he does not want or does not believe
11. **Awareness of personal degeneration**—the client's awareness of his own physical and mental failings
12. **Rejection**—feelings of being forgotten, of significant others not caring, and perceiving the ridicule and dislike of others
13. **Unknown duration**—feelings that the confinement will never end and that time drags

and acceptance of death and the acceptance that life goals may remain unfulfilled.

Stressors that arise out of the social milieu can be divided into several categories related to the social structure and aging. These include retirement, loss of social roles and status, social isolation, relocation, role reversal, and institutionalization. It is not, however, necessarily the event itself that becomes a stressor, but the associated disruptions that accompany or surround the event. For example, the retirement event or the thought of retirement may not be a stressor. However, retirement may mean a change in relationships with family members; an increase in contact with certain family members; a confrontation with self, perhaps for the first time; a lack of economic resources to pursue lifetime aspirations; and a loss of peer and collegial relationships. These changes may constitute the stressors. With institutionalization of the elderly, Phillips (1976) found at least thirteen independent categories of stressors existed for these individuals in both the long-term and the short-term care setting. These are listed and defined in Table 11-3. The same is true of any social event or social structure that has an impact on an elderly person. It is the personal consequence of the event more than the event itself that creates a stressor.

At least three sources of cultural stressors exist for the elderly person. These are age-graded expectations, negative cultural attitudes and values, and the cultural change. The first are certain behavioral expectations in every society that are culturally prescribed based on age alone. For example, parenthood is culturally determined in our society as appropriate between the ages of 20 and 40. If a man should become a father at age 85, he is exhibiting behavior contrary to that appropriate to his age. This may constitute a stressor. All cultures determine the appropriate ages for childhood, adulthood, parenthood, termination of education, termination of employment or work, and death. The person who flouts these normative prescriptions may be faced with unexpected stressors that arise out of not "acting one's age" (Neugarten and others, 1968). Second, negative cultural attitudes and values exist in our society regarding the aging process that are stressors for some people. For example, physical aging is difficult to face in a society that places high value on physical prowess and youthful beauty. Also, becoming a full-fledged member of a minority group that holds little power, authority, or status in this culture, such as the aged, may be a stressor. Third, cultural change may serve as a stressor. Our society is becoming increasingly technologic and fast moving. The world with which many elderly individuals are familiar has essentially disappeared with changing values, standards of behavior, and language. As a result, many elderly persons are chronically exposed to cultural shock as a stressor. As with social stressors, however, it is not the presence of these three factors that determines whether the event is a stressor or not, but the individual's perception of the event and its personal significance.

Alarm phase

During the alarm phase, there is the balancing of the individual's personal resources and liabilities (cognitive component), as influenced by the individual's current experiences (experiential component) and by the individual's perception of the aging condition. Each of these has an important and independent effect on the way any given stressor will affect the behavior of the elderly person.

Many diverse stabilizing forces that arise from individual's personal/interpersonal, social, and cultural milieus constitute the individual's personal resources. Antonovsky (1979), for example, identifies the following as personal resources (generalized resistance resources):

1. Material resources, such as money, financial security, and housing
2. Knowledge and intelligence
3. Functional coping strategies, particularly flexible, farsighted, and rational ones that have worked in the past
4. Social supports, social networks, and social ties
5. Cultural stability
6. Forms of magic and superstitious beliefs
7. Religion, philosophy, arts, or a stable set of answers
8. Preventive health orientations

Health and mobility may be major resources for an elderly person, just as may an accumulated store of wisdom. Clearly, a strong sense of identity that enhances feelings of self-esteem, self-worth, and personal integrity is an important personal resource.

According to Antonovsky (1979), one of the most important personal resources is a strong sense of coherence, "a global orientation that expresses the extent to which one has pervasive, enduring though dynamic feelings of confidence that one's internal and external environments are predictable and there is a high probability that things will work out as well as can be expected" (p. 185). A personal sense of coherence mobilizes, augments, and supersedes any of the other personal resources available to the individual. This sense of coherence is distinct from both a sense of control, which denotes the person's feelings that he has the absolute capacity to affect the outcome of an event, and from the Pollyanna notion that life will hold no frustration or failure.

Quite the contrary may even be true. Life may well be seen as full of complexities, conflicts, and complications. Goal achievement may be seen as contingent on an immense investment of effort. Moreover, one may be fully aware that life involves failure and frustration. The important thing is that one has a sense of confidence, of faith, that by and large, things will work out well. Not that things will have a Hollywood happy ending. This is why the proviso "as can reasonably be expected" is added. A strong sense of coherence includes a solid capacity to judge reality (Antonovsky, 1979, pp. 126-127).

The sense of coherence is determined by experiences, previous successes with tension management, past participation in the shaping of outcomes, and past abilities to balance conflicts, stressors, and resources. A strong sense of coherence permits the effective mobilization of other resources in the time of stress. It is probably the sense of coherence that has a major impact on why some individuals react severely and adversely to stressors, whereas others meet these same stressors and grow and learn in the process.

Personal liabilities also arise from the individual's personal/interpersonal, social, and cultural milieus. They are, in many ways, similar to stressors, as described previously, and may be directly opposite resources. For example, lack of material resources, lack of knowledge, inadequate coping strategies, lack of social supports, cultural instability, and lack of a belief system are personal liabilities, as are illness, lack of mobility, and physical disabilities. A poor self-identity is a liability, as is a weak sense of coherence. Unresolved past conflict, unfulfilled goals and aspirations, and past injustices and failures that still haunt the individual are also personal liabilities. The more lacking the individual is or perceives himself to be, the less ability he has to combat stressors and use his resources.

The experiential component of the alarm phase is more difficult to clearly define. Feeling states, processes, and bodily perceptions comprise the experiential component. These help to determine the affective tone perceived by the individual and his perceptions of personal resources and liabilities. The experiential component may be best explained by use of an example. If the stressor is death of a spouse, the initial experiences of the individual may be anxiety (feeling state), loneliness (feeling state), grief (process), sleeplessness (bodily perception), palpitations (bodily perception), and nausea (bodily perception). These reactions do not constitute either crisis or chronic stress by themselves. Rather, they are simply *normal*, individual reactions to the reality of the death of a spouse. They may, however, predispose to crisis or tension either because the individual perceives these reactions as so frightening and unfamiliar that he attaches another meaning to them, such as going crazy or finding symptoms of cancer, or because the individual permits these experiences to color the way he performs the cognitive task of weighing resources and liabilities. In addition, it is possible that certain of the processes, feeling states, or bodily perceptions existed prior to the stressor, influencing the way the alarm is handled. Taking grief as an example, it is widely acknowledged that multiple, almost perpetual losses are associated with aging. These include loss of peers, loss of economic stability, loss of parents, and loss of siblings and confidants, which may cause the elderly client to be in a state of chronic grief. This chronic grief is then superimposed on the grief experience that occurs in response to the death of his spouse. Very often, the "presetting" of experience occurs as a result of the client's perception of and reaction to the aging condition. Table 11-4 contains the feeling states and processes commonly and often continually experienced by elderly people.

Table 11-4. Feeling states and processes commonly experienced by elderly individuals

Experiential concept	Definition and theoretical considerations	Experience
Grief	A normal and natural reaction to the real loss of a highly valued person or object. Grief is both universally experienced and self-limiting. The resolution of grief following a loss is a necessary task for self-development and is related to the client's ability to establish important connections with other people (Mereness and Taylor, 1978).	Feelings of shock and disbelief initially. Denial, anger, anxiety, and isolation are not uncommon. Developing awareness of the loss, characterized by sadness, depression, guilt, and identification with the lost person. Restitution, characterized by acceptance of the loss and appreciation of the lost person for what they really were. (Adapted from Engel, 1962; Kubler-Ross, 1969.)
Separation	The process that must be completed in order that a significant object to which the client is attached, devoted, or has a personal investment can become detached. Separation is also a reaction to loss, whether the loss is temporary or permanent, planned or unplanned, of short duration or prolonged (Jasmin and Trygstad, 1979).	Protest stage: feelings of anxiety, anger, and ambivalence. Despair stage: feelings of guilt, sadness, fear, panic, barrenness, hopelessness, vulnerability, and relief. Detachment stage: feelings of acceptance and peace. (Adapted from Bowlby, 1973; Jasmin and Trygstad, 1979.)
Rejection	A state that is created whenever the client feels that he is not included or not with those separated from him because he is unsatisfactory, unworthy, or objectionable. Rejection is often experienced when the client feels he has lost his love object because of his own deficiencies. Feelings or rejection are directly related to self-esteem.	Feeling forgotten, ignored, or ridiculed. Feelings of anger, guilt, sadness, and vulnerability. Expressions of self-depreciation and worthlessness.
Loneliness	Two types of loneliness may be experienced either independently or together. First is existential loneliness, or "an intrinsic and organic reality of human life, in which there is both pain and triumphant creation emerging from a long period of desolation" (Roberts, 1976, p. 138). Second is loneliness anxiety, or the fear of being alone and alienated from self (Roberts, 1976). Both of these may have a here-and-now component and a future component.	Feelings of anxiety and panic, desperation, despair, and desolation. Expressions of a void in the client's life, sadness, and doubts about his ability to survive. Feelings of estrangement from self and others.

Table 11-4. Feeling states and processes commonly experienced by elderly individuals—cont'd

Experiential concept	Definition and theoretical considerations	Experience
Hopelessness	A state that is associated with rigid and inflexible thoughts and feelings. The central notion of hopelessness is the feeling of entrapment. Hopelessness means the feeling of impossibility, futility, and no future (Lynch, 1965; Roberts, 1976).	Expressions of the desire to give up, of futility, and of meaninglessness. The client complains of no energy and no motivation. He is incapable of identifying or desiring a future goal.
Helplessness	A state that is associated with an external orientation toward control and power. The central notion is that the self is vulnerable and unable to affect the outcome of the situation, no matter what the action. Helplessness may be learned and experienced as a means of getting and keeping people close when they would otherwise be distant (Roberts, 1976; Shea, 1970).	Expressions of letting go, of letting others decide and act. The problems and feelings are usually externalized rather than seen as a part of the client himself.
Powerlessness	Like helplessness, a state in which there is "the expectancy or the probability held by the individual that his own behavior cannot determine the outcome or the reinforcement he seeks" (Roberts, 1976, p. 118). Powerlessness arises from loss of personal control, loss of control over the environment, and lack of knowledge. Powerlessness can be fostered from the outside by powerful others, including caregivers. Alienation from self is a dominant theme with powerlessness (Roberts, 1976).	Expressions of passivity and dependency, either verbally or behaviorally. The client will not take the initiative to make decisions or choices and will let happen what will. Powerlessness is often displayed by increasing egocentrism.
Anxiety	"Pyschological response to specific stressors: threats to self-concept, independence, or control" (Jasmin and Trygstad, 1979, p. 55). The stressors that arouse anxiety are frequently not recognized by the anxious client. Often there is simply the feeling of apprehension and a sense of impending doom that the client cannot associate with any single factor in his life.	Activation similar to stress activation, including narrowed perceptions, decreased problem solving, and sense of being "on." Physically, the client will display tremors, perspirations, dilated pupils, increased gastrointestinal motility, dry mouth, and paleness. Anxiety can be acute or chronic (Jasmin and Trygstad, 1979).
Ambivalence and conflict	A feeling state characterized by the presence of both positive and negative feelings, which are simultaneously experienced. "Ambivalence is a type of confusion" (Jasmin and Trygstad, 1979, p. 169). Ambivalence is often associated with feelings of anxiety and psychic discomfort.	Expressions of vacillation, inconsistency, hesitancy, and instability. Erratic and uncharacteristic behaviors are associated with ambivalence. The client may express feeling split or puzzled. Physical responses are similar to anxiety, often including insomnia and fatigue (Jasmin and Trygstad, 1979).

Although a client is personally involved with changes in his own being and his own aging, he is also exposed to certain universal notions about the nature and effects of age changes. These universal notions can be called the aging condition. The aging condition is physiologically, socially, and culturally determined. It involves and yet supersedes the individual. Universally, aging is characterized by the "increasing vulnerability of an organism progressing through its life span" (Hendricks and Hendricks, 1977, p. 27). Physiologically, the aging person is assumed to demonstrate loss of physical stamina, loss of recuperative powers, loss of mobility, and loss of adaptability to environmental stressors. As a result, the notion arises that the aging client is less able to use his body to exert control over his environment and to influence people in his environment. Superimposed on the physiologic aging process are other types of losses that similarly increase the vulnerability of the aging individual. The elderly are frequently faced with sudden and radical changes in living situations and life-styles. Inherent in the aging conditions, then, is a vulnerability that causes the individual to feel more or less defenseless, lacking the reserve to cope with physical and emotional assaults.

Although there are universal notions about what constitutes the aging condition, it is the way the client perceives and personalizes these notions that affects his ability to react to stressors. When he has internalized weakness and vulnerability as a part of his self-concept, he is less likely to perceive his personal resources. When he is constantly confronted with the deficits of aging and few of the benefits, he is likely to be in a chronic state of grief, loneliness, anxiety, and isolation, which interferes with his ability to solve problems and constructively adapt to change. The interplay of these three components—the individual's perception of the aging condition, the cognitive component, and the experiential component—determines whether a stressor will result in adaptation, resolution, and growth or crisis or chronic stress.

Crisis

Crisis can be defined as a "state of psychic disequilibrium" (Ebersole, 1976, p. 270). Akin to the catastrophic state described in Chapter 2, crisis occurs when a stressor is perceived as an insurmountable obstacle (Caplan, 1961) that threatens to overwhelm the ego (Aguilera and Messick, 1978), and render the individual unable to behave according to his essential capabilities (Goldstein, 1939). Crisis results "from the interaction of an event with the individual's or family's coping mechanisms, which are inadequate to meet the demands of the situation, combined with the individual's or family's perception of the event" (Mereness and Taylor, 1978, p. 468).

On the other hand, crisis can be viewed as a "catalyst" that challenges the person's previous coping styles, evokes new responses, and stimulates development and maturation. With or without intervention, there are three possible resolutions to a crisis state. First, the individual may reintegrate at a higher level of functioning; second, the individual may reintegrate at the same level of functioning; and third, the individual may reintegrate at a lower level of functioning or regress (Mereness and Taylor, 1978).

Most crisis theorists agree that crisis is an acute state that is short-lived, self-limiting, and usually resolved within the period of 4 to 6 weeks. This, however, may not be exactly true for the elderly. Since many extraneous factors complicate crisis for the elderly and because elderly people have a lifelong history of dealing with crisis that may alter the intensity of their reaction, it may be more useful to consider Bloom's (1963) conceptualization of crisis with respect to the elderly. Bloom states that crisis is a state of disequilibrium with a *slow resolution* and a known precipitating event. For many elderly persons, even identifying the precipitating event may be difficult. The

Fink crisis model (1967), which is based on Bloom's conceptualization, describes the process of crisis resolution in terms of an extended time rather than mere weeks. Although originally designed to describe the process through which individuals cope with the crisis of permanent, sudden disability, the Fink model may be particularly helpful in understanding crisis as it is experienced by the elderly.

Fink (1967) acknowledges five states in the crisis resolution process. They are: (1) precrisis, (2) shock (stress), (3) defensive retreat, (4) acknowledgment (renewed stress), and (5) adaptation. Precrisis is characterized by rigidly organized, stereotyped behavior that may be considered by those around the person to be appropriate under the circumstances. During the precrisis stage, the individual experiences a sense of numbness and depersonalization. He appears to those around him as docile and submissive. When he perceives the reality of what for him is a real danger and threat to his person, he enters the shock stage. During the shock stage, the stress surrounding the crisis event is perceived as overwhelming. The person experiences panic, anxiety, and helplessness and appears to be totally disorganized. His behavior no longer makes sense to him or to those around him as he relinquishes his ability to reason, plan, or even understand the situation. Confusion is an outstanding characteristic of this stage. The shock stage of crisis is self-limiting because the individual is unable to maintain the energy levels required for such intensity of reaction for long periods.

The shock stage of crisis gives way to defensive retreat as the individual attempts to reestablish himself as the individual he was precrisis. He attempts to reinforce his old values and his old habits to maintain his sense of control over the situation. The person's thinking and behaving become quite rigid as he denies the personal impact of the event and uses his old defense system to deal with the crisis.

Because the human organism is constantly striving for continued growth and development, time alone may account for the individual's movement into the acknowledgment stage, or he may reach this stage because his reinforcement system fails to support the continuation of the old defenses. During acknowledgment, there is renewed stress and anxiety. Very often the person expresses self-deprecation, depression, mourning, and an attitude of bitterness over the loss. He again suffers a sense of disorganization as his defenses break down. Confusion may recur at this point. Later in the acknowledgment stage, a slow feeling of reorganization is sensed as the individual begins to learn new defenses and to develop new coping styles. The person begins to realize that "what has been lost is not the whole picture; what still remains may be recognized as the resources of the future" (Fink, 1967, p. 595).

In the adaptation stage that follows, the individual tries out his new self, his new coping styles, and his new defense system. There is a gradual lessening of anxiety and depression and the development of goal direction with future orientation. Slowly, the individual may begin to see the crisis in a positive light and begin to acknowledge the learning he has achieved through the crisis.

As with other staged models, this model cannot be used or accepted without acknowledging certain conditions. First, the movement through these stages is essential to crisis resolution, but the time required to do so and the way it is accomplished are highly individual. Some people move quickly and others move slowly. Some individuals fail to reach resolution at all. A certain number of individuals use suicide as a means of failing to reach crisis resolution. Among elderly men, suicide is not an uncommon response to crisis. A certain number of individuals decompensate during crisis resolution into a psychotic depression or a prolonged confusional state and fail to resolve the crisis. It may be that the elderly who decompensate are those who are most devoid of personal resources and those whose precrisis coping styles were most inadequate. The most common points in the cycles for decompensation are during the "stress" phases of shock and acknowledgment. A number of individuals have such strong denial systems that they are unable to move out of defensive retreat. Fink (1967) believes that it is virtually impossible to pull a person out of defensive retreat, that this step must be made by the person himself. Presenting stark reality to a person in defensive retreat serves only to cause the person to entrench himself deeper in his withdrawal and denial in an effort to reduce stress and preserve his very being. Individuals who fail to move out of defensive retreat are probably those who Mereness and Taylor (1978) believe complete crisis resolution at a lower level of coping than they began. Often, these people *appear* confused. They are probably the same elderly persons who become recluses, refusing to leave their homes, participate in society, or change their life-style in line with reality.

The literature identifies two types of crisis, both of which affect the elderly person: maturational and situational. The events that precipitate situational crisis have already been discussed under stressors. The stressors that precipitate maturational crisis have not been fully developed. A maturational crisis is precipitated when the person enters into a new developmental stage that necessitates the mastery of new tasks or when the person has a sudden change in social status. Some of the maturational stressors encountered by the elderly are: the anticipation of one's own death; the reduction in status, influence, and power that accompanies the loss of life roles and retirement; role reversal with spouse or children accompanying the serious illness of a spouse or one's own serious illnesses; the realization that life goals remain unfulfilled; and the onset of human isolation. Resolving the conflicts that surround these events is an unavoidable task for most elderly persons. When the conflicts are perceived as unresolvable and events unmasterable, however, the disequilibrium that results is termed a maturational or identity crisis.

Among the elderly, the symptoms of crisis may not be as obvious as with younger people, nor may crisis be as easily recognized. Many elderly persons are reluctant to admit they are viewing their situation as insurmountable. Instead of focusing on the feelings and emotions that are accompanying a stressor, many elderly individuals focus on the details of the situation as a way of avoiding the underlying feelings. Physical symptoms of a crisis among the elderly may range from multiple, vague physical complaints to classic anxiety symptoms such as tightness in the throat, a choking sensation, shortness of breath, weakness, muscle tension, and trembling. Elderly people in crisis may become increasingly withdrawn from other people. Paranoia and confusion that ranges from mild to gross disorientation may be present (Ebersole, 1976). A wide range of emotions may constitute the feeling state of crisis, including massive free-floating anxiety, depression, and fear (Mereness and Taylor, 1978).

Oberleder (1970) suggests that at least some of the memory loss, confusion, disorientation, and inappropriate behavior seen among aging people diagnosed as having organic brain syndrome may be directly attributable to crisis states that are not necessarily recognized in that light.

> Memory loss and disorientation might be employed selectively as a reality-denial defense or as a part of an ego-preserving delusional system. Incontinence might represent a substitute gratification for frustrated sexual or aggressive drives. Incoherent speech might be a disguised way of communication as it is in schizophrenia. Delusions and hallucinations might serve as restitutional defenses as they do in all mental disorders. "Senility" itself, if one thinks of it as pathological psychological aging, might be a systematic defense reaction to an ego crisis . . . (p. 111).

Undoubtedly, at least some of the confusional behaviors of the elderly represent either various stages of normal crisis resolution, as specified by Fink (1967), or decompensation during crisis resolution, as suggested by Oberleder (1970).

Chronic stress or tension

Colloquial English tells us that the psychologic implications of chronic stress and tension have probably always been known. For example, a person may say, "I am sick with worry," "I am sick at heart," and "He died of a broken heart." Selye (1973), however, was one of the first scientists to clearly identify the relationships among stress, physiologic changes, and psychologic changes. Since that time, extensive work has been to explore the relationship betwen chronic stress and clinical disease (Antonovsky, 1979; Hurst, Jenkins, and Rose, 1979; Simonton, Matthews–Simonton, and Creighton, 1979). The general format of Selye's general adaptation syndrome (GAS) is quite simple. Fig. 11-2 identifies the various stages with their outcomes. Within the model, the individual first responds to a general stressor with a generalized alarm response, during which there is an assessment of the situation and a mobilization of both psychologic and physiologic resources. The dominant physiologic theme during alarm is catabolism, with the breakdown of stored energy sources. Selye (1973) is very clear that not every stressor has negative implications. Rather, stressors are essential for the individual to survive, grow, and maintain alertness and interest. The initial response to a stressor is very often increased attentiveness; increased alertness; feelings of energy, elation, and happiness; and increased problem solving. Growth, learning, and adaptation are possible outcomes for the alarm stage. If the stressor is prolonged, the alarm response yields to the stage of resistance, which is essentially a reconstructive stage. Anabolism is the dominant theme as the individual attempts to restore his physiologic and psychologic equilibrium. Should the individual fail at resistance, the resistance yields to exhaustion or disease. If the individual is completely overwhelmed, death may be the result (Selye, 1973; Jasmin and Trygstad, 1979).

The negative aspects of stress occur when the person is chronically exposed to multiple stressors or when the stressors have no apparent resolution. This is often the case among the elderly. In addition, Selye (1970) believes the aging process itself is physiologically stressful, causing the individual to be less able to resist the stressors. When stressors are prolonged and the stress state becomes chronic, the person experiences physiologic and psychologic damage. He becomes less able to focus, discriminate, solve problems and remember (Jasmin and Trygstad, 1979). These diminished mental abilities may result in actions that resemble confusion to outsiders, as well as feelings of confusion for the individual. Interestingly enough, the physical picture with chronic stress can be quite deceiving, not suggesting a stress reaction at all. We usually associate sympathetic nervous system activation and its accompanying symptoms, such as tachycardia, hypotension, tremors, anorexia, diarrhea, insomnia, and rapid respirations, with stress. However, with prolonged stress, the physical response may include hypertension, bradycardia, slow respirations, blurred vision, and incontinence. The person may report such feelings as loneliness, sadness, helplessness, and hopelessness rather than anxiety or fright (Jasmin

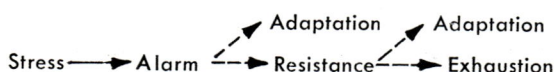

Fig. 11-2. General adaptation syndrome. (Adapted from Jasmin, S., and Trygstad, L. N.: Behavioral concepts and the nursing process, St. Louis, 1979, The C. V. Mosby Co.)

and Trygstad, 1979). An observer could well be misled into believing that the slowness and confusion displayed are the result of organic brain syndrome or acute depression rather than a reaction to prolonged, chronic stress, particularly if this is the first contact with the stressed person. Having misdiagnosed the problem, the observer could conceivably make no further attempt to assess or to intervene against chronic stress.

Summary

Confusion can be a decompensating reaction to either crisis or chronic stress. Confusion can also be present at various points in the stressor resolution cycle, such as during the alarm phase, during crisis, and during chronic stress. Although a stressor does not necessarily produce an adverse reaction or confusion, it is possible that when the stressor is applied for long periods or is a part of a total picture that includes multiple, continuous stressful assaults, the end result is confusion. In addition, a stressor can produce growth, adaptation, and resolution. Very often the person who experiences even strenuous stressors concludes the experience at a higher level of adaptation and coping than when he began. This is possible no matter what occurs following a stressor. Even if the person displays total decompensation and a complete inability to function in his usual way, there may be a return from this state. Therefore, even if the confusion *appears* hopeless, if it can be traced to multiple, prolonged stressors or to the inability to resolve crisis, the probability of reversing the confusion may be promising.

Following are stressors that cause clients to be at high risk for confusion:
1. Loss of natural supports, from death, separation, or rejection
2. Loss of social supports, from relocation, separation, confinement, retirement, or death of social acquaintances
3. Loss of economic supports, from retirement, inflation, illness, death of spouse, victimization, or economic reversal
4. Role reversal, from illness, disability, death of significant others, or the client's own illness or disability
5. Threat to body integrity or body image, from disability, physical deterioration, acute illness, or chronic illness
6. Discontinuity with usual life-style, from hospitalization, institutionalization, confinement, or relocation
7. Confrontation with the client's own vulnerability, aging, and death because of maturation

Fourth-level assessment

The goal of this fourth-level assessment is to identify those psychosocial stressors disrupting the pattern and meaning of the elderly person's existence that potentially may or actually cause confusion. Such an assessment requires that the caregiver is able and willing to explore the client's frame of reference using an accepting and permissive approach.

Interestingly, the role of the professional caregiver in this process is a role similar to that often performed for us by our intimate and loving friends. Since many elderly individuals have lost their initimate friends, the professional caregiver may be placed in this role, becoming a *skilled* friend and confidant. This is not to say that the caregiver will be as skilled as a geropsychiatrist, psychiatric social worker, or psychiatric nurse, whose skill *may* be needed, but often these professionals are unavailable in the settings when elderly people need help. Therefore, the role of skilled friend involves an availability and willingness to use genuine caring, self-disclosure, therapeutic listening, shared intimacy, and mutual trust to explore feelings, share perceptions, validate experiences, and identify alternatives. The atmosphere should be intimate enough to facilitate sharing and permissive enough to allow for the verbal and often physical expression of both positive and negative thoughts and feelings without fear of reprisal. A list of additional reading at the end of this chapter are provided for the reader interested in expanding knowledge regarding the counseling role.

> **Fourth-level assessment for stress**
>
> Current and past stressors
> Relationship to the aging condition
> Dominant affective tones
> Dominant thought content
> Current resources
> Current liabilities
> Potential outside resources and their acceptability
> Suicide potential

Although the last of these, suicide potential, may not be considered as relevant to confusion as some other factors, since many caregivers may not think of suicide as a potential problem among the aged, it is discussed here because, as Miller (1977) points out:
1. The suicide rate for elderly men is about four times the average national suicide rate, increasing dramatically through the eighth decade of life
2. A large percentage of older suicidal men are under the care of a health care provider immediately preceding their suicide, indicating it may be possible to prevent many suicides among the elderly
3. Confusional episodes and suicide seem to be related
4. Suicide *attempts* are uncommon among the elderly; when an elderly person has made the decision to commit suicide, he rarely shares it with anyone and proceeds to complete the act deliberately and successfully

Each of the assessment areas are considered separately in this section. It goes almost without saying that the assessment areas are not explored as if making a grocery list, one after the other and in order, nor are the suggested questions used verbatim. Each assessment of each elderly client is a unique experience. The assessment will move only as fast and as far as the client desires. Not only is self-disclosure a painful, sensitive, and intimate process requiring sensitivity and caring, but the nurse may be assuming a precarious position by taking the role of skilled friend. First, the nurse is assuming intimacy with a person with whom she is probably not intimately acquainted. Second, she is assuming a nurturing role with a person who may be twice her own age. In addition, many elderly persons have spent an entire lifetime repressing the negative feelings that accompany negative events, priding themselves in their own ability to survive and deal with adversity. Answering these questions may bring floods of emotions that may frighten the client and be viewed by him as intrusion. The cues for how the *skilled* friend proceeds during such a process must arise from the client himself and from the intuition and knowledge of the friend.

Tables 11-2 and 11-3 list some of the potential stressors to which an elderly person may be exposed. In addition, illness, accidents, malnourishment, fears, maturational conflicts, social events, and cultural realities may serve as stressors for the elderly. All of these are, however, generic stressors, meaning they are *potential* stressors for every elderly person. Identifying which of these generic stressors the client has actually experienced may require the input of the client, his family members, and his friends. Then, discovering if the actual event is a stressor or not requires determination of the significance and the client's perception of the event.

The following statements and questions may be helpful in eliciting this perspective. The death of a friend is used here as an example:
1. Tell me about your friend.
2. Tell me about the death of your friend.
3. How does the death of your friend affect you and your life?

4. What roles did your friend serve in your life?
5. What role did you serve in his?
6. What changes in your life does the death of your friend mean?
7. How do you feel about your friend?
8. How do you feel about the death of your friend?
9. Is your friend replaceable?

As the helper in this situation, you must be willing to accept all answers. They may not be the answers that are expected, nor may they be socially acceptable or nice. He may, for example, have hated his friend as much as he loved him, or he may have used his friend unmercifully. His feelings may be neither noble or selfless. You must be willing to accept the answers as expressions of unique personal feelings, not judging or blocking the expressive process with your own feelings.

Each elderly client has a unique relationship to the aging condition or to what he sees as the dilemmas of aging. His feelings about his place in the process are important: whether he sees himself as weak, vulnerable, and alone; or strong for having lived long and mastered such situational conflicts as dependence versus independence and giving versus taking. The following statements and questions may be helpful in determining this relationship:

1. Tell me about what aging is like.
2. Tell me about what your aging has been like.
3. How is it for you to be 72 (or 85 or whatever)?
4. What are your major problems with getting older?
5. What are your major joys with getting older?
6. What is the ideal old person like?
7. How are you like that person?
8. What feelings does the ideal old person have about getting older?
9. What feelings do you have about getting older?

Again, the answers to these questions may be neither nice nor noble; they just are.

These answers represent the unique relationship of one older client to the dilemmas he faces in aging.

The client's dominant affective tones are determined by how he has experienced what has happened to him. Affective tones include happiness, loneliness, rejection, sadness, guilt, grieving, challenge, and peace. The perception of bodily processes that are alien and frightening may be an important aspect of the client's affective tone. For example, sleeplessness often has affective implications that supersede the simple fact of not sleeping at night. For some individuals, sleeplessness may mean loneliness, sadness or fear. For others, sleeplessness may mean peace, as they pursue a solitary activity that would be otherwise interrupted during the day.

The content of the following questions may be helpful in eliciting information about the client's affective tones:

1. How is it for you most of the time?
2. Name an emotion that best describes you most of the time. Name another.
3. How would you describe your life?
4. What are you feeling right now?
5. How do you perceive your body lately?
6. Does your body act differently now than it used to? How so? How do you feel about that?

The answers to these questions are often encountered without specifically asking the questions. For example, during an exploration of a stressor, relevant bodily changes and dominant affective tones may be easily revealed in that context. In addition, affective tones are often portrayed far better than they are verbalized. A sad look or a clenched fist reveals more about what a client is feeling than the words he speaks.

The client's dominant thought content or the thoughts that recur and preoccupy him often tell much about what he is experiencing. For example, if he says he thinks about the death of his wife most of the time, he is revealing something about where he is in the grieving process, about his loneliness and sadness, or about his thoughts of his own death. To determine which of these is correct for the individual depends on further exploration. If he remarks that he worries that someone is poisoning his food, he is saying something else about himself. The exploration of thought content can reveal such possible experiences as delusions, hallucinations, suicidal thoughts, and obsessional thoughts. It can expose the client's current state of mind in relation to his situation. Answers to the following may be helpful for eliciting this kind of information:

1. Tell me what you think about most.
2. Do you worry? What kinds of things do you worry about?
3. Do you have thoughts that you just can't seem to get rid of? What are they like?
4. Lots of people have what they think are real crazy thoughts. Do you ever have thoughts that you think are real crazy? Would you talk about them?
5. Do you have daydreams? What kinds of things do you daydream about?

The exploration of such thoughts may tell you more of what the client experiences on a daily basis than even he might realize.

The exploration of current resources helps the client focus on his real or potential sources of strength. The intent is to identify the stabilizing forces in the client's life, his usual and successful coping styles, and his current life supports. The exploration of past events the person has coped with successfully may be a very important part of this assessment process. The answers to the following questions may be helpful:

1. Tell me about times when you were most successful. How did you do it?
2. Tell me about the people currently in your life who help you the most. What kinds of things do they help you with?
3. What are your greatest personal resources?
4. What kinds of things make you strong?
5. What kinds of things give you comfort? How accessible are these to you?
6. What kinds of things have you done in the past when things have gone wrong? How did they help?
7. Tell me about your happiest time. What about it made you happy?

People who have lived to be old are survivors. They have experienced personal tragedy and joy many times and have managed to cope and maintain their personal sense of integrity and worth. Sometimes, it is very difficult for any person who is faced with what appears to be continual adversity to keep personal strengths and abilities in mind. A review of resources and strengths may help the client reconnect with his innate abilities.

The assessment of current liabilities needs to focus on *real* liabilities only. Those which are imagined or feared may be important later, but during this initial assessment, focusing on these imagined liabilities may be so overwhelming as to be immobilizing. The following questions may elicit helpful answers:

1. What would you say is your greatest weakness right now?
2. What things interfere with your living today?
3. If you could change one thing that bothers you the most right now, what would it be?
4. When you got up this morning, what was the hardest thing you knew you had to face today?

Liabilities may be present in the form of economic problems, health and mobility problems, or problems with daily living. The client himself must identify which are the most significant to him.

It is also important to assess potential outside resources and their acceptability to the client. In most situations and in most communities, there are at least some resources available to the elderly client. These resources might include homemaker, home health, congregate eating, home-meal delivery, friendly visitor, or telephone reassurance services. Even many small rural communities have centers for the elderly that provide a variety of services. Most communities have churches that are willing to provide a certain amount of volunteer time to elderly people. Most institutions have arrangements with volunteers who can be used in creative ways. With the current federal emphasis on mental health, few communities lack access to mental health centers, where skilled professionals offer services to elderly people. Even if the client is totally devoid of personal support systems, it is often possible to mobilize some outside resources that will take the place of the extended family in meeting his physical and social needs. Of course, the other issue is the acceptability of the identified services to the elderly person. Therefore, not only do these outside resources need to be identified and the eligibility requirements determined and matched to the client, but his ability and willingness to accept these services must be assessed as well. The mobilizing of outside resources without the input of the elderly client leads only to disaster.

Suicide is not a spontaneous event (Miller, 1977); it requires thought, planning, and problem solving. The factors that precipitate suicide are identifiable, cumulative, and synergistic. In others words, the suicidal client usually experiences many stressors that he perceives as overwhelming before he decides to end his life. Often, the actual event that precipitates a suicide may be viewed as "minor" by an outside observer, but that event may truly be the "straw that breaks the camel's back" (Miller, 1977). Miller identifies thirteen factors that are often associated with geriatric suicide; interestingly, these same factors were identified earlier as stressors associated with crisis, chronic stress, and confusion among elderly people. They are:
1. Addiction to drugs or alcohol
2. Loss of the will to live
3. Loss of independence
4. Loss of status
5. The insults of aging, such as loss of hair, teeth, and mobility
6. Loss of income
7. Loss of self-confidence
8. Loss of self-esteem
9. Pathologic family relationships
10. Loss of a spouse
11. Loss of employment and retirement crisis
12. Mental and emotional problems
13. Multiple physical problems

It should also be remembered that certain elderly people who commit suicide do so during a confusional episode or during a bout of panic that is also accompanied by confusion.

There are striking differences between suicidal elderly and younger people, both in the motives and the way the suicidal intent is demonstrated. The suicidal motives of many young people are varied, often including elements of a desire for help or a punishment for another person. The actual desire to end life may be a secondary or tangential motive for the young, while it is the primary desire of most suicidal elderly people. Although suicide is often masked in the romantic terms of "joining a dead loved one," elderly people are, by and large, deadly serious about completing the act and terminating what is for them an absolutely intolerable existence. Most do not openly discuss or "threaten" suicide. Rather, they give subtle cues that only the perceptive individual may recognize. For example, an elderly client may signal his intent by suddenly making a will or settling his affairs. He may begin to give away personal items that have been significant and precious to him over the years. Often, a previously depressed elderly client becomes quite animated prior to committing suicide, acting and planning as if he is going on a long-desired trip. Strange acts that are not characteristic of the individual may be the clue to suicidal intent. For example, a person who has always expressed a hatred for firearms may suddenly purchase a gun.

Depression is a dominant theme in geriatric suicide, with its symptoms of chronic sleeping problems, reliance on alcohol or drugs, feelings of hopelessness and helplessness, and a general slowing of the physical and mental being. The most common events associated with suicide are the death of a spouse and the admission to a nursing home. Immediately before and after these events are particularly high-risk times (Miller, 1977). In addition to active suicide, passive suicide, such as starving to death and alcohol intoxication, are common among the elderly. When any of these signs are present, the following may be helpful questions in determining the suicide potential:

1. Do you ever think of dying?
2. Have you ever thought of taking your own life?
3. When you think of dying, under what circumstances do you imagine your death?
4. How would you take your own life?
5. When would you do it?
6. Do you have a plan?

Even though most elderly people do not freely *offer* the information that they desire to take their own life, if asked, many will freely share the information. The immediacy of the problem can be determined by the type of plan the individual describes. For example, "I would take my life in my bedroom during the evening with a gun that is in my nightstand. I've thought about doing it this weekend," represents an emergency situation; without intervention, this episode probably will terminate in suicide. Whereas, "I would take my life by driving off a cliff, even though I don't own a car," represents a more distant but still serious threat. Miller (1977)) cautions that one question should *not* be asked when assessing the suicide potential: Why do you want to commit suicide? Not that the answer is unimportant, but during an assessment of the suicide potential, the answer to this question serves only to divert the assessor's attention from the immediate issue, which is: Is this person going to commit suicide and how concrete is the plan?

The suicide potential for many older individuals represents a *real* problem that requires assessment to determine the risk involved and then immediate emergency attention. Miller (1977) offers excellent insights and a bibliography for studying this problem.

These eight areas of assessment should be helpful in determining the way an elderly client perceives the pattern and meaning in his life. Obviously, when he is severely depressed, regressed, or confused, the assessment process will be abbreviated and modified. During those times, some of the desired information may need to be obtained from close friends, family members, or acquaintances. Gathering information from these sources, however, provides only guidelines. It is no substitute for validating the information and determining its significance with the client himself. During acute confusional episodes, it might be necessary to simply convey to him that you are aware that many areas of his life are difficult to face and deal with and that you are willing to talk when he is. Exploration of the problems with him may have to wait until he is more lucid and more able to speak for himself.

One final point of summary concerns the peculiar issue of sharing the information gathered during an assessment. When the information concerns vision or nutritional status, there is no question about the need to pass it on to all concerned with the care. However, when an elderly client shares intimate information about himself, he may assume that the trust between the client and the caregiver is sacred. If this is not so, the client needs to know, so he can decide what and how to share. If the information gathered has life-threatening implications, such as a high suicide potential, the client should understand that the information *must* be passed on to those people who can help him. One approach is to tell the client that you, the caregiver, consider the information too important not to pass on; then ask how he would prefer the sharing to be done. He can choose if he will share it with others, if you can, or if you and he together will share it. If the information is not life threatening, ground rules for sharing need to be clear and explicit. If the setting can support intimate, consistent one-to-one relationships that are sacred and confidential, that understanding should be verbally stated. In this case, the contents of the assessment are not shared or charted, except superficially. Only approaches that would be helpful in dealing with the client should be shared. If the one-to-one relationship is confidential but you need the consultation of others to help the client, the nature of the consultation should be clear to the client. If the situation does not support one-to-one relationships and a team of people has verbal or printed access to the information gathered, the client should know. Nothing destroys a trusting relationship quicker than when one person in the exchange does not understand the rules and holds a false assumption that is then violated by the indiscriminate or unexpected sharing of information.

Prevention

The following suggestions may help to prevent some of the confusion that arises whenever stressors disrupt the pattern and meaning in the client's life experience.

1. *Manage stressors.*

a. Help the client identify life patterns from which stressors arise and the reactions he has to these patterns. The life review process and keeping a journal of daily experiences may help the client identify consistent life patterns that produce stressors. For example, he may find that money management has been a problem throughout his entire lifetime, and it is currently connected with the stressors he is experiencing. He may never have budgeted his money, which did not present a significant problem to him until now, when he is on a limited income. A life review may also help him determine that one of his interaction patterns, for example, putting others on the defensive, produces stress. The isolation he is experiencing is directly related to this pattern. This process may help the client assume control and responsibility for impinging stressors. He can identify those stressors that he can either control, avoid, or limit.

b. Help the client learn to balance his stressors. Very simply, stressors come in three varieties: those that exhilarate, challenge, and give enormous satisfaction and pleasure; those that frighten, overwhelm, and confuse; and those that fall in between. Each person faces essentially two tasks; first, determining what dominant category a stressor falls in (it may fall into all of them); and second, learning to arrive at a balance so the stressors on the two ends of the continuum do not become excessive. Ways to balance stressors include physical activity and exercise; stable patterns, routines, and rituals; relaxation and meditation; creative endeavors; physical comfort; sensual pursuits; being with people; and being alone. You can help an elderly client identify how tension is most comfortably released, how seemingly negative stressors can produce pleasure, and in what areas stability is absolutely essential. You can also help him determine ways stability can be provided in the setting by establishing stable physical routines or providing for stable social relationships. The crux of stress management and prevention of confusion is not the elimination of stressors, but the balancing of stressors.

c. Help the client prepare for stressors through anticipatory planning. When we consider what might happen to us and "live" through some of the emotions encountered during a stressful situation, we can more easily deal with the experience when it actually happens. To avoid the potential trap in this approach, anticipatory planning must be separated from rumination and worry. Planning involves problem solving and the identification of personal options and alternatives. Neither of these are involved in worry. For example, if the client is concerned about the death of his spouse, being helped to think about what the death will feel like, what changes will be involved in his life, how he will manage these changes, and what material and social resources are available to him is anticipatory planning. Exclusive concentration on the pain that will be involved in that separation is worry and rumination. Most individuals need to be helped by others to avoid this trap and gain the benefits of planning.

2. *Deal with the perception of aging and the experiential component of stressors.*

a. Help the client gain an understanding of the relationship between how he sees aging and how he sees himself as an individual. Many clients have difficulty seeing the relationship between what they think about the world and what they feel about themselves. Probably one of the most beneficial ways of understanding this relationship is through group work, where the client can be exposed to the feelings and thoughts of others while expressing his own. In a group, the client can share his perceptions of the world and of himself within that world. He can be helped to see that his ideas and perceptions are not unusual and that others with the same ideas cope in ways similar to or different from his way. These groups do not have to be formalized "therapy" groups. Many elderly people accomplish this task independently by joining in simple social activities, which often result in shared feelings. Such activities can be structured around any commonly shared interest among several people. For rather isolated individuals, a group facilitator initially may help in the movement toward intimate levels of discussion.

b. Help the client identify and anticipate his patterned responses to stressors, whether these be emotional or bodily reactions. We respond to stressors in ways that have been patterned throughout our lifetime. The client can be helped to identify these experiences and anticipate his own reactions by keeping a journal that includes stressful events and the personal experiences associated with them. He can look at his life with this focus and use the information to alleviate some of his anxiety.

3. *Deal with the cognitive component of stressors.*

a. Explore and reinforce lifelong resources. The questions presented in the assessment section may start this exploration process. Problem solving must begin with the client asking, Who am I? What do I have? What can I do? and What have I done in the past? The life review is a technique that can be used to help the client focus on the strengths and resources he has had and still has at his disposal. During the life review, however, you must consciously tune into the ways the client has used his resources in various situations to help him discover if these resources are still feasible. You must reinforce and support the client's use of his resources. For example, he may have always been quite skilled in social exchanges because of his outgoing and gregarious nature. Faced with the stressors in his current situation, however, he may have forgotten that meeting new people and establishing new relationships has always been quite easy, satisfying, and rewarding. It may be possible for you as caregiver to identify this strength and help the person find ways this strength can be used now. It may be necessary to help the client overcome certain obstacles, such as a hearing loss, in order to use this past resource. In addition, he may need support during the process, such as being accompanied to social functions until he has rediscovered his old skills and is comfortable using them in a new situation.

One of the most effective ways of reinforcing the client's strengths is helping him maintain those skills that have given him pleasure in the past. These skills can include recreational, occupational, or self-maintenance tasks, such as demonstrated by the nursing home resident in Fig. 11-3. The client may also have to be helped to relearn some of the self-maintenance skills he has lost, as pictured in Fig. 11-4.

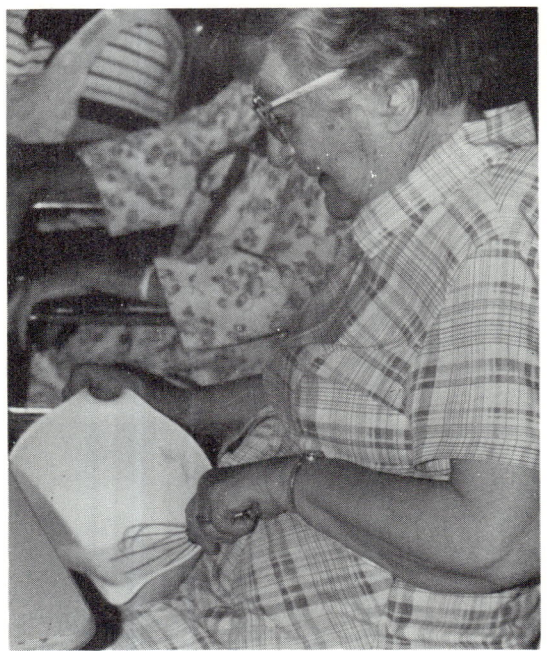

Fig. 11-3. Maintaining life patterns. (Photograph by C. D. Falk.)

Fig. 11-4. Relearning old skills. (Photograph by C. D. Falk.)

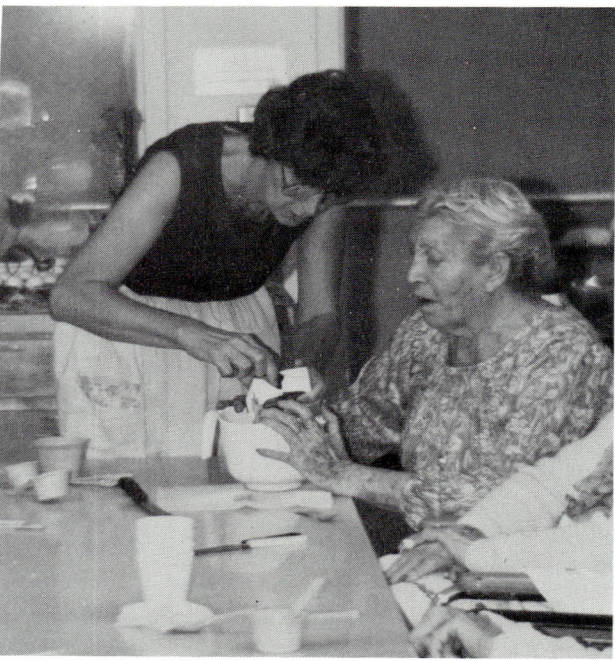

b. Help the client identify coping strategies that are both inside and outside his repertoire of problem–solving skills. We each develop habitual coping skills that are used frequently throughout our lifetime. In spite of the many possible coping skills, we learn to confine ourselves to the few we think work best for us. Ryan (1979) states that we usually equate coping with the strict problem–solving approach, which views coping as if it is a rational process. Problem solving involves gathering all the facts in a practical manner, identifying all the alternatives, and then rationally making decisions. We can easily slip into condemnation of coping styles that do not use this approach, despite the fact that coping and decision making are almost never simple, straightforward, or totally cognitive. Following the work of Antonovsky (1979) and Vroom and Yetton (1973), Ryan (1979) suggests there are many coping strategies, such as thinking about, sharing, determining who and what to share, writing down, and talking out. Introducing these to the client in a positive light may be helpful.

We also tend to think of positive decisions as being exclusively decisions for action. Ryan (1979) believes this is not necessarily true, listing such alternatives to action decisions as retreating, restraining, tolerating, redistributing, and letting others decide. Suggesting alternative coping strategies to the client and giving positive reinforcement for their use may be an important part of preventing the confusion that arises from coping with multiple stressors.

c. Help the client learn to confine his assessment of liabilities to the present time. The client may tend to focus on past failures, perhaps because of depression, or to focus on possible future difficulties, which may never arise as a result of his anxiety.

Neither of these is desirable. For example, the client's statement, "I have always had difficulty making friends because I am shy," allows a diversionary tactic to creep into the process. More to the point is the client's statement, "I am feeling shy right now." Or the client may identify a hearing loss as a real liability, then wander into all of the possible consequences of the hearing loss that make his situation impossible. A hearing loss *is* a real liability, but a consequence such as "I can't make a new friend because I can't hear" clouds the issue. The statement, "I am afraid that my hearing loss will keep me from communicating," is a feeling that accompanies the liability and should be expressed. The trap occurs when the feeling is confused with imagined consequences; together, they make the situation appear insurmountable. This distinction is difficult to make without careful listening and practice. Liabilities and the feelings associated with them need to be identified, but care and thought are required to avoid mixing liabilities and feelings with logical or illogical consequences.

4. *Prevent crisis.*

a. Teach anticipatory planning strategies. After the client has become acquainted with what is stressful for him, it is important to use anticipatory planning around those stressors. For example, if finances are a major stressor, planning for the income and output of money is obviously helpful. When retirement means a major financial change, anticipating and planning for that change many years in advance help eliminate the crisis nature of the situation. If hospitalization is a major stressor, learning to identify the support systems available while in the hospital is helpful, for example, identifying who can be telephoned and when, who is able to visit, what sources of transportation are available, how the hospital bill will be handled, and who within the hospital structure can serve as resources. Obviously, it is not possible to plan for every possible contingency, but anticipating the major life changes is important, whether these changes are pleasant, such as planned retirement or a vacation, or unpleasant, such as institutionalization or a death.

b. Help the client identify ways of maintaining social networks and replacing social losses. It may be difficult for the client to realize that his immediate family cannot serve as his sole social support. Following the death of a spouse, the death of friends, and the loss of colleagues, the elderly client may have his social circle diminished to a point where only his children remain to meet all his social and emotional needs. The intensity of this situation leads to frustration and disappointment for the parent and "burnout" for the children. Elderly people can be helped to realize that replacing social losses is essential for their continued well-being, self-esteem, and independence.

5. *Manage stress.*

a. Help the client establish daily routines that permit stress release, stress encounter, and relaxation.

b. Help the client plan and use relaxation training to manage stress and tension. Relaxation training programs are available from several sources; Jasmin and Trygstad (1979) and Simonton, Matthews–Simonton, and Creighton (1979) present general formats that can be used. One example of a relaxation program appears in Appendix D. The goal of all relaxation training is the reduction of body tension and of mental rumination on worrisome and distracting topics. These may be difficult concepts for people who have spent their entire lives using one dominant thought pattern—worry. For example, when meditation was suggested to one elderly gentleman as a possible intervention for his chronic–stress–related joint and back pain, his response was, "I meditate all the time. I meditate on the problems I have with my son and don't get anywhere." In spite of this misconception, meditation and relaxation involve the freeing of troublesome thoughts from the mind by concentrating on some pleasant or pleasurable experience. This experience may be a bodily process, such as slow, rhythmic breathing or the warmth and heaviness of the limbs, or it may be a pleasant image, such as lying by the beach and watching the waves roll in or sitting by a stream in the forest and watching the sunlight. Many people use the image of the sunlight filling them as a pleasurable focus that is comforting and energizing. The more pleasurable sensations that can be combined, such as seeing the sunlight and feeling its warmth, the more relaxation is possible. Relaxation involves letting go and permitting these thoughts and experiences to become dominant rather than working to make them actually happen. By practicing and providing time each day, the client can use the relaxation state to meditate and solve problems on a symbolic and subconscious level. Elderly people experiencing many stressors should be introduced to this concept and, after they determine its acceptability, helped to plan their activities so periods of therapeutic relaxation are possible.

c. Help the client to identify his physical or psychologic stress signs and to plan for stress release. Stressors create unpredictable bodily reactions. As Antonovsky (1979) and Simonton, Matthews–Simonton, and Creighton (1979) have indicated, many illnesses are related to stressors and the inability to release the tension and conflict associated with stressors. Many people do not know this. For example, one elderly nurse who recently lost her husband went to her physician because of low back pain and bowel changes. After a thorough physical, it was determined that these bodily experiences were stress-related. The nurse later stated, "I knew stress could cause headaches, but I never knew it could cause back pain and bowel changes. I thought I had something seriously wrong with me." It is possible to identify lifelong bodily reactions to stress and learn to prevent acute stress reactions by heeding such bodily signs.

Intervention

The nursing objectives for intervention are as follows:
1. To provide support during acute confusional episodes
2. To help the client by alleviating the total number of stressors
3. To help the client deal with his percep-

tions of aging and the experiential component of the stressors
4. To help the client deal with the cognitive component of a disruption of pattern and meaning
5. To help the client deal with acute crisis using crisis intervention techniques
6. To help the client deal with chronic tension or stress through stress reduction techniques

1. *Provide support during acute confusional episodes.*

As already stated, problem solving and self-expression are limited during acute confusional episodes. Therefore, interventions during these times may be largely confined to the provision of support. Support in this case means therapeutic listening, empathetic touching, and thoughtful caring. Special attention must be given to the client's safety, security, and physical needs. In addition, you should be especially sensitive to nonconfused moments so these can be appropriately and consistently reinforced. The most likely time for the staff to fall into the pattern of inadvertently reinforcing aberrant behaviors is during acute confusional episodes. This must be consciously avoided so the client "discovers" that being not confused is far more pleasant and reinforcing than being confused. Nonconfused moments are the times when the assessment and interventions can be instituted to help alleviate the situation.

2. *Alleviate stressors.*

a. Help the client gain understanding of the stressors impinging on him. Stressors arise from the personal, social, and cultural milieu of the client (Fig. 11-1). The initial step is the assessment, during which you and the client identify all the significant stressors in the situation. The second step is helping the client determine where these stressors arise from, why they are happening, and exactly what they mean to him. For example, if the death of a friend is one stressor, the client needs to have an understanding of all things that friend meant to him and of the feeling he has regarding their loss. The roles played and the services the friend performed need to be identified so the client can realistically deal with the stressor.

b. Act to reduce the total number of stressors present. There may be stressors impinging on the client that you as caregiver can directly reduce with little or no help from the client. For example, in the institutional setting, multiple stressors are under the control of the nurse, such as the disruption of personal routines, lack of warmth, lack of privacy, pain management, and lack of consistency among the staff. During the initial phases of intervention, while the confusion is still a dominant problem, you should act to reduce the stressors under your control by consistently and conscientiously providing for the client's physical, safety, and security needs. The temperature can be regulated, food provided that the client likes, pain managed, personal routines established by which rituals are preserved, and attention paid to privacy. Later, as the client becomes involved in identifying other significant stressors, both you and the client can determine ways to decrease the total number of stressors. For example, perhaps isolation is a significant stressor. You may need to actively provide a means for the significant other still in the community to visit regularly, whereas the client may choose those ways within his setting that are his most desirable and acceptable ways of reducing isolation. The reduction of stressors is essential for the reduction of the confusion the client is experiencing and demonstrating.

3. *Deal with the client's perceptions of aging and the experiential component of the stressors.*

a. Help the client gain access to and express feelings he may not recognize. The tension that surrounds the suppression or denial of feelings may be immobilizing. The client needs to be helped to identify his positive and negative feelings about what he is experiencing and who he is as an aging person. He also needs to be shown how to supersede the "should" in his experience ("I should feel grateful" or "I should love") and arrive at what he truly feels in a situation (Aguilera and Messick, 1978). The questions presented in the assessment section may be a first step in this process, but frequently, the client feels reluctance to express suppressed feelings and requires gentle and thoughtful help to express exactly what he is experiencing. There may be multiple risks perceived in expressing feelings, and many people have spent an entire lifetime suppressing their "bad" feelings. This obstacle may need to be overcome. It should be emphasized that feelings are neither "good" nor "bad" and that having certain feelings does not make a "good" or a "bad" person. Feelings simply are; they must be experienced and expressed. The more energy expended in denying and suppressing feelings, the more conflict and tension build. As Oberleder (1970) found, sometimes the release experienced by the elderly person in the expression of feelings is enough to permit him to begin solving problems and finding other expressions of his experiences besides confusion.

b. Validate with the client the "normalcy" of his experiences and emotions. When a client feels angry after the loss of a loved one, wanting to throw his dinner tray across the room or strike out at the people who are trying to help him, he begins to question his rights to these feelings and whether he is a "normal" person for feeling the way he does. This tension and conflict can contribute to the experience of confusion. During group work, one of the most astounding occurrences for many participants is discovering the common nature of feelings. When the client feels isolated, it is easy for him to perceive that he is the only person who ever felt the way he does. Verbalizing a thought or a feeling provides the opportunity for validation that the feeling is shared by many of his circumstances. With a confused client, this validation must often come from the one-to-one experiences with his caregiver. Later, as his situation is more tolerable and he has found that one person whom he trusts will see his experiences as "okay," he may be able to join in a group process, with other elderly participants validating his feelings by sharing the experiences with him.

c. Explain bodily reactions the elderly person is perceiving. At least some of the anxiety and panic that stressed people experience is directly related to anxiety about their unexplained and unfamiliar bodily experiences. As caregiver, you can help explain these reactions and validate the "normalcy" of the experiences by giving information and sharing thoughts and feelings.

4. *Deal with the cognitive component of a disruption of pattern and meaning.*

a. Explore and reinforce the client's strengths and resources.

b. Explore the client's liabilities and help him express his feelings about them. Again, confine the exploration of liabilities to the present time.

c. Explore the client's alternatives. The identification of resources and liabilities is partly tied to the exploration of situational or life alternatives. However, a separation must be made to emphasize that there are always more alternatives than the client is able to realize himself. Sometimes, the affective tone of the situation masks all the possibilities available to the client to make the situation better or at least different. For example, a hearing loss may cause him to become so narrowed in this scope that he perceives only one alternative: a hearing loss means discontinuation of social relationships. This client needs someone who will give information regarding, for instance, audiologic examinations, the feasibility of a hearing aid, the possibility of learning speech reading or sign language, and the availability of other amplifying devices. In addition, he needs someone to explore other situational alternatives based on his strengths. For example, if his eyesight is keen, written communication is an alternative; if he has full range of motion, communication involving pantomime is possible;

if his finances are adequate, an audiologic examination will provide no financial burden; and since he may have many significant others, their help can be elicited to establish a means of communication and to facilitate the forming of new relationships. Acceptability of alternatives must always be a dominant theme in this exploration. Determine, with the client's help, specific actions that will ameliorate his problems.

5. *Deal with crisis.*

The following are steps in crisis intervention, as adapted from Aguilera and Messick (1978), who should be referred to for a better understanding of this process.

  a. Help the client gain an intellectual understanding of the crisis.

  b. Help the client discuss his present feelings, of which he may not be aware.

  c. Explore coping mechanisms used in the past and still salient.

  d. Help the client reopen his social world.

  e. Help the client function in groups that focus on grief work and crisis intervention (Oberleder, 1970). Oberleder found that crisis resolution may be a slow process among elderly people, and the precipitating factors that surround crisis in the elderly are usually shared experiences. Consequently, he suggests crisis work be done in groups whenever the individual is able to function at a group level. Group activity may be helpful both in crisis resolution and in anticipatory planning for new crisis events.

6. *Deal with chronic tension or stress.*

  a. Help the client identify and understand the sources of stress.

  b. Help the client gain a sense of control over the multiple stressors that impinge on him. When the client feels that the forces that shape his experience are totally unpredictable and totally out of his control, managing the stress is almost impossible. If, however, the stressors become demystified, with the client assuming conscious responsibility for those possible for him to control, the stress is more tolerable. In addition, if the client can learn to avoid or limit intense stressors that he cannot control, he is taking conscious responsibility for his stress state. For example, physical stressors may be fairly easy to control. Pain can be managed, and hunger and thirst and incontinent episodes can be prevented with conscious thought and the cooperation of others. The client may have no control over the behavior of his daughter, which he finds tremendously stressful. He can, however, be helped and supported to limit contact with his daughter to a tolerable amount of time and can begin to work with his emotions that surround his daughter's visits. Although it is neither possible nor desirable to eliminate all stressors from an individual's life, it is possible to help the individual control and limit stressors to the point that the state of chronic tension is avoided.

Outcome criteria of successful nursing intervention against stress

1. The client is able to identify his personal sources of stress.
2. The client is able to alleviate or avoid events that are excessively stressful for him, when possible.
3. The client can recognize and express his feelings regarding aging and his life events.
4. The client is able to identify the relationship between his feelings and the events that impinge on him.
5. The client reports and demonstrates a reduction in his anxiety level.
6. The client reports and demonstrates a reduction in crisis feelings and behaviors.
7. The client can demonstrate his ability to use stress reduction techniques in his everyday life.
8. The client is no longer confused.

Summary

Certainly, the preventions and interventions suggested are not exhaustive.

Through creativity, interaction, and thought it may be possible to identify many others that would be beneficial in dealing with the confusion that arises from the disruption of pattern and meaning by stressors. The use of this framework should be helpful in identifying the point the elderly client is at in the stress situation and helping him determine the most appropriate ways of proceeding.

SOCIAL INTERACTION AND CONFUSION

Stressors are not the only problem encountered by elderly people in relation to the disruption of pattern and meaning in their lives. The social environment also can be a contributing factor to confusion.

Social interaction is the vehicle by which people in society meet most of their higher-level needs. Through relationships with others, a person is able to define himself and his roles and determine the plans and actions that will afford him the most rewards for the least overall cost. This is true for the young and old alike. For the young person, however, the sources of social interaction are almost limitless because of the mobility and personal resources that build and maintain relationships. The situation is different for the elderly. As the elderly person becomes frail, his relationships with other significant people are often characterized by dependence. As a result, these relationships become crucial to the survival of the individual and the maintenance of his self-concept and ego. The context of social interaction has a direct influence on whether or not some elderly people will become confused.

Interaction through social exchange—the imprisonment model

Social interaction can be defined as "an exchange of rewards (or punishments) between at least two persons" (Homans, 1961, p. 378). In Homans' view, social interaction conforms to, first, an operant paradigm and, second, an economic paradigm. As with other operant paradigms, this one involves a discriminating stimulus immediately followed by a behavioral response. The response is followed by a positive or negative reinforcement that determines the likelihood of the behavior being emitted again under similar circumstances following a similar stimulus. The social element of this paradigm is that the behaviors are rewarded or punished by the behavior of another person, and the exchange is characterized by the chaining of human behaviors in such a way that one individual's behavior alternately stimulates and reinforces the other's.

Homans' description differs from the description offered by Skinner for animal behavior because of a component added to the paradigm called "expectations." This cognitive-affective component mediates between the stimulus and the response, permitting the individual to decide between at least two courses of action. Following a stimulus, an individual is capable of deciding the behavior that will assure him of the greatest rewards (Homans, 1961).

An economic paradigm enters the picture of social exchange with Homans' presentation of the law of distributive justice, "which refers to a person's expectations of the rewards due to him and costs which he may incur—the proportion of his rewards to his costs: that these should be seen to be distributed in a fair ratio to each other" (Chadwick–Jones, 1976, p. 161). In other words, as in the marketplace, a person expects that his rewards and costs will be proportional to the other's rewards and costs. When the law of distributive justice is violated, the result is anger and resentment.

Social exchange can then be viewed as the interaction between two people during which, all things being equal, each person rewards or punishes the other person and at the same time attempts to accrue rewards and profits for himself (in the form of warm sentiments, good feelings, and instrumental services) and to minimize his own punishments or costs (in the form of bad feelings and exploitation).

In some relationships, however, all things are not equal. People have differential access to resources, including status, money, esteem, and prestige, as well as different capabilities to provide instrumental services. There can be an imbalance in the social exchange that can be termed "power." "From this perspective, power is synonymous with the dependence of Actor A upon Actor B. It is based in the inability of one of the partners in the social exchange to reciprocate a rewarding behavior" (Dowd, 1975, p. 587). The person who is less dependent and is perceived as contributing the most to the relationship has the power advantage. A powerless person must comply. When the dependent person has no choice about continuing the relationship, as in situations such as prisons, the armed forces, or health care facilities, the other person has what is called "fate control." This is the situation "where one person has power over another, and is in a position to allocate rewards to himself, irrespective of the choice of action by the other" (Chadwick–Jones, 1976, p. 35). The "fate control" situation can be converted into a situation where the other person has "behavior control," when "the person with the greater influence does take into account the actions and payoffs of the other, and arranges that these are improved providing they correspond with his own preferred outcome" (Chadwick–Jones, 1976, p. 37). When the dependent person has no choice about his interaction with the other person, the person with the power advantage develops a monopoly on rewards and the potential to shape the behavior of the other person.

According to Dowd (1975), the aging condition predisposes the elderly person to just such a situation. As the person ages, he has less access to power resources and progressively less ability to perform instrumental services. In fact, with his increasing physical infirmities, he begins to require more and more in the form of instrumental services, and he experiences a decrease in his potential to supplement his social ties and extend his power base. Dowd (1975) also suggests that as the imbalance in power increases, the older person begins to display more and more compliant behavior in an effort not to alienate the few people who provide him with rewards and services.

Using these principles of social exchange, the imprisonment model (Fig. 11-5) (Phillips, 1976) was formulated to describe a process by which some elderly clients, with no other identifiable etiology for their confusion, enter an institutional setting and subsequently become confused. The behaviors described in the model are those of a client and of one or more caregivers who share common perceptions of and expectations for him. The model operates according to Homans' principles and is based on the assumption that confusion, under certain circumstances, is learned or shaped behavior. The following definitions and principles apply to the model:

1. A *discriminating stimulus* or the cue that begins a behavioral chain can result from the behavior of another person or from the situational context. In the imprisonment model, the client's need for help and the nurse's role requirements are the usual cues that initiate an interaction. However, a discriminating stimulus may occur simply because the nurse and the client are in the same place at the same time.

2. *Expectations* mediate between the perception of the discriminating stimulus and the behavioral response. In a black-box fashion, expectations serve to screen incoming stimuli and permit both parties to consciously or unconsciously choose a behavioral response. Through the mediation of expectations, client and caregiver will always act to maximize their profits and minimize their costs. In the imprisonment model, expectations of the client are shaped by the degree to which imprisonment is felt. The client perceives imprisonment as strong, insurmountable psychologic, physiologic, or social forces operating to constrain his freedom, shape his behavior, and limit his behavioral alternatives. Any of

298 *Confusion: prevention and care*

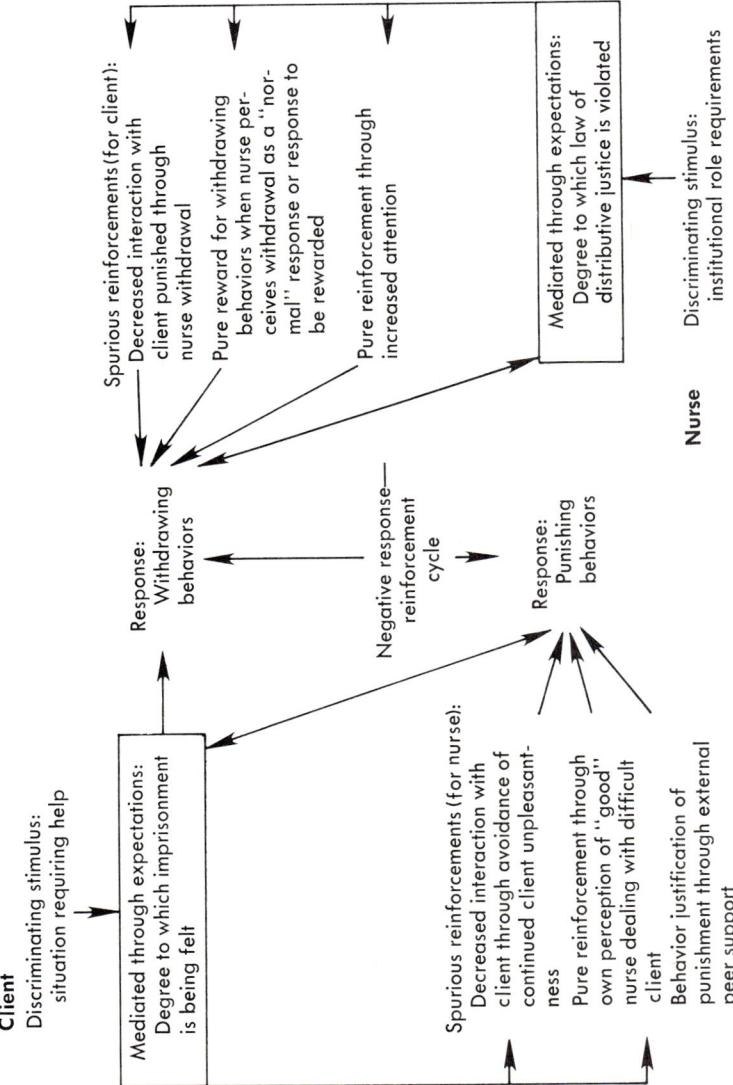

Fig. 11-5. Negative social interaction in the institutional setting—the imprisonment model.

the stressors identified in Tables 11-2 and 11-3 may contribute to the perception of imprisonment. The expectations of the nurse are indexed by the degree to which she feels the law of distributive justice has been violated or the degree to which she feels her costs, in terms of time, energy, or commitment, are greater than the client's.

3. The *responses* of both client and nurse are behaviors displayed under the given circumstances. The responses of each constitute the primary reinforcements for the other person in a negative response–reinforcement cycle. Thus, the withdrawing behaviors of the client are negatively reinforced by the punishing behaviors of the caregiver, and vice versa. The client's withdrawing behaviors are any behaviors that make him socially inaccessible to the nurse, such as apathy, hostility, anger, lethargy, or confusion. The punishing behaviors of the nurse are any behaviors or threats of behaviors that inflict a penalty on the client, such as angry words, rough handling, slowness in obtaining pain medication or answering a light, or leaving the breakfast tray slightly out of reach. Such responses influence the likelihood that the client will repeat his withdrawing responses in the future.

Since the interaction between the client's responses and the nurse's responses are in a negative mode, a word must be said about negative reinforcement. Under usual circumstances, when both parties have options about their relationship, negative reinforcement will lead to the extinction of the punished behavior, avoidance of punishment through behavior alteration, or termination of the interaction. However, in this model, neither party has a choice about the relationship, particularly the client. The nurse is bound by her job to provide services but, at the same time, can barter with her coworkers to decrease her time with the client and distribute the negative reinforcement among the staff members.

The nurse has the power advantage, with a greater access to outside supports and reinforcements. The client must rely on the caregiver to supply services and reinforcements on a regular basis. Particularly if the client has few visitors and few remaining family members, the nurse has a virtual monopoly on reinforcements; this is the "behavior control" situation previously described. In addition, behavioral alteration may not be as viable an option as maintaining the negative behaviors when spurious reinforcements arise that positively reinforce the negative behaviors.

Following the model in Fig. 11-5, it can be seen that for both parties, the discriminating stimulus is mediated through expectations in the form of new discriminating stimuli in a feedback loop. In addition, a negative reinforcement cycle is established between the behavior response of the client and the behavior response of the nurse.

4. *Spurious reinforcements* are those positive rewards that arise unexpectedly and help maintain the negative behaviors. Some people might think of these as "secondary gains." At least three spurious reinforcements are available to the client as a result of the nurse's behavior. First, as the nurse withdraws from the client, there is less chance of social interaction with a punishing person. For example, because the nurse remains out of the room longer, the client has less exposure to angry words or rough handling. Second, pure positive rewards may be obtained when the nurse begins to reinforce the withdrawing behaviors as if they were "normal" or appropriate to reward. For example, the nurse expects that all older persons are confused. When the client talks incoherently or calls for his mother, the nurse interprets this as normal for his age and situation and spends increasing amounts of time with him in the name of "therapy," ignoring or not perceiving appropriate behaviors. This is reinforcement for aberrant behavior. Third, since the client has so few sources of social reinforcement, even punishing behaviors may be perceived by him as rewarding. Like the child who learns to seek punishment for attention, as opposed to no attention at all,

the elderly person may seek a relationship with the caregiver at any cost.

For the nurse, at least three sources of spurious reinforcement exist, two of which arise from the client's behavior and one from an outside source. First, as the client withdraws, the nurse feels punished for being a "bad nurse" or simply from being exposed to unpleasantness. Decreased interaction with the client means she can avoid this punishment. Second, some pure positive reinforcement can arise from caregivers who define their "good nurse" role in terms of dealing with the difficult client no one else wants. Thus, the more the client withdraws, the more attention and therapy the nurse directs at him. The third source arises from the external environment of the nurse, from the peer support she receives from her co-workers. When the client becomes labeled as difficult by most of the caregiving staff, there is a great deal of sympathy and support given to the person who must care for him. The nurse can display a punishing behavior, such as not answering the light, and then justify this behavior by commiserating with her co-workers that the client is confused or hostile.

So as not to leave the impression that these behaviors of the nurse or the client are calculated or deliberate, let us consider one research project that explored the effects of imprisonment on a technically nonimprisoned sample of college-aged adults. Honey, Banks, and Zimbardo (1973) constructed a prison simulation experiment in which healthy students were randomly assigned the roles of "prisoners" and "guards." There was no difference identified between the "prisoners" or the "guards" during extensive psychologic, preexperiment testing. Both groups maintained their assigned roles throughout the duration of the simulation, and neither group was instructed in how to perform their roles. It was left to the subjects themselves to determine the rules for proper behavior. The "guards" became increasingly aggressive and punitive as the simulation progressed and ultimately reported enjoying their power. The "pri-soners" displayed extreme emotional depression, crying, rage, and acute anxiety. "Model prisoners," those who were most cooperative and compliant, displayed passivity, dependence, and flattened affect. All prisoners reported a loss of personal identity. After 5 days, the simulation had to be ended prematurely by the researchers because the emotional displays were far beyond those expected or considered safe. Therefore, in an imprisoning situation, it would seem that each party begins to play his role as he defines it. There is probably not a predisposition of the people in charge to punish nor a predisposition of "prisoners" to become compliant and passive. This same observation was supported in the prisoner-of-war situation. "Most SS men never wasted a minute of free time in mistreating prisoners . . . Such behavior is alien to sadists who enjoy mistreating others" (Bettelheim, 1977, p. 237). Imprisonment behaviors, therefore, are probably the result of strong social forces rather than psychologic predispositions.

The following example should help make clear how the imprisonment model operates in the institutional setting. The client needs to get out of bed (discriminating stimulus). Sensing imprisonment (expectations of the client), he may respond negatively with an angry, "No, I don't want to get out of bed," or may simply stare at the nurse, giving no response (withdrawing behaviors). The nurse, who feels that the client is able to get out of bed and is not trying (expectations of the nurse), may respond with an angry remark or a stern sarcastic comment (punishing behavior). During the transfer, the client cries and whines, and the nurse becomes increasingly frustrated and irritated. The nurse transfers the client quickly, a little bit roughly, and without the teaching cues that would make the transfer smoother (these series of behaviors represent the negative response-reinforcement cycle). Each response is mediated through the expectations of the person and confirms for the client that imprisonment is present and for the nurse that the client is violating the law of distributive justice. This confirmation itself constitutes a form of positive reinforcement. As soon as the transfer is over, the nurse flees from the room (a release from punishment that is a spurious positive reinforcement). She goes immediately to the nurse's station, where she discusses the exchange with her co-workers. They agree with her that the client is difficult and that her behavior was appropriate under the circumstances (behavioral justification is a spurious reinforcement). She begins to arrive at an internal definition of herself as a "good nurse," because she is appropriately handling a difficult client (spurious reinforcement). When the nurse leaves the room, the client is left to sit in the chair, alone. As the time in the chair increases, he becomes more and more uncomfortable (more punishment). However, interestingly, this long wait in the chair also has positive aspects. The longer the nurse stays out of the room, the less the client is exposed to her punishment. In addition, the more unpleasant the transfer, the less likely the nurse is to want to get the client out of bed very often (this is a spurious reinforcement to both parties). As the client sits in the chair, he cries and becomes more upset. His cries give way to screams. The nurses immediately respond to these screams since they disrupt the nursing unit. The client is, therefore, given attention for aberrant behavior; whether or not the attention is pleasant is of no consequence, it is attention nonetheless (spurious reinforcement).

According to the imprisonment model, the behavior the client learns to display becomes some form of withdrawal, whether in the form of apathy, disinterest, lack of motivation, incoherent speech, wandering, or frank disorientation. The client becomes increasingly socially inaccessible by maximizing the behaviors that will assure him the greatest rewards. As stated in Chapter 1, social inaccessibility is one of the chief diagnostic indicators used by nurses to identify the presence of confusion. In addition, the shaping of behavior can occur rapidly. The more individuals who inadvertently share in the reinforcement process or the more complete the monopoly held by the caregivers, the faster the behavior is shaped (Homans, 1961). Since the actual reinforcement schedule is not usually consciously shared by the nursing staff, its strength and rate of positive reinforcement are variable and unpredictable. This type of schedule is by far the most effective in shaping the behaviors of all those involved in the interaction process.

The imprisonment model is not the only sociologic explanation for the confusion seen among elderly people. The common thread running through all such models is that some part of the social environment interacts with the individual's perceptions to create a situation in which confusion is a viable alternative. For example, in the social breakdown model (Kuypers and Bengtson, 1973), social labeling as "old" results in self-labeling, which leads to a definition of self as inadequate and incompetent. The end result of this social process is confusion. Since this theme appears in many works, the social environment must be considered an active part of the problems encountered by elderly individuals as they move in and out of confusional states.

High-risk factors

The factors that cause an individual to be high risk in this interaction process are not different from the stressors presented in Tables 11-2 and 11-3. The focus, however, is on the social environment and the effect of social interaction during all of these stress events. Retirement, for example, is a stressor, but in addition, retirement has a direct effect on the way others interact with the retired individual. Institutionalization and the loss of a loved one are stressors, but in the social sense, depending on the values and attitudes of the individuals interacting, they also set up certain patterns of interaction that significantly affect the self-esteem and sense of identity of the elderly individual.

> **Fourth-level assessment for confusion related to social interaction**
>
> Nature of the social interaction
> How and why interaction is enacted
> Expectations of the people in the exchange
> Attitudes of the people in the exchange
> Reinforcement cycle that has been established
> Spurious positive reinforcements available in the situation, or the secondary gains

Aware observation is the single most salient assessment technique for the social environment and behavioral exchanges. Using this technique requires a detached, analytic approach whereby the caregiver stands back and observes, makes notes and analyzes, then stands back and observes again. It requires becoming an uninvolved bystander to the actions and using heightened sensitivity and creative "figuring out." Only after the interaction patterns are thoroughly understood can any concrete actions be taken to change the situation. After that, prevention or intervention is fairly straightforward.

Prevention and intervention

It is possible to apply direct preventions and interventions to a social system as if it were an individual. It may not, however, be possible to be as precise as when dealing with stress. The prevention and intervention suggestions in this section are, therefore, more global and conceptual in nature than those previously presented. In addition, they are combined here because essentially they are the same, with only the time of application being different. In order to prevent confusion, the measure is applied for those who are at high risk prior to a confusional episode. In order to intervene for confusion, the measure is applied during a confusional episode. The nursing objectives are as follows:

1. To change the reinforcement pattern so that reinforcements are obtained for adaptive, productive behaviors rather than withdrawing ones
2. To eliminate, as much as possible, the sources of spurious positive reinforcement
3. To open communication about the staff's and client's expectations and attitudes about behavior in order to facilitate change
4. To review the social structure to determine who has the power and how power is exercised; then act to redistribute power by promoting the active decision making of the client and increasing his power base

1. *Change the reinforcement pattern so that reinforcements are obtained for adaptive, productive behaviors rather than withdrawing ones.* As has been stressed repeatedly in this book, when aberrant behaviors are being reinforced, the result is catastrophic. The client learns to behave in ways that are counterproductive and maladaptive. A great deal of confusion arises simply out of not knowing how to "be" in a situation, but when the definition of how to be turns out to be "crazy" or "confused," a real problem arises. It is possible to reverse these patterns by careful and thoughtful attention to what is being reinforced, by whom, and how.

2. *Eliminate, as much as possible, the sources of spurious positive reinforcement.* Again, the same principle applies; however, spurious reinforcements are often more difficult to identify than more obvious reinforcements. Sensitive observation of the staff and the client during interaction and immediately afterward holds the key to the identification. The objective must be to somehow make productive and adaptive behaviors far more interesting and appealing than confused behaviors.

3. *Speak openly about expectations and attitudes in order to facilitate change.* Both the caregivers and the client need to explore and express their expectations and attitudes in a given situation. This is often easier to accomplish with the caregivers, who can use team meetings to focus on expectations,

express feelings, and share attitudes. Sometimes, opening the subject helps facilitate the group expression of expectations that are revealing and surprising. Understanding and change can follow such expression. For the confused client, it may be quite difficult and even inappropriate to explore expectations until the confusional episode is passed. The client, however, at some point needs the opportunity to consider what expectations he has in the situation, as well as his attitudes about the setting and aging itself.

4. *Review the social structure to determine who has the power and how power is exercised; then act to redistribute power by promoting the active decision making of the client and increasing his power base.* In the institutional setting the power base of the client is automatically reduced by virtue of his dependence on the staff for instrumental services, sources of reinforcements, and alternatives. This situation can continue, with the likelihood that the client would be more prone to confusional episodes, or the situation can be carefully considered to determine the points at which the power advantage can be assumed by him. This is somewhat more difficult, but not impossible, to do in the acute care setting, which is usually based on an almost military-like power structure. In the long-term care setting, there is no reason why clients cannot be helped and encouraged to assume the power they have, even though this may be thought to be disruptive to the setting. When medical crisis is not the issue, disruption is all right. Some of the most obvious places where power is easy to transfer to the client are in the choice of how and when daily routines will be accomplished and the choice concerning social interaction and social activities. Helping the elderly client to perform some "work" functions within the organization adds to the power obtained by performing instrumental services. Clients can, for example, be helped to answer telephones, assemble charts, feed other patients, and fold linen. Each of these is a service to the institution and helps the elderly person obtain a more favorable bargaining position. Many clients somehow know this and create their own power with no support and encouragement. These are often the "good" clients who are liked, well cared for, and respected.

Last, but not least, is the issue of monopolies on rewards. The more concentrated the sources of rewards are in one or two individuals, the more power is available to those people. Careful thought should be given to ways in which clients can increase their social networks, not only because of the reasons already discussed, but also because many social supports decrease the likelihood of a monopoly and increase the client's power base.

Outcome criteria of successful nursing intervention against confusion related to social interaction

1. The client's adaptive and productive behavior is consistently and positively reinforced.
2. The client's behavior is adaptive and productive most of the time.
3. The client's sources of spurious positive reinforcement for negative behaviors are no longer present.
4. The client demonstrates the ability to identify and use his power sources in positive ways.
5. The client is no longer confused.

SUMMARY

In this chapter, basically two ways have been presented in which the pattern and meaning of an older person's existence can be disrupted, ultimately leading to confusional episodes. The first concerned stressors that interfere with the individual's personal milieu, and the second concerned the social structure or environment that interferes with his perception of meaning. Both of these are amenable to prevention and intervention.

The assessment ideas and suggestions for prevention and intervention are summarized in the charts that follow.

CHAPTER 11 SUMMARY
Disruption of pattern and meaning in the elderly
Confusion related to stressors

Fourth-level assessment	Prevention	Intervention

Stressors
Relationship to the aging condition
Dominant affective tones
Dominant thought content
Current resources
Current liabilities
Potential outside resources and their acceptability
Suicide potential
	1. Manage stressors.
	  a. Help the client identify life patterns from which stressors arise and the reactions he has to these patterns.
	  b. Help the client learn to balance stressors.
	  c. Help the client prepare for stressors through anticipatory planning.
	2. Deal with the perception of aging and the experiential component of stressors.
	  a. Help the client gain an understanding of the relationship between how he sees aging and how he sees himself as an individual.
	  b. Help the client identify and anticipate patterned responses to stressors, whether these are emotional or bodily reactions.
	3. Deal with the cognitive component of stressors.
	  a. Explore and reinforce lifelong resources.
		1. Provide support during acute confusional episodes.
		2. Alleviate stressors:
		  a. Help the client to gain an understanding of the stressors impinging on him.
		  b. Act to reduce the total number of stressors present.
		3. Deal with the client's perceptions of aging and the experiential component of the stressors:
		  a. Help the client gain access to and express feelings he may not recognize.
		  b. Validate with the client the "normalcy" of his experiences and emotions.
		  c. Explain bodily reactions the elderly person is perceiving.
		4. Deal with the cognitive component of a disruption of pattern and meaning.
		  a. Explore and reinforce the client's strengths and resources.

CHAPTER 11 SUMMARY
Confusion related to stressors—cont'd

Fourth-level assessment	Prevention	Intervention

	b. Help the client identify coping strategies that are both inside and outside his repertoire of problem-solving skills.
	c. Help the client learn to confine his assessment of liabilities to the present time.
	4. Prevent crisis.
	  a. Teach anticipatory planning strategies.
	  b. Help the client identify ways of maintaining social networks.
	5. Manage stress.
	  a. Help the client establish daily routines that permit stress release, stress encounter, and relaxation.
	  b. Help the client plan and use relaxation training to manage stress and tension.
	  c. Help the client identify his physical or psychologic stress signs and plan for stress release.
		b. Explore the client's liabilities and help him express his feelings about them.
		c. Explore the client's alternatives.
		5. Deal with crisis (adapted from Aguilera and Messick, 1978).
		  a. Help the client gain an intellectual understanding of the crisis.
		  b. Help the client discuss his present feelings, of which he may not be aware.
		  c. Explore coping mechanisms used in the past and still salient.
		  d. Help the client reopen his social world.
		  e. Help the client function in groups that focus on grief work and crisis intervention (Oberleder, 1970).
		6. Deal with chronic tension or stress.
		  a. Help the client identify and understand the sources of stress.
		  b. Help the client gain a sense of control over the multiple stressors that impinge on him.

Continued.

CHAPTER 11 SUMMARY
Confusion related to social interaction

Fourth-level assessment	Prevention/intervention
Aware observation with: Nature of the social interaction How and why interaction is enacted Expectations of the people in the exchange Attitudes of the people in the exchange Reinforcement cycle that has been established Spurious positive reinforcements available to both parties in the exchange	1. Change the reinforcement pattern so that reinforcements are obtained for adaptive, productive behaviors rather than withdrawing ones. 2. Eliminate, as much as possible, the sources of spurious positive reinforcement. 3. Speak openly about expectations and attitudes in order to facilitate change. 4. Review the social structure to determine who has the power and how power is exercised; then act to redistribute power by promoting the active decision making of the client and increasing his power base.

REFERENCES

Aguilera, D. C., and Messick, J. M.: Crisis intervention: theory and methodology, St. Louis, 1978, The C. V. Mosby Co.

Alpugh, P., and Haney, M.: Counseling the older adult, University Park, 1978, University of Southern California Press.

Antonovsky, A.: Health, stress, and coping, San Francisco, 1979, Jossey-Bass Publishers.

Baizerman, M., and Ellison, D. L.: A social role analysis of senility, Gerontologist **11**:163-170, 1971.

Bengtson, V.: The social psychology of aging, Indianapolis, 1973, The Bobbs-Merrill Co., Inc.

Bettelheim, B: The informed heart, New York, 1971, Avon Books.

Bloom, B. L.: Definitional aspects of the crisis concept, J. Consult Psychol. **27**:498-502, 1963.

Bowlby, J.: Attachment and loss: separation, vol. 2, New York, 1973, Basic Books, Inc.

Caine, L.: Widow, New York, 1974, William Morrow and Co., Inc.

Caplan, G.: An approach to community mental health, New York, 1961, Grune and Stratton, Inc.

Chadwick-Jones, J. K.: Social exchange theory: its structure and influence in social psychology, London, 1976, Academic Press, Inc. Used with permission. Copyright by Academic Press, Inc. (London) Ltd.

Dowd, J. J.: Aging as exchange: a preface to theory, J. Gerontol. **30**:584-595, 1975.

Ebersole, P. P.: Crisis intervention with the aged. In Burnside, I. M., editor: Nursing and the aged, New York, 1976, McGraw-Hill Book Co.

Engel, G. L.: Psychological development in health and disease, Philadelphia, 1962, W. B. Saunders Co.

Fink, S. L.: Crisis and motivation: a theoretical model, Arch. Phys. Med. Rehabil. **48**:592-597, 1967.

Goldstein, K.: The organism, New York, 1939, American Book Co.

Hendricks, J., and Hendricks, C. D.: Aging in mass society: myths and realities, Cambridge, 1977, Winthrop Publishers.

Holmes, T. H., and Rahe, R. H.: The social readjustment rating scale, J. Psychosom. Res. **11**:213, 1967.

Homans, G. C.: Social behavior: its elementary forms, New York, 1961, Harcourt, Brace and World, Inc.

Honey, C., Banks, C., and Zimbardo, P.: Interpersonal dynamics in a simulated prison. Unpublished manuscript, 1973, Stanford University.

Hurst, M. W., Jenkins, C. D., and Rose, R. M.: The relation of psychological stress to onset of medical illness. In Garfield, C. A., editor: Stress and survival: the emotional realities of life-threatening illness, St. Louis, 1979, The C. V. Mosby Co., pp. 17-26.

Jasmin, S., and Trygstad, L. N.: Behavioral concepts and the nursing process, St. Louis, 1979, The C. V. Mosby Co.

Kubler-Ross, E.: On death and dying, New York, 1969, Macmillan Publishing Co.

Kuypers, J. A., and Bengtson, V. L.: Competence and social breakdown: a social-psychological view of aging, Hum. Dev. **2**:37-49, 1973.

Lynch, W. F.: Images of hope Baltimore, 1965, Helicon Press.

Mereness, D. A., and Taylor, C. M.: Essentials of psychiatric nursing, St. Louis, 1978, The C. V. Mosby Co.

Miller, M.: Suicide among the elderly: the final alternative. Unpublished manuscript, 1977, Arizona State University.

Neugarten, B. L., Moore, J. W., and Lowe, J. C.: Age norms, age constraints and adult socialization. In Neugarten, B. L., editor: Middle age and aging, Chicago, 1968, University of Chicago Press, pp. 22-28.

Oberleder, M.: Crisis therapy in mental breakdown of the aging, Gerontologist **10**:111-114, 1970.

Phillips, L. R.: The imprisonment model. Unpublished manuscript, 1976, University of Arizona.

Roberts, S. L.: Behavioral concepts and the critically ill patient, Englewood Cliffs, N.J., 1976, Prentice-Hall, Inc.

Ryan, S. A.: Personal communication about the Ryan coping model, 1979.

Selye, H.: Stress and aging, J. Am. Geriatr. Soc. **28**:669-680, 1970.

Selye, H.: The stress of life, New York, 1976, McGraw-Hill Book Co.

Shea, F.: Hopelessness and helplessness, Perspect. Psychiatr. Nurs. **2**:32, 1970.

Simonton, O. C., Matthews-Simonton, S., and Creighton, J.: Getting well again, Los Angeles, 1979, J. P. Tarcher, Inc.

Topalis, M., and Aguilera, D. C.: Psychiatric nursing, St. Louis, 1978, The C. V. Mosby Co.

Vroom, V. H., and Yetton, P. W.: Leadership and decision making, Pittsburgh, 1973, University of Pittsburgh Press.

SUGGESTIONS FOR FURTHER READING IN THE AREA OF COUNSELING AND HELPING ELDERLY PEOPLE

Burnside, I. M., editor: Nursing and the aged, New York, 1976, McGraw-Hill Book Co.

Butler, R. N., and Lewis, M. I.: Aging and mental health, St. Louis, 1977, The C. V. Mosby Co.

Gray, J., and DeFelice, L.: Emotional crisis: how to cope, how to recover, Washington, N.Y., 1976, Ashley Books, Inc.

Okun, B. R.: Effective helping: interviewing and counseling techniques, North Scituate, Mass., 1976, Duxbury Press.

Powell, J.: Why am I afraid to tell you who I am? Niles, Ill., 1969, Argus Communications.

Powell, J.: The secret of staying in love, Niles, Ill., 1974, Argus Communications.

12

CARE OF THE CLIENT WHOSE CONFUSION RESULTS FROM ALTERATIONS IN NORMAL PHYSIOLOGIC STATES

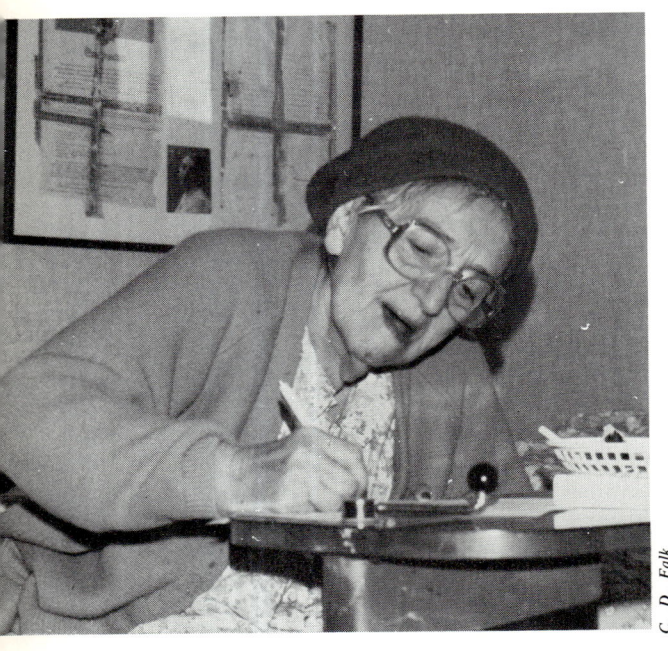

C. D. Falk

This chapter is concerned with nursing the elderly client with alterations in normal physiologic states, such as comfort maintenance (pain avoidance), sleep, activity, and elimination. Most of these are cyclic in nature and are developed around the circadian rhythms. In Chapter 2, the conceptual framework dealt with the holistic model of man. The interaction of man (as an open system) with the biosphere has resulted in reactions to light and dark, to magnetic changes, to barometric changes, and to temperature changes, as well as to the periodicity of seasons. The body's capacity for self-regulation, by which it adapts to the natural phenomena, is taken for granted. It also has its own internal feedback system that reacts to conditions within the body.

In Chapter 2, three principles were given to explain man's organization. These were later discussed in relation to their importance to confusion in the elderly. These principles are:

1. A part not functioning in accordance with the whole tends to be brought into harmonious function with the system.
2. If a position in the whole is perceived by the organism as unfilled, the organism will tend to fill it.
3. An open system will be perceived by the organsim, will cause disquiet, and will be closed by the organism.

This chapter attempts to work with the concept of altered physiologic function in relation to the three principles and their effect on the efforts of the person to retain identity. Identity is a highly personal phenomenon. Three *identials* have been defined: the name, the body, and the life history. This chapter is concerned with the body, which cannot be separated from the life history.

The identity as related to body is frequently spoken of as body image and is usually described in terms of structure. Butler and Lewis (1977) suggest using the mirror to diagnose and obtain information about the person's body image. Rich data can be collected in a short time as the older client reacts to the external appearance of his body. *Function is also an important factor in the individual's body image. The internal environment of the body has sent such constant messages that they are not recognized except when deviant.* The older person recognizes weariness or fatigue, for "feeling good" is accepted as the true state of the body. Sleep rhythms have been established through life, and insomnia or sleeplessness is a sign of *dis*-ease. Probably no cycle is as taken for granted as elimination. Bladder and bowel filling and emptying have a personal pattern, with cues that are unmistakable. Interruptions, such as inability to empty the bladder or constipation, are immediately recognized as *dis*-ease. Pain is the most commonly dealt with sign of a change in the body's image. Living is not painful; pain represents threat. Using the three principles, it is apparent why each of the altered physiologic functions leads to chaotic behavior when the open system is not under the client's control, as when he has a catheter or colostomy or if he cannot control his pain or his sleep pattern.

Vernon (1968) states that we rely on the body to behave reliably, sensibly, and meaningfully.... "We can predict more or less correctly what will happen; and, more important still, we know what is the most effective way of reacting to it" (p. 39). Any distortion or deficiency in the sensory mechanism can produce confusion. As stated in Chapter 2, the constants in the world, on which the older person has based his decisions and actions, change; the same must be said for the body. If the change is gradual, adaptation occurs. The "me-ness" of the client is his body's own action and reaction, its feedback mechanisms that keep him in touch with his every part, where it is, and what it is doing at all times. The feedback mechanism is so much a part of our constant being that it is not recognized until it challenges our sense of its reliability and meaning. Vision is never fully appreciated and understood until there is lack of vision.

The work in biofeedback has opened a way of becoming aware of our inner world before the event of *dis*-ease. The use of biofeedback after disease has resulted in control over such autonomic nerve functions as blood pressure and pulse, as well as return of skeletal muscle function in stroke (Shiavi and others, 1979). By its definition and description, the extent of the body's feedback system and the conscious and unconscious control over it are finally being used by individuals of all ages. For the elderly the potential is great. Autogenic training and relaxation offers control over their bodies when control seems to be slipping away and when the deviant messages from the body are used by caregivers to label the person senile.

CONFUSION SECONDARY TO CHANGES IN ELIMINATION

Bowel function is established before birth, as demonstrated by meconium-stained amniotic fluid; it ends with sphincter relaxation and final emptying at death. The urinary bladder empties freely until the individual recognizes bladder sensations and uses them to control emptying, some time after the first year of life. Control over elimination is learned so early that few people can remember the process, and after control is established, there is reasonable expectation that elimination will be conducted in the manner and in the places

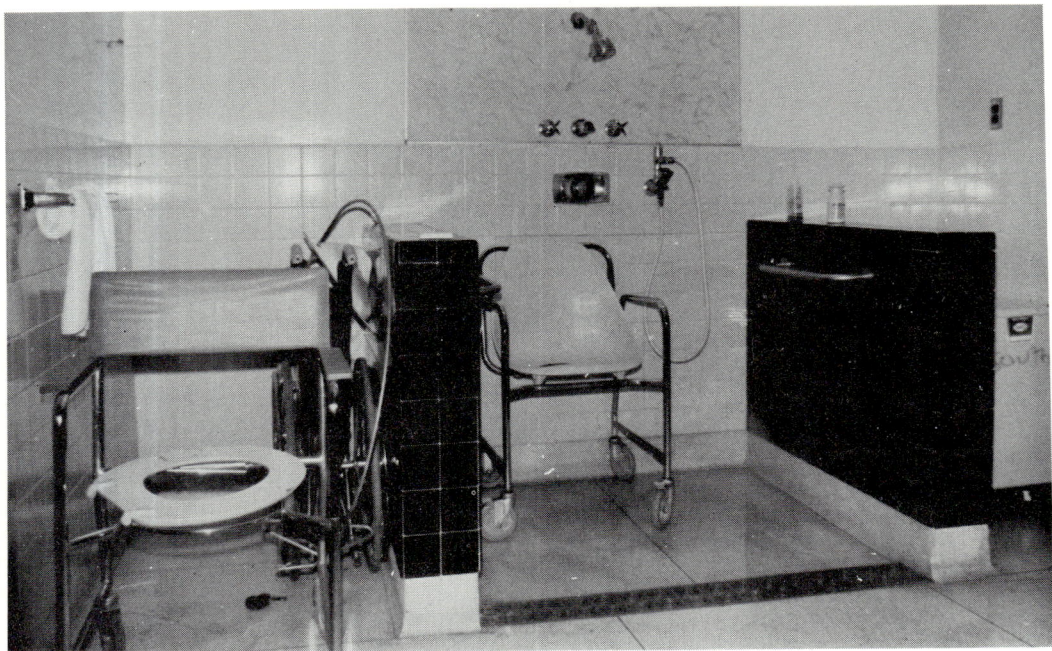

Fig. 12-1. Privacy in the bathroom or for toileting may be nonexistent in the institutional setting. (Photograph by C. D. Falk.)

prescribed by culture. Body rhythms and the feedback mechanism, once established, continue throughout life; culture has an impact on how elimination is conducted and on the individual's perception of the elimination process as natural, disgusting, or even shameful.

The childhood teachings of the generation now reaching 65 and of those over that age were part of the Victorian period when sex and elimination were tabooed subjects; often, the two were associated. The very taboo may have resulted in a rebellion in the opposite direction, but mother's teachings continue to guide reaction to the organs of elimination, especially when the older person is dependent on others for personal care. Elimination in our culture is a private and personal matter, but this is not always true in the health care setting (Fig. 12-1).

> **Fourth-level assessment for confusion secondary to inability to empty bladder**
>
> Abdominal palpation to determine bladder level
> History, if obtainable from client; rapid onset of symptoms, both urinary and confusional
> Inability to urinate in usual position or in required position if illness prevents standing
> Drug profile: drugs with anticholinergic effects (atropine-like drugs) or ganglionic blocking agents (for hypertension), whose action causes urinary retention and constipation; narcotics and tranquilizing drugs
> Situational factors: lack of privacy; strange surroundings
> Surgery in the pelvic area that may have interfered with nerve supply

Inability to empty the bladder

The full bladder is an emergent situation. The elderly male is concerned with his inability to urinate when prostatic enlargement interferes. Acute confused states in elderly males should always be investigated for a full bladder and drug reaction—not in that order, but simultaneously and immediately.

Signs and symptoms include restlessness, which proceeds to agitation, lack of output, bizarre behavior, and a palpable bladder above the symphysis pubis. Palpation is not always possible in an obese abdomen. History and behavior are important cues.

The elderly male with prostatic enlargement (more than 50% of men over 50 and 75% of men over age 70 have some degree of prostatic enlargement) is a high-risk candidate, as is the elderly person taking large doses of atropine-like drugs or tranquilizers. Men and women who have had pelvic surgery may be unable to void. The older client who misses his privacy or who does not understand the arrangements for emptying the bladder in a recumbent position may have a full bladder.

Prevention is part of good nursing care. Awareness of lack of output is essential. Bladder filling should correspond roughly to intake. For the elderly person in an acute care unit, the matter should be discussed frankly and arrangements made for frequent checking, for the need to void should occur every few hours. If intravenous fluid is being given, there is a positive check on the amount of intake. The nurse, who anticipates the need, establishes a nonembarrassing relationship with the elderly client so he can express his needs before restlessness or agitation provides certain clues. First-time hospitalized elderly clients will almost always retain childhood taboos when the dependent role is assumed. The nurse is the one who should make the situation a normal one; she should not consider this first-time and learning person as a routine matter.

The nursing objective for intervention is to reestablish a normal bladder-emptying pattern. When the bladder is full there is only one treatment: emptying—by natural means when possible and by intrusive procedures such as catheterization or surgery if required. The confusion must be treated by the emergency means discussed in Chapter 8. After the relief afforded by one emergency intervention, the cause must be reviewed and treated. It may require adjustment of drug dosage, change in activity status, or further intrusive measures. The underlying consideration is that the client's ability to take care of his normal functions is no longer under his control. His feedback system is frustrated. Nursing intervention should be guided toward assisting the client regain control—if not over the whole process, at least over part. He needs to have his dependable world reestablished.

The client who wanders the halls in the acute care unit at night is hunting for a toilet. Most elderly people have nocturia not once but several times a night. If fluids are encouraged and the client has more intake than usual, the kidneys excrete the extra fluid at night while he is in a horizontal position. The client who has any sedation may not be oriented on awakening to anything except the need to empty his bladder. He will always get out of bed and walk toward light, which is usually in the hall. He does not stop to clamp tubings or lower bed rails, and rarely does he remember to press the call button. The client in the hall should be taken to the toilet as the first step back to bed. This area is discussed in Chapter 8.

Outcome criteria of successful nursing intervention against inability to empty bladder

1. Normal emptying pattern of the bladder is reestablished.
2. The client or his caregiver can use any artificial aids safely.
3. The client or his caregiver can give the early signs of an inability to empty bladder and knows the steps to take in obtaining help.

Constipation and impaction

The elderly person has probably been "tinkering" with his bowel habits for years. Easy access to laxatives and the emphasis on "regularity" have focused attention on the bowel. For many people the impulse that signals the full rectum has apparently been lost through this personal "tinkering" with the system. For others, bowel elimination is based on a certain diet, regularity of habit, and activity. Change in any of these as a result of illness may lead to slower transit through the gastrointestinal tract. Drugs may mask the signals from the rectum. The fecal mass dehydrates and impaction of feces results. One breakdown in the feedback system is the cause, but a second breakdown can result from actions taken to remove impaction.

Signs and symptoms of constipation and impaction include the lack of bowel emptying or a small, frequent loss of stool around the large fecal mass. Malaise, restlessness, agitation, confusion with a very short attention span, inability to note detail in the environment, and unproductive activity usually follow.

Fourth-level assessment for confusion secondary to constipation or impaction

Bowel movement record (dependable history)
Record of cathartics
Behavior: restless, distractible, unable to organize, inattentive to detail and agitated
Manual examination of rectum for impaction
Dehydration
Food intake

At risk is any older person whose living habits change abruptly with reduced activity, less fluid intake, or less food intake, or who is given drugs that reduce the motility of the intestine. The patient in the acute care unit whose ambulation is restricted or curtailed is also vulnerable. Older people who have a lifetime habit of inducing rapid emptying of the bowel have lost their natural rhythms.

Prevention is easier than cure. A careful history will include information on the bowel habit, unless the elderly person is too confused to give reliable information. In the home the administration of cathartics is a clue, but a rectal examination may be necessary to establish the fact, with prediction and prevention used to prevent occurrence. It is often too late when the nurse makes the first contact. Prevention involves a review of the total life-style and any recent changes that could lead to inactivity, loss of appetite, or use of new and different drugs. Adequate fluid intake is essential. Stool softeners or bulky substances such as Metamucil may be given. The rectal area should be examined for fissures or hemorrhoids that may cause pain and inhibit defecation. Grief and depression often lead to reduced bowel activity through a reduction in activity and food intake. Constipation and impaction may be predicted as a secondary process to many treatable causes.

Nursing objectives for intervention are:
1. To treat the immediate need of relieving the full rectum
2. To investigate associated and contributing factors
3. To assist the client or his caregiver to initiate a preventive program

The fecal mass should be removed as carefully and painlessly as possible, with the elderly person in a supported position, well draped, and in a good light. This may involve preparation over a period to soften the mass. The procedure is strange and can be very frightening unless preceded with careful explanation and slow, careful actions.

No impaction or constipation occurs in isolation. There are contributing factors probably more in need of treatment than the bowel condition itself. This means a review of recent events that precipitated the impaction or of a concurrent event still in progress, such as immobilization for a fractured hip. A little detective work may uncover a causal factor that no amount of remedial work at the site of the impaction will change.

Recurrence can and will happen unless the life matrix is altered for prevention. This demands carefully assessing the lifestyle and conferring with the client or his caregiver over what are reasonable alterations. No one makes a radical departure from a previous pattern of daily existence without causing strains in another area. The client must feel that change will be helpful in order to participate with any degree of enthusiasm. Confusion secondary to an impaction may be treated by adequate hydration when the impaction is secondary to dehydration. Medications may have to be reviewed and reconsidered.

Outcome criteria of successful nursing intervention against constipation or impaction

1. The impaction or constipation is relieved.
2. The client is no longer confused.
3. A teaching plan has resulted in the client or the caregiver reorganizing the factors in his environment that contributed to the impaction.
4. The client or his caregiver is committed to a regimen of prevention.

Incontinence

Incontinence of bladder and bowel is the inability to control their emptying. This ranges from stress incontinence in the older woman to the dribbling that may persist after a transurethral prostatectomy. Stress incontinence occurs when the bladder pressure is increased beyond a certain point, either because of a large amount of urine or from external pressure such as coughing, sneezing, straining, or heavy lifting. Urine enters the proximal third of the urethra and may escape at that point; it is not under the voluntary control of the client. For the older woman with relaxed pelvic musculature, perineal exercises may help in prevention or in relief; surgery is done with mixed results.

The signs and symptoms of incontinence are the actual evidence of loss of urine or feces and the behavior of the client, who may be masking embarrassment. Often, elderly people will deny that they have been incontinent, even if it is obvious.

Fourth-level assessment for incontinence

Loss of urine or feces in situations other than through approved elimination devices
Stained or wet clothing or beds
Washed underwear discovered
Embarrassed conduct that can be almost irrational; refusal to participate in social activities or to leave room; withdrawal

---

Almost any older person is at risk, but those at high risk are diabetic clients with neuropathy, which affects the nerves from the pelvis; those with various other neurologic problems that affect older persons more than others, such as stroke or parkinsonism; and women with relaxed pelvic muscles. Older men, after transurethral prostatectomy, are also vulnerable.

Prevention is based on keeping the bladder and bowel empty so that incontinence does not occur. This means frequent toileting. For the dependent person or the wheelchair-bound, bowel training can be established to prevent fecal incontinence, but at the price of vigilance and careful observation by the caregiver. Urinary incontinence is not so easily prevented. Attempts at control by limiting fluids often cause dehydration and are not advised. Frequent emptying to prevent the accumulation of urine in the bladder to the point that a small amount of pressure causes its involuntary expulsion is the best solution, time consuming as it may be. Since confusion and incontinence seem to be found together, controlling his confusion often helps the elderly client to more ably plan for prevention of incontinence. For the dependent client, the caregiver can often gauge the amount of time from intake to urinary output after careful observation and intervene at the appropriate time. Often, controlling disease processes such as urinary tract infection provides protection.

Intervention is based on the following objectives:

1. To prevent the occurrence of incontinence
2. To provide protection for clothing
3. To prevent social isolation

Bowel and bladder training should be instituted to prevent recurrences. The problem is never solved, but good training often helps the nurse match her timing with the client's natural body rhythms. Stress incontinence is rarely mentioned in textbooks and even more rarely between client and caregiver, for it is a matter of embarrassment the client feels is too personal to share. The older woman with a cough is a fair candidate for this experience, and it is best handled matter-of-factly by both caregiver and client. It is best for the caregiver to assume that stress incontinence is found in the older woman and to handle it as an expected phenomenon. The cough may be important to remove secretions from the chest. Intervention to teach productive coughing and to reduce the chest secretions helps to treat incontinence.

Providing protection for clothing should aim toward the minimum needed. Wearing a sanitary pad may be sufficient rather than going to the "rubber pants" stage. Reference to "diapering" is to be deplored in the care of the elderly. Frequent, scrupulous cleaning of the genital area is required to prevent the odor of stale urine, which repels family and visitors.

Example. Mrs. S., age 89, prepared her bed in the nursing home each afternoon by putting on layers of newspapers, a plastic cover, and some commercial bed protectors. She was terribly embarrassed by a wet bed each night and tried to reduce the need for a sheet change during the night.

Social isolation is prevented by reducing the client's shame and the avoidance by others because of the odor of stale urine or feces. The confusional type of behavior that results is often a crisis response that yields to relief of the situation. Shame leads to panic and social isolation.

Example. Miss K., age 70, was the daughter of a Presbyterian minister and had attended church every Sunday of her life. A friend who gave her a ride to and from church was in a hurry to leave. Miss K. did not have a chance to go to the toilet, which she always did immediately after services. This day, as she stood near the curb waiting for her friend, she suddenly began urinating. Her friend, who saw the puddle when she drove up, was shocked and critical. Miss K. never went to church again.

Incontinence leads to withdrawal, and withdrawal to isolation.

Outcome criteria of successful nursing intervention against incontinence

1. The client or his caregiver has undergone a bowel and bladder training program.
2. The client or caregiver knows the mechanisms in stress incontinence and the principles applied to the client's own situation.
3. The client has been assisted in finding the minimum protection for his clothing, and supplies have been provided or social agencies contacted to help in purchase of supplies if funding is needed.
4. The caregiver and client are comfortable in discussing the situation and planning together for amelioration of incontinence.
5. The client and caregiver have discussed methods of preventing social isolation. Referral to community agencies is made as needed.

CONFUSION SECONDARY TO INTERFERENCE WITH NORMAL FEEDBACK MECHANISMS
Intubation

Tubes in the body orifices are unnatural devices that interfere with the body's own feedback system. There are constant messages that have either no meaning or a very threatening meaning. The communication or feedback is contradictory, and the client is powerless to respond in the natural pattern that has always worked for him. There is loss of control over very elementary physiologic processes, such as eating, voiding, or even breathing. Explanations are required and must be repeated over and over again. The message must be consistent, using the same words each time and giving the same message. The major question the nurse answers, regardless of how it is stated, is, "Am I ever going to have control over this function again? And if not, *can I depend on others to take care of this situation for me?*" The individual who does not have the answer to this question will panic, and confusion often results. The client's question must be answered.

The indwelling catheter gives a sensation of pressure that is interpreted as a need to void. This is an irrelevant message, since the bladder is drained and contracted. Explanations are often useless in overcoming the body's own inner feedback.

In addition to having lost control over a most personal function and as one 83-year-old man described, "my most delicate organ," catheter insertion is usually done at a time of crisis and with arcane rituals that shroud the procedure in an aura of mystery. The sterile technique, particularly the gloved hands and the cleaning of the area surrounding the meatus with applicators and cotton balls, tends to remove confidence in ability to ever regain control. There are further instructions regarding what not to do, but little is said about what can be done. There is excitement when the client attempts to explore his own body, with frenzied instructions not to pull the catheter out followed by hand restraint.

The indwelling catheter is never a comfortable object. However, part of discomfort is "not knowing." The client should have a chance to fully explore a nonsterile catheter, including seeing fluid run through it and the retaining balloon expanded. He should be given extremely simple explanations of sterility that focus on the fact that precautions are made to prevent introducing infection to him; otherwise, the rubber gloves and cleaning are interpreted to mean he is the "dirty" object. For some men whose previous experiences and education has included venereal disease, the process may quickly be associated with gonorrhea or syphilis. The client's questions should be examined for such implications. Clients usually speak in metaphor about such matters, and the mind must be sensitized to the actual meaning of remarks that do not make sense in themselves. Clients must be reassured if such an association is made.

Long, involved explanations should be avoided. When an anxious client is being given new information, his attention span is limited. Three ideas are the limit, and testing after each idea will determine its impact. It is very important to keep uppermost the idea that the intrusive procedure violates the body's own feedback system and that according to principle number one mentioned earlier, the new way of functioning must be brought into harmonious function with the system. A catheter represents an open system, and it will cause disquiet until it is closed. The closure is evidenced by the behavior that caregivers label as confusion. Nursing care demands this be anticipated.

The artificial bowel opening

Colostomy and ileostomy will be treated by the client in the same way as the indwelling catheter. Lack of control over one of the earliest of controlled functions causes anxiety and confusion until the client masters his own care. For the elderly person who is shocked and frightened by the artificial opening, independent care may never be achieved. Having spouses and others care for the artificial opening offers no meaningful feedback for the client. Unless the feedback principles are taken into consideration in planning the learning experience, the process of trying to teach colostomy care may exacerbate the confusion. The body image has been violated and the feedback system has been interrupted; connections with life history must form the basis for working with the client. Mystique should be avoided.

CONFUSION SECONDARY TO SLEEPLESSNESS

The causes of sleep have not been explained and the function is unclear. It is, however, one of the body cycles, and the need for sleep and activity is part of the feedback system. The older client has the same need for sleep as the infant; however, he meets it in far different ways with individual patterns established during his life. Each person has a favorite body position that leads to sleep—right side, left side, arms under head, right knee angled and left knee straight—the combinations are endless. No one sleeps naturally in a semi-Fowler's position, except to take naps. The body has a "feel" for the right condition conducive to individual sleep. Violation of the feedback system that indicates when the proper position has been assumed results in sleeplessness.

Dependence on others for the sleep preparation rituals violates the body's feedback system. The normal pattern is interrupted. Each person has a personal ritual for preparing to sleep. For some, the process may take hours—a bath, snack, reading until drowsy and so on. For others it is a short, but still ritualistic, catering to the body's demands. When this is altered by illness and dependence on the convenience or pleasure of others, the result is sleeplessness. Behavior exhibited by the client in an effort to meet his sleep needs without the usual preparation and position can result in "sundown syndrome," the confusion that occurs at night.

The bed itself contributes to feelings of strangeness. Almost everyone complains that they do not sleep well the "first night in a strange bed." Factors preventing usual sleep include a difference in the foundation, firmness of the mattress, material used for sheets, weight of blankets, and pillow softness and width. The comfortable pillow supports the head in line with the spinal column. This requires that its width be equal to the distance from the shoulder to the ear. Many older people with cervical arthritis take their pillows with them to ensure a night's sleep in a strange place. The width of the bed may inhibit sleep, and if one is accustomed to sleeping with another, the absence of the sleeping partner may be severely felt. In addition, there are the noises and lights of strange places, and in the institution, sharing a room with a stranger. The miracle is that sleep occurs at all. Using the knowledge of body feedback, which is negative in many of the instances already cited, the nurse can work with the client to induce a night's sleep. The most comforting thing is human understanding. Understanding for the nurse must include her knowledge of the body's cycles, rhythms, and feedback systems.

CONFUSION SECONDARY TO PAIN

Pain is a subjective experience perceived by the client in two ways: its discomfort and its meaning. The discomfort can be thermal, chemical, mechanical (pressure), and electrical. Meaning comes from a lifetime of experience. It can be a very emotional experience influenced by age, sex, cultural background, psychosocial factors, environmental factors, and expected response (Karb, 1979). Being old is not painful, although there is a great deal of pain associated with some of the infirmities of aging, such as degenerative arthritis. Many elderly people have developed a strong religious faith, in which ability to suffer pain demonstrates their belief. There are diametrically opposed reactions to pain in different people. However, pain is a primary stimulus. It serves to distract the attention of the client from the world around him, narrowing his perceptual field to a pinhole vision of reality. It is this reaction to a world where pain marks the boundaries that leads a caregiver to label the client's mental status as confused. Perhaps it would be better to indicate that he has a limited view of reality and is responding to the only world he knows.

Appropriate nursing intervention requires an assessment of the pain and an effort to determine its cause. Pain must be relieved. Pain from thermal causes yields relatively easily to correcting the cause, whether it is excess cold or heat. Mechanical causes are often less easily solved, especially when the therapeutic regimen demands a certain position, as with a fracture. Changes of position with relief of pressure and exercise of unused or stiff joints may help. Often, reducing sensory overload or clearing up the mysteries helps. Pain in the abdomen is tolerated more easily when the client learns that it is not from cancer, but from some less threatening problem. Mental and physical relaxation is one of the most important relief measures, but relaxation may be impossible if pain is severe enough to force it to the center of consciousness. In such events, analgesics are important. For the elderly surgical patient, relief of pain often relieves the confusional state (Grant, 1978; Williams and others, 1979). When moving the elderly patient in pain, time should be taken to explain what will happen to him and how he can help and to listen to what he thinks will reduce the pain of movement. Individuals who scream when moved need treatment for the pain, not for the screaming. Painful areas of the body should be supported; movements should be slow and coordinated. Isolation from things that have meaning can reduce the tolerance to pain. Nursing has many pain-relieving measures in its repertoire.

SUMMARY

Interference with the natural body rhythms and feedback mechanisms for elimination, sleep, and comfort have been discussed in relation to the chaotic and confused behavior that often results. The client is trying to find meaning and predictability in his own internal world, the body that represents himself. The nurse can help maintain identity by assisting with restoration of control over body functions or by helping the client find meaning when control has been lost and the feedback system is frustrated.

SUGGESTIONS FOR FURTHER READING
Pain

Jacox, A.: Assessing pain, Am. J. Nurs. **79**(5): 895-900, 1979.

Karb, V. B.: Pain. In Phipps, W. J., Long, B. C., and Woods, N. F., editors: Medical-surgical nursing: concepts and clinical practice, St. Louis, 1979, The C. V. Mosby Co., pp. 343-360.

McCaffery, M.: Nursing management of the patient in pain, Philadelphia, 1972, The J. B. Lippincott Co.

McCaffery, M., and Moss, F.: Nursing intervention for bodily pain, Am. J. Nurs. **67**:1224-1227, 1967.

Feedback and systems theory

Putt, A.: General systems theory applied to nursing, Boston, 1978, Little, Brown & Co.

Body rhythms and the circadian cycle

Luce, G. G.: Body time, New York, 1971, Random House.

REFERENCES

Butler, R. N., and Lewis, M. I.: Aging and mental health, ed. 2, St. Louis, 1977, The C. V. Mosby Co.

Engel, B. T.: Using biofeedback with the elderly. Presentation at the State of the Art Seminar on Aging Research, Oct. 1, 1976, NIA Gerontology Research Institute on Aging, Baltimore, Md.

Grant, M.: Pain, confusion and analgesics in young

and elderly orthopedic patients. Presentation at WICHE Research Conference, Portland, Ore., 1978.

Karb, V. B.: Pain. In Phipps, W. J., Long, B. C., and Woods, N. F., editors: Medical surgical nursing: concepts and clinical practice, St. Louis, 1979, The C. V. Mosby Co.

Shiavi, R. G., and others: Efficacy of biofeedback therapy in regaining control of lower extremity musculature following stroke, Am. J. Phys. Med. **58** (4):185-194, 1979.

Vernon, M. D.: The psychology of perception, Baltimore, 1968, Penguin Books, Ltd.

Williams, M. A., and others: Nursing activities and acute confusional states in elderly hip-fractured patients, Nurs. Res. **28** (1):25-35, 1979.

13

CARE OF THE PATIENT WITH A TRUE DEMENTIA

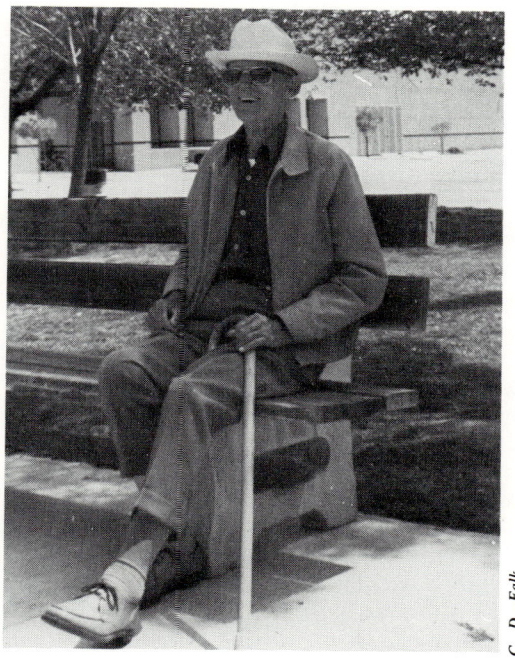

COURSE OF THE TRUE DEMENTIAS

Case study: Bill. (*As told by a family member*.) In 1966, Ann and Bill were moving into their newly built home. During the building process, Bill had taken the responsibility of measuring for carpets, linoleum, and furniture placement. Ann noticed that his measurements were faulty. During that year, Bill had begun to complain that he was having difficulty on the job. He was a member of a scientific team with the responsibility for writing research reports. He complained that he was having difficulty putting his thoughts on paper. Even in speech, he was having difficulty finding the words he wanted to use. He found that on some days he was unable to open the office safe, even though he had opened it every day for 10 years. Gradually, dealing with money and making change was becoming difficult for him, as well as driving the car. Bill was alternately anxious and depressed about what was happening to him, but he continued to work and tried to maintain as normal a life as he could. Bill was 57 years old.

In November of the next year, Bill was seen by a psychiatrist. Previously, his family doctor, whom he had been seeing with regularity, had been assuring him that nothing was wrong except that he was experiencing the stresses of growing older. However, after a diagnostic workup by the psychiatrist, the diagnosis was confirmed—Alzheimer's disease. Ann was told by the psychiatrist that Alzheimer's disease is "premature aging or premature senility." The psychiatrist stated that Alzheimer's disease is characterized by progressive physical and mental deterioration for which there is no cure. Ann was informed that her husband would lose one ability after another and finally would require custodial care.

During those early years, Bill was plagued by a constant fear of rejection and ridicule by those he loved. This did not happen. Those around him treated him with love and patience. Ann constantly tried to reassure him and slowly took over all household duties, such as handling money, shopping, and making arrangements for repairs. Bill's family helped with whatever they could do, visiting often. Work was finally impossible, and he had to quit. When he was home all the time, Bill's sisters began to "sit" with him on a regular basis to give relief to his wife. Slowly, the psychiatrist's prediction was becoming true.

For the next 5 years, Bill remained at home. He became more and more limited. He lost his ability to find his way around his house. He became incontinent, not through loss of bowel control, but because he was unable to find the bathroom. His sight was affected. At dinner, he would ask for more food when the left side of his plate was still full. When his plate was turned around, left to right, he would thank his wife for providing more food. He said he saw things crawling on the walls. One week he wanted to know who the man at the door was when he saw his own reflection in the glass of the storm door. He "admired" pictures on the wall where there were no pictures. Finally, he lost track of whether it was day or night and was likely to roam around the house for hours at night while Ann tried to get some rest after hectic days.

In February of 1972, hospitalization became necessary. He was becoming progressively belligerent and aggressive. When agitated, he was likely to march out into the busy street, unconcerned for his own safety. He would even get up at night and wander into the street. Ann couldn't watch him 24 hours a day by herself, and he was admitted to a general hospital for evaluation. Three weeks later, Bill was admitted to a state mental hospital.

For the next 7 years, until his death, Bill resided at the state mental hospital. Ann visited twice weekly, without fail, although she doubted after the first 3 years if he knew who she was. Her visits were ritualistic—on each visit she took pureed foods to him and, when he was well enough, wheeled him around the hospital. She took along toilet articles, oiled and combed his hair, cleaned his fingernails, creamed his skin, and talked on and on whether he answered or not. Brothers and sisters visited once a month for the next 5 years, but visits were cut considerably when he became too ill. The physical and psychologic strain of his illness became almost intolerable for his close family members.

Nursing staff became quite attached to Bill. They and the other residents on the unit fondly referred to him as "the professor" and his nursing care was, for the most part, exemplary.

Despite this, his physical condition progressively deteriorated. Bill became emaciated and finally bedfast. In spite of all efforts, decubitus ulcers developed over his bony prominences, probably resulting in part from his nutritional status. During 7 years of institutionalization, Bill had pneumonia three times and continual bladder infections. He was readmitted to the general hospital for his infections several times. Each time he was treated aggressively with antibiotics and returned to the state hospital.

In the last year of his life, Bill was unable to communicate coherently. He laid in bed and "bellowed like a bull" on and on, keeping the nursing unit in an uproar. Finally, some 12 years after diagnosis, Bill died, succumbing at last to one of his many infections.

This story illustrates the course of a "true" senile dementia. In this chapter, diseases characterized by cerebral atrophy that are progressive and "irreversible" in nature will be discussed. It should be emphasized that probably only a small proportion of the people who receive a diagnosis indicating an organic, irreversible process actually fall into that category; "senile dementia" as used in this chapter refers *only* to those people. We will explore disease processes, pathologic findings, diagnostic procedures, assessment protocols, and treatments beneficial to those with true senile dementia. We hope to make clear in this chapter that although senile dementia, like the dying process, may be irreversible and progressive, the *living* involved during the process can still be hopeful, filled with good feelings and moments of satisfaction. When the attitudes of those around the client and the client's environment are manipulated in a positive way, the likelihood is that his life experiences will be positive.

THE "TRUE" SENILE DEMENTIAS

In spite of the looseness with which health professionals use "chronic brain syndrome," "organic brain syndrome," and "senile dementia," there are a limited number of individuals who actually qualify for these diagnoses because of pathologic processes characterized by organic brain and behavioral change. Symptoms of the true dementias traditionally include memory disturbances, usually most marked early in the disease by impairment of recent memory; deterioration of intellectual functioning; emotional changes, including withdrawal, retarded speech and movement, and feelings of depression and inadequacy; personality changes; changes in language; and a wide range of neurologic and extrapyramidal signs (Miller, 1977). The prevalence of true senile dementia is unknown, since, as we have implied throughout this book, only a small proportion of the total number of people who receive a so-called organic diagnosis (including arteriosclerotic brain syndrome, chronic brain syndrome, organic brain syndrome, and senile dementia) are probably actually affected by an "irreversible" phenomenon. However, Kay and others (1970), using stringent criteria, report an overall prevalence in about 6.2% of the population over 65 years of age, with the bulk of the occurrence being among those over 80 years of age. It is interesting to note that in the 1964 report of Kay, Beamish, and Roth, "the subjects diagnosed with senile dementia and living at home were just as likely to be severely impaired as those who were institutionalized. This finding suggests the importance of factors other than the disease itself that predispose to institutionalization, such as lack of social supports and economic status (Miller, 1977).

Traditionally, the dementias of aging have been divided into two categories distinguished by the age when onset occurs. Those appearing before the age of 65 have been considered "presenile," and those appearing after the age of 65 have been considered "senile." In the presenile group are Alzheimer's disease, Pick's disease, Huntington's chorea, Jakob-Creutzfeldt disease, normal pressure hydrocephalus, and neurosyphilis. Of these diseases, Pick's disease, Huntington's chorea, Jakob-Creutzfeldt disease, normal pressure hydrocephalus, and neurosyphilis are relatively rare (Miller, 1977). In the group of dementias that occur to people over 65 are senile dementia of the Alzheimer type (Terry, 1978) and arteriosclerotic dementia (Miller, 1977). The Alzheimer lesion accounts for over half of the identifiable pathology of senile dementia, with vascular or arteriosclerotic disease accounting for less than 20% of the cases. According to Miller (1977), "the diagnosis of arteriosclerotic dementia is only justified where there is evidence of multiple strokes producing sudden exacerbations in the condition as opposed to the relatively smooth and steady decline found in most cases of dementia" (p. 5).

Certain controversies have always surrounded the diagnosis of a "true" dementia. Today, it is generally thought that the Alzheimer's lesion is the chief pathology of most dementias of aging, senile and presenile alike (Terry, 1978). However, controversy surrounds the issue of whether the Alzheimer's disease associated with those under 65 constitutes one or two disease entities. In 1969, the Ciba Foundation held the first Alzheimer's Symposium in London. In the proceedings of that symposium, it is fairly clear that those participating were comfortable distinguishing between *Alzheimer's disease* as a presenile, focal cerebral disease and *senile dementia* as a separate, less specific form of cerebral atrophy that occurs late in life. In 1977, a Workshop Conference on Alzheimer's disease–senile dementia was held in Bethesda, Md. Even though many of the participants were the same, the span of 8 years had changed attitudes. In the proceedings of the 1977 workshop, the participants were far less willing to speak of these two entities as separate diseases, each with separate characteristics and etiologies. In spite of the incidence of the Alzheimer's type of dementias of aging being bimodal, with the age of onset between 40 and 54 and 70 and 84, most participants were unwilling to commit themselves to a two-disease model. Rather, it was suggested that the two be considered and described by using the following terminology: Alzheimer's disease–senile dementia of the Alzheimer's type complex, or the AD-SD complex. This terminology will be used in this chapter.

Another question arises: Are the dementias of aging an extension of or an accelerated version of the normal aging process? On the one hand, the Alzheimer lesion is found on postmortem examination of aging brains among people who are asymptomatic and "normal." On the other hand, some mild physical and mental deterioration seems to accompany the normal aging process. This deterioration is similar to that seen in the dementias of aging but differs in degree. It is currently accepted that the dementias of aging are pathologic processes superimposed on the normal age changes, that cerebral atrophy is not associated with "normal" aging, and that the dementias of aging reflect abnormal aging (Miller, 1977; Katzman, Terry, and Bick, 1978). In reference to mental symptoms, Kral (1978) states that a limited amount of forgetting is a normal part of aging, but this forgetting, which he terms "benign senescent forgetfulness," is different from that seen in the AD-SD complex. The former is an expression of normal physiologic aging of the human brain, and the latter is an expression of cerebral pathology.

The amount of research devoted to the dementias of aging prior to this decade has been minimal. However, it may be beneficial to consider each of the dementias separately, discussing what is known about each and their unique characteristics. The discussion will be divided into (1) the AD-SD complex, (2) other presenile dementias, and (3) other senile dementias.

The AD-SD complex

The Alzheimer's dementias are progressive and degenerative. They are characterized by brain atrophy, particularly in the temporolimbic structures, and certain morphologic brain changes, including cerebral atrophy, neurofibrillary tangles (the Alzheimer's lesion), and "senile" plaques (Sourander and Sjogren, 1970). "These changes occur in the isocortex and allocortex of both cerebral hemispheres and are sometimes seen also in the subcortical grey matter and occasionally the brain stem" (Sourander and Sjogren, 1970, p. 11). These characteristic brain lesions have been fairly extensively studied, but their actual significance is not clearly understood. The concentration of neurofibrillary tangles is correlated to the presence of dementia, with $r=.75$ (Ingvar and others, 1978). In addition, regional cerebral blood flow for patients with the AD-SD complex is restricted in the temporal-parieto-occipital region of the brain. The EEG of patients with the AD-SD complex is usually severely abnormal and becomes progressively worse during the course of the disease (Ingvar and others, 1978).

The usual age of onset for Alzheimer's disease (presenile version) is between 40 and 54. The usual age of onset for senile dementia of the Alzheimer's type is between 70 and 84. Kay and associates (1970) demonstrate that the overall prevalence of the disease increases from 2.3% among those 65 to 69 and 2.8% among those 70 to 74 to 22.0% among those 80 or older. The prognosis of a person diagnosed as having the AD-SD complex is poor. Wang (1978) reports that observed survival after a confirmed diagnosis ranges between 6 and 7 years. Cause of death for those with the AD-SD complex is not clear. Libow (1978) suggests the following possibilities: pneumonia and other infections (the incidence of which he believes is overestimated); neglect by physicians and nurses (benign neglect); family desire to not resuscitate or perform "heroics"; incorrect diagnosis that leads to inappropriate treatment of an underlying pathology; death by an organic brain mechanism related to the Alzheimer's lesion that is yet unknown; overmedication; malnutrition and dehydration; a systemic disease as yet unknown that produces both Alzheimer's dementia and death; and "voodoo" type of death that occurs when the patient "gives up."

The cardinal symptoms of the AD-SD complex include:

1. *Progressive aphasia*, which ranges from simple word-finding difficulties early in the disease to a completely noncommunicative state late in the disease
2. *Progressive apraxia*, which is demonstrated early in the disease by an inability to reproduce pictures in perspective and late in the disease by an inability to perform purposeful activity or to perceive meaning in objects and events
3. *Progressive agnosia*, which usually begins with difficulty recognizing pictures of objects and objects themselves and ranges to an inability to recognize body parts late in the disease
4. *Progressive mnemic disturbances*, beginning with simple problems involving the ability to remember recent events and ranging to profound difficulties with all forms of memory later in the disease

Other intellectual abilities that are progressively affected are reasoning, problem solving, judgment, ability to manipulate numbers, and attention span. Personality changes, emotional lability, and progressive physical deterioration usually accompany the disease process, as do certain neurologic signs, such as astereognosis, loss of a normal reaction to pain, and some abnormal reflexes. Some authors (Sourander and Sjogren, 1970; Constantinidis, 1978; Roth, 1978) believe that the earlier the disease is seen, the more rapid the onset, the quicker the deterioration, and the more serious the disease course. Thus, the presenile version of the AD-SD complex may be viewed as a more malignant form of the disease.

Freemon (1977) describes the types of early complaints that patients with the AD-SD complex present when they are first seen for diagnosis. Two clinical pictures are dominant. He describes these as almost "pure" forms, although most patients display symptoms of both pictures rather than simply one or the other. The first clinical picture is characterized by apathy and withdrawal. Usually, the patient presents himself to the physician as lacking affect, and his family reports occasional emotional outbursts. The patient does not speak unless he is spoken to, and the family reports that the patient "is not quite himself." The second clinical picture is characterized by memory losses and what can be termed a "cocktail party" personality. The patient primarily denies a memory loss and is able to converse on a wide variety of philosophic topics. However, on close assessment, it is apparent that he is completely unable to relate the specifics of what he is discussing. When pressed for actual facts, he is unable to provide them.

Sourander and Sjorgen (1970) relate some of the symptoms seen in the AD-SD complex to brain damage in the region of the temporal lobes and their limbic structures. These symptoms constitute the Klüver-Bucy syndrome and are fairly common as the disease progresses. They include:

1. Visual agnosia, as described before, particularly apparent by the patient's inability to recognize the faces of those significant to him and his own face in the mirror
2. Hyperorality, which is manifested by the patient's tendency to examine and touch objects with his mouth
3. Hypermetamorphosis, which is displayed by the patient's tendency to touch everything in the environment with his hands
4. Loss or diminution of emotions, most usually displayed by apathetic withdrawal or seemingly "dulling" or "taming" of the emotions
5. Hypersexuality, although infrequent, may be displayed by almost violent homosexual, heterosexual, or autosexual activity
6. Profound changes in dietary habits, usually displayed by an uncontrollable appetite and the inability to determine appropriate things to eat. Some pa-

tients must be watched closely, because they attempt to eat flowers, clothing, and other nonfood objects in the environment.

In terminal stages of the AD-SD complex, the patient is usually noncommunicative and assumes an almost "vegetative" state. These patients are usually cachexic, with extreme and rapid decreases in body weight. The weight loss seems unrelated to the amount of food intake or to cancer. The patient becomes prone to dehydration, decubitus formation, and bowel problems. Incontinence is present, usually preceding the terminal stages of the disease. Nursing problems are those associated with the care of a totally dependent, immobilized person during the terminal stage.

Seizure activity, both grand mal and petit mal, is not unusual. Sourander and Sjogren (1970) have observed that grand mal seizures usually occur during the last 6 months of life, with minor seizures much akin to fainting spells occurring much earlier in the disease. Masticatory seizures are also common, manifested by rhythmic chewing, lip smacking, tasting, and lip licking, and are often accompanied by the loss of consciousness. The causes of death, as stated before, are not clearly understood (Sourander and Sjogren, 1970).

Etiology of the AD-SD complex is unknown. Research, however, has revealed some rather interesting risk factors that are related to the complex; further study may lead to the determination of cause. The risk factors listed in the proceedings of the 1977 Workshop Conference on Alzheimer's disease–senile dementia, by Katzman, Terry, and Bick (1978), are:

1. *Genetic risk factors*. It is well known that the incidence of the disease is increased for near relatives of patients. Jarvik (1978) reports from the Slater and Cowie data (1971) that the risk of the AD-SD complex in the general population is around 1%, whereas the risk of the siblings of an AD-SD complex patient is 3.8% and the risk for the patient's parents is 10%. Constantinidis (1978) and Sourander and Sjogren (1970) have reported similar incidences among relatives of patients. There is also a known correlation between Down's sydrome and the AD-SD complex. Many persons with Down's syndrome develop the disease, and frequently, the two diseases are found in the same families. Constantinidis (1978) has proposed a dominant gene transmission theory for cases between generations and a recessive gene theory for cases within a generation. Although researchers believe the genetic factors interact with environmental factors to produce the disease, the genetic factors alone and chromosomal abnormalities warrant further investigation (Katzman, Terry, and Bick, 1978).

2. *Increased brain aluminum concentrations*. Patients with the AD-SD complex have a several-fold increase in the amount of aluminum found in the brain tissue. This amount seems to be related to the number of neurofibrillary tangles present in the brain. In addition, it is known that aluminum poisoning of the central nervous system leads to other progressive encephalopathies with symptoms similar to the AD-SD complex. However, the role of aluminum in the body, its mode of excretion, and the way in which it is deposited in brain tissue are poorly understood, and the exact significance of increased aluminum levels in the AD-SD complex is unknown (Crapper, Karlik, and deBoni, 1978).

3. *Latent viral infections*. It has been suggested that the AD-SD complex is related to some type of a slow, viral brain infection. However, the results of experiments in which the brain tissue of AD-SD complex patients has been innoculated into nonhuman primates and other mammals have been inconclusive. Most of these experiments have not produced disease. Wisniewski (1978) reports that when tissue of two patients with familial Alzheimer's disease were innoculated into nonhuman primates, a disease was induced with symptoms similar to Alzheimer's disease. On autopsy, however, the animal's brain tissue showed no resemblance to Alzheimer's. Actually, the tissue was more consistent with

the picture presented by Jakob-Creutzfeldt disease, which has a substantiated viral origin. Nonetheless, the area of viral infection certainly warrants further investigation.

4. *Immunologic factors*. Two research studies have contributed to the idea that the AD-SD complex may be immunologic in origin. First, there is a direct correlational relationship between serum immunologic levels and tests of cognition (Eisdorfer, Cohen, and Buckley, 1978). Although to date this finding is nothing more than an association and not a cause-and-effect relationship, the relationship appears curvilinear. For normal healthy elderly people, the serum immunoglobulin levels are low and the cognitive test scores are high. As the immunoglobulin levels increase, there is a concomitant decrease in test scores. At a certain point, the test scores and the serum immunoglobulin levels continue to decrease, with the result that at both ends of the scale the serum levels are low. This suggests two possible hypotheses (Eisdorfer, Cohen, and Buckley, 1978). Either the relationship is truly curvilinear, with both ends of the scale being a part of the same continuum, or there are two independent processes operating. In this latter case, it may be that normal people have relatively low levels of serum immunoglobulin and respond with increasing amounts to stressful conditions; exactly the reverse is true for the AD-SD patient. Eisdorfer, Cohen, and Buckley (1978) suggest that even though serum immunoglobulin levels are crude measurements, the findings are promising as an area for new research. In addition, they point out that these findings do not preclude the possibility of viral infection causing the changes in serum immunoglobulins.

The second research finding involves the discovery of brain-reactive antibodies in aging animals and humans (Nandy, 1978). It may be that the neuronal loss found among aging people and those with the AD-SD is related to an autoimmune reaction. It is postulated that this autoimmune reaction is humoral in type, which roughly means the body perceives a portion of its own tissue (in this case, brain tissue) as antigenic and produces antibodies to destroy the "foreign" material. Glenner, Ein, and Terry (1972) suggest that the senile plaques found in the brains of people with the AD-SD complex are actually phagocytized and degraded antigen-antibody complexes that have been deposited in the brain. Although this area appears promising, the research supporting this hypothesis is scant.

5. *Neurotransmitters*. On postmortem examination of the brains of AD-SD complex patients, Davies (1978) found the activity of choline acetylase and acetylcholinesterase significantly reduced in several brain regions. The regions most affected by this reduction are the hippocampus, midtemporal gyrus, parietal cortex, convex frontal cortex, and orbital frontal cortex. Since the cortical cholinergic system involves neurotransmission and is concerned with the speed and efficiency with which nerve impulses move between cortical neurons, decreases in activity in critical regions of the brain could account for some of the symptoms seen in the AD-SD complex. It is not known, however, whether the decreases observed are the result of a primary deficiency or of an underlying pathologic process, such as a viral infection or an autoimmune reaction. In addition, the study of neurotransmitters following death is difficult. It is not known to what degree neurotransmitters retain their stability during the postmortem period or to what degree the type and time of death affects the amount of neurotransmitters present at death. Nevertheless, neuropharmacologic investigations of the cortical choline system and other neurotransmitters, some of which may be unidentified, will be further studied in the future as a possible cause of the AD-SD complex.

To summarize, in spite of the Alzheimer-type dementia of aging being first described by Alois Alzheimer in 1906, little knowledge has been gained in the intervening years. Until the last 15 years, little research effort or money has been focused on the AD-SD complex. This is partially because a high degree of sophistication in equipment and laboratory techniques is necessary to perform brain research, and these have only begun to be available. In addition, little interest in gerontologic research in any form has been generated until the last 20 years. The investigation of the AD-SD complex is still in its infancy. Researchers and clinicians are still struggling to determine the origin of the disease, the potential for treatment, reversal, and prevention, and the proper modes of management during the disease course. More information is needed on differential diagnosis, with even more concise descriptions of the disease process. With the new upsurge of interest, it may be possible in the future to give the proper attention that clients with AD-SD complex so sorely need (see Appendix A).

Other presenile dementias
Pick's disease

In many ways Pick's disease is almost indistinguishable from the AD-SD complex. Differentiation, however, is made by many researchers and clinicians based on postmortem neuropathology and early clinical symptomatology. Like the AD-SD complex, Pick's disease is characterized by cerebral atrophy, but the atrophy is usually confined to the frontotemporal regions of the cerebral cortex and may be mild in comparison to the atrophy seen in the AD-SD complex (Ingvar and others, 1978). McHugh (1971) states that Pick's disease is microscopically characterized by the "Pick cell," which is a degenerated neuron swollen into a ballooned form. These Pick cells are found in the atrophied areas of the cortex. In addition, senile plaques and neurofibrillary tangles characteristic of the AD-SD complex may be found in other portions of the brain. In Pick's disease, the regional cerebral blood flow is most reduced in the frontal and anterior temporal regions of the brain (Ingvar and others, 1978).

Clinical symptomatology is often described as focal in nature, using the words "frontal lobe syndrome." The early symptoms of Pick's disease include insidious but profound personality changes, such as emotional blunting, disinhibition, lack of insight, and lack of social awareness (Ingvar and others, 1978; Roth, 1978). Early in the disease, intellectual and language functions may not be affected at all. As the disease progresses, however, more global deterioration may be noted (Roth, 1978). Memory disturbances begin to appear, as well as language disturbances. These language disturbances usually include progressive and expressive aphasia, mutism, or rapid voluble speech. Spatial abilities seem to remain fairly well intact throughout the course of the disease, and the EEG remains essentially normal (Ingvar and others, 1978). Physical and mental deterioration is progressive.

The usual age of onset for Pick's disease is in the mid-fifties. By comparison, the incidence of Pick's disease is far less frequent than the AD-SD complex. Jellinger (1976) reports that only 2.3% of the subjects in his sample had the neuropathologic configuration of Pick's disease, whereas the AD-SD complex was confirmed in 52.8% of the cases. Terry (1970) stated in the 1969 Ciba Symposium on Alzheimer's disease that he estimated Alzheimer's disease was about one hundred times more common than Pick's disease in New York. The geographic distinction was made because some authors have reported a far higher incidence of Pick's disease in Sweden than in other places (Sourander and Sjogren, 1970). Prognosis for a person with a diagnosis of Pick's disease is poor, with an expected life span of about 7 years after diagnosis (Miller, 1977). A higher incidence of Pick's disease has been reported among relatives who have died with the disease, indicating that there may be a genetic predisposition (Miller, 1977).

Huntington's chorea

This disease is a progressive, degenerative disease characterized by both physical and mental deterioration. The major neuropathology of Huntington's chorea is marked atrophy of nerve cells in the caudate nuclei, the putamen, and the pallidum. As the disease progresses, there may be atrophy of the frontal regions of cerebral cortex (Curtis, Jacobson, and Marcus, 1972). The most outstanding characteristic in the early stages is choreitic movements. Usually, intellectual impairments and emotional disturbances denoting dementia are seen slightly later, but this pattern may be reversed (Yahr, 1971). Albert (1978) categorizes the dementia seen in Huntington's chorea as subcortical, although he acknowledges that cortical lesions are also seen with this disease. A subcortical dementia is most typified by personality changes, ranging from apathy to violent emotional outbursts, memory disorders, inability to solve problems and process information rapidly, and impaired concept formation. With the pure subcortical dementias there are no language disturbances. However, because cortical lesions are sometimes found with Huntington's chorea, language disturbances may eventually be present.

The usual age of onset for Huntington's chorea is between 35 and 50. There is a confirmed genetic basis, with the disease transmitted by a dominant autosomal gene. The disease may be transmitted by either sex and affects both sexes equally. It is transmitted from the affected person to the offspring; usually, those in a family who are asymptomatic do not carry the disease (Yahr, 1971). Because of its familial nature, the differential diagnosis of dementia related to Huntington's chorea is usually not difficult to make. The life span of a person diagnosed with this disease is about 15 years (Yahr, 1971).

Jakob-Creutzfeldt disease or Cruetzfeldt-Jakob disease (CJD)

CJD can be distinguished from other presenile dementias by several factors. First, its onset is extremely rapid. As described by McHugh (1971), the patient first notices motor or sensory disturbances. There may be combinations of any of the following symptoms: visual disturbances, hearing disturbances, decreased muscle strength, and difficulty with coordinated movements. The patient deteriorates rapidly. Within weeks he may be experiencing blindness, deafness, severe ataxia, and hemiplegia and may be displaying myoclonus and tremors. The onset of dementia is concurrent and equally as rapid. The dementia includes progressive language, emotional, and intellectual disturbances, depending on which regions of the cerebral cortex are affected. The patient may deteriorate within 4 to 8 months, becoming totally bedfast with decerebrate symptoms

Second, the neuropathology involved is distinctive. There is destruction of neurons in the cerebral cortex. The astrocytes hypertrophy and proliferate, and many become vacuolated and filled with cellular debris. There is disruption of the regular cellular structure of the cortex and an "overgrowth" of glia or the supporting tissue of the brain. As a result of these changes, the cerebral cortex takes on a sponge-like appearance. The cerebellum and the basal ganglia may be involved in the pathologic changes as well (McHugh, 1971; Gibbs and Gajdusek, 1978).

Third, some of the most exciting research done to date on the dementias of aging has been done with CJD. It is one of the few dementias of aging for which a documented viral agent has been identified. The brain tissue of CJD patients has been inoculated into primates, resulting in similar symptoms and similar brain changes after an incubation period between 11 and 14 months. Gajdusek and others (1977) report that of their 122 CJD patients whose brain tissue was inoculated into primates at least 3 years ago, 70% have transmitted the disease. They are in the process of attempting to isolate the causative organism from the brain tissue of the affected primates. These two researchers also report that the CJD virus has been found in the lymph nodes, lungs, liver, kidneys, and cerebrospinal fluid of human patients. Identifying a virus as the causative agent for CJD, however, does not mean that either prevention or treatment is available. These are still being studied.

The prospect of CJD being transmitted by a slow virus brings to mind the possibility of person-to-person transmission of the disease. There is absolutely no reason to suspect, at this point, that personnel are being exposed to the risk of infection during the course of administering nursing or medical care (Gajdusek and others, 1977; Gibbs, 1978). However, they caution that during invasive procedures, such as biopsies and spinal taps, care should be taken to terminally disinfect the equipment, and good technique should be used during the procedure. Reasonable care also needs to be taken with specimens. They recommend autoclaving the equipment to completely inactivate the viral agent. In addition, Gajdusek and others (1977) recommend that those who perform postmortem examinations of CJD patients should wear scrub suits, double gloves, and face masks and that these should be terminally sterilized or destroyed after the procedure. Care must be taken with specimens taken during the autopsy, as well as with the instruments and the autopsy space.

The question of human-to-human transmission has also been raised by those who question the possibility of hematogenic spread of the infection (Maneulidis, Gorgacz, and Manuelidis, 1978). These authors believe it is conceivable that there is danger of the disease being spread by the transfusion of human blood from an infected, asymptomatic donor to a recipient, but this has not been demonstrated clinically. Duffy and others (1974) report the apparent human-to-human transmission by the transplantation of a cornea from an asymptomatic infected person to a recipient. As more is known about CJD, there will be more definitive information along these lines.

Like the other presenile dementias of aging, the incidence of CJD is actually very low. CJD is far less common than the AD-SD complex, Pick's disease, or Huntington's chorea. The usual time of onset for CJD is during middle age; however, cases of CJD have been reported among people as young as 20. The course of the disease is unrelentingly downward, and the expected outcome is death. However, the current research being conducted on CJD holds promise for understanding not only this dementia of aging, but several others as well.

Normal pressure hydrocephalus (NPH)

First described in 1965 (Adams and others, 1965; Hakim and Adams, 1965) NPH affects about 5% to 6% of the patients who have a presenile dementia (Katzman, 1978). Katzman projects that between 4,000 and 14,000 people in the entire United States are affected by the disease. The cardinal symptoms of NPH are a wide-based gait disturbance, disturbances of intellect, memory, and emotions, and urinary incontinence unaccompanied by embarrassment (Freemon, 1977). Frontal lobe signs may also be present, including emotional blunting and abnormal reflexes.

In differentiating NPH from the presenile version of the AD-SD complex, it is important to know that the gait disturbance is usually the first sign of NPH, whereas memory disturbances usually appear first with the AD-SD complex (Katzman, 1978). In addition, many of the patients with the AD-SD complex have severely enlarged ventricles similar to those with NPH. However, when patients with the AD-SD complex are treated with shunting, the results are not favorable, and Katzman (1978) believes that the risks involved in the misdiagnosis of NPH and incorrect surgical intervention are great. As a result, the need for more precise medical diagnostic procedures is evident.

Neurosyphilis (also dementia paralytica or general paresis)

If primary syphilis is untreated or inadequately treated, a certain number of patients will display the complication known as neurosyphilis or dementia paralytica. This complication appears from 2 to 30 years following the primary lesion and usually occurs between the ages of 30 and 60. Neurosyphilis affects more men than women, at a rate of about 3:1. Dementia paralytica is a true dementia in that the usual presenting symptoms are impaired memory, faulty judgment, paranoia, and disturbed emotional displays. In addition, the patient usually displays abnormal reflexes, fine and course tremors, dysarthria, and occasionally, convulsive disorders (Dodge, 1971).

The pathology involves cerebral atrophy that is most pronounced in the frontal and anterior temporal lobes of the brain, with characteristic deposition of iron pigments. The presence of spirochetes can usually be demonstrated in the cerebral cortex (Curtis, 1972). The spinal fluid of persons with neurosyphilis is always abnormal, and in most cases spinal fluid reacts positively to a reagin text for syphilis. Dodge (1971) states that about 90% of the patients will have a positive blood serology as well.

Early identification and treatment of the person with neurosyphilis result in an arrest of the disease process. However, if not treated early, the resulting dementia resembles the other presenile dementias in every way. The patient becomes progressively impaired intellectually and physically. Terminal stages are characterized by physical debilitation and a bedridden state. Untreated, this disease is usually fatal within 3 years of onset (Dodge, 1971).

Other senile dementias
Arteriosclerotic dementia or Multiinfarct dementia

Multiinfarct dementia is present in 10% (Heyman, 1978) to 20% (Terry, 1978) of the patients over 60 who display the symptoms of dementia. In addition, another 18% of these patients have a "mixed" form of dementia, displaying the pathology of both the AD-SD complex and multiinfarct dementia. Although the differential diagnosis between these two diseases is at times difficult, many authors think the differentiation can be made based on presenting symptoms and history of onset. Roth (1978) believes arteriosclerotic dementia is characterized by an abrupt onset and specific neurologic signs. Sudden onset of aphasia, agnosia, and apraxia, for example, usually indicates multiinfarct dementia, not the AD-SD complex. Focal symptoms, such as constructional apraxia, acalculia, and alexia with an otherwise well-preserved intelligence, also usually indicate multiinfarct dementia. Preservation of social behaviors and personal habits in the presence of isolated memory and intellectual losses is associated with this dementia, whereas both of these are progressively impaired in the AD-SD complex. In addition, multiinfarct dementia may have an intermittent course rather than the steadily progessive deterioration seen with the AD-SD complex. Hypertension is a usual and significant finding with multiinfarct dementia (Roth, 1978). A great number of the patients with this dementia display concurrent motor deficits that are usually not seen with the AD-SD complex (Scheinberg, 1978). In short, the problem of multiinfarct dementia occurs with strokes or cerebrovascular accidents rather than with the mystifying causes of AD-SD complex.

The neuropathology seen in multiinfarct dementia is multiple cystic infarcts called lacunes scattered throughout the regions of the brain (Scheinberg, 1978). These infarcts are thought to arise from emboli released from other sites in the body; they result in the death and softening of brain tissue. The actual cause of the dementia itself is not clearly understood. Lacunes are seen in the brains of people who are asymptomatic for dementia but who have hypertension and arteriosclerotic disease (Fisher, 1965; Heyman, 1978). In the Fisher study, 10% of the 1000 people autopsied had lacunes, but only about one fifth of these had any sign of dementia. It may be, however, that the area or the volume of infarcted tissue is related to the dementia and not to the simple presence of lacunes (Roth, 1978; Terry, 1978).

That multiinfarct dementia is intimately related to both cerebrovascular accidents and hypertension cannot be overemphasized. From the standpoint of prevention, the treatment of hypertension is essential. Although not studying multiinfarct dementia in particular, Eisdorfer (1977) showed a relationship between untreated hypertension and intelligence among elderly persons. With a diastolic blood pressure over 105 mm Hg, there was a significant decline in intelligence over 10 years for those subjects between 60 and 69 years of age. No such decline was noted among the normotensive subjects, and a slight increase in intelligence was noted for those who were slightly hypertensive. It would seem that treating severe hypertension may be as important for the prevention of this one dementia of aging as it is for the prevention of cerebrovascular accidents.

Current medical therapies for the dementias of aging

With the new research interest in the dementias of aging, new forms of therapy have been devised that have shown some success. A few of these will be briefly discussed.

Chemotherapy

Among the most frequently used medical therapies for the dementias of aging are drugs. These drugs basically fall into four categories: vasodilators and anticoagulants, psychotropic agents, nootropic agents, and experimental drugs.

Vasodilators and anticoagulants. There is evidence that with the normal aging process there is a decline in cerebral blood flow (Scheinberg, 1978). When one of the dementias is superimposed on this normal occurrence, the blood flow may be diminished even more. However, the timing of the diminished blood flow in the disease course differs, depending on the diagnosis. With arteriosclerotic dementia, the probability is that the reduction in blood flow precipitates the dementia. Hence, the reduced blood flow is noted early in the disease. With the AD-SD complex, there is evidence that the reverse is true, with reduced blood flow secondary to the neuronal changes (Terry, 1977) and seen much later in the disease course. There has never been a question about the use of vasodilators or anticoagulants among those with documented arteriosclerotic dementia. The success of this treatment with this group of patients has been noteworthy (Fine and others, 1970; Young, Hall, and Blakemore, 1974; Miller, 1977). However, controversy exists regarding the use of these drugs with the AD-SD patient, since a primary reduction in blood flow is not the cause of the disease. Nevertheless, Ball and Taylor (1967) demonstrated a positive effect with the use of vasodilators with a nonspecified group of dementia patients, some of which undoubtedly had the AD-SD complex. Walsh, Walsh, and Melaney (1978) have shown the positive effects of using anticoagulants with both types of dementia. In the future, the use of these drugs with both types of dementia patients may be quite common.

Psychotropic agents. Among elderly people, the psychiatric symptoms associated with dementia respond well to a chemotherapeutic approach. Major tranquilizers, such as chlorpromazine and thioridazine, and minor tranquilizers, such as diazepam and chlordiazepoxide, can be used to treat agitation, irritability, and aggression. The insomnia displayed by many patients with dementia responds well to methyprylon, methaqualone, or even diazepam. Depression, which is the most common psychiatirc problem among the elderly and which often mimics dementia, responds well to antidepressants such as doxepin. Lethargy and apathy sometimes respond to psychostimulants, such as methylphenidate or pentylenetetrazol, but these often produce anxiety, restlessness, and insomnia. They may even aggravate or induce psychotic symptoms among those patients who did not previously have them. For these reasons, the use of psychostimulants is questionable.

Caffeine may be as good as any of the psychostimulants in treating lethargy and does not appear to have any of the problematic side effects of the other drugs. For psychotic symptoms, elderly people respond quite well to major tranquilizers; however, they are more prone to the side effects of postural hypotension and tardive dyskinesia than younger patients. The use of these drugs must be carefully monitored. (For an excellent discussion of the use of psychotropic agents with the geriatric patient, please refer to Lehmann [1977] and to Chapter 9 in this book.)

Nootropic agents. This group of drugs is the so-called mind-acting drugs. One in the group, piracetam, has been used successfully in clinical trials to reduce confusion, improve "demented" behavior, and improve mental performance by selectively acting on the telencephalic integrative mechanism of the brain. Piracetam appears to have no toxic side effects and few effects on arousal levels, autonomic functions, and psychomotor behavior (Lehmann, 1977). Others in this group are Hydergine, centrophenoxim, and naftidrofuryl. These are thought to increase glucose metabolism in the brain, increase cerebral blood flow, and improve brain cellular metabolism. Although relatively new, these drugs hold great promise for the future treatment of confusional states among the elderly (Lehmann, 1977).

Experimental drugs. Substitute therapy for decreases in neurotransmitters is the primary focus of investigations with experimental drugs. Currently, the administration of L-dopa has been attempted as a treatment for the AD-SD complex, with varying degress of success (Drachman and Stahl, 1975; Kristensen, Olsen, and Theilgaard, 1977). The administration of choline substitutes has been attempted by many groups of researchers, again with varying degrees of success (Kolata, 1979). Even though the success in improving behavior and decreasing confusion has been variable, these drugs may offer exciting new therapies for the dementias of aging in the future.

Individual psychotherapy

Much has been said about the benefits of psychotherapeutic group work with patients with the dementias of aging. Little appears in the literature about the benefits of individual psychotherapy. Walsh, Walsh, and Melaney (1978) report a great deal of success with the use of individual psychotherapy in combination with anticoagulant therapy. They suggest that such therapy sessions should be focused on the life review.

This approach constitutes a mental form of "physiotherapy" that stimulates areas of the brain that have not been used for sometime by the patient. In the past, many mental health workers have avoided the patient with a dementia of aging on the premise that they cannot reverse or ameliorate an organic process. With the new chemotherapeutic agents combined with individual psychotherapy, different rates of success may be seen.

Surgical intervention

As indicated previously in this chapter and in Chapter 9, there has been success with "shunting" procedures on patients who have normal pressure hydrocephalus. Surgical intervention with other forms of the dementias of aging has not been as successful.

Hyperbaric oxygen

Exposing patients with symptoms of a dementia of aging to 100% oxygen at a pressure of 2.5 atmospheres over a period of 15 days has been shown to be effective in the treatment of the symptoms (Jacobs and others, 1969). However, the response to this treatment is transient, and the treatment is poorly received by many patients. Some experiments have resulted in no responses at all. Although investigations continue in this area, this treatment may not hold as much promise as some of the others.

Although presently chemotherapy holds great promise for the future, the treatment of patients with the "true" dementias of aging remains basically a nursing problem. The nursing treatments found to be helpful will be discussed in the rest of this chapter.

PROVIDING A FACILITATIVE ENVIRONMENT FOR THE ELDERLY PATIENT WITH A TRUE DEMENTIA

The course of the true dementias is a progressive deterioration of the ability to remember, to communicate, to make judgments, and to be independent in daily living. Although some theories have been expressed as to cause, they are not helpful enough to propose any treatment. The result is a patient with a diagnosis that has no available treatment at this time. The caregiver cannot offer cure, but care is needed in increasing amounts over the remainder of the patient's life. We term this care *providing a facilitative environment*. It is based on the concept that care will be provided at the time it is needed and will be of the quality and quantity that will enable the patient with true dementia to live to the best of his abilities at any of the stages of his disease. The course of the disease may be progressive deterioration, but it starts mildly, and its progression may be delayed by appropriate supportive action or hastened by events that add stress to the patient already bewildered at the failure of his own mind.

We have been concerned throughout this book with the need for accurate assessments, prevention of confusional states, and intervention of nursing actions that aid in recovery. We have dealt with physiologic

---

Guidelines for providing a facilitative environment for the elderly patient with true dementia

1. Make change very slowly. The patient must be well prepared for any physical, emotional, drug, nutritional, personnel, or geographic change.
2. Keep the patient ambulatory as long as possible with daily exercise routine, including a walk in the sunshine.
3. Maintain a routine. A dependable world and a structured existence and environment are essential.
4. Provide social stimulation without overload. Maintain communication through every possible channel.
5. Avoid crowds or large spaces without boundaries. Avoid sensory overload.
6. Assist in organizing the personal aspects of the client's affairs—safekeeping of treasures, obtaining legal aid of attorney or ombudsman, and setting up file of personal papers.
7. Monitor use of health measures, including good nutrition, attention to mouth and teeth, and adequate shoes. Avoid the use of drugs.
8. Do not expect the patient to understand or participate in complex activities or conversations.
9. Maintain positive input, such as reinforcement for any worthy act, to maintain the patient's self-esteem and encourage self-participation in activities of daily living.
10. Ensure that information is available to the patient about the time and place landmarks that provide reality (Fig. 13-1)—calendars with huge figures, clocks with all numbers for the hours, reality boards for institutions, and reminders of special events such as birthdays, anniversaries, and holidays.
11. Make bowel and bladder control consistent, using a routine. As the patient's mind becomes more hazy, use clothing with simple fasteners, or elastic waistbands for pants.
12. Support the family, who in turn support the patient, by simple reinforcement of their efforts with a special commendation. Respite care from the daily watching may enable them to care for the patient in the home and visit him in the institution long after internal rewards have ceased to exist.

problems, sensory problems, and stress-related problems. This chapter is concerned with a state that cannot be prevented and for which the goal is to prevent complications. However, the patient with true dementia has the same sensory, physiologic, and stress-related problems of any other older person, and acute confusional states may be superimposed on his developing true dementia. There is no skill, attitude, or knowledge referred to in this book that does not apply to the elderly patient with true dementia. He may survive an acute confusional state and continue on the relentless course of the true dementia. At some point family, friends, employer, or coworker will recognize that he is no longer able to function as before. At that time the facilitative environment will have to be initiated to allow him to live independently or semiindependently for an extended period.

The second part of this chapter is concerned with the caregiver's role in providing the facilitative physical and social environment during the four stages of the course of the true dementias. These stages are marked by the patient's increasing difficulty in maintaining an independent existence and his increasing need for help from others. The early, advanced, later, and terminal or final stages require a total adjustment of life-style, affiliations, personal habits, health care monitoring, and exercise-rest patterns, including time in the sunshine and sleep at night. During each stage the patient is studied in relation to his family and their ability to cope with the increasing burden of care and understanding.

General principles have been given throughout this book that also apply to the elderly patient with a true dementia, but in the guidelines on p. 332 specific information is added for this special person and his particular circumstances.

Early stage of dementia

Quayhagen (1977) has identified the observable behaviors in the early stages of dementia as:
1. Difficulty in focusing attention on important events
2. Declining interest in the environment and present affairs
3. Indifference to ceremonies and courtesies of social life
4. Forgetting to use nouns in speech (may not be able to recall)
5. Vague, uncertain, and hesitant in initiating action

The patient with a family

At this stage the patient who has a family member or living arrangement that is fairly protective can manage. His behavior may bewilder the caregiver since often a strong, decisive person becomes unable to manage

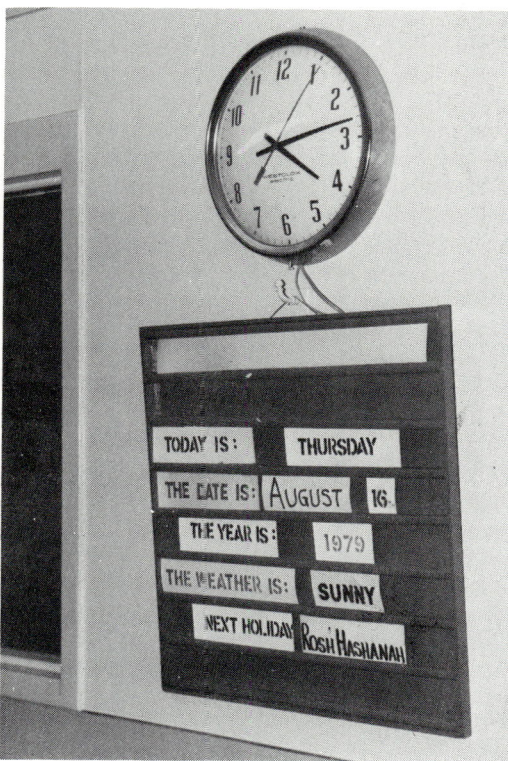

Fig. 13-1. Reality board and highly visible clock. (Photograph by C. D. Falk.)

his own affairs. The nurse should assess the strengths of the family to cope with the behavior and reinforce the members who must accept an additional burden of care. When she comes into the home where the care is shared by several, it is wise to help the family plan a division of labor; Chapter 14 suggests a *primary caregiver* and a *secondary caregiver*. One person must have the responsibility for making the final decisions about the patient and must hold this position with the cooperation and consent of the others. Often the nurse, as an outsider, can help arrange a network of services. It is essential at this time to make sure that proper legal authorities are contacted to handle finances, endorse and sign checks, and make necessary payments. Families have much hesitancy in approaching this. Often, by talking with the patient the nurse realizes he is concerned about managing his affairs, and she can speak directly to him about the legal needs and assist in initiating action. It is important to be sensitive to the metaphoric language used by the patient in speaking of threatening matters.

The family should be approached very honestly about the prognosis. It is the physician's responsibility to make a diagnosis and confer with the family. The elderly spouse should be kept informed as the patient moves from one stage to another. If the physician shirks this duty, the nurse must help the family understand. The family members should be assembled to face the reality together so family strengths can be identified and used for planning. The slowly developing crisis ahead will tax the emotional and physical assets of all members, as shown in the case study at the beginning of this chapter.

The person observed in the early stages of true dementias should have his medical and social service record flagged. Prevention can prolong this stage for some time. Often, however, the person comes to the attention of health caregivers through an automobile accident, a health problem caused by neglect in such everyday practices as eating, or a simple injury or infection, any of which may have magnified the problem.

The patient who lives alone

For the elderly person who lives alone, the nurse will have to assess the total situation, determining what friends are available and which neighbors will watch; setting up routines to maintain health status; and finally, providing organizing mechanisms in the patient's life. Bills have to be paid, records kept, checks cashed, and money spent. Early in the disease, such organization can be a shoe-box file system with separately marked shoe boxes for insurance policies, tax receipts, bills, and letters. A heavy, black marking pen can be used to make a list on a large piece of cardboard of names, addresses, and telephone numbers most likely to be needed. This should be hung above the telephone, which is also placed in an accessible position (Fig. 13-2), and triplicate lists placed in two other prominent places and in the purse or wallet. An identification bracelet with name, address, and telephone number is an appropriate gift. Identification and phone number must be fastened onto the ambulatory patient. The purse or billfold should be checked for adequate identification data, including any medical diagnoses and medications.

The elderly person living alone and showing signs of the early stage should be known to the police, fire department, and mail carrier. Often, working through the patient's friends or family makes it possible to set up the legal processes that will take over when necessary. A community agency conservator should be aware of such matters as bank accounts, income sources, safety deposit boxes, and important papers and property. Someone has to take the responsibility of making arrangements when the patient slips into the more advanced stage. Libow and Zicklin (1973) propose the penultimate will (the next-to-last will, to be used in life when the patient is unable to function) as a means to protect the mentally deteriorated elderly.

Care of the patient with a true dementia 335

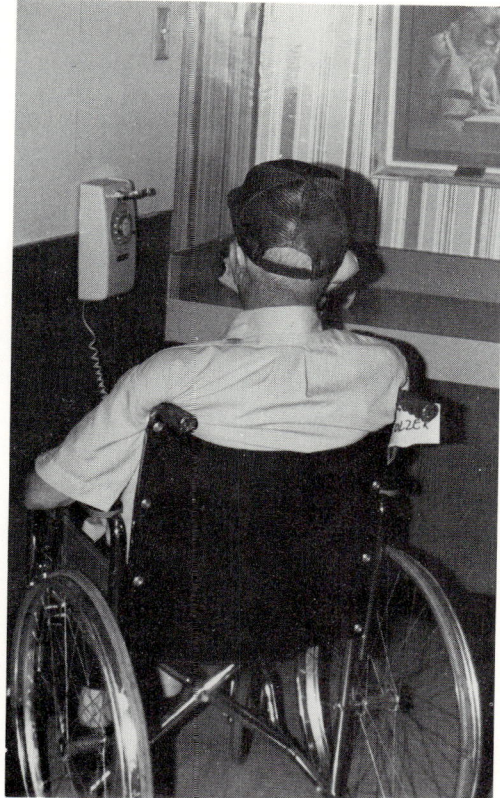

Fig. 13-2. Placement of telephone facilitates its use. (Photograph by C. D. Falk.)

This is made when a person is in possession of all his faculties. It should name the person who is to take charge if and when incapacitation occurs. No elderly person should be without one.

The home should be assessed for safety factors, including such items as visibility of the wall thermostat, provision for night lighting, arrangements for cooking, fire hazards, and number of cubbyholes and hiding places. Elderly people in the early stages of dementia have a habit of putting things away in safe places that can never be located. Logical safe places include the insides of books, covered dishes, and dresser drawers. Setting up a file system helps, even if shoe boxes or pocketed notebooks are used to separate papers. Everyone has important papers that need to be accessible in a safe place.

Advanced stage of dementia

Behaviors observed in the advanced state include:

1. Shows obvious defects in memory, retention, and recall
2. Hesitates in response to questions
3. Displays disorientation as to time; confuses night and day
4. Complains of neglect
5. Resents interference of younger people (Quayhagen, 1977)
6. Loses important papers; loses way home in familiar community; forgets to pay bills; lets housekeeping chores slip and newspapers pile up; does not dispose of garbage; and does not take medications
7. Forgets appointments, usual organizational meeting dates, and holidays and birthdays
8. Loses possessions and claims that they have been stolen; may name person who took them
9. Unable to retain simple directions
10. Neglects use of health and hygiene measures

The patient in the home

The person in the advanced stage of a true dementia who is living at home is no longer a simple problem. The family usually feels stress and often falls apart rather than pulling together in the face of progressive deterioration. Family members must assume some kind of 24-hour guard to ensure that poor judgment does not cause the patient to perform some act that will endanger himself and others. Matches are hidden from the cigarette smoker, the kitchen stove is checked often for lighted or unlit burners, and nights become nightmares as the patient forgets where he is and what time it is. He may walk away from home during this time. He is often disheveled and forgets to change his clothing, take baths, or tend to grooming needs. Such health care as dental visits and shoe repair are overlooked until noted by family members.

Families need social agencies to help cope during this period when they tend to become exhausted and angry. The nurse may be able to marshall the resources to create a helping network for the family. Hirschfield (1978) studied 30 families living with an older person diagnosed as suffering from chronic brain syndrome with mild to severe mental impairment. She found that in those families where the impaired member was able to give some positive meaning to the caregiver, regardless of cognitive decline, family life seemed tolerable. Where the impaired person was seen as a burden only, the stress was overwhelming. Families coped by use of internal rewards such as, "She smiled at me today," or "I think he knows who I am," which gave a sense of being loved and needed by the impaired person. And they valued external rewards such as a comment by the visiting nurse, "You take wonderful care of him."

Families who find the patient a burden are less likely to watch his fluid intake, nutrition, and activity needs. These families should be helped either to find relief in their situation or to decide to place the patient in an institution. The latter is not easy, and Chapter 14 goes into the problems that arise. Conway (1978) tells the story of the family confronted with this decision and of the anguish when the patient is institutionalized but unwilling to leave his family. She believes that long after the patient has adjusted, the family is still struggling with guilt. For the elderly person in the advanced stage of dementia, care at home may be almost impossible.

The patient who lives alone

For the elderly person living alone in the advanced stage of true dementia, living is too costly in mental and physical terms. Stories of recluses are told in newspapers, and neighbors bear a sense of guilt as they realize the elderly confused person they had not seen died or become ill from inability to care for basic physical needs. When hospitalized, personnel recognize that the patient can no longer take care of even simple needs. Unfortunately, relocation is often the final straw that sends the patient into the later stage or final stage, but there is no alternative. He cannot live alone.

The later stage of dementia

Behaviors observed in the later stage include:
1. Disorientation as to place; wanders aimlessly, gets lost, and loses way to bathroom
2. Loses possessions
3. Disorientation as to person; forgets personnel, misidentifies personnel as familiar person, may not recognize familiar person, develops illusions
4. Deterioration in motor ability; writing deteriorates to illegible scribble; problems in dressing, eating, and getting to the toilet
5. Sexual exposure; immodesty (Quayhagen, 1977)
6. No time sense; cannot recall meals or earlier event in day
7. Communication difficulties; incoherent, forgets words; nonverbal language principal means of communication (Bartol, 1979)

The patient in the home

The patient in the home now needs total care from his caregivers. Inability to attend to the physiologic and health demands of the body often means the person is bedridden. The family can still offer the patient support through social interaction, touch, and sensory stimulation. Their own rewards will be fewer, and care becomes more of a burden. The chance of illness from infection or pneumonia increases; nutritional problems are very likely unless the nurse is able to assist the family in setting up a plan for meeting all physiologic needs. If the caregiver is an aging spouse, the nurse becomes one of a team to support the decision to change the burden of care to an institution. The move to an institution subtracts from the advantages the familiar surroundings offered. While the patient was in his own home, the home environment was a *facilitative component* of care. For the patient in the advanced or later stages in an institution, the facilitative environment is both social and physical but may become a liability that can push the patient into the more advanced stage if he is relocated.

Example. The 70-year-old woman was barely able to manage her activities of daily living in a home she shared with a younger woman who took care of all the homemaking duties. When the younger woman had surgery, the 70-year-old, who was in the advanced stage of true dementia, was taken to a nice personal care home. She had a private room and many comforts, with her family pictures and memorabilia of her past surrounding her. She went into the later stage of true dementia almost immediately and had to be moved to a secure unit because she made no adjustment whatsoever. She no longer recognized the younger housemate. The transition took less than 10 days.

The move to the institution may result in an early death. On the other hand, for the recluse who is starved and neglected, the institution may offer return to a much better state of being. The advanced and later stages do not have clearly differentiated boundaries. The environment of the institution is the critical element in maintenance; medical treatment has almost nothing to offer at this point, except when physiologic problems are encountered, such as cardiac problems, infections (especially in the urinary tract), and injuries requiring treatment. At this stage, as in earlier ones, the geriatric nurse practitioner is the best primary care provider. She is interested in prevention and finds this patient a challenge.

The long-term care unit as a design for living

The patient in the advanced stage of dementia needs an environment with a minimum of complexity. Any new place offers a dilemma—its mastery may be impossible and "relocation" panic results. Huge, open spaces are frightening to the patient; he needs boundaries that are easily visible. He has come from an architectural arrangement of space in the home where rooms are clustered together and units are small. Architecturally, long-term care units resemble the impersonal space of a motel or airport rather than a home. The equipment (Fig. 13-3) and the long halls with doors on either side leading off into what may seem infinity tax the ability of the patient with true dementia to orient himself. He will tend to withdraw to his room or get lost as he wanders trying to find a landmark. Halls should be short with clearly defined ends, and signs should be painted on the walls with arrows pointing to central areas such as the dining room. Color should be used freely as a means of orientation, with each hall a different color and each door a distinctive color. Wall space should be broken by murals or wall decoration.

The patient in the advanced stage of true dementia still needs physical activity, which is best provided by walking if formal exercise programs are not provided. He will take the initiative, for walking is a lifelong measure used to reduce tension. Too many institutions have not provided for this need, except to allow wandering the long halls. An outdoor patio with see-through fences should be adjacent to an outside door the patient can feel free to use. The patio needs shrubbery to offer privacy, with seating hidden from view. Walking in the sunshine is important for everyone, but for the patient with dementia, it provides an orientation to time and seasons that keeps him from slipping into the next stage so rapidly. The long halls of the average long-term care unit have no relation to the dark, hot, cold, rainy, or sunny world taken for granted by those who use it every day.

Institution blandness (Fig. 13-4) and repetition are found in rooms and bathrooms, which seem to have come off of assembly

338 *Confusion: prevention and care*

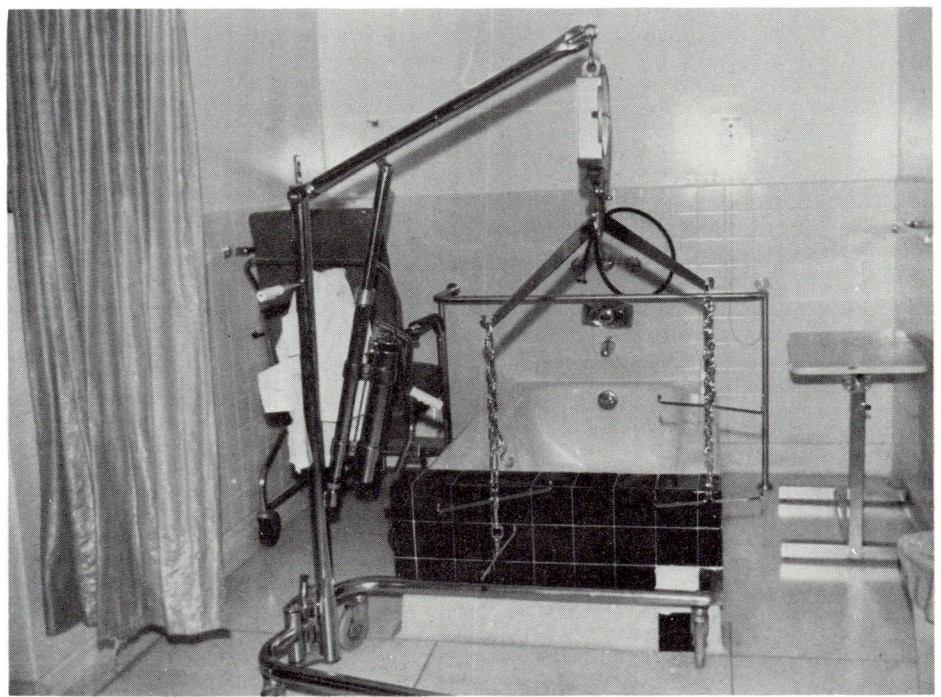

Fig. 13-3. Institutional equipment can be impersonal and worse, terrifying. (Photograph by C. D. Falk.)

Care of the patient with a true dementia 339

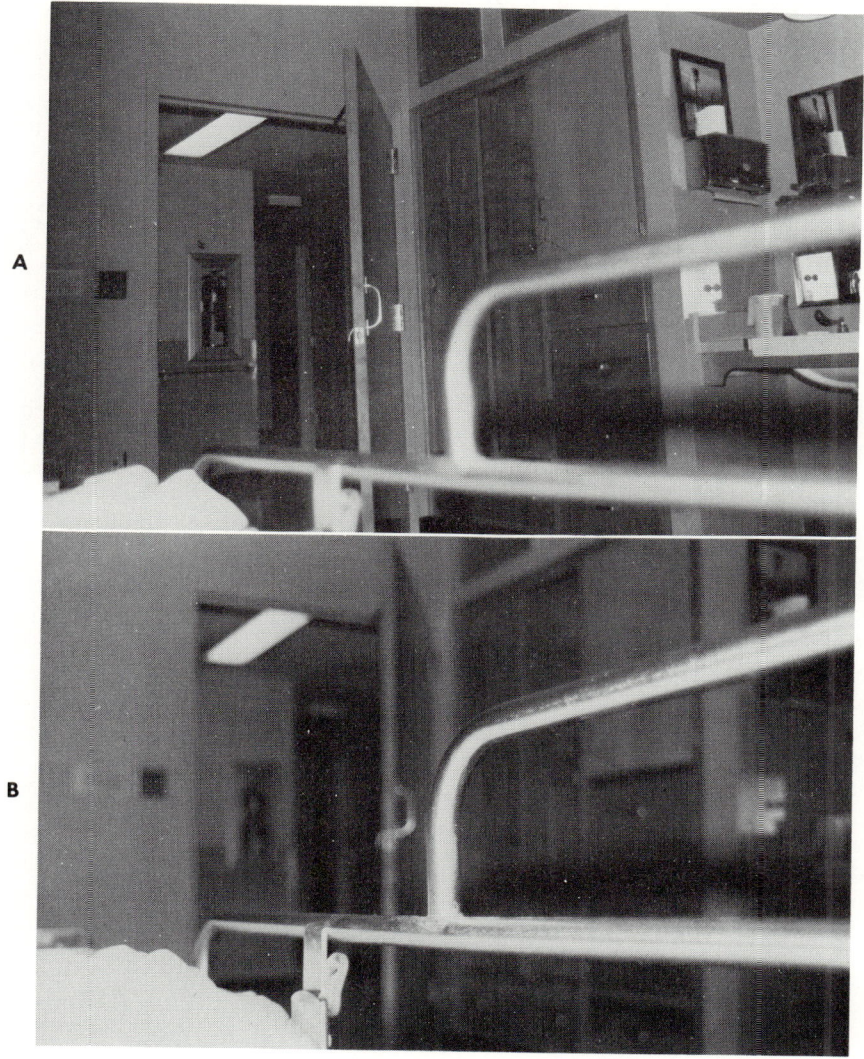

Fig. 13-4. A, Institutional blandness is turned into a prison by the addition of bars, **B**. (Photographs by C. D. Falk.)

lines. Contrast in bathrooms should be provided either by painted walls and colored tile or by highly colored linen and soap. Small tables should be provided for meals to allow eye contact with others and to prevent the confusion of crowds and noise. Piped-in music is distracting when it is continuous; five minutes of music per hour may be pleasant. Small dayrooms are preferable to huge, barny lounges with many people.

Territoriality and privacy. Relocation as a cause of confusional states in the elderly must not be overlooked (see Chapter 11), and consideration of the patient's territoriality in the semiprivate room must not be neglected. If he is transferred from his home to an institution, hospital, or nursing home, the patient is undergoing an environmental change that may be crucial to his mental status. Each person has an invisible bubble of space around himself that he keeps inviolate. When he can control his space, he moves away from those who would invade the invisible bubble, or he may invite a special person to share it with him. In addition, each person has existed in a society by defining his private territory throughout his life. He has a special place for his toothbrush, his clothing, a favorite chair, even a space to the right or the left of the family dining table. Such territoriality reduces ambiguity, confusion, and indecision by providing the person with previously determined areas in which the routines of life can be carried out. The personal space goes with the person as he moves about, but the private territory should ensure that property rights will be respected even when the owner is absent. Altman (1975) says that personalization and ownership are designed to regulate social interaction and to help satisfy various social and physical motives.

The confused elderly patient will lose his territory and may not know how to stake out new claims in a new setting. It is necessary for strangers with good intentions to invade his personal space to assure themselves that he is free from life-threatening problems. Bauer (1979) found that elderly residents felt anxiety when their drawers were rifled or their chair taken out of the room. Less anxiety occurred from invasion of personal space by professional personnel, as long as it was on legitimate treatment matters. Institutional routines may prevent a patient's caregiver from understanding the intrusion on the personal space, while lack of knowledge of the need for private territory may cause disregard for the staked-out space. Personal possessions should remain inviolate while the elderly patient is away. Each person on admission to a new facility should be given space and possessions if he has not brought his own. The bed should be marked with the patient's name if it is the greater part of his new private territory. Towel racks, comb, toothbrush, and all personal items should have his name clearly printed on them, and his name on the door should be readable without glasses.

Example. The old man wandered through the halls, unable to find his room, which looked like every other room in the institution. The nurse took some red tape and asked him to put a design on his door, which he did, making a triangle. He brought people to "his" door saying, "This is my address."

We all have some space where we can be alone, where we can close the door against intrusion and have the silence to observe and deal with ourselves without the distraction of others. Altman (1975) believes that privacy permits one to carry out self-evaluation, a fundamental process in attaining self-understanding and self-identity. He considers self-identity to be central to human existence, "For a person to function effectively in interaction with others requires some understanding of what the self is, where it ends and begins, and when self-interest and self-expression can be exhibited." (For further reading on the architectural and social designs of facilitative environments, we recommend the work of Synder [1973, 1975, 1978] and Snyder and Ostrander [1974].)

Sexual activity. When Dr. Mary Calderone, executive director of the Sex Information and Education Council of the United States (SIECUS) (1976), was asked if there was a difference between the sexual interests and activities of normal and disturbed elderly patients, she replied that there was no difference in terms of sexual interest, but in terms of expression there could be a great difference. The confused elderly patient may not observe the rules of privacy that are part of our culture; we cannot understand or forgive his instigating a sexual approach or his masturbating in public. Yet he has the same needs to reduce sexual tension that he has always had and will use the same methods. The staff can help the patient in expressing his sexual needs by giving him privacy. This has to be a deliberate action in which the staff accepts the need and are willing to grant the patient a closed door without leering or making jests about behavior inappropriate "at that age." Elderly confused patients have sexual needs and *rights*. Sexual needs fall in the same category as any of the other body drives and functions that must be met. The public environment of the institution and the confused mind of the patient prevent the normal expression. Female patients are particularly misunderstood. The male confused patient is called a "dirty old man," but a nice grandmotherly looking woman is denied the right to be a sexual being. She should have privacy as well. Both need to have affection, which is part of sexuality. Often "good feelings" from happy social interaction help to relieve sexual tension.

The wanderer. The advanced and later stages of true dementia are characterized by the patient's aimless wandering and being lost, unable to find his way back to "home base." The physical being is much more active than the mind and requires motor activity that tends to reduce agitation, although it is usually seen as a sign of agitation. When an institution has long halls, moving from one part of the building to another is seen as wandering by the staff, when actually it may be needed to reduce the physical tension since there is no other place to move about. An exercise program can reduce tension and help prevent the wandering. Wandering is confused behavior and should be handled quietly by one person who walks alongside the patient for a short distance, falling into step with him and speaking to him by name in a conversational tone. This tends to distract the patient from his goal or purpose, and soon the two can turn in the same direction and walk back to the home base. A second staff member may be in the vicinity, but under no circumstances should the two confront the patient together as a threatening gesture.

The primary caregiver. The patient with true dementia should have one person who knows him and acts as his advocate and resource. A primary caregiver should be designated on admission to a facility. This person should be the liaison with the family for the institution and should be part of any care planning. The patient should know that this person is his personal representative and that he can depend on that representative. For the patient who has no family, the personal representative may be forced into the role of "professional relative." This does not displace the legal representative, who may be a conservator who cares for the business and financial matters or a guardian who makes all decisions regarding the patient, but in institutional matters, the primary care person will represent the patient unable to think and speak for himself.

Group therapy. Group therapy in the care of the elderly with the true dementias applies to three different categories of groups. The first is the patient group, in which the patients are brought together in small groups for either socialization or the working out of a common problem, for example, a mutual disability such as grief. The second group is the families of the elderly patients who are sharing a similar experience and who need the support of others who understand; all receive support from a well-led group. The third group is the caregivers who are not family members. Caring for persons with progressive disorders is an experience that demands renewal and support for the caregiver. The term burnout is being used to describe the exhaustion of the caregivers who have used their physical and emotional resources day after day without the rewards of success that occurs with patients discharged from the intensive care units or surgical wards. This third group will be discussed in Chapter 15.

FOR THE PATIENT. Social isolation is one of the personal problems of the patient with true dementia. He may be of two types: withdrawn and apathetic or outgoing and effusive. Each is an expression of the bewilderment he undergoes when he realizes he is losing control over mind, body, and lifestyle. In this situation he can no longer rely on a dependable self or world. Therapeutic techniques have been developed for use with small groups. The more common and better known are remotivation therapy, reality orientation and training, reminiscing therapy, socialization groups, and groups with special focus, such as music, art, books, poetry, or current events.

Other groups focus on shared problems, such as widow-to-widow programs for those who share recent mourning, stroke groups, or exercise groups that focus on restoration of special functions.

Groups are usually planned for a small number of patients who indicate a willingness to experiment. The same group meets at a special time each week and has a designated leader who serves as a catalytic agent and often as a motivating force to enable the group to change from four to six individuals surrounded by their high, stone walls to a cohesive group who reach out to each other both figuratively and literally. Burnside (1973) has always emphasized the use of touch in her work and has brought small treats of cookies and beverages. Ebersole (1978) has stressed the use of life history as a focus to stimulate people to begin sharing experiences and then moving to the present. The Folsom and Taulbee (1978) work on reality orientation and training has led to the use of reality boards in many institutions (Fig. 13-1). Garber (1965) speaks of remotivation therapy as creating a bridge between the patient's self-perception and perception of others.

Wolanin (1977) has described the remedial effect of group work as the Cinderella effect. The isolate becomes a member of a group and experiences, for a short time, a return to his status as a person whose being and opinion are valued. The magic is brought into focus by the patient's response during the therapy to a charismatic leader and group. Unfortunately, as with Cinderella, the clock strikes 12, and the leader leaves or the group is disbanded. The patient returns to his former status. There have been some remarkable exceptions, but since much of the group work is done on an experimental basis, evidence of permanent change is often lacking. Often, the wonderful work initiated by inspired and inspiring leaders is turned over to unenthusiastic personnel who may use the group work as an end rather than a means to the end of continued and lasting improvement in self-esteem and social functioning of group members.

Music, art, and poetry are dependent on a talented leader who believes in what he is doing and who commits himself to the process. Familiar music brings back happy memories, poetry allows the elderly person to say in metaphor what is often hard to say in direct everyday language, and a product of one's own hands gives a sense of achievement. During the advanced and later stages of dementia affected persons can still participate in some group.

(For the principles of group work and techniques which have been tested, the reader is referred to Burnside, 1978.)

FOR THE FAMILY. The family needs to share their grief over institutionalization of a loved one. Separation from family is a form of premature death. In the case study at the beginning of this chapter, the sisters and brothers grieved for the brother they had lost long before his death. His wife continued her visits, under conditions of hardship, long after the man she had known as a companion was only a nonresponsive body. This loss and grief does not have the dramatic quality of final rites, the ritual of the funeral, and the interment or cremation of the body. It is a continuing grief not alleviated by time, for the end has not come. Few people are able to share the burden of the loved ones whose visits are less and less rewarding as deterioration takes place. Only another person who has shared the experience can understand. This is the basis for group work. The group acts as a surrogate family who shares the same family experience. The members can accept the anger at what fate has imposed, the tears and desperation, and even the suicidal impulses the family member may face. There have been a few successful groups where the leader was able to set the group in motion and step back. Such allow the family member to find the strengths needed to continue visiting and giving affection to a patient unable to respond in rewarding ways. Each family is isolated in its grief and loss. At the institution they may come together as a group of people with a common burden.

The institution has the responsibility of initiating the group formation. The principal problem is communication. When the patient can no longer communicate on a meaningful level, the family member finds it very difficult to visit and face the effort of trying to talk with someone who does not seem to remember from one minute to the next or even to recognize them. The shared experience, which is the basis for communication, is absent. We do not know to what degree the patient is able to understand at any stage of this illness, but who is to say that his inability to communicate represents the real person, who may still be struggling inside. Hayter (1974) warns us that we do not know how much the patient comprehends and that we must always talk with him as if he understands. The family needs our help in continuing the unilateral communication.

Communication

Hayter (1974) believes the patient tries desperately to communicate but cannot find the right words. He may not have verbal ability but responds to kind gestures and sincerity. She quotes one patient as saying, "You can tell by the way a person touches you if he really cares about you." The teaching that nurses find successful with others does not work with the patient suffering true dementia. He may require constant reminders during a meal to continue eating. Later in the course of the disease, he may have to be prodded to take the first step, for example, a spoon placed in his hand as a reminder to eat. Hayter recommends always accompanying all nonverbal activity with appropriate verbal direction.

The hard part of the communication is waiting for a reaction. Time between giving a direction and its execution may seem endless. Hurried personnel are more likely to act quickly and perform the action themselves, rather than giving the patient a chance to be involved. Take time to wait, and often the action will reward the wait. If the patient is nonresponsive to communication, test by asking a simple question, then wait for the answer until you are sure that he has gone on to something else. Ask only one question at a time. Many patients appear to not hear or understand, yet given time, which is rarely done, they make an appropriate reaction. Bartol (1979) gives guidelines for nurse or family communication in dementia. She advises simple sentences with short words and no pronouns. If you repeat a statement or a question, repeat it exactly. She also recommends the use of self-humor by caregivers. If done naturally, the use of humor brings much-needed laughter, a dimension often lost in such settings.

Bartol (1979) is very interested in the patient's nonverbal substitution for the words that no longer come easily. She has studied how the patient uses his body position to indicate his messages. She suggests that the eyes alone can tell the nurse about discomfort, pain, anger, hostility, and misunderstanding, either through eye contact or avoidance of eye contact. Frustration and anger have their own body movements, from increased motor activity to shaking fists. Bartol suggests decreasing the environmental stimuli by decreasing demands on the frustrated patient, maintaining a calm manner, being sure the messages sent are congruent, and asking, "What is the patient trying to tell me by this behavior?" (p. 25).

An important aspect of the patient's nonverbal behavior is his "nonlistening" behavior. If he does not give you his full attention, stop and try later. Bartol identifies the nonreceptive behaviors of the patient that tell the nurse to go away; for example, when he walks away, closes his eyes, or uses other avoidance behavior.

"After the survival needs, the need to communicate is the most important in the hierarchy of human needs. It marks out the thin line that separates the person from the non-person state. Self-esteem is based on meaningful communication on a verbal and non-verbal level" (Wolanin, 1976, p. 409).

(For indepth reading concerning communication with the patient who has the true dementias we recommend Bartol, 1979).

Activities of daily living

In the earlier stage problems in activities of daily living begin with simple carelessness, forgetfulness, and lack of attention to details of grooming. As the patient's condition deteriorates, inattention to the personal habits—forgetting to bathe, brush teeth, and eat—become obvious signs. Day and night are confused; sleep patterns change. Health activities are forgotten. Elimination, nutrition, and fluid intake will have to be monitored carefully, for the patient does not respond to the cues that normally motivate him: thirst, hunger, and signals to defecate. The problem of remembering to go to the toilet will result in the patient becoming more and more incontinent. Hayter (1974) thinks this is an inability to remember socially acceptable ways of elimination. Clothes are changed when soiled and stained by food. The patient must have someone plan and give his personal care. Exercise should be part of the daily program to prevent the stasis problems of inactivity. Passive intervention will change to active intervention when the patient's conditon demands spoonfeeding, initiating bowel and bladder programs, and assisting the patient from bed to ambulatory activities. This marks the end of the later stage and the approach to the final or terminal stage.

The final or terminal stage of dementia

Observable behaviors in the final or terminal stage include:
1. Incontinence of urine and feces
2. Severe motor control impairments, with loss of ability to walk or make purposeful acts
3. Visual hallucinations
4. Extreme psychomotor retardation
5. Somnolence (Quayhagen, 1977)
6. Inability to communicate
7. Inability to recognize family
8. Little or no response to stimuli
9. Susceptibility to infections and injury
10. Marked loss of weight unrelated to caloric intake
11. Little or no human characteristics

The terminal phase may be very short—as long as an infection requires to close down the body processes—or it may be prolonged by exquisite care, such as that given to the patient in the case study at the beginning of the chapter. It rarely is very long, however, and may be triggered by a rapid change in some aspect of the patient's physiologic or emotional status. No one dies of the true dementias; rather, the patient dies from infections, injury, starvation, or fluid and electrolyte imbalance. In the case study, the patient was admitted to acute care settings and treated intensively for his urinary infections, but his emaciation would have eventually taken his life. Care during this stage is the care of the totally incompetent person who must rely on nursing care for his every need. Families are often able to maintain the patient for long periods by loving care with professional guidance. On the other hand, the family with few resources or dependence on one person for all the caregiving cannot cope with the intensive demands of this period. Few nursing homes are staffed to give the constant care the terminal stage requires.

We will not go into the supportive care of the terminally dependent person's physiologic needs when we can only maintain his vegetative existence. Although it is tempting to forget the patient is a person, the assumption must be made that the unresponsive body and mind are receiving the messages sent to them by gentle touch, warm hands, kind voices, refreshing cold drinks, soothing warm baths and massage, dry clean beds, and the comfort of position changes.

The family that has needed support throughout the first three stages of true dementia needs recognition of their anticipatory grief during the patient's terminal stage. For many elderly spouses the last stage is a mixed blessing: there is relief that there need be no more suffering and mental anguish; on the other hand, there is the impending loss of this person as a central focus in life. The spouse or family member is facing bereavement, although it would seem the loss is well prepared for and expected. This is not the time however, to decrease the level of support for the family.

If the family and staff have made the first three stages of dementia as meaningful and satisfying for the patient as possible, they can approach the end of his life with no regrets. There were limits to what could be done, but having given care when it was needed should be a source of comfort and solace. The final care should be an epilogue to the supportive efforts of all involved during the course of the dementia.

CHAPTER 13 SUMMARY
The true dementias

True dementias are characterized by pathologic processes and behavioral changes, including memory disturbances; deterioration of intellectual functioning; emotional changes, including withdrawal and retarded speech and movement; personality changes; language difficulties; and a wide range of neurologic and pyramidal signs. The two divisions by onset are the presenile, including Alzheimer's disease, Pick's disease, Huntington's chorea, Jakob–Creutzfeldt disease, and neurosyphilis; and the senile, including the senile dementias of the Alzheimer type and arteriosclerotic dementia.

Cardinal symptoms of Alzheimer disease–senile dementia complex are (1) progressive aphasia, (2) progressive apraxia, (3) progressive agnosia, and (4) progressive mnemic disturbance.

Stages of disease	Signs	Nursing intervention
Early	Shows declining interest in affairs. Has problem identifying people. Displays indifference to courtesies and rituals. Appears vague, uncertain, and indecisive. Forgets nouns.	Assist family in preparing for increased care; suggest legal assistance and help with organizing affairs. Monitor health habits, especially nutrition. Support family; refer to community agencies for assistance.
Advanced	Displays obvious defects in memory, recall, and retention. Hesitates in responding to questions. Is disoriented as to time; confuses night and day. Resents interference; complains of neglect. Loses important papers; forgets to keep appointments, pay bills, and cash checks. Forgets birthdays; has trouble with calculations. Unable to retain simple directions. Neglects health and hygiene.	Assess coping ability of family to maintain the vigilance required. Assist in rallying resources of community to aid of family. Monitor health status. Assist in relocation when that is the best alternative.
Later	Is disoriented as to place. Wanders aimlessly. Misidentifies people. Motor ability deteriorates. Loses time sense; cannot recall meals. Displays communication problems; incoherent use of nonverbal language.	Support family in the home if care is given there; teach family supportive care. Provide a facilitative environment in the institution to keep the patient ambulatory as long as possible and to maintain his existence as a person. Stress communication by touch and sensory stimulation.
Final or terminal	Experiences incontinence. Cannot communicate verbally. Undergoes deterioration with weight loss and loss of motor ability to vegetative state. Terminal stage is usually ended by infection or physiologic crisis, such as malnutrition or dehydration.	Provide care for a completely dependent person. Support the family undergoing anticipatory grief. The assumption cannot be made that the patient's mind is not functioning, so communications by touch and sensory change should be included as part of care to the end.

REFERENCES

Adams, R. D.: Recent observations on normal pressure hydrocephalus, Schweiz. Arch. Neurol. Neurochir. Psychiatr. **116**:7-15, 1975.

Adams, R. D., and others: Symptomatic occult hydrocephalus with "normal" cerebrospinal-fluid pressure, N. Engl. J. Med. **273**:117-126, 1965.

Albert, M. L.: Subcortical dementia. In Katzman, R., Terry, R. D., and Bick, K. L., editors: Alzheimer's disease: senile dementia and related disorders, New York, 1978, Raven Press, pp. 173-180.

Altman, I.: The environment and social behavior, Monterrey, Calif., 1975, Brooks-Cole.

Ball, J. A. C., and Taylor, A. R.: Effects of cyclandelate on mental functions and cerebral blood flow in elderly patients, Br. Med. J. **3**:525-528, 1967.

Bartol, M. A.: Non-verbal communication in patients with Alzheimer's disease, J. Gerontological Nurs. **5**(4):21-31, 1979.

Bauer, J.: Intrusion of personal and territorial space: a source of anxiety in institutionalized elderly persons. Master's thesis, University of Arizona, 1979.

Burnside, I. M.: Touching is talking, Am. J. Nurs. **73**(12):2060-2063, 1973.

Burnside, I. M., editor: Working with the elderly, group processes and techniques, North Scituate, Mass., 1978, Duxbury Press.

Calderone, M.: Interview. In Managing the disturbed elderly in family practice, vol. 2, Fort Washington, Pa., 1976, McNeill Laboratories.

Constantinidis, J.: Is Alzheimer's disease a major form of senile dementia: clinical, anatomical, and genetic data. In Katzman, R., Terry, R. D., and Bick, K. L., editors: Alzheimer's disease: senile dementia and related disorders, New York, 1978, Raven Press, pp. 15-25.

Conway, J. M.: The guilt factory, Newsweek, May 22, 1978.

Crapper, D. R., Karlik, S., and de Boni, U.: Aluminum and other metals in senile (Alzheimer) dementia. In Katzman, R., Terry, R. D., and Bick, K. L., editors: Alzheimer's disease: senile dementia and related disorders, New York, 1978, Raven Press, pp. 471-486.

Curtis, B. A., Jacobson, S., and Marcus, E. M.: An introduction to the neurosciences, Philadelphia, 1972, W. B. Saunders Co.

Davies, P.: Studies on the neurochemistry of central cholinergic systems in Alzheimer's disease. In Katzman, R., Terry, R. D., and Bick, K. L., editors: Alzheimer's disease: senile dementia and related disorders, New York, 1978, Raven Press, pp. 453-460.

Dodge, P. R.: Syphilitic infections of the central nervous system. In Beeson, P. B., and McDermott, W., editors: Textbook of medicine, 1971, W. B. Saunders Co., pp. 235-240.

Drachman, D. A., and Stahl, S.: L-Dopa handling vid demens: extrapyramidal dementia and levodopa, Lancet **1**:809, 1975.

Duffy, P., and others: Possible person-to-person transmission of Creutzfeldt-Jakob disease, N. Y. J. Med. **299**:692-693, 1974.

Ebersole, P.: Establishing reminiscing groups. In Burnside, I. M., editor: Working with the elderly, group processes and techniques, North Scituate, Mass., 1978, Duxbury Press.

Eisdorfer, C.: Stress, disease and cognitive changes in the aged. In Eisdorfer, C., and Friedel, R. O., editors: Cognitive and emotional disturbance in the elderly, Chicago, 1977, Year Book Medical Publishers, Inc., pp. 27-44.

Eisdorfer, C., Cohen, D., and Buckley, C. E. III: Serum immunoglobins and cognition in the impaired elderly. In Katzman, R., Terry, R. D., and Bick, K. L., editors: Alzheimer's disease: senile dementia and related disorders, New York, 1978, Raven Press, pp. 401-408.

Fine, E. W., Lewis, D., Villa-Landa, I., and Balkemore, C. B.: The effect of cyclandelate on mental function in patients with arteriosclerotic brain disease, Br. J. Psychiatry **18**:739-745, 1968.

Fisher, C. M.: Lacunes: small, deep cerebral infarcts, Neurology **15**:774-784, 1965.

Freemon, F. R.: Evaluation and treatment of patients with dementia, J. Natl. Med. Assoc. **69**:307-310, 1977.

Garber, R. S.: A psychiatrist's view of remotivation, Ment. Hosp. **16**:210-221, 1965.

Gajdusek, D. C., and others: Precautions in medical care of and in handling materials from patients with transmissible virus dementition (Cretzfeldt-Jakob disease), N. Engl. J. Med. **297**:1253-1255, 1977.

Gibbs, C. J., Jr.: Discussion. In Katzman, R., Terry, R. D., and Bick, K. L., editors: Alzheimer's disease: senile dementia and related disorders, New York, 1978, Raven Press, p. 576.

Glenner, G. G., Ein, D., and Terry, R. D.: The immunoglobulin origin of amyloid, Am. J. Med. **52**:141-147, 1972.

Hakim, S., and Adams, R. D.: The special clinical problem of symptomatic hydrocephalus with normal cerebrospinal fluid pressure: observations on cerebrospinal fluid hydrodynamics, J. Neurol. Sci. **2**:307-327, 1965.

Hayter, J.: Patients who have Alzheimer's disease, Am. J. Nurs. **74**(8):1460-1463, 1974.

Heyman, A.: Differentiation of Alzheimer's disease from multi-infarct dementia. In Katzman, R., Terry, R. D., and Bick, K. L., editors: Alzheimer's disease: senile dementia and related disorders, New York, 1978, Raven Press, pp. 109-110.

Hirschfeld, M. J.: Families living with chronic brain syndrome. Paper presented at the International Congress of Gerontology, Tokyo, August 1978.

Ingvar, D. H., Brun, A., Hagberg, B., and Gustafson, L.: Regional cerebral blood flow in the dominant hemisphere in confirmed cases of Alzheimer's disease, Pick's disease, and multi-infarct dementia: relationship to clinical symptomatology and neuropathological findings. In Katzman, R., Terry, R. D., and Bick, K. L., editors: Alzheimer's disease: senile dementia and related disorders, New York, 1978, Raven Press, pp. 203-212.

Jacobs, E. A., Winter, P. M., Alvis, H. J., and Small, S. M.: Hyperoxygenation effect on cognitive functioning in the aged, N. Engl. J. Med. **281**:753-757, 1969.

Jarvik, L. F.: Genetic factors and chromosomal aberrations in Alzheimer's disease, senile dementia, and related disorders. In Katzman, R., Terry, R. D., and Bick, K. L., editors: Alzheimer's disease: senile dementia and related disorders, New York, 1978, Raven Press, pp. 273-277.

Jellinger, K.: Neuropathological aspects of dementias resulting from abnormal blood and cerebrospinal fluid dynamics, Acta Neurol. Belg. **76**:82-102, 1976.

Katzman, R.: Normal pressure hydrocephalus. In Katzman, R., Terry, R. D., and Bick, K. L., editors: Alzheimer's disease: senile dementia and related disorders, New York, 1978, Raven Press, pp. 115-124.

Katzman, R., Terry, R. D., and Bick, K. L., editors: Alzheimer's disease: senile dementia and related disorders, New York, 1978, Raven Press.

Kay, D. W., Beamish, P., and Roth, M.: Old age mental disorders in Newcastle-upon-Tyne, I. A study of prevalence, Br. J. Psychiatry **110**:146-158, 1964.

Kay, D. W., and others: Mental illness and hospital usage in the elderly: a random sample follow up, Comp. Psychiatry **11**:26-35, 1970.

Kolata, G. D.: Mental disorders: a new approach to treatment? Science **203**:36-38, 1979.

Kral, V. A.: Benign senescent forgetfulness. In Katzman, R., Terry, R. D., and Bick, K. L., editors: Alzheimer's disease: senile dementia and related disorders, New York, 1978, Raven Press, pp. 47-52.

Kristensen, V., Olsen, M., and Theilgaard, A.: Levodopa treatment of presenile dementia, Acta Psychiatr. Scand. **55**:41-51, 1975.

Lehmann, H. E.: Use of medication to prevent custodial care. In Eisdorfer, C., and Friedel, R. O., editors: Cognitive and emotional disturbance in the elderly, Chicago, 1977, Year Book Medical Publishers, Inc., pp. 129-138.

Libow, L. S.: Epidemiology—excess mortality and proximate causes of death. In Katzman, R., Terry, R. D., and Bick, K. L., editors: Alzheimer's disease: senile dementia and related disorders, New York, 1978, Raven Press, pp. 315-322.

Libow, L. S., and Zicklin, R.: The penultimate will: its potential as an instrument to protect mentally deteriorated elderly, Gerontologist **13**:440-442, 1973.

Maneulidis, E. E., Gorgacz, E. J., and Maneulidis, L.: Viremia in experimental Creutzfeldt-Jakob disease, Science **200**:1069-1071, 1978.

McHugh, P. R.: Dementia. In Beeson, P. B., and McDermott, W., editors: Textbook of medicine, Philadelphia, 1971, W. B. Saunders Co., pp. 102-107.

Miller, E.: Abnormal aging: the psychology of senile and presenile dementia, London, 1977, John Wiley & Sons.

Nandy, K.: Brain-reactive antibodies in aging and senile dementia. In Katzman, R., Terry, R. D., and Bick, K. L., editors: Alzheimer's disease: senile dementia and related disorders, New York, 1978, Raven Press, pp. 503-512.

Quayhagen, M. P.: Confusion in the elderly. Workshop presented at Vail, Colo., August 1977.

Roth, M: Epidemiological studies. In Katzman, R., Terry, R. D., and Bick, K. L., editors: Alzheimer's disease: senile dementia and related disorders, New York, 1978, Raven Press, pp. 337-339.

Scheinberg, P.: Multi-infarct dementia. In Katzman, R., Terry, R. D., and Bick, K. L., editors: Alzheimer's disease: senile dementia and related disorders, New York, 1978, Raven Press, pp. 105-108.

Slater, E., and Cowie, V.: The genetics of mental disorders, London, 1971, Oxford University Press.

Snyder, L. H.: An exploratory study of patterns of social interaction, organization and facility design in three nursing homes, Int. J. Aging Hum. Dev. **4** (4):319-333, 1973.

Snyder, L. H.: Living environments, geriatric wheelchairs and older person's rehabilitation, J. Gerontological Nurs. **1** (5):17-20, 1975.

Snyder, L. H.: Environmental changes for socialization, J. Nurs. Administration **8** (3):44-50, 1978.

Snyder, L. H., and Ostrander, E. R.: Research basis for behavioral programs, New York State Veteran's Home, Oxford, N. Y., Ithaca N. Y., 1974, NYS College Department of Human Ecology, Department of Human Ecology, Department of Design and Environmental Analysis.

Sourander, P., and Sjogren, A.: The concept of Alzheimer's disease and its clinical implications. In Wolstenholme, G. E. W., and O'Connor, M., editors: Alzheimer's disease and related conditions, London, 1970, J. & A. Churchill, pp. 11-31.

Taulbee, L. R.: Reality orientation: a therapeutic group activity for elderly persons. In Burnside, I. M., editor: Working with the elderly, group processes and techniques, North Scituate, Mass., 1978, Duxbury Press.

Terry, R. D.: Discussion. In Wolstenholme, G. E. W., and O'Connor, M., editors: Alzheimer's disease and related conditions, London, 1970, J. & A. Churchill, p. 35.

Terry, R. D.: Aging, senile dementia, and Alzheimer's disease. In Katzman, R., Terry, R. D., and Bick, K. L., editors: Alzheimer's disease: senile dementia and related disorders, New York, 1978a, Raven Press, pp. 11-14.

Terry, R. D.: Ultrastructural alterations in senile dementia. In Katzman, R., Terry, R. D., and Bick, K. L., editors: Alzheimer's disease: senile dementia and related disorders, New York, 1978b, Raven Press, pp. 375-382.

Terry, R. D., and Wisniewski, H. J.: Structural aspects of aging of the brain. In Eisdorfer, C., and Friedel, R. O., editors: Cognitive and emotional disturbance in the elderly, Chicago, 1977, Year Book Medical Publishers, Inc., pp. 3-9.

Walsh, A. C., Walsh, B. H., and Melaney, C.: Senile-presenile dementia: Follow-up data on an effective psychotherapy-anticoagulant regimen, J. Am. Geriatr. Soc. 26:467-470, 1978.

Wang, H. S.: Prognosis in dementia and related disorders in the aged. In Katzman, R., Terry, R. D., and Bick, K. L., editors: Alzheimer's disease: senile dementia and related disorders, New York, 1978, Raven Press, pp. 309-314.

Wisniewski, H. M.: Possible viral etiology of neurofibrillary changes and neuritic plaques. In Katzman, R., Terry, R. D., and Bick, K. L., editors: Alzheimer's disease: senile dementia and related disorders, New York, 1978, Raven Press, pp. 555-558.

Wolanin, M. O.: Nursing assessment. In Burnside, I. M., editor: Nursing and the aged, New York, 1976, McGraw-Hill Book Co.

Wolanin, M. O.: The Cinderella effect, an administrative challenge, Concern care aging 3 (3):8-12, 1977.

Wolstenholme, G.E.W., and O'Connor, M.: Alzheimer's disease and related conditions, London, 1970, J. & A. Churchill.

Yahr, M. D.: The choreas. In Beeson, P. B., and McDermott, editors: Textbook of medicine, Philadelphia, 1971, W. B. Saunders Co., pp. 183-185.

Young, J., Hall, P., and Blakemore, C. B.: Treatment of the cerebral manifestations of arteriosclerosis with cyclandelate, Br. J. Psychiatry 124:409-440, 1974.

14

THERAPEUTIC INTERACTION WITH FAMILIES OF THE CONFUSED ELDERLY

Lee B. Maxey

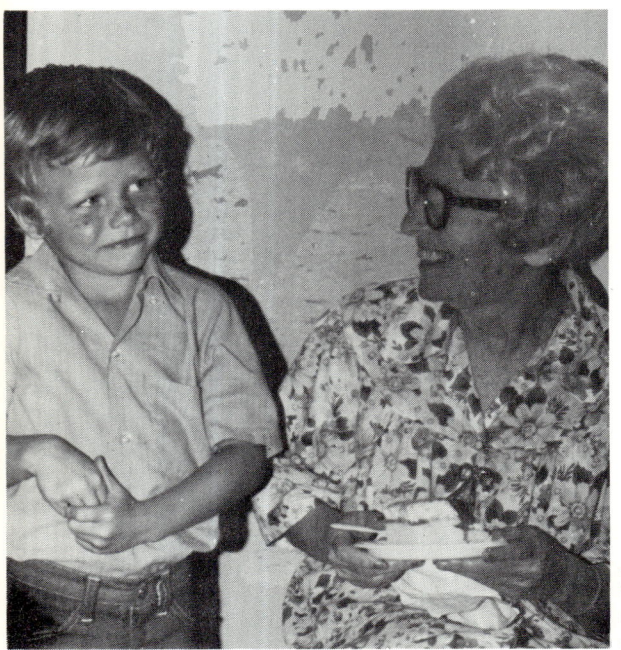

DEVELOPMENT AND CHANGE OF THE FAMILY SYSTEM

In examining the impact of confusion in elderly persons on their families, it is helpful to gain some perspective through a brief discussion of the historic development of the family as an institution in human society and the general functioning of the family as a system in our own society.

Man is the most social of animals. Anthropologists indicate that the development of organized human behavior sets man apart from other animals and has allowed him to alter (and often control) major portions of his environment. The earliest form of organized human behavior probably centered around the family and subsequently, around kinship-based groups. It was necessary at some point in the early development of our ancestors to form an organized group that could effectively provide a protective environment and ensure the survival of the relatively helpless human infant. The survival value of the family in performing this task was probably proved sometime during the early dawn of our race, more than 2 million years ago. The family as an established human institution, complete with a clear division of labor based on sex, was present by the time "modern man" appeared between 50,000 and 100,000 years ago.

Little is actually known of human social organization prior to the domestication of plants and animals. However, this major human discovery allowed man to settle in large numbers in one spot, thereby increasing the size and effectiveness of organized social groups. Cities could not exist prior to the domestication of plant and animal life because enough food could not be accumulated to support large concentrations of people. The earliest settlement yet discovered where plants and animals were clearly domesticated dates back about 10,000 years BC. The world population at that point is estimated to have been less than 1 million. During the next 10,000 years the human population expanded to 100 million. Mechanization, industrialization, and modern technologic advances during historic times have pushed the species population to over 3 billion souls (Katz, 1978, pp. 6-7).

Paralleling and supporting this spectacular ability of the race to control and manipulate environmental resources has been an increasing complexity in human social organization. From loosely knit hunting and gathering groups existing prior to the domestication of plants, man has progressed from nomadic and settled tribal groups, to agrarian-based nation-states, to modern nations, to supernational organizations such as the United Nations, international cartels and businesses, and international banks, laws, and military alliances. But of all the organized human groups now existing or recorded in human history, the nuclear family is probably the oldest and most enduring. It is present in virtually all human societies, in one form or another, since each man or woman must have two biologic parents and, therefore, a family. One can draw a parallel with atomic physics in which the "atoms" of society are seen as each individual and families are the "molecules" holding society together.

Each family is attached to many others with one or more "bonds" to form more complex groups of society similar to "compounds." Religious sects, political parties, hospitals, community agencies, social clubs, professional organizations, businesses, and the military are examples of such complex groups.

Although the nuclear family exists in innumerable forms in the more than 2,000 known human societies, no one can dispute that every society has established some form of nuclear family system for the protection and rearing of children and the passing on of the tools of culture to them in order to ensure the ultimate survival of the race. Each human culture has created, over thousands of years, its own unique family system that can both incorporate and adjust to all of the social complexities engendered in that specific social system. To tamper with or change so complex a "molecule" as the family system is to toy with the very foundations not only of society, but of our own individual identities as well, since it is within the matrix of the nuclear family system that the "electrons," "protons," and "neutrons" of our own individual personalities are formed.

In examining society in the United States, we can see a distinct historic change over the past 80 years in the traditional agrarian-based extended family system. In the traditional extended family many relatives and friends were available to provide care to the aged, and the aged filled specific support and functional roles within the family system. However, with increasing industrialization and the technologic revolution of the past 50 years, there have been massive internal migrations of people from rural areas to the larger urban centers where jobs were available (Goode, 1974). By 1976 only a little over 4% of the 88½ million employed Americans were working in agricultural pursuits (World Almanac, 1977). This population shift has fragmented the extended family system so that there is less support available to the elderly than prior to 1900. Congruent with this weakening of family ties has been the development of a dispersed four-generational extended family in which medical technology is managing to keep grandparents and great-grandparents alive (Califano, 1978). In all of man's previous 2 million years of existence this is unprecedented on a society-wide scale. Previously, two-generation families were the norm because people seldom lived long enough to become grandparents. However, family systems did provide very specific roles and tasks for the elderly whenever three-generation families were present, and grandparents were a scarce and valued commodity.

In most societies the elderly were venerated and respected, for they passed on the oral history, traditions, and customs of society to succeeding generations. Even among Eskimo and Tasmanian groups, where older people were left in the wilderness to die of exposure when they could no longer contribute to the tribal economy, they were still venerated. In addition, everyone openly accepted the prescribed suicidal aging role in order that the young might survive in a harsh environment. Historically in all societies, since the bulk of the families possessed only two generations, there was always a maximum amount of support available for the few members of the third generation who might survive. Surviving members of the fourth generation were extremely rare historically and, consequently, family systems in general have not had to develop supportive roles to incorporate frail fourth-generational elderly into the family system until this century.

While these factors have weakened the ability of the nuclear family to care for their aged members, two significant demographic variables have increased the care burden placed on today's families. They are the rapidly rising percentage of very old or "frail" elderly among the aged population and the accompanying increase in the elderly segment of the total population (estimated to reach 30½ million by 2000 AD).

These recent increases in the elderly population have resulted from rapid technologic and medical advances that allow us to prolong the human life span for large numbers of aging individuals. The increasing entry of women into the labor force has further reduced family resources in the provision of care to elderly members, since adult daughters and daughters-in-law have historically been the primary care providers to the elderly (Brody, 1978). It is clear that, since people are living longer, more and more of the adult children of aged parents have reached their fifties or sixties and are beginning to experience crises precipitated by their own aging needs at the same time that the demand is greatest on them for provision of care to their 70-, 80-, and 90-year-old parents. Thus, the family itself is aging and is becoming increasingly dependent on outside resources to assist in the care of elderly members. It is estimated that 30% to 40% of all elderly over 65 require at least some form of outside service in order to function, and the elderly as a group require more services than younger adults because of the increasing loss of independence in personal functioning associated with the aging process (Brody, 1978). Also, as the aged population expands, the proportion of men to women decreases because of the shorter life expectancy for men in our society.

The nuclear family is still the most resilient and appropriate institution human society has developed for the provision of care to elderly people. Yet, increasing fragmentation of both the nuclear and the extended family has led to a greater number of elderly living alone, because (1) they have outlived their spouses and occasionally their children, (2) their families often cannot care for them in the same household, or (3) they have never married (a distinctly new option for larger numbers of women during this century). In spite of these factors, a 1966 National Health Survey study of home care indicated that 80% of the home care provided to aged persons 55 and older was given by family members residing in the household (Brody, 1978).

The implications of this discussion for the confused elderly and the nuclear family system must be considered. The same factors that influence the general elderly population and their families will more severely affect the confused elderly and their families. More and more often, family members find they do not have the time or energy to provide the resources and services required by aging relatives. The demands confused elderly place on nuclear family systems are even greater because of the lower levels of personal functioning at which most confused elderly people operate.

The confused elderly will be more likely than other elderly persons to become involved with public support systems and institutions as a result of their greater dependency needs and the inability of the immediate family to supply the extensive and complex personal care they require. In addition, families of confused elderly experience greater strain on emotional, financial, and other resources in attempting to provide care to confused elderly members.

As a result of the geographic dispersal and social fragmentation of the extended family mentioned before, when we examine familial support available to the aged individual, we find we are usually dealing with one or more nuclear family systems. The "nuclear family" has been defined by Murdock (1949), Bott (1957), Nimkoff (1965), Satir (1972), Coser (1974), Lee (1977), and many others to consist of a man, a woman, and their offspring.* It is important to examine the developmental process through which the nuclear family system passes as its members grow older.

*For a complete discussion of definitions for the nuclear family, extended family, family of orientation, and family of procreation, see Murdock, G.P.: Social structure, New York, 1949, The Free Press.

There are three basic developmental stages through which a nuclear family passes over time (Fig. 14-1). In each of these stages the focus of familial relationships and interactions is different. If you think of yourself, you will remember that as a child and adolescent you belonged to your *family of orientation*. This nuclear family probably consisted of you, your parents, your siblings (brothers and sisters), and perhaps one or two attached members (such as grandparents, uncle, or aunt). However, the primary focus of this family system for you was on your parents and siblings. As a young adult your familial focus shifted to the marriage (or mating) relationship and your *family of procreation*. In this second stage your spouse and your children received the bulk of the time and energy you allocated to the family. In the third stage of nuclear family development there are usually two or more *families of orientation* for you, as this is (or will be) your major period of aging. During this period your concerns, energy, and time will be divided between your spouse (if alive) and the families of your children.

In looking at the nuclear family through this simple framework we can begin to examine deviations in this normative process and assess the impact of specific factors (such as confusion) on the elderly and their families. Obviously, many families may not follow this pattern exactly. For example, homosexual couples or childless couples will skip stage II (the family of procreation) and move directly from stage I to stage III. They must replace the absent *families of orientation* with surrogate support systems outside their own nuclear family system if they are to receive support in old age, perhaps by utilizing extended family members or friends and their families. For the single-parent families now very prevalent in our society because of the ever-increasing divorce rate, stage II becomes a much more exacting period of life. It requires a much greater outlay of energy and time by placing the single parent in the posi-

354 Confusion: prevention and care

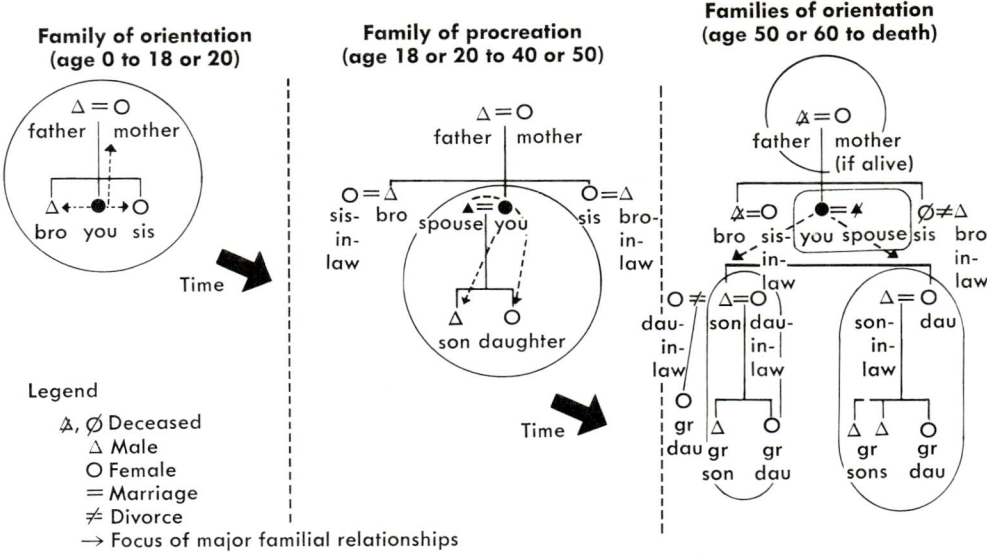

Fig. 14-1. Developmental cycle of the nuclear family (late 20th century). (Used with permission of Lee B. Maxey, M.S.W.)

tion of maintaining the double role of both "breadwinner" and "parent" to the children. There may well be less availability of care and support to aging grandparents from single-parent families in the future. A confused elderly grandparent will place excessive demands on such families, necessitating increasing amounts of intervention from support systems outside the family. In addition, aging single parents are more likely to face the losses associated with growing old alone without the support of a spouse. As they grow older they may shift increasing demands to their *families of orientation* (stage III). In many instances the ever-increasing divorce rates may well increase the number of elderly parents an adult child must help, since stepparents have also become an increasingly prevalent phenomena.

Another problematic situation appearing with increasing frequency among the elderly is that of the professional or single older man or woman who, for various reasons, never married and has no children or relatives on whom to rely for support. Many of these people have devoted most of their lives to jobs or professions and, on retiring or reaching old age, find themselves without purpose and, more seriously, without familial support systems to fall back on during times of crisis. Many of these people have been unable to establish intimate family relationships in their own lives and may have actually bypassed Erikson's stage of intimacy during adulthood (Erikson, 1963). Living relatives for such people will be siblings, nephews, nieces, distant cousins, or parents, all facing aging problems themselves or busy caring for closer elderly relatives. This group of "aging singles" is particularly at risk because these persons face the aging process alone with no familial support systems, and many may be poorly equipped socially and psychologically to seek the necessary help they require from community resource systems. Such people will face loneliness and isolation unless they find a way to tap the currently fragmented public resources available or natural support systems such as friends and neighbors. In summary, there is good reason to be concerned that the increasing fragmentation and changes over the past 80 years within the traditional nuclear and extended family systems in the United States have and will continue to contribute to a parallel increase in the amount of support and care required from community and institutional resource systems. This situation will be aggravated by the rapidly increasing proportion of elderly to younger persons in our society. One important implication is that the role played by helping professionals in providing care to the elderly will also increase proportionately as more families are able to manage less and less of the complicated care required by family members reaching their seventh, eighth, and ninth decades of life (Califano, 1978).

THE AGING PROCESS AND THE IMPACT OF AGING LOSSES ON THE FAMILY SYSTEM

In examining human aging, we see that there are two major developmental processes at work within any individual. These are (1) organic and (2) psychoemotional growth and development. Impinging on and greatly affecting the course of both processes is (3) the environment within which each individual must exist (Fig. 14-2). In referring back to our model of individuals as "atoms" and families as "molecules" of society, families can be placed in the environment with all other social groupings, while each individual in society experiences both the organic and the psychoemotional aspects of aging from birth to death.

Organic growth is finite in that it begins with fertilization of the egg by the sperm and ends with death. This process may vary in length for any individual, but the process itself holds true for us all. Early growth of the human fetus and infant is incredibly rapid. Physical growth continues to somewhere around the age of 24 or 25 (Goldman, 1971). At this point in time body cells cease to replace themselves at the same rate at which they are dying, and we begin to die, or age. The process continues until our death and affects all body systems. This is the natural organic growth and aging process, and it is with this process that the medical profession has been primarily concerned (Rossman, 1971).

Psychoemotional growth is not finite in character as is organic growth. It begins at a point during the ontogenetic development of the fetus but takes a quantum leap after birth as the result of the geometric increases in environmental stimuli as compared to the highly protective and circumscribed fetal environment. Psychologic, emotional, and intellectual growth can continue on an upward gradient until death (and theologians argue that it continues after death) unless it is severely interrupted by organic or environmental factors. The many highly functional (that is, "active," "alert," "happy," "curious," and "lively") elderly who are "aging gracefully" today are examples of this process. Nearly everyone has encountered such individuals, who have managed to preserve, intact, their natural psychoemotional growth process and their own personal identities during the concurrent organic aging process.

Psychoemotional growth was observed by Erikson (1963) in his description of the various developmental stages of the individual. His work indicates that each of us establishes an internal personal identity during infancy and childhood. This period is characterized by the development of increasing psychologic and social independence that occurs in conjunction with rapid organic development. Both processes progress within the protective confines of the nuclear family system. Adolescence is a period of testing for this carefully accumulated independence and thus becomes a transition period for breaking away from the nuclear family of orientation and entering into adulthood. During young adulthood we all seek to establish the educational and vocational skills required for occupational competence that we will use to support our

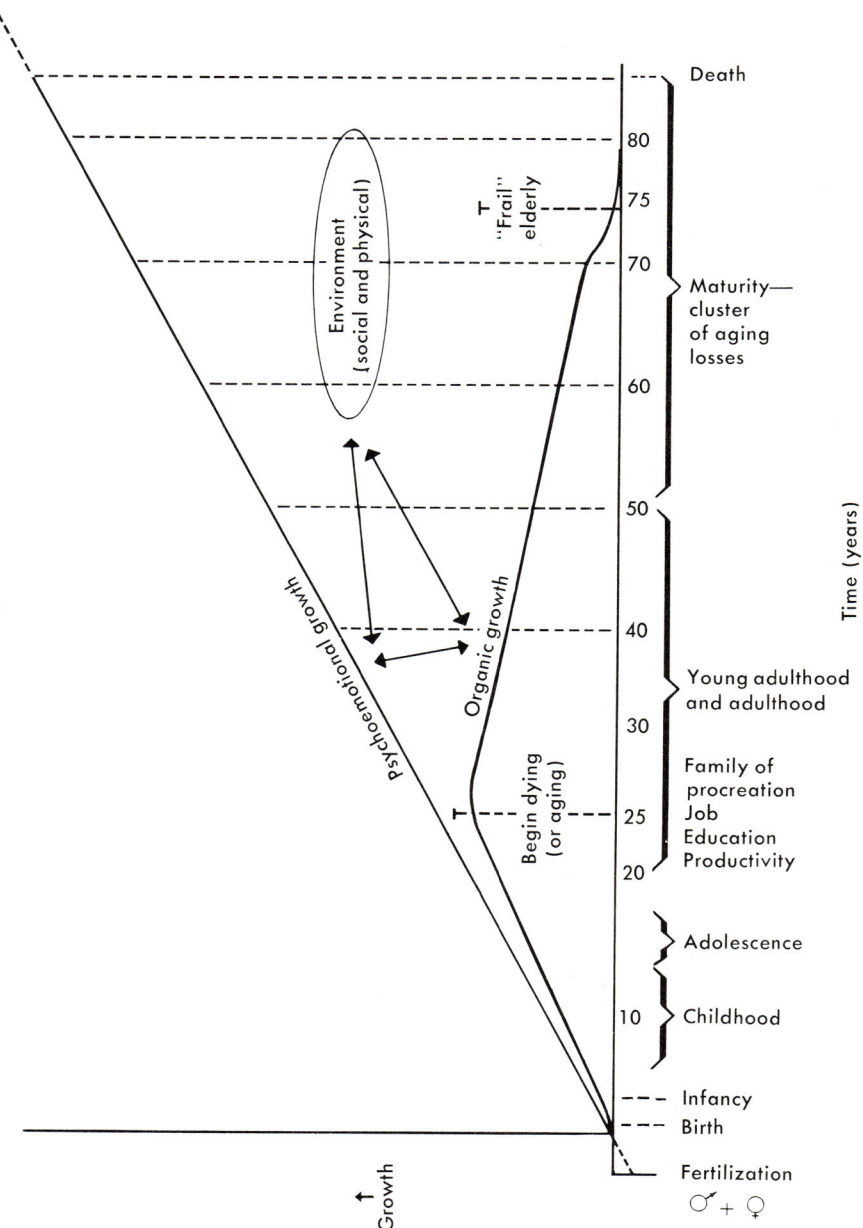

Fig. 14-2. Individual aging process. (Used with permission of Lee B. Maxey, M.S.W.)

future families of procreation. Adulthood is usually the time of greatest productivity and the period in which we raise the members of the next generation. It is during this phase of our lives that our independence as a total organism reaches its greatest development. It is also during this period that psychoemotional development must reach a sufficient point of stability, independence, and growth so that it can support us during our years of rapid organic decline and increasing personal dependence on others. The interplay between organic and psychoemotional functioning and environmental factors during the first half of life determines, to a great extent, our later ability to adjust to the increasing loss of independent functioning encountered as we age. Each of us will cope with aging and its accompanying losses and conflicts in the same manner we previously coped with life. We will employ the same patterns of thinking and acting or reacting that we established in passing through the periods of infancy, childhood, adolescence, and adulthood.

It is important to examine this interplay among the environment, organic growth and aging, and psychoemotional growth in order to begin to understand how people cope in an individual fashion with the losses encountered in growing old. The majority of us have only just begun our families of procreation when we begin aging. If we or our family have encountered no major organic or environmental losses at that point, such as major diseases, death, congenital or genetic defects, social deprivation, mental illness, or severe physical injury, then we will probably spend the next 20 years or so successfully raising our family of procreation. However, it is the process of learning to cope effectively with the losses we all encounter during our early lives that allows us to continue the natural, psychoemotional growth that will carry us through the period of aging losses successfully.

Since the aging process is actually a process of increasing loss of personal independence, it is the struggle to maintain independence that will occupy much of our attention during our declining years. This process is, in effect, a mirror image of earlier development in which we continually attempted to increase our independence of outside support and decrease to a minimum level our dependence on others. In essence, life is a series of personal conflicts with which we must individually cope in order to maintain our own feelings of personal fulfillment and self-worth. Each time we resolve a life conflict, we attain personal satisfaction. Unfortunately, when we reach maturity and begin to lose the ability to master many of the unresolveable cluster of conflicts presented by aging, we also begin to lose the independent ability to meet many of our own needs. This is doubly frustrating because we have spent a lifetime painstakingly developing the behavior patterns we use to resolve such life conflicts.

In our society, many of us enter the aging process never realizing that the sheer magnitude and number of losses we encounter may well overwhelm our established coping patterns and force us to seek help from others.

Individuals and their families must recognize that many of the changes and losses of aging may be too difficult to resolve totally within a personal or familial resource system or that such losses are final and impossible to resolve in any way other than to simply accept their reality and adapt to them psychologically and emotionally. Carlson (1978), in her discussion of loss, emphasizes the great importance of continuity and predictability to everyone's life. She indicates, for example, that in the Buffalo Creek disaster (described by Titchner and Kapp, 1976) in which 4 000 people lost their homes, 90% of the victims experienced disabling psychiatric symptoms and life-style changes within 2 years. Although this was a heterogeneous group and not, specifically, an aged population, a comparison can be made. Many aged people do eventually lose their homes in addition to experiencing a series of disastrous losses.

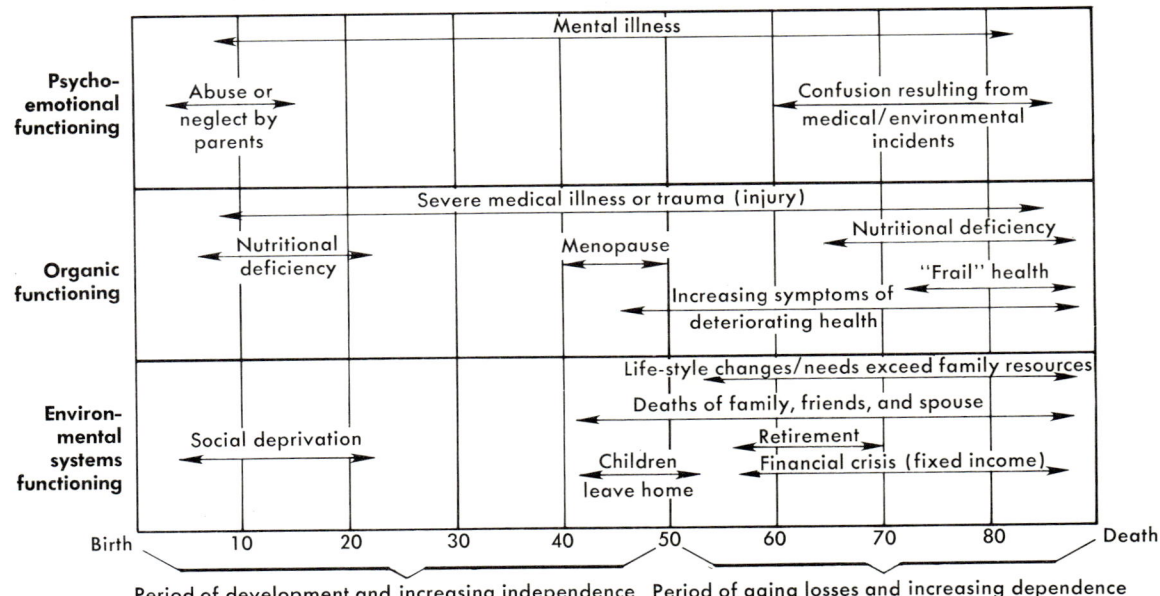

Fig. 14-3. "Clustering" of aging losses and the effect on psychoemotional, organic, and environmental systems. (Used with permission of Lee Maxey and Mary Jane Hattsteadt.)

The difference is that aging losses *may* be more predictable.

There is seldom just one precipitating cause or loss contributing to dependency among the aged. Rather, there is almost always a clustering or series of losses that may occur over several years or even decades, and each loss in the series, whether environmental, organic, or psychoemotional, almost invariably contributes to the next one. This clustering of aging losses and the impact of such losses on the organic, psychoemotional, and environmental systems functioning of the individual is depicted in Fig. 14-3.

There is a specific psychodynamic process that occurs to an individual and subsequently, to the family system, when significant aging losses take place (Fig. 14-4). Any major loss of aging will precipitate a severe emotional reaction, such as anxiety or depression, that is usually accompanied by some form of identity crisis for the individual involved. This is because a decrease in independent personal functioning is almost always a factor in any "aging" loss. Such losses often dictate a change in life style that can result in financial, legal, medical, or psychologic crisis. Recovery from this situation requires a restructuring in the individual identity of the affected elderly person, as well as an accompanying shift and restructuring of any close, supportive relationships, especially those in the family. For example, if an elderly person becomes confused or is widowed, all family members must adjust to the identity loss and subsequent personality changes suffered by the affected individual. Older people experiencing such losses will fall back primarily on their closest support system for help—the family; secondarily on other

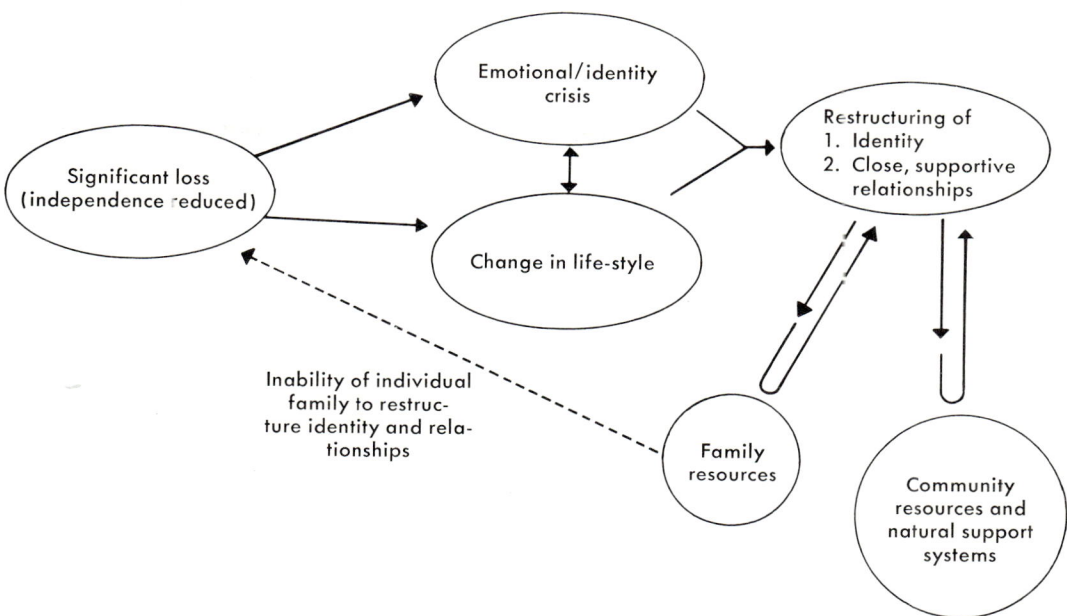

Fig. 14-4. The psychodynamics of loss in aging. (Used with permission of Lee B. Maxey, M.S.W.)

natural support systems—friends, neighbors, and distant or affined relatives; and last on community resource systems. If, as is often the case, the family is unable to provide the necessary resources to care for an elderly person or if they are unable to or avoid utilizing outside community resources and natural support systems, then the family itself may become "overloaded" and unable to restructure relationships with an "at risk" elderly member. This can result in the breakdown of family relationships and an additional loss of support for the elderly person.

Family members who fail to provide care to an aging relative often experience feelings of guilt, frustration, and helplessness. Should these feelings become too intense, they may well overwhelm family members and cause them to withdraw or avoid an elderly member whose situation appears hopeless and unresolvable. The effect of this withdrawal on an elderly person is that of a second major loss that essentially blocks his access to the family as a supportive resource during a crisis period. The result is increased vulnerability for the elderly family member. Should this situation occur in a heavily kinship-based family system or where ethnic values require that children must care for their aging relatives, for example, in Jewish, Hispanic, Indian, Oriental families or first- or second-generation immigrant groups, then the feelings and resulting emotional conflicts become magnified.

In short, the identity crisis suffered by an individual during a significant aging loss or during a series of losses will almost always precipitate a crisis within the family. The family is the major support system available to the aging member, and all family members will have to restructure their roles and relationships with an aging member in crisis. As Spiegel (1957), Ackerman (1958), Bell (1963), Jackson (1968), Haley (1971), Satir (1972), and others have pointed out, familial relationships and role prescriptions are complementary and interdependent on one another; a crisis with one family member affects his relationships with all other members. There is a drain on existing family resources, and the family role structures may shift, especially in health or emotional crises.

During aging, health or emotional crises or losses invariably occur. Most families find that there are no general role prescriptions in our society for caring for the elderly in a three- or four-generation family. The role of "parenting your parent" is a new development to which families must adjust, and this role usually falls on the adult children or grandchildren of aged individuals. Children or grandchildren must shift and readjust their lifelong roles and relationships to their aging parents or grandparents from that of *child*/parent to that of *caregiver*/parent. This shift must include a readjustment for the children in their personal identities if they are to be successful in restructuring their supportive roles with aging parents or grandparents. The role shift for spouses is similar—from that of mate/mate to that of caregiver/mate—and engenders similar role conflict.

This process is essential to consider when dealing with the confused elderly because the identity loss suffered by such a person is more global and severe and will produce a much greater impact on significant others. Identity loss associated with confusion is more severe since in our society, illness, stigmata, or visible physical and behavioral handicaps are difficult for most people to accept because such handicaps are devalued and considered threatening, abnormal, or negative in nature (Goffman, 1963). Our culture tends to emphasize youth, perfection, and beauty as the normative state for everyone. The television and advertising industries have ingrained this concept into the conscious and unconscious minds of children and adults for the past 20 years. Partly as a result of this national value system, much role confusion results among family members when one of their number becomes ill or handicapped or exhibits unusual and difficult behavior patterns such as confusion or mental illness. This role confusion can be aggravated when the affected family member is elderly because of the absence of clear familial role prescriptions for dependent parents and grandparents. If the older person is also confused or disoriented, with the attendant loss of familiar personality and behavior patterns, then the situation is usually perceived as hopeless and irreconcilable by family members. This often necessitates seeking assistance outside the familial resource system.

Unfortunately, most people whose parent becomes confused view him as "ill" or, more specifically, as a "patient." Categorizing a person as an "identified patient" may be appropriate from a medical viewpoint for the nurse or the physician, but it is actually not appropriate for family members to stereotype an elderly person in this fashion. Such stereotyping places family members in the position of mixing two distinct roles, that of "caregiver" with that of "relative," while at the same time feeling helpless to actually change or control the situation for the affected family elder. When family members place themselves in the position of being totally responsible for resolving the lives of and caring for aging relatives, they assume an impossible task. Many people feel that they *must* care for the parents or grandparents who raised them, and there is often a natural tendency to utilize child-rearing patterns. When faced with the problem of how to "parent a parent," many people revert to the only tried-and-true patterns of caring for dependent people they know—the ones they learned in rearing their own children or as children themselves. This is inappropriate with the elderly because they possess an intact identity and do not wish to give up the personal independence they see slowly slipping away as they become more dependent on others. Good child-rearing techniques are designed to foster increasing independence and to create a stable identity in the child through limit-setting and direction. Such techniques usually cause older adults to feel patronized and infantilized by the very people to whom they *must* turn for help during an aging crisis.

The use of such techniques with confused elderly, though sometimes temporarily effective, usually becomes much too burdensome and exhausting financially and emotionally for any family or family member to maintain over a prolonged period. Should confusion be a temporary condition, there is the risk that family members will continue to relate to the older confused person in an infantilizing manner, actually prolonging or supporting the confused condition longer than necessary. It is this "role confusion" and "identity crisis" among family members themselves that must be addressed to ensure that an elderly confused person receives his maximum support.

Another major problem encountered by families with a confused elderly member are the feelings of anxiety, fear, depression, and grieving experienced when an older member exhibits confusion. The actual loss experienced by the family is the loss of the personality, either permanently or temporarily, of the confused individual. If confusion is permanent, the family can experience a loss greater than death because it is not a final loss. They see their loved relative daily and must repeatedly experience the frustrations of observing the accompanying childlike, bizarre behavior. Yet they remember the person as he was: vigorous, productive, and able to function as a complete person. It is always very difficult and often impossible for close family members to accept at an emotional level the daily behavior patterns of a permanently confused close relative. Many such people feel as if they are witnessing a "living death" each time they see the affected person they love. They seem to reexperience the "death" or loss of the confused person's personality with each encounter, even though the person continues to function physically. This paradoxical situation increases the role confusion around "parenting a parent" already encountered by family members and leaves many with unresolved feelings of conflict, helplessness, and guilt. Nor is this an unrealistic assessment, since destruction of or damage to brain cells or "partial brain death" is a common cause of confusion. Should permanent confusion occur with an elderly member, it is advisable for families to explore community or institutional resources for the daily care of the affected person in order to protect the emotional stability of close family members. Otherwise, family members may be placed at emotional risk themselves.

Less severe, but more common than permanent confusion, are the variety of temporary confusional states discussed previously in this book. In most instances, when an elderly member of the family is stricken with confusion, it is an episodic or temporary state. Here the family may encounter sporadic confusional episodes of varying duration over a nonspecific period of time. Often, the condition may be present over several years or even a decade or more. It may also be progressive, with episodes occurring more frequently or lasting longer and longer with each occurrence. The effect is like that of an irregularly flashing neon light, since there is often little or no predictability to the episodes. The inability to predict such episodes places a severe strain on close family members and can increase appreciably their internal anxieties and tensions. Feelings of anger, frustration, guilt, and anxiety may become mixed and interfere in their relationships with the affected elderly person, both during and between confusional episodes. Such situations of temporary confusion are more amenable to effective intervention from natural and community resource systems outside the family than are permanent confusional states.

In most families one or two people usually assume the role of "caregiver" or "rescuer" toward an elderly relative in crisis. As is well known in family systems theory, all family members tend to assume specific roles toward one another in their ongoing relationships. These roles will be complementary in nature but may not necessarily be healthy or helpful to all parties. Unfortunately, the effect of such assumed familial role prescriptions can often be to shift or skew the bulk of the care burden onto only a segment of the close family. Geography, finances, medical crisis, and other factors can further skew the care burden so that only one or two members of the nuclear or extended family are attempting to help an older relative through the losses of aging. It is most important in such situations that intervention from outside resources be sought in order to share and distribute the burden of care among familial, natural, and community support systems so existing familial resources are not exhausted and family members are not burnt-out emotionally. This is doubly important in order to avoid the common guilt feelings attendant on failure to care for an aging relative or parent as well as to prevent the aging individual from experiencing another major loss in the aging process, that is, support from important significant others in the family.

INTERVENTION AND TREATMENT APPROACHES TO THE CONFUSED ELDERLY PERSON AND HIS FAMILY

Since our ultimate concern must be to help the confused older person function to his full potential and, concurrently, to help the family system function as effectively as possible in maintaining that older person at his maximum level of functioning, we must look carefully at practical methods of intervention that will help achieve these goals.

It is a well known fact that prevention is the ideal solution to any health problem. Unfortunately, very few people in the helping and health care professions have managed to develop prevention-oriented screening programs for confusion, and none exists on a large enough scale to be effective for many individuals and their families. This situation is difficult to understand when one realizes that almost all of those who suffer from confusion have been hospitalized, often by their families, at one time or another for some kind of medical evaluation or condition. The discharge planning process is often inadequate in most acute care facilities, yet this is where preventive intervention and planning should occur with elderly patients and their families. Prevention-oriented programs for the elderly should be located in the institutions these people frequent, such as hospitals. The personnel responsible for discharge planning (social workers, nurses, and physicians) should be key people in prevention-oriented programs. In actual practice, most hospital staff physicians do not play a major role in the patient discharge process after treating the patient; they simply make a recommendation to other discharge planning personnel who are responsible for developing and implementing the discharge plan. Medical care then reverts to the family doctor or previous attending physician in the community. Frequently, there is little or no communication between physicians and other discharge-planning personnel during the discharge process, resulting in disruption in the continuity of care received by the elderly patient.

Many factors can contribute to this disruption; one major variable is the insular nature of the hospital as an institution in our society. In the United States hospitals tend not to function as a part of the continuum of care within the larger community. Their budgets rarely provide significant funding for discharge planning, and the general philosophy of care is not oriented toward interdependence and continuity in the provision of care as with other community services.

As a result, patients are often "dumped" into the community with little or no appropriate after-care planning or follow-up contact. There is also a tendency among a significant number of health professionals to exhibit the attitude that older people do not merit the same amounts of energy and time, or care, that younger populations should receive. The rationale for this tendency to "shelve" the older population seems to rest on the opinion that they have already lived out their lives and will soon die. This attitude contributes heavily to the lack of preventive care and the disruption in continuity of care to the elderly and confused elderly in hospitals and in the other community agencies.

We are beginning to realize that, "in total dollars," short-term, crisis-oriented acute care is becoming a much more expensive form of health care to the aged than long-term care. The emphasis should be on preventive models of care. Unfortunately, treatment takes place where money for funding is allocated, and most of the money for care to the aged population is in categorical funding programs. Few of these programs emphasize preventive intervention.

Because prevention is seldom, if ever, practiced with the aged and their families, the elderly person almost always appears on the doorstep of a caregiver or community agency in a state of crisis. The financial, physical, and emotional resources of the individual and his family have generally been depleted. Family members who have assumed the role "caregiver" are emotionally and physically drained. Often, they have been trying to cope with a confused or elderly relative or spouse in maladaptive ways. The elderly spouse of such a person often cannot find the energy to seek help or has no idea where to look for help in the community. Spouses and family members are commonly caught up in the paradoxical roles of "relative" and "caregiver" and divert excessive energy to this internal struggle. Families do not abandon the confused elderly member if outside support can be found (Dobrof and Litwak, 1977). Frequently, however, community resources are unavailable or inaccessible to the elderly.

Another obstacle the elderly face in the United States is a general lack of community resources. This condition stems from a series of problems that include: (1) lack of physical access to resources, especially in rural areas where long distances and limited programs are the rule, because of poor or no transportation and the distance to service providers; (2) the categorical and short-term nature of most funding for aged programs and the assumption that local communities can or will pick up and continue such programs; (3) interagency competition and lack of coordination in implementing programs that lead to fragmentation, duplication, and inaccessibility of services; and (4) the overwhelming emphasis of categorical funding on secondary and tertiary health care intervention at the expense of primary preventive intervention models.

Without widespread preventive intervention programming, the next best effort to bridge the gap is to utilize education in disseminating information about preventive health care for the elderly and confused elderly. The prime target groups in this effort must be (1) professional and paraprofessional caregivers to the elderly, who should receive training in preventive intervention, referral, and health care techniques; (2) the elderly themselves, who should receive training in self-help care and be familiar with available local support services; and (3) the families of elderly people, who should receive training in the vulnerability to confusion of family members who encounter aging losses and be familiar with local support services and preventive health care techniques.

Health care professionals such as nurses, social workers, physicians, and psychologists are a major source of such information and must assume a major role in intervention with the confused elderly and their families. Such professional caregivers must provide assessment and intervention in several basic areas while helping confused elderly people. The first step in providing care is to determine at which point on the behavioral continuum the elderly client is functioning. How confused is he? Is the confusion temporary or periodic in nature, or is it permanent? This should be determined through medical and psychosocial records, various mental status evaluations, questioning of family members or others who have lived with the client or who are familiar with him on a daily basis, about his personal history and behavior patterns, and direct observation of the person's behavior.

The second step is to analyze the care and support systems available to the client. These are: (1) the nuclear and extended family; (2) natural support systems such as neighbors, friends, the church, fraternal lodges or organizational memberships, and occupational or professional associates; and (3) community agencies and resources providing services to the elderly. Contact with key individuals in each of these support systems should then be initiated to determine precisely who is committed to the provision of care to the affected individual and the extent of that commitment. Both the quality and the quantity of care available must be explored. The level of care appropriate to the behavior of the confused client should be sought, and such care should encompass the unmet medical, psychoemotional, and environmental needs of the individual.

After evaluating the nature of the elderly client's confusion, his care needs, and the resources available to meet those needs, it is necessary to designate the amount and nature of care to be provided by specific persons or entities in the available support system. A *primary care manager*, such as a family member, agency/community professional, or legal guardian, should be specified to coordinate the various aspects of the confused person's existence. This care manager may sometimes provide limited care or support, but his primary responsibility must be to ensure that the confused individual receives necessary medical, financial, legal, social, and emotional support from available resources. *Secondary care managers* are those people within the family, the natural support system, and the community service network who are designated to provide the bulk of the care required by the confused elderly client. Ideally, the primary care manager is a close family member. However, he must be heavily supported by secondary care providers, and he must recognize the necessity of limiting his responsibility for direct care interventions with the confused individual.

This approach involves a rational attempt to appropriately distribute the complex, taxing care required by the confused elderly. It acknowledges that such care is indefinite for the permanently confused and institutionalized elderly and will be continuing for elderly who live in the community but are subject to periodic or temporary confusion. It also recognizes that, although the family may be primary in the care of the confused elderly, it is necessary that outside support systems such as institutions, community agencies, churches, neighbors, and friends assume direct caregiver roles with the confused elderly client in order to help maintain the integrity of the family unit and to avoid placing the confused client or members of his family at greater risk. The comparative scarcity of resources demands that a careful and pragmatic approach be employed in assessment and intervention when helping families cope with the overwhelming needs of a confused elderly member.

ADAPTIVE AND MALADAPTIVE PATTERNS OF FAMILY ADJUSTMENT TO AGING, LOSS, AND CONFUSION IN ELDERLY MEMBERS

At this point we will examine two examples that illustrate adaptive and maladaptive family responses when confusion and other aging losses are encountered in an elderly member. Both of these case illustrations have been taken from a population of institutionalized elderly living in a nursing home environment. In each case, the elderly client described requires skilled nursing care and will undoubtedly remain in the institution until death.

Case study: Sarah and Mrs. A. (maladaptive response). Sarah was admitted to the nursing home with a diagnosis of left hemiparesis and aphasia after suffering a cerebrovascular accident. She was 85 at the time of admission and was accompanied by her 54-year-old daughter, Mrs. A. She had been transferred from a nearby nursing home where she had been for 1 month.

Sarah immigrated to this country from Lithuania in 1896 at age 2. The family settled in Chicago where she lived until age 85. She married, raised a family, and was widowed in 1977 at age 83.

Mrs. A. had wished to move to a southern climate for 8 years because she suffered from arthritis in her joints. However, her 60-year-old husband, a physician with a successful practice, had resisted the move. In 1979, at Mrs. A.'s insistence, Sarah moved with her to a southwestern city 2,000 miles from Chicago. She suffered a stroke 6 weeks after her relocation.

After Sarah's stroke, Mrs. A. suffered severe anxiety, depression, and feelings of guilt for having precipitated her mother's condition with the relocation. When Sarah was initially placed in the nursing home by her physician, Mrs. A. was unable to establish positive working relationships with any of the staff. Mrs. A. appeared daily, often several times, to visit her mother. She would clean Sarah's room, criticize the nursing staff's care of her mother, make unreasonable demands that the physical therapist make her mother walk, and demand that nursing staff provide care her mother did not require. In short, she attempted to assume responsibility for all aspects of her mother's care. During admission, Mrs. A. was told her mother's care would not be coverable by Medicare. Yet, when informed of this after admission, she demanded a financial adjustment, claiming she had not been informed. Several weeks after the admission Mrs. A. demanded a room change for her mother, but when another room was offered to her a month later, she refused it. The week after her mother's admission, Mrs. A. was seen twice by the social worker for personal counseling. These sessions revealed serious marital difficulties between Mrs. A. and her husband, but she did not return for further counseling. Mrs. A.'s disruptive behavior and the venting of her anxieties on staff finally led both her and the institution to the conclusion that she could not handle the situation alone, 2,000 miles from the rest of her family. A conference was arranged with Mrs. A. to coincide with a pending visit by her husband, and she was asked to bring him along. The purpose of the meeting was to determine who would care for Sarah. At the conference it was pointed out that Mrs. A. was assuming the "caregiver role" with her mother, the very role she was paying the nursing home a great deal of money to maintain. Because Dr. A. was less anxious and easier to communicate with, the group was able to reach an agreement that Dr. and Mrs. A. should make a decision as to whether or not they would relocate Sarah to a nursing home in Chicago. It was also agreed that should Sarah stay, Mrs. A. would seek staff assistance and relinquish her caregiver role to the staff. This decision was reached in May. Subsequently, Mrs. A. did relinquish much of Sarah's care to the staff, was able to establish more stable relationships with most staff members, and seemed less anxious about her mother. Two months later, in July, Mrs. A. moved her mother to a nursing home in Chicago and rejoined her husband. She sent a brief but grateful letter to a staff member thanking the home for their help but criticizing the new nursing home in Chicago.

This case illustrates quite clearly the role confusion suffered by an adult child in attempting to "parent a parent." In addition to maintaining the caregiver role for her mother and failing to distribute part of the care burden to the institution, Mrs. A. was unable to extricate herself from this role because of her severe feelings of guilt for precipitating her mother's condition. Mrs. A. did not know that relocation of the frail elderly can be disastrous, nor was she fully aware that moving her mother related heavily to her own dependency on her mother and that this was also closely associated with marital problems between herself and Dr. A.

The case of Mrs. A. is a classic example of a chronic situation that occurs in institutions whereby a family member who is at emotional risk becomes a care management problem rather than the client.

In addition, support from the spouse of an adult child can be *the* crucial factor in adaptive coping with the aging crisis of a parent. The absence of Dr. A. during Sarah's initial crisis period placed an extreme burden on Mrs. A. with which she could not cope. Resolution of Sarah's care situation was really dependent on Dr. and Mrs. A. reaching some kind of agreement about their problems and on Dr. A.'s support of Mrs. A. in helping her mother. Previously, Dr. A., a very busy man, had left the care of Sarah entirely up to Mrs. A. because Sarah was "her mother."

The presence of a previous pathologic situation within the nuclear family can severely impair the ability of the family to cope with aging crisis in parents and grandparents. Mrs. A.'s letter to the staff criticizing her mother's final placement would indicate that her feelings of guilt and her role confusion in caring for her mother were still unresolved.

Case study: Molly and Mrs. B. (adaptive response). Molly began to experience symptoms of confusion at about age 50. After raising her family, she worked for the welfare department in Los Angeles for a number of years. Her inability to function forced her to quit working at age 59. Molly continued to live alone in Los Angeles until she was 74. She was helped by one of her daughters (Mrs. B.'s sister) who lived 30 miles away. Mrs. B. often helped her sister to support Molly. At that time Molly was suffering from angioneurotic edema, which required prompt treatment in the emergency room of a hospital. On one of her trips to the hospital she got lost looking for her car and her daughter. Mrs. B. was eventually contacted in an adjoining state.

Mrs. B. decided to relocate her mother from Los Angeles to her own city, finding Molly an apartment within 1 minute's walking distance from her own home. Mrs. B. had discussed her mother's move with Mr. B. and their two boys (ages 21 and 14), and received their full support. She established a daily routine for monitoring her mother that was shared among the family members. This routine included several daily visits of brief duration. During the visits the water, stove, and electric lights were turned off by the visiting family member. Mrs. B. and the family also devised a clever technique, using masking tape and telephone instructions, to supervise her mother's daily medications. This became necessary when her mother began stashing her medications around the apartment. In this system, Mrs. B. would tape various pills together under a table or in some unobtrusive place where Molly could not find them. She would then call Molly when it was time for the medication and give her very precise instructions where to find and how to take the pills.

Molly's physician eventually suggested that Mrs. B. place Molly in an adult day-care program for 6 hours daily, 5 days per week. This gave the family some respite from the constant care they were providing. Molly liked the day-care program very much. During Molly's residence in the apartment, Mrs. B. made every effort to keep her mother "happy and comfortable." Discovering her mother liked dolls and musical toys, Mrs. B. began to take her mother to a children's store regularly to allow Molly to play with and buy the toys. Mrs. B. also discovered that her mother enjoyed outings to zoos and pet stores. Molly accompanied the family to church and joined them on holidays and other occasions. In taking her out, Mrs. B. found it important not to tire her mother with long outings, as Molly's attention span was limited. She also found that focusing on a single activity was better than a multiple-activity outing.

There was strong support for Mrs. B. from her husband and sons throughout this process. They were able to recognize her need to help her mother, and they shared in the process. At one point, when Mrs. B. had to travel to an adjoining state to help a sick relative for an entire month, Mr. B. and the sons took care of Molly. During this process Mr. and Mrs. B. recognized that their primary and major commitment was still to each other and their children and not to Molly. But they worked as a team with outside resources to maintain the specific commitments they felt toward Mrs. B.'s mother. The B. family has spent many hours over the years in long discussions between parents and sons regarding aging, confusion, and Mr. and Mrs. B.'s wishes regarding their own care, should they require it. Mrs. B. is also very active in the church and has derived a great deal of support from her personal religious convictions and her church.

At one point the family placed Molly in a nursing home for 2 weeks while they went on vacation. Returning to take her mother home, Mrs. B. said she felt as if she were "taking a kitten and depositing it in the middle of the jungle." She began to realize that her mother was exceedingly vulnerable, uncomfortable, overwhelmed, and overstimulated by the normal work-a-day activities of the outside world. This experience led Mrs. B. to place her mother in a long-term care institution. In seeking support from the physician, Mrs. B. encountered resistance. Molly's doctor was of Cuban extraction, and his cultural values were opposed to putting the elderly in nursing homes. He became angry with Mrs. B. when she suggested her plan for Molly, making her feel guilty and uncomfortable about her decision. She changed physicians immediately and placed her mother in a skilled nursing home.

At the point of Molly's placement, Mrs. B. felt that her mother had ceased to exist as a full personality, saying, "My mother is not my mother now," and "It has been necessary for me to learn how to become a good mother to her." This engendered a long period of slow and difficult loss for Mrs. B. that was sometimes so painful to her that she has no wish to recall it and prefers that such memories remain "buried."

However, Mrs. B.'s adjustment to her mother living in the nursing home has been excellent. Molly lives on a locked unit where she can wander safely at will and does not need to be tied or "restrained" to a chair. There are plenty of nursing staff to help her through the routine tasks of daily living. Mrs. B. has established an open, communicative relationship with the nursing staff. She visits her mother regularly and has gotten to know the other residents and their families on the unit. She is helpful to everyone she meets. Mrs. B. gauges her visits according to Molly's condition and on her own ability to tolerate such visits. She visits quite frequently when Molly is ill and requires more one-to-one attention or care, such as feeding. She will then taper the visits off as her mother recovers. This is supportive not only to the nursing staff and Molly, but also to Mrs. B., as this physical care is often all she can do to help her mother. However, it is carefully coordinated with staff, and Mrs. B. does not attempt to perform or monitor all care to her mother.

Mrs. B. has found that her mother's attention span may last only a few seconds or minutes and that, rather than confronting her, it is easier to go along with her whims and thoughts since Molly can always be redirected to a specific task as soon as the thought passes. Mrs. B.'s primary concern with her mother is that she is well cared for in a "good" environment and that the family knows she is as safe and comfortable as possible. When taking Molly on brief outings, Mrs. B. has observed that the "protective structure" of the unit is very reassuring to her mother. When they return to the unit, Molly visibly relaxes and lines of tension leave her face. At first, Mrs. B. took Molly on outings to the church every Sunday. However, all outings have had to be discontinued, as they are overwhelming and overstimulating to Molly at this point. Mrs. B. finds that as much nonverbal communication as possible, including kissing, holding hands, hugging, and eye contact, is necessary to hold Molly's attention; verbal communication usually does not work and is often very confusing to both Mrs. B. and Molly. The many stages of adjustment have been difficult for Mrs. B. and the family as they have experienced her mother's progressive confusion, deteriorating personal functioning, and movement to higher and higher levels of daily care.

There are several significant factors that stand out in this family's adaptive response to permanent confusion in an elderly member. The nuclear family members were exceedingly supportive of the affected elderly person, of one another, and of the adult child, Mrs. B. The family also sought appropriate help from the church, the physician, and other community resources, utilizing all support systems over the course of Molly's deterioration and institutionalization. Sharing of the caregiver role was never an issue with this family, and distribution of the care burden was effectively accomplished with outside resources over many years. Primary management and coordination of care were assumed by Mrs. B., but she was careful to protect her own health by relying on secondary care managers such as her church and friends, her husband and children, her mother's neighbors, her physician, and community agencies. This judicious and rational use of family, natural and community support systems allowed Mrs. B. to provide appropriate care to her confused mother for 20 years and to avoid institutionalizing her mother for 10 years.

Mrs. B. has found the experience to be at times painful and difficult and has often sought emotional help and sustenance from her husband and her personal faith. Had it not been for this emotional and psychologic support, she probably would have been unable to cope with her mother's confusion. Each situation will be very different for every family. Although Mrs. B. was fortunate enough to have very strong personal religious convictions she could rely on for emotional sustenance, for the many people today who might lack such religious convictions, it may be necessary to seek counseling from outside resources.

Perhaps the greatest struggle Mrs. B. herself has encountered has been the realization that she must arrange her relationships with her mother and her own family in order of importance and that her children and husband take priority whenever she must make a choice. It is a double-bind situation that automatically sets up guilt feelings with Mrs. B., no matter what her choice may be. This is because she feels strongly that she must care for both her family and her mother at the same time. As a result, Mrs. B. experiences feelings of guilt many times when she returns to the nursing home to visit her mother. Establishing a routine visiting schedule incorporated into family activities relieves this double bind and enhances the visits to the institution.

The presence of open, fulfilling, and supportive relationships can greatly increase the ability of the family to cope adaptively with severe losses and crises encountered with older family members.

SUMMARY

Medical technology in this century has significantly extended the human life span. This has led to the development of a new four-generational family system in which there are no traditional role prescriptions for "parenting" aging parents and grandparents. The effect has been that of "aging" the nuclear family system and, at the same time, greatly increasing the numbers and proportion of elderly persons in the general population.

The nature of the aging process itself leads to a series or clustering of losses in personal independence that increases the dependence of more and more elderly on familial, natural, and community support systems. The coping patterns aging people have developed during earlier stages of life will greatly influence their ability to adapt to such losses. The aging process involves psychologic, emotional, and environmental factors in addition to the obvious organic breakdown of the human body. When confusion is one of the losses of aging, it involves a personality loss and aging crisis for the affected individual and precipitates a concurrent and often severe identity crisis among close family members. Familial relationships must be restructured after intrapsychic adjustments have been made by family members. The utilization of extrafamilial resources is almost always necessary in the provision of care to the confused elderly, and the designation of primary and secondary care managers is important.

Prevention is the preferred approach to the aging person and his family, but hospitals and other community and governmental agencies have failed to provide adequate preventive programs. Consequently, careful and appropriate assessment and intervention by health professionals are a necessity in helping families perform this task.

ACKNOWLEDGMENT

Mrs. Mary Jane Hattsteadt, R.N., M.A., provided significant contributions in time, expertise, and work in conceptualizing this chapter. Many of the ideas were previously developed jointly by her and the author for public education purposes. Were it not for her astute help, this chapter might not have been written.

REFERENCES

Ackerman, N. W.: Psychodynamics of family life: diagnosis and treatment of family relationships, New York, 1958, Basic Books, Inc., Publishers.

Bell, R. R.: Marriage and family interaction, Homewood, Ill., 1963, Dorsey Press, pp. 16-23.

Bott, E.: Family and social network, ed. 2, New York, 1957, The Free Press.

Brody, E. M.: The aging of the family, Ann. Am. Acad. Political Social Sci., July 1978, pp. 13-27.

Califano, J. A., Jr.: The aging of America: questions for the four-generation society, Ann. Am. Acad. Political Social Sci., July 1978, pp. 96-107.

Carlson, C. E.: Loss. In Carlson, C. E., and Blackwell, B., editors: Behavioral concepts and nursing intervention, Philadelphia, 1978, J. B. Lippincott Co., pp. 72-83

Coser, R. L., editor: The family: its structures and functions, ed. 2, New York, 1974, St. Martin's Press.

Dobrof, R., and Litwak, E.: Maintenance of family, ties of long-term care patients: theory and guide to practice, U.S. Department of Health, Education and Welfare, Publication No. (ADM)77-400, 1977.

Erikson, E. H.: Childhood and society, ed. 2, New York, 1963, W. W. Norton & Co.

Goffman, E.: Stigma, Englewood Cliffs, N.J., 1963, Prentice-Hall, Inc.

Goldman, R.: Decline in organ function with aging. In Rossman, I., editor: Clinical geriatrics, Philadelphia, 1971, J. B. Lippincott Co.

Goode, W. J.: The role of the family in industrialization. In Winch, R. F., and Spanier, G., editors: Selected studies in marriage and the family, New York, 1974, Holt, Rinehart & Winston, pp. 87-96.

Haley, J., editor: Changing families, New York, 1971, Grune & Stratton, Inc.

Jackson, D., editor Therapy, communication and change, Palo Alto, Calif., 1968, Science and Behavior Books.

Katz, S. H.: Anthropological perspectives on aging, Ann. Am. Acad. Political Social Sci., July 1978, pp. 1-13.

Lee, G. R.: Family structure and interaction: a comparative analysis, New York, 1977, J. B. Lippincott Co.

Murdock, G. P.: Social structure, New York, 1949, The Free Press.

Nimkoff, M. F.: Comparative family systems, Boston, 1965, Houghton Mifflin Co.

Rossman, I.: Clinical geriatrics, Philadelphia, 1971, J. B. Lippincott Co.

Satir, V: Peoplemaking, Palo Alto, Calif., 1972, Science and Behavior Books.

Spiegel, J. P.: The resolution of role conflict within the family, Psychiatry **20**:1-18, 1957.

Titchner, J. L., and Kapp, F. T.: Family and character change at Buffalo Creek, Am. J. Psychiatry **133**(3):295-299, 1976.

World Almanac, 1977, U.S. labor force, employment and unemployment, p. 128.

BIBLIOGRAPHY

Anderson, M., editor: Sociology of the family, New York, 1971, Penguin Books.

Andrews, G., and Tennant, C.: A scale to measure the cause of life events, Aust. N. Z. J. Psychiatry **11**(3):163-167, 1977.

Andrews, G., Tennant, C., Hewson, D., and Schonell, W.: The relation of social factors to physical and psychiatric illness, Am. J. Epidemiol. **108**(1):27-35, 1978.

Andrews, G., Tennant, C., Hewson, D., and Vaillant, G. E.: Life event stress, social support, coping style, and risk of psychological impairment, J. Nerv. Ment. Dis. **166**(5):307-316, 1978.

Bell, J. E.: Family therapy, New York, 1975, Jason Aronson, Inc.

Bell, R. R.: The impact of illness on family roles. In Falta, J. R., and Deck, E. S., editors: A sociological framework for patient care, New York, 1966, John Wiley & Sons, Inc., pp. 177-190.

Blumberg, R. L., and Winch, R. F.: Societal complexity and familial complexity. In Winch, R. F., and Spanier, G., editors: Selected studies in marriage and the family, New York, 1974, Holt, Rinehart & Winston, pp. 97-113.

Braidwood, R. J.: Prehistoric men, ed. 6, Chicago, 1963, Chicago Natural History Museum Popular Series, Anthropology No. 37.

Brown, B. B.: Social and psychological correlates of help-seeking behavior among urban adults, Am. J. Community Psychol. **6**(5):425-439, 1978.

Butler, R. N.: Why survive? being old in America, New York, 1975, Harper & Row Publishers, Inc.

Butler, R. N., and Lewis, M.: Aging and mental health: positive psychological approaches, St. Louis, 1973, The C. V. Mosby Co.

Caldwell, J. R.: New roads to yesterday: essays in archaeology, New York, 1966, Basic Books, Inc., Publishers.

Childe, G. V.: Man makes himself, New York, 1951, Mentor and Signet Books, The New American Library of World Literature, Inc.

de Beauvoir, S.: The coming of age, New York, 1973, Warner Paperback Library.

Fell, J.: Grief reactions in the elderly following death of a spouse: the role of crisis intervention and nursing, J. Gerontological Nurs. **3**(6):17-20, 1977.

Glasser, W.: The identity society, New York, 1972, Harper & Row Publishers, Inc.

Goode, W.: Readings on the family and society, Englewood Cliffs, N.J., 1964a, Prentice-Hall, Inc.

Goode, W., editor: The family, Englewood Cliffs, N.J., 1964b, Prentice-Hall, Inc.

Gould, R. L.: Transformations: growth and change in adult life, New York, 1968, Simon & Schuster, Inc.

Haley, J., and Hoffman, L.: Techniques of family therapy, New York, 1967, Basic Books, Inc., Publishers.

Hamilton, J. W.: The significance of object loss in individual response to accidental trauma, Comp. Psychiatry **18**(2):189-199, 1977.

Hirsch, E. A.: Some thoughts concerning the life cycle, Bull. Menninger Clin. **41**(3):255-265, 1977.
Jacobs, S., and Ostfeld, A.: An epidemiological review of the mortality of bereavement, Psychosom. Med. **39**(5):344-357, 1977.
Krader, L.: Formation of the state, Englewood Cliffs, N.J., 1968, Prentice-Hall, Inc.
Kubler-Ross, E.: Death, the final stage of growth, Englewood Cliffs, N.J., 1975, Prentice-Hall, Inc.
Kutscher, A. H.: Death and bereavement, Springfield, Ill., 1974, Charles C Thomas, Publisher.
Laing, R. D.: Knots, Middlesex, England, 1970, Penguin Books.
Laing, R. D.: The politics of the family and other essays, 1971, Vantage Books.
Life and death and medicine (special issue), Sci. Am. **229**(3):22-169, 1973.
Lurie, E.: Limits to informal support systems of the elderly. Paper presented at the Western Gerontological Society Meeting, San Francisco, Calif., May 1, 1979.
Marris, P.: Loss and change, New York, 1974, Pantheon Books, Inc.
McAdams, R.: The evolution of urban society, Chicago, 1966, Aldine Publishing Co.
McGreehan, D. M., and Warburton, S. W.: How to help families cope with caring for elderly members, Geriatrics **33**(6):99-100, 102, 106, 1978.
Mead, M.: Changing patterns of parent-child relations in an urban culture, Int. J. Psychoanal. **38**:369-378, 1957.
Moulthrop, H. E., and Toxborough, J.: Know your community resources: network support for the aged: the viable alternative to institutionalization, J. Gerontological Nurs. **4**(6):64-66, 1978.
Otten, J., and Shelley, F. D.: When your parents grow old, New York, 1976, Funk & Wagnalls, Inc.
Sahlins, M. D.: Tribesmen, Englewood Cliffs, N.J., 1968, Prentice-Hall, Inc.
Schmuck, R.: Sex of sibling, birth order position and female dispositions to conform in two-child families, Child Dev. **34**:913-918, 1963.
Service, E. R.: The hunters, Englewood Cliffs, N.J., 1966, Prentice-Hall, Inc.
Sheehy, G.: Passages, New York, 1977, Bantam Books.
Shock, N. W.: Perspectives of the aging process. In Simon, A., and Epstein, L. J., editors: Aging in modern society. Psychiatric research reports of the American Psychiatric Association, 1966.
Shorter, E.: The rise of the nuclear family. In The making of the modern family, New York, 1975, Basic Books, pp. 205-268.
Shneidman, E. S., editor: Death: current perspectives, Palo Alto, Calif., 1976, Mayfield Publishing Co.
Shulman, K.: Suicide and parasuicide in old age: a review, Age Aging **7**(4):201-209, 1978.
Silverstone, B., and Hyman, H. K.: You and your aging parent, New York, 1976, Pantheon Books.
Spiegel, J. P.: Cultural strain, family role patterns and intrapsychic conflicts. In Howells, J., editor: Theory and practice of family psychiatry, New York, 1971, Brunner/Mazell, Inc., pp. 367-389.
Spuhler, J. N., editor: The evolution of man's capacity for culture, Detroit, 1965, Wayne State University Press.
Steury, S., and Blank, M. L., editors: Readings in psychotherapy with older people, U.S. Department of Health, Education and Welfare, Publication No. (ADM)77-409, 1977.
Sullivan, H. S.: The psychiatric interview, New York, 1970, W. W. Norton & Co., Inc.
Tobin, S. S., and Lieberman, M. A.: Last home for the aged, San Francisco, 1976, Jossey-Bass Publishers.
Toffler, A.: Future shock, New York, 1971, Bantam Books.
Towle, C.: Personality development. In The learner in education for the professions, Chicago, 1954, University of Chicago Press.
Turner, R.: Family interaction, New York, 1970, John Wiley & Sons, Inc.
Wallace, A., and Fogelson, R.: The identity struggle. In Boszormenji-Nagy, I., and Framo, J., editors: Intensive family therapy, New York, 1965, Harper & Row Publishers, Inc.
Watzlawick, P., Bevin, J., and Jackson, D.: Pragmatics of human communication, New York, 1967, W. W. Norton & Co., Inc.
Wheelis, A.: The quest for identity, New York, 1958, W. W. Norton & Co., Inc.
Whitehead, T.: Confusing causes of confusion, Nurs. Mirror **147**(12):29-30, 1978.
Wolf, E. R.: Peasants, Englewood Cliffs, N.J., 1966, Prentice-Hall, Inc.

15

SUMMING IT UP: THE CAREGIVER'S URGENT NEEDS

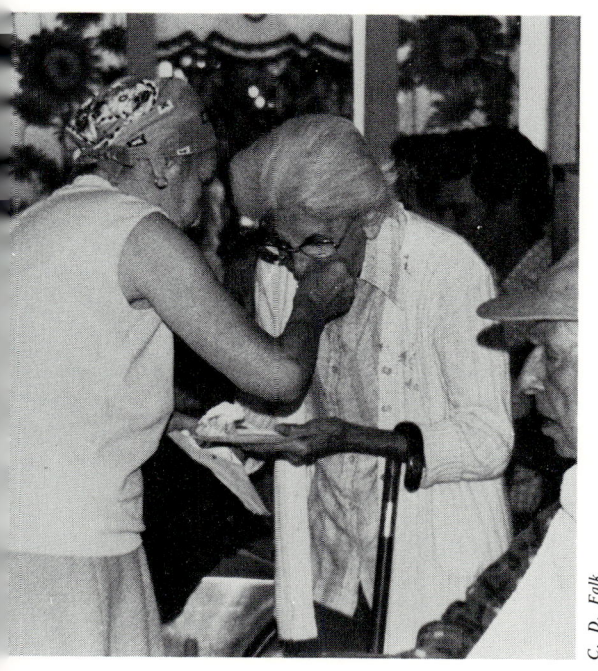

C. D. Falk

Care of the older person by a younger one presents role reversal—the younger person as caregiver and the older one as a dependent recipient of care. The view of the aged as dependent, frail, and in need of assistance has not been incorporated into our attitudinal and value systems. It has resulted in a stereotyped approach to the care of the aging person. The younger nurse who has not experienced aging can only make inferences, so she is forced to act according to fixed ideas. This chapter confronts the problems of stress and strain experienced by the caregiver when caring for the confused aged. It affects all professional persons who tend to avoid the care by hasty contacts and decisions based on preconceived ideas.

Example. The student nurse came to her instructor about 89-year-old Mr. L., who had a diagnosis of organic brain syndrome. He seemed quite well oriented to her and in touch with his reality. Thinking that she had missed something in her assessment, she asked the physician the basis of his diagnosis. "I asked him who the president is, and he doesn't know," was his reply. The student went back to Mr. L. and asked him who the president was. His reply, "At 89 years of age, what the hell difference does it make."

The physician had diagnosed on the basis of his stereotype and a standard test that did not take into consideration that the patient was a migrant worker, had never voted in his life, and did not have access to information. Such action is frequently found in relation to the elderly when the professional caregiver is not acquainted with the life history and culture of the elderly. They do not find such contacts rewarding and tend to avoid them.

The confused elderly are found everywhere: in airports, social security offices, rental offices, hospital beds, and nursing homes. They are reacted to on the basis of their age and the attitude and stereotypes held by caregivers. We noted that on an orthopedic ward, when there were three confused elderly patients with hip fracture at the same time, tension increased among the staff. There are no scales to measure such tension, but nurses "blew up;" short answers were the rule, work was disorganized, and deadlines unmet. In analyzing the chaotic situation it would seem that when the dependable world of the caregiver changes, she becomes tense and stressed; more fatigue was expressed at an earlier hour. The strain of trying to predict the unpredictable behavior in the confused elderly took its toll of the caregiver's strength and energy.

Staff in long-term care units where there are large numbers of confused elderly have various mechanisms for handling the stress of care. Infantilization of the elderly is one such mechanism. Comments such as, "She is the cutest thing," are heard. Women's hair is decorated with ribbon bows, dolls are given to patients, and in general the need to treat this older person as a child is demonstrated. Another form of denial is "gallows humor," in which the client and his family are mimicked and mocked. Staff tend to work in pairs, with social interaction occurring between staff members rather than with the patient, who becomes a part of the furniture. Coffee breaks are prolonged and sick days are taken frequently. Staff turnover may reach the 100% level during a year. This is an indication of the strain staff members express when caring for elderly people who do not react or communicate in predictable patterns. There are other causes for these behavioral responses, but the emphasis centers on stress and client unpredictability.

INTERNAL REWARDS

It is frustrating to go home after a day of working with elderly people and know that at no time during the day was a task really finished. The feeling of guilt can be pervasive as the nurse realizes she has not given good or even adequate care. The reason may be that she does not know how to set realistic goals or to recognize small gains. Conflict may arise because of a need to care for the elderly in the way she would like to be cared for and the lack of time, knowledge, and skill to do it. Rewards come from knowing that one has done a great job, an acceptable job, or at least one performed as well as possible under the circumstances. What leads to the nurse's knowing that she has accomplished one of the three? How can the nurse who must "pass medicines" live with the fact that she missed opportunities to give the human kindness that the client needed more than a cathartic? And how can she reconcile the fact that no one could have used the time any more efficiently than she, but still there was not enough?

We cannot answer these tough questions, nor can any one at this time, but the following suggestions are offered for assisting the caregiver to get the internal rewards that will enable her to continue with a frustrating job.

1. Peer group sharing should occur whether sanctioned within the work situation or not. The caregiver must be able to measure her efforts against some kind of yardstick. Peers often tend to be more realistic than administrators but can also provide slipshod shortcuts. Peer group sharing should be an in-service activity that leads to constructive suggestions.
2. The more knowledge one has, the greater the number of options available when routines are interfered with or delayed. Ritualized care does not promote the challenge to thinking and acting that more knowledge offers. There should be adequate orientation and staff development for the caregiver who works with the confused elderly. This approach would allow for greater prediction and reduce the strain of uncertainty.

3. Only skilled practitioners should care for the confused elderly. The competent staff member does not experience the stress of the uncertain person. Interactional skills are required by all levels of personnel, from janitor to physician. Special training should be provided for those who will work with the agitated or aggressive client.

If we handle a situation well and know that we have functioned at a high level of competence, the inner satisfaction is highly rewarding. We place staff at a disadvantage when we ask them to assume responsibilities for tasks they cannot perform adequately because of lack of training, insight, or emotional readiness. *We set them up for failure.* The result is an unhappy, frustrated staff member who will probably leave soon and affect the morale of other staff members. This behavior, in turn, adds to the problems of the confused client. Inner rewards can be negative; they may even be interpreted as punishment.

Suggestions have been made to solve some of our social problems by having people work in long-term care units with the elderly. Some have even been so drastic as to suggest using such service as an alternative to a jail sentence. Others have used jobs of caring for the elderly as a means of taking mothers with little children off welfare roles. *We question the wisdom of such programs. Those who care for the confused elderly should do so by informed choice,* with full knowledge of the physical and emotional strains inherent in working with people whose behavior is not easily understood and often not predictable.

EXTERNAL REWARDS

Good work should have recognition. Rewards that reinforce satisfactory performance will often produce greater effort. This should not be used in a manipulative way but should give honest praise for worthwhile achievement. There are many ways of offering external rewards—a pat on the back and the words "well done" cost nothing and mean much. Other recognitions may include a bonus, raise in pay, or a picture and story on the bulletin board or in the house organ. The staff member may be held up as a role model and asked to demonstrate some special technique she used to improve care. A recognition day was planned in one institution to honor employees' special achievements. Administration members cannot afford to overlook outstanding achievement, but they must also recognize the day-in and day-out performance of the competent worker whose performance is taken for granted. Determination of ways in which external rewards can be given is limited only by the imagination.

"Burnout"

The most expensive employee is the new one. Yet the problem of employee burnout ensures a constant loss of oriented and trained personnel and a stream of new employees taking their place. The problem of employee burnout is being widely discussed today; its recent naming and definition have resulted in problem-solving attempts to achieve a solution. The unsupported caregiver, who is mentally and physically exhausted from day-to-day contact with clients she cannot understand, may have such an intolerable feeling of failure that she has to leave the job. Employee turnover in the long-term care units should be studied to determine ways of decreasing turnover arising from employee burnout, or low employee morale.

Elongated shadow

Emerson is quoted as saying that institutions are the elongated shadow of a single man. The institution with a high employee turnover rate must see whose shadow it is and determine the attitudes held by the one who casts the shadow. Often, indifference to the elderly or the emphasis on aspects of the institution other than good quality care originates at the top. An institution is no better than the person who represents authority. Good administration is more than day-by-day operation; it includes responsibility for the growth and welfare of the employees. It is here that external rewards originate and policies and procedures resulting in internal rewards are controlled.

Organizational activity that leads to better administration practice

In the United States there are many organizations for providing long-term care with programs for their members that assist in developing their knowledge, attitudes, and skills. For the nurse there is a newly organized group for long-term care unit personnel, the Council of Nursing Home Nurses, organized by the gerontologic nursing division of the American Nurses' Association. A number of nursing home organizations exist that provide continuing education and group meetings for exchange of ideas and information. Most organizations have a publication with articles designed to update the knowledge of the membership. Every caregiver should belong to at least one organization and keep abreast of at least one publication geared to the interest and needs of those working in long-term care.

The American Geriatric Society has a broad-based membership. The Gerontological Society has scientific sessions annually with sections devoted to a number of scientific disciplines. Membership includes subscriptions to the *Journal of Gerontology* and the *Gerontologist*, which report research about the elderly. The Journal of Gerontological Nursing is published by the Charles B. Slack Publishing Co., and *Geriatric Nursing* is published by the American Journal of Nursing Co.

Every medical center has a library usually open to interested persons. A number of gerontology centers connected with universities offer help to those who request it. Publications by the Public Health Department and Institutes of Aging (Department of Health and Human Services) offer a wide spectrum of resources. Each state has a state Office of Aging, and every community should have access to a regional council on aging. Lack of information cannot be blamed on lack of resources.

CONTINUING EDUCATION

In-service education and short-term courses should be available for everyone, including the janitor, who can be extremely influential in the care of the elderly. He may represent the sole male link with an outside world for the male residents. His importance should not be minimized.

Example. The Mexican-American janitor was the only one who spoke Spanish with three old men. Each morning they waited near the employee's entrance for Carlos to speak to them in their language and tell them of the outside world. The time he spent was noticed by his employer, who fired him for "goofing off and talking to patients." The three old men began fading and withdrew. They retreated into their former shells and did not even speak with one another. Carlos had been a strong therapeutic influence.

The cook who prepares a dish that a dying patient has wanted to taste one more time feels an internal reward. The cook first has to realize that this is acceptable conduct, that taking the time will not be deducted. This comes from in-service education regarding the needs of the elderly and the policies of the institution. It is concern about continued growth of employees that increases the quality of their performance and leads to internal rewards. The organizational activity and resources lead to comprehensive in-service material, which should lead to personnel development and better quality care.

The care of the confused elderly is a human service that cannot be mechanized or computerized; it is quintessentially human interaction. The best education model is the example of an expert. No one will learn through texts or visual aids alone. There must be a role model who is respected and successful in dealing with the complex care of the confused elderly. Everyone's body of knowledge and skills is used in giving care to the aged, and one important quantity may still be missing—the innovative and imaginative use of self by the committed caregiver.

IMPLICATIONS FOR RESEARCH

Throughout this book there have been implicit problems for research. Several groups of nurses are studying confusion in the elderly; psychologists are studying the phenomenon, and biomedical studies are being made. We believe the day-by-day care of the confused elderly person must be studied in a way that can be translated into practice by the practitioner. Explicit in this is the need to study personnel and administrative practices that give support to the caregiver, whose constant contact with the confused elderly leads to behavior that may either deny the situation and the personal feeling of defeat or lead to infantilization and depersonalization of the elderly. With the increase of confused elderly in their own homes, in hospitals, and in long-term care units, the problems of caregiver burnout deserve intensive study. The caregiver may be the family member or the person hired by an institution; both need study.

Design of long-term care units as facilitative environments also must be more thoroughly researched. Economics and convenience rather than the effect on the elderly person have often dictated architectural design and furnishings. Administrators and architects should realize the environment itself provides a therapeutic influence on the elderly.

The nursing practitioner as a primary health caregiver deserves testing as a resource to predict and prevent confusion in the elderly (Appendix A). This will demand legislative action, political strategies, and a change in the present Medicare system of paying the physician as the primary medical caregiver. It also will involve a concept of preventive care versus curative medicine.

Which interactions are therapeutic and what makes them so are problems that must be studied. We have seen the miracles that follow one person's interaction and the failures of another person who apparently replicated the technique and principles involved.

We are only beginning to turn our research interest to the unglamorous, and sometimes repulsive, confused elderly person. It is a frontier that must be penetrated by providers of direct care who have research skills. There has been a great deal of research by those who do not have direct contact with the confused elderly. Now we need to learn from the caregivers who have worked closely with them and who have insights that can lead to researchable solutions to the problems still facing all of us.

APPENDIX

CONFUSION IN THE ELDERLY: A PROTOCOL TO DETERMINE ACUTE ORGANIC BRAIN SYNDROME VERSUS CHRONIC ORGANIC BRAIN SYNDROME*

Darlene J. Anderson

This protocol is to be used with clients presenting with confusion. Memory loss may be actual or spurious. The purpose of this protocol is to facilitate the early recognition of the acute, potentially reversible states of confusion, such as those caused by infection, malnutrition, heart failure, or drug intoxication, and eradicate the cause before they progress to become chronic irreversible states. This protocol will include physiologic as well as functional acute episodes.

Important parts of a history and physical examination that should be explored are enumerated with rationale given for each part. Flow sheets have been devised that will point toward the determination of whether the confusion is of a chronic or acute nature. Pertinent objective data are outlined with ranges of normal and abnormal and explanations of possible interpretation of abnormal findings. An assessment of various disease entities in the categories ''you cannot afford to miss'' as well as a plan (by no means all inclusive) discussing possible management alternatives are also included.

What you cannot afford to miss

Acute organic brain disease resulting from:
1. Infections
2. Metabolic disorders
3. Cardiovascular disorders
4. Drugs
5. Cerebral dysfunction
6. Sensory deprivation
7. Environmental changes

---

* For the geriatric nurse practitioner

SUBJECTIVE DATA

If possible, the history should be obtained first from the client, *allowing ample time for response to questions.* (Do not mistake expressive aphasia for confusion.) Second, a family member or close associate should be questioned to confirm findings and elicit any behavioral changes. Avoid inducing paranoia in the client by preventing this second person from speaking in whispers or tones not audible to the client. Other history sources could include social workers and past medical records.

Age _____
Mode of onset
   How long has confusion been present? _____
   When does confusion occur? _____

YES	NO		YES	NO	*Character of confusion*
☐	☐	Early morning?			Orientation to:
☐	☐	Between meals?	☐	☐	Person
☐	☐	Daytime?	☐	☐	Place
☐	☐	Nighttime?	☐	☐	Time
			☐	☐	Capable of simple calculation?

Years of completed schooling _____

YES	NO	*Aggravating factors*
☐	☐	Head trauma? If yes, when _____
		Fractures? _____
		Skull films? _____
☐	☐	Recent alcohol intake? When _____
☐	☐	Recent alcohol discontinuance? When _____
☐	☐	Recent drug intake? When _____
☐	☐	Recent drug discontinuance? When _____
☐	☐	Recent change in environment? Relocation? _____
☐	☐	Recent change in job? _____
☐	☐	Recent change in relationships? _____
☐	☐	Recent change in family? _____
☐	☐	Recent change in friends? _____
☐	☐	Recent change in memory? _____
☐	☐	Recent medical disease? _____
☐	☐	Recent surgical disease? _____
☐	☐	Recent neurologic disease? _____
		Recent loss of:
☐	☐	Spouse
☐	☐	Significant other
☐	☐	Pet
☐	☐	Treasured possession
☐	☐	Does client eat alone?

Who prepares meals? _____
What does diet consist of? _____

Continued.

SUBJECTIVE DATA—cont'd

Associated symptoms

YES	NO		YES	NO	
☐	☐	Change in attention span?	☐	☐	Decline in intellectual functions?
☐	☐	Change in ability to concentrate?	☐	☐	Blurred vision?
☐	☐	History of seizures?	☐	☐	Diplopia?
☐	☐	Poor control of emotions?	☐	☐	Hallucinations?
☐	☐	Fear for existence/paranoia?	☐	☐	Lethargy?
☐	☐	Melancholia?	☐	☐	Stupor?
☐	☐	Pessimism?	☐	☐	Changes in sensation?
☐	☐	Weakness?	☐	☐	Gait changes?
☐	☐	Numbness, tingling?	☐	☐	Drooling?
☐	☐	Paresthesias?	☐	☐	Slurred speech?
☐	☐	Headache?	☐	☐	Breathing problems?
☐	☐	Fever?	☐	☐	History of falls?
☐	☐	Vomiting?	☐	☐	History of syphilis?
☐	☐	Smoker?	☐	☐	Inappropriate behavior?

Past medical history (give date of onset if known and who diagnosed)

YES	NO	
☐	☐	Chronic obstructive pulmonary disease _____
☐	☐	Cardiac disease _____
☐	☐	Cerebrovascular accident _____
☐	☐	Hypertension _____
☐	☐	Diabetes _____
☐	☐	Anemia _____
☐	☐	Peptic ulcer disease _____
☐	☐	Depression _____
☐	☐	Renal problems _____
☐	☐	Hyperthyroidism _____
☐	☐	Hypothyroidism _____
☐	☐	Injuries _____

Medications

YES	NO		YES	NO	
☐	☐	Barbiturates	☐	☐	Tranquilizers
☐	☐	Antidepressants	☐	☐	Amphetamines
☐	☐	Adrenal steroids	☐	☐	Atropine
☐	☐	Belladonna	☐	☐	Alcohol
☐	☐	Salicylates	☐	☐	Antihypertensives
☐	☐	Diuretics	☐	☐	Sedatives
☐	☐	Hypnotics			
☐	☐	Ingestion (accidental or deliberate) of household or industrial cleaners?			
☐	☐	Fumes from zinc welding or mixture of cleansing agents?			

Past treatment

YES	NO	
☐	☐	Previous neurologic examination:
		Date _____
		Findings _____
☐	☐	Dynamic brain scan: Findings _____
☐	☐	Electroencephalogram: Results _____
☐	☐	Spinal tap: Findings _____
☐	☐	Skull films: Findings _____
☐	☐	Computerized axial tomography: Findings _____

Coping mechanisms
Cultural background _____
Frequency of past medical visits _____
Recreation _____
Pattern of handling stress _____

YES NO *Review of systems* (elaborate positive findings)
☐ ☐ Nausea/vomiting _____
☐ ☐ Diarrhea _____
☐ ☐ Anorexia _____
☐ ☐ Weight gain _____
☐ ☐ Weight loss _____
☐ ☐ Sense of smell _____
☐ ☐ Sense of taste _____
☐ ☐ Voiding/bowel movement patterns _____
☐ ☐ Retention of urine _____
☐ ☐ Impotence _____
☐ ☐ Joint aches _____
☐ ☐ Headache _____
☐ ☐ Nasal stuffiness _____
☐ ☐ Vision disturbances _____

OBJECTIVE DATA

Vital signs
Weight _____ Height _____ Temperature _____ Respiration _____
Right blood pressure and pulse: Sitting _____ Standing _____ Lying _____
Left blood pressure and pulse: Sitting _____ Standing _____ Lying _____

YES NO *General* (appearance and affect)
☐ ☐ Do clothes match?

YES NO *Skin*
         No examination _____
☐ ☐ Lesions
☐ ☐ Bruises
☐ ☐ Spider hemangiomas
☐ ☐ Jaundice

YES NO *Eyes*
         No examination _____
         Acuity _____
☐ ☐ PERRLA (Pupils equal, round,
         react to light and accommodation)
☐ ☐ Nystagmus
☐ ☐ Extraocular movements
☐ ☐ Visual fields full
         Deficit _____
☐ ☐ Funduscopic examination
☐ ☐ Arteriovenous nicking
☐ ☐ Exudates
☐ ☐ Hemorrhage
☐ ☐ Cataracts

YES NO *Neck*
         No examination _____
☐ ☐ Stiffness
☐ ☐ Bruits
☐ ☐ Thyroid enlargement
☐ ☐ Radiation of murmurs
☐ ☐ Lymph node enlargement
         Character and quality
         of pulses _____
         _____

YES NO *Head*
         No examination _____
☐ ☐ Bruits
☐ ☐ Battle's sign
☐ ☐ Asymmetry
☐ ☐ Bossing

YES NO *Ears*
         No examination _____
         Weber's test _____
         Rinne test _____
☐ ☐ Cerumen occlusion
☐ ☐ Otitis

Continued.

OBJECTIVE DATA—cont'd

YES NO *Nose*
         No examination _____
☐   ☐   Nasal stuffiness

YES NO *Mouth*
         No examination _____
☐   ☐   Edentulous
☐   ☐   Tooth decay
☐   ☐   Gum disease
☐   ☐   Buccal lesions
☐   ☐   Tongue normal

YES NO *Throat*
         No examination _____
         Position of uvula _____
☐   ☐   Tonsils present

YES NO *Chest*
         No examination _____
☐   ☐   Rales
☐   ☐   Rhonchi
☐   ☐   Breath sounds
             Present _____
             Diminished _____
             Absent _____
☐   ☐   Egophony

YES NO *Heart*
         No examination _____
         Point of maximal impulse _____
         _____
☐   ☐   Murmur
         Describe _____
☐   ☐   Rub
☐   ☐   Peripheral pulses
☐   ☐   Gallop
☐   ☐   Pedal edema

YES NO *Extremities*
         No examination _____
☐   ☐   Cyanosis
☐   ☐   Edema
☐   ☐   Temperature
☐   ☐   Vibratory sense diminished
☐   ☐   Proprioception intact

YES NO *Abdomen*
         No examination _____
☐   ☐   Masses
☐   ☐   Liver-Kidney-Spleen palpable
☐   ☐   Ascites
☐   ☐   Bruits

YES NO *Rectum*
         No examination _____
☐   ☐   Occult blood
☐   ☐   Masses

YES NO *Neurologic examination*
         No examination _____ (Explain abnormal findings)
☐   ☐   Cranial nerve deficit (Explain results of examination [+ or −])
         _____ I _____ II _____ III _____ IV _____ V _____ VI
         _____ VII _____ VIII _____ IX _____ X _____ XI _____ XII
☐   ☐   Decreased motor function, range of motion, muscle strength
☐   ☐   Sensory deficits _____
         Deep tendon reflexes (Grade 0 to 4+)
☐   ☐   Diminished
☐   ☐   Hyperactive
☐   ☐   Babinski's sign
☐   ☐   Romberg's sign
☐   ☐   Finger-to-nose testing intact
☐   ☐   Heel-to-shin testing intact
☐   ☐   Stereognosis
☐   ☐   Fasciculations

The neurologic examination should be extended when trying to determine organic brain disease. The following tests are extensions of that examination. Their interpretation and rationale will be given under *Objective rationale* later in this protocol.

Mental status questionnaire (MSQ) (Indicate correct response with [+], incorrect response with [−].)

PLUS   MINUS
____   ____   1. What is the name of this place? or Where are you now?
              Answer given _____
____   ____   2. Where is this place located? _____
____   ____   3. What day is it? _____
____   ____   4. What is today's date? _____
____   ____   5. What year is it? _____
____   ____   6. How old are you? _____
____   ____   7. When were you born? (month) _____
____   ____   8. When were you born? (year) _____
____   ____   9. Who is the president of the United States? _____
____   ____   10. Who was president before him? _____

Face-to-hand test (Indicate correct response with [+], incorrect response with [−].)

The client is touched simultaneously on the cheek and the dorsum of the hand (according to the following sequence) and asked to indicate where he was touched. The test is first done with the eyes closed and then open.

Repeat the first four trials (trials 7 to 10 are the same as 1 to 4). Only steps 7 to 10 are considered significant in determining the degree of altered brain function.

PLUS   MINUS   PLUS   MINUS
____   ____   1. Right cheek—left hand   ____   ____   6. Both hands
____   ____   2. Left cheek—right hand   ____   ____   7. Right cheek—left hand
____   ____   3. Right cheek—right hand   ____   ____   8. Left cheek—right hand
____   ____   4. Left cheek—left hand   ____   ____   9. Right cheek—right hand
____   ____   5. Both cheeks   ____   ____   10. Left cheek—left hand

YES NO   *Testing recall*
☐   ☐   Remembers three unrelated things

YES NO   *Testing basic language skills*
☐   ☐   Names common objects such as pencil, clock, pillow, book, and chair
☐   ☐   Matches printed and written words with pictures
☐   ☐   Reads some simple words, both printed and written
☐   ☐   Reads and follows written simple commands such as "Tap right foot"
☐   ☐   Follows simple verbal commands such as "Stand up" or "Shake my hand"
☐   ☐   Follows complex verbal commands such as "Left hand on right knee" or "Look at the ceiling and raise your arm"

YES NO   *Testing attention and concentration*
☐   ☐   Subtracts 7 from 100 and continues subtracting by 7
☐   ☐   Repeats a series of digits at the rate of 1 digit per second and adds another digit in each series until 8 digits are reached
☐   ☐   Reverses a series of 4 digits

YES NO   *Testing for abstract reasoning*
☐   ☐   Correctly explains how similar objects are the same, such as an orange and an apple, a cat and a mouse, and paper and coal

Continued.

OBJECTIVE DATA—cont'd

YES NO *Testing for judgment*
☐ ☐ Correctly answers such questions as (1) What would you do if you lost a library book? (2) Why is it better to give to an organized charity than to a street beggar? and (3) Why should criminals be put in jail?

YES NO *Testing sensory perception and coordination*
☐ ☐ Writes own name on a page of blank paper on request
☐ ☐ Copies simple figures, including a circle, square, cross, diamond, and a few dots

YES NO *Evaluating mood*
☐ ☐ Do you get pretty discouraged, depressed, and blue?
How do you feel? _____
☐ ☐ Do you ever feel life is not worth living?
☐ ☐ Have you ever considered suicide?
How would you do it? _____
What would happen after you were gone? _____

Assessment _____

Laboratory tests to aid in differentiating acute and chronic organic brain syndrome (OBS)

Complete blood count with mean corpuscular volume, mean corpuscular hemoglobin, and mean corpuscular hemoglobin concentration
Urinalysis
Serum glucose, fasting blood sugar, and 2-hour postprandial
Electrolytes
Blood urea nitrogen and creatinine
Thyroid function
Liver function
Serum levels of barbiturates, bromides, and digitalis
Vitamin B_{12} and folic acid
Fluorescent treponemal antibody absorption
Chest x-ray
Electrocardiogram
Venereal Disease Research Laboratories test (VDRL)
Electroencephalogram
Skull x-rays
Spinal tap
Dynamic brain scan
Computerized axial tomography scan
Cisternography

SUBJECTIVE DATA RATIONALE

How long has confusion been present? Abrupt onset is usually indicative of an organic cause. Slow, progressive onset is more indicative of a degenerative cause. Confusion may be the first sign of myxedema, pneumonia, prostatism or urinary retention, and diabetes.

When does confusion occur? Confusion in the early morning or between meals may denote hypoglycemia. Daytime confusion is usually indicative of a bilateral cerebrovascular accident. It may also result from nighttime hypnotics because the drug is not fully excreted in the elderly. Nighttime confusion, more often than not, is innocuous. However, sedatives and hypnotics can be a factor.

Orientation to person, place, and time. Acute disorientation is commonly found in many kinds of inflammatory, toxic, metabolic, or traumatic brain disease. Disorientation for place and person implies more profound degenerative cerebral disorder.

Capable of simple calculations. Inability to calculate is a sensitive index of dominant parietal lesions and diffuse cerebral disease. It may be present in depression and anxiety.

Years of schooling completed. This must be taken into consideration in testing arithmetic skills.

Head trauma. Consider cerebral contusion, midbrain hemorrhage, and subdural hematoma as causes for confusion.

Recent changes in job, family, friends, and environment. Relocation or dislocation of environment can produce paranoia in the elderly. The elderly have less readily adaptive capacities and can suffer confusion as a result of abrupt changes in daily routines and the environment—the danger of "transfer trauma."

Recent loss of spouse, significant other, pet, or treasured possession. This can lead to a depressive reaction that is sometimes easily missed and labeled an "organic" cause of confusion.

Eating habits and diet. Consider malnutrition as a cause of confusion. Elderly are particularly susceptible to vitamin B deficiencies.

Associated symptoms

Changes in attention span, ability to concentrate, intellectual function, ability to control emotions or trouble expressing thoughts. Do not assume the client with behavior disturbances has significant cerebral damage before testing him. Much can be done to help the client adapt by improving his mood and behavior. Poor memory may be caused by depression. Defects in grasp and comprehension may suggest acute OBS. These symptoms may have an organic or functional etiology. The client who *states* that his memory is poor or his concentration is less often does well on MSQ test and other mental status tests. When good performance on testing is evident, you must think of depression as the cause of confusion. Acute onset of these changes points to metabolic or drug-induced changes. Insidious onset is more likely from a progressive degenerative process. In organic disease involving the cerebral structure, emotional lability is quite common. Depression is characterized by drowsiness and falling asleep in the evening, waking by bedtime, falling asleep without trouble, and perhaps awakening in the early morning feeling anxious or worried.

History of seizures. Seizures may begin many months after a severe head injury that causes fractures or penetration of the skull. In the older patient with no history of previous seizures, cerebral tumor is a possibility. Cerebrovascular accident must be considered in patients over 60 with a sudden onset of focal paralysis. Convulsions with no focal or general history of infection or evidence of embolic focus elsewhere are often diagnosed as the result of tumor. Infection (meningitis, encephalitis, or brain abscess) must be considered, especially if stiff neck, fever, chills, headache, and localized neurologic abnormalities are present. Diastolic blood pressures of greater than 140, with headache, blurred vision, stupor, and hypertensive history, point to hypertensive encephalopathy.

Blurred vision/diplopia. Temporal arteritis may present with sudden blindness. Cataracts must be considered in the elderly. Other disturbances of vision can include hemorrhage into the retina or vitreous, vascular disturbances such as embolus of the retinal artery, thrombosis of the retinal vein, or spasm, which is encountered in arteriosclerosis and uremia. Glaucoma, retinal detachment, and iritis are other conditions that can disturb vision. Exophthalmic thyroid disease can produce diplopia resulting from pressure. Diabetes, intracranial aneurysms, brainstem disease, and myasthenia gravis are other possible causes for blurred vision/diplopia.

Fear for existence/paranoia, melancholia, pessimism, hallucinations, and inappropriate behavior. Psychoneurosis is rarely seen in late life; a practical rule is that all mental illness in late life results from structural disease or depressive reactions. Paranoia may be caused by hearing loss. Visual hallucinations are most frequently seen in toxic states. Hallucinations may occur in any of the sensory modalities, but they are most common in the auditory sphere. Usually, illusions appear in confused states and are toxic in origin. It takes mental capacity to elaborate a psychosis or psychoneurotic behavior. Coercive, exploitive, paranoid reactions are seen only when the brain syndrome is no more than moderate.

Lethargy. Lethargy often is associated with depression and may be a cause of confusion in the elderly. Also consider medications, including Aldomet, reserpine, sedatives, tranquilizers, antidepressants, and antihistamines. Lethargy may also be a nonspecific manifestation of numerous disease entities; for example, upper respiratory tract infection, meningitis, anemia, cardiorespiratory failure, and low-grade infections such as urinary tract infection and tuberculosis.

Stupor. A diabetic client taking insulin or oral hypoglycemic agents may be in a coma without lateralizing neurologic signs. Stupor may be secondary to a severe systemic infection such as pneumonia/bacteremia. (Often the temperature does not elevate in the elderly with pneumonia.) Other possible causes of stupor include metabolic and endocrine disorders, brain abscess, chronic and acute renal failure, cerebral infarction, brain tumor, and shock.

Changes in sensation. Sensory examination may be difficult and of questionable reliability. Testing, therefore, should be made as objective as possible and the reliability of the observation noted. Comparison with corresponding parts of the body will provide the best control. Motor or inconstant sensory impairment has no significance unless found with other more clearcut signs of trouble. Pinpricks will be felt at the thalamic level, but the number, location, size, and pressure of multiple simultaneous pinpricks will be interpreted as a function of the parietal cortex. In peripheral nerve lesions, the sensory loss will be in the cutaneous distribution of that nerve. Light touch with wisps of cotton is to be identified where the touch is felt and is a test of discriminatory (parietal lobe) function. Deep pain is lost or decreased in lesions of the dorsal columns and dorsal roots, such as in tabetic neurosyphilis and diabetic pseudotabes. Loss of joint position sense may be indicative of such disease entities as neurosyphilis, diabetes, or postinfectious polyneuritis.

Gait changes. Ataxia of gait may indicate low pressure hydrocephalus. Awkward or shuffling gaits could be caused by osteoarthritis or Parkinson's disease. Spastic hemiparesis is indicative of upper motor neuron disease. Foot drop usually is secondary to lower motor neuron disease. Sensory ataxia is manifest in a positive Romberg test, and the gait is unsteady and broad based. Fractured hip is another possible cause of gait changes. If the gait is staggering, unsteady, and wide based with exaggerated difficulty on the turns and the client cannot stand steadily with feet together and eyes closed or open, there is disease of the cerebellum or associated tracts.

Weakness, drooling, and slurred speech. If onset is acute with weakness on one side of the body, suspect cerebrovascular accident.

Headache. Hypertensive headache is not generally produced until the diastolic blood pressure is greater than 120.

Fever. Temperature-regulating mechanisms are less reliable in the elderly. Older patients do not work up the high temperatures usually expected in acute infections. The conventional temperature chart is of limited value; charts of subnormal ranges are much better. Pyrexia may be late in appearing or may never appear, and the temperature rarely goes above 103°F (39.4°C). Do not wait for fever to diagnose pneumonia—the patient may die first. Tachypnea and tachycardia are much better indicators of chest infection and should be acted on with promptness. High, swinging fever in an old person most often indicates a hidden localization of pus, such as in a lung or perinephric abscess.

Vomiting. This is a fairly nonspecific factor. However, a common culprit in the elderly is digitalis intoxication. Also to be considered is alimentary malignant disease or uremia. Functional bowel distress, such as gastrointestinal symptoms of functional origin with no demonstrable anatomic changes to account for them, may be a factor. These are related to such stressors as emotional tension, distress of elderly living, and fear of disease and death.

Breathing problems. The elderly are not short of breath unless more than moderate exertion is involved, such as running or walking at a fast rate or doing a task requiring heavy muscular exertion. The normal aged person has no persistent cough or sputum production, unless he is a smoker. The diseases of the lungs of increased prevalence in old age are tuberculosis, lung cancer, chronic bronchitis, and emphysema.

History of falls. Modest doses of minor tranquilizers, such as Valium, Librium, and meprobamate, become cumulative readily in the aged and contribute to falls. Also suspect are vascular problems. "Drop attacks" involve compromised blood supply through basilar arteries.

History of syphilis. Effects of previous syphilitic infection are fairly rare in the elderly. However, dementia paralytica may first show itself after age 65 if the primary infection has occurred in middle age. It presents in the elderly as epilepsy of late onset, with tremor, particularly of tongue and extremities, slurred speech, depression, and progressive dementia with delusions not always grandiose. Pupils show no reaction to light, there is a positive Babinski's sign, cerebrospinal fluid is abnormal with increased cells and protein, and the serologic test is positive.

Numbness, tingling, and paresthesias. This may result from diabetic neuropathy or direct nerve injury. Smoking can also be a factor.

Past medical history rationale

Chronic obstructive pulmonary disease. Maximum oxygen uptake, ventilatory volume, and vital capacity progressively diminish with age. Lung volumes increase owing to diminution in elastic recall. Acute symptoms of OBS are precipitated by cerebral hypoxia.

Cardiac disease. Thirteen percent of acute OBS is caused by congestive heart failure. Arrhythmias impair the cerebral blood supply.

Cerebrovascular accident. Infarction may be precipitated by even minimal reduction of blood flow, with decreased blood pressure, decreased cardiac output, anemia, or increased viscosity of blood. In completed or continuing cerebrovascular accidents, investigate to exclude occult hemorrhage, myocardial infarction, blood dyscrasias, dehydration, or acute reduction in blood supply.

Hypertension. Hypertensive encephalopathy impairs the cerebral blood supply.

Systolic hypertension in the elderly is now thought to be a compensatory mechanism to shunt adequate blood to the head in the presence of loss of elasticity of the aorta, and systolic blood pressures of less than 160 to 170 should probably not be treated.

Diabetes. In adult-onset diabetes, the onset is usually gradual and mild. Any aged individual with renal disease, retinopathy, neuropathy, or peripheral vascular disease should be suspect, especially if obese and with a positive family history. The greatest concern in management has to do with the high incidence of complications rather than with the diabetes itself, which is generally managed with little difficulty.

Anemia. Anemia is *not* a normal concomitant of aging. Anemia and other disorders of the hematopoietic system in an elderly patient require the same evaluation as in a younger person.

Peptic ulcer disease. Incidence is about the same in elderly as in younger populations. Bleeding is more serious in the elderly and requires prompt, aggressive management.

Depression. This has been discussed in other parts of this protocol.

Renal problems. Fluid and electrolyte imbalance and toxic states disrupt the cerebral metabolic process.

Hyperthyroidism. In the older person, many of the landmarks of typical thyrotoxicosis are missing or can easily be confused with other diseases common at this period of life. In the elderly the following symptoms may help make the correct diagnoses: the nervousness of hyperthyroidism is continuous, that of the normal elderly is paroxysmal; tremors seen in aging individuals are coarse, not fine as in hyperthyroidism; and normal aging skin is alternately hot and cold and alternately moist and dry, but is continuous in thyroid disease. The older client with an excellent appetite who is still losing weight must also be investigated for diabetes and other nutritional diseases. The tachycardia of hyperthyroidism does not disappear during sleep or after rest. Therefore, in borderline cases, a test with an antithyroid compound that controls the cardiac irregularity or the tachycardia, as well as other manifestations, confirms the diagnosis, for antithyroid compounds will have no perceptible influence on hypertension or arteriosclerotic heart disease. Serum protein-bound iodine is not affected by age per se, therefore, an elevated serum protein-bound iodine is bona fide evidence of increased thyroid activity in the older individual.

Hypothyroidism. It is easy to confuse this with a vitamin deficiency (particularly of vitamins A, B, and C), severe anemia, and chronic nephritis. Weakness, coarseness, and dryness of the skin, sensitivity to cold, slowness of thought and speech, and memory impairment are also seen in elderly who are not myxedematous, thereby clouding the diagnostic picture. Capillary permeability, which is not affected by aging per se, is elevated with all patients with myxedema. Serum protein may be normal or high, but albumin fraction is disproportionately elevated. The complete blood count shows secondary anemia, and the protein-bound iodine is low.

Injuries. Generally, injurious effects have more potential for complications because of the decreased compensatory mechanisms. The first treatment is prevention.

Medications

Generally, you must suspect that the altered biochemical environment has affected the excitability of the neurons in those cases where OBS is precipitated by drugs.

Barbiturates, hypnotics, and sedatives. Administration of barbiturates on a regular basis will perpetuate problems because the cerebral cortex is being depressed. Nighttime hypnotics will probably have some effect on the client's cognitive daytime functioning because the drug is not completely excreted in an older person.

Tranquilizers. Thorazine and Mellaril have their effect on the subcortical level.

Antidepressants. In elderly clients with endogenous depression, imipramine appears to be less effective, while the response obtained with the use of amitryptyline is the same for persons of all ages. Monoamine oxidase inhibitors should be used with caution in the elderly, for they are capable of potentiating other drugs and inducing hypotension.

Amphetamines. It is not true that elderly do not use them. Problems are the same as those of younger users.

Adrenal steroids. Their use in the elderly should be reserved for cases where inflammation is extremely severe and painful. They can cause electrolyte imbalances, fluid retention, osteoporosis, reactivation or initiation of peptic ulcer disease, and calcium loss. They may affect protein catabolism.

Atropine. This drug must be used with caution because of the increased incidence of borderline glaucoma. It can produce blurred vision from decreased internal secretion. In the elderly there is a decrease in the effect of atropine on the heart and an increase in the effect to the eye and bladder.

Belladonna. This can increase constipation problems.

Alcohol. The depressive action on the central nervous system can mimic OBS.

Salicylates. Generally, these are used safely and effectively in the elderly. If there is decreased renal function, however, there is the possibility of central nervous system disturbances signaled by deafness, tinnitus, vertigo, and confusion. Gastrointestinal bleeding and decreased prothrombin time may also be precipitated.

Antihypertensives. Vigorous antihypertensive treatment in the elderly is not recommended. Thiazide diuretics are the drug of choice, with awareness of their potential for precipitating hypokalemia and increasing the blood sugar levels. Alpha-methyldopa, guanethidine, or ganglionic blocking agents should be used only when high blood pressure has failed to respond to milder therapy.

Diuretics. The thiazide diuretics, furosemide and ethacrynic acid, have a greater tendency to produce potassium loss. They can also yield photosensitivity, pancreatitis, sodium and potassium depletion, and precipitate uric-acid levels. The loss of potassium is of greater concern in the elderly who may be receiving a digitalis preparation. All potent diuretics cause an increase in the blood urea nitrogen. Triamterene reduces potassium excretion but can cause hyperkalemia and ensuing drowsiness.

Past treatment. The findings and results of all past treatments are necessary and important parts of the data base to assist in the determination of whether the client presenting with confusion has an acute process or a progressive, chronic disorder.

Coping mechanisms. The cultural background and pattern of handling stress are often helpful clues when considering etiology of confusion. The frequency of past medical visits is sometimes a good indicator of those who are overly concerned with somatic complaints.

Review of systems. Many of these points have been mentioned in other portions of this protocol.

OBJECTIVE DATA RATIONALE

Skin: Recognition of normal and abnormal changes in geriatric skin is difficult. Lesions range from normal pigmentation changes to carcinoma. Jaundice is a common manifestation of hepatobiliary disorders in the elderly. An estimate is that half the cases of jaundice result from cancer of the pancreas and hepatobiliary tract and half result from benign disorders including choledocholithiasis, cirrhosis, drugs, hepatitis, and hemolytic jaundice.

Head:
  BRUITS: Indicate cerebrovascular insufficiency.
  BATTLE'S SIGN: Can indicate trauma.
  BOSSING: May be present in Paget's disease.

Eyes: Good vision is considered to be 20/20. Fair to adequate—20/40 to 20/70. Poor—20/100 or less.

NYSTAGMUS: A lesion in the posterior lobe of the cerebellum is more certainly diagnosed if intention tremor in the limbs or one side of the body is accompanied by a jerking type of nystagmus on looking to the same side.

FIELD OF VISION AND FUNDUSCOPIC EXAMINATION: Macular degeneration occurs primarily in older people and leads to loss of central vision—the vision that is sharpest and clearest. Peripheral vision is unaffected.

Ears:

WEBER'S TEST: Lateralization to one ear needs further investigation.

RINNE TEST: Normally air conduction is greater than bone conduction.

OTITIS: Middle ear infection in the elderly may be an indication of more serious disease, for example, diabetes and benign tumors of the nasopharynx such as polyps or cancer.

Nose:

NASAL STUFFINESS: This may be drug induced and may indicate allergy. Pale, boggy mucosa and polyps may be seen on physical examination.

Mouth:

TOOTH DECAY, GUM DISEASE, BUCCAL LESIONS, AND EDENTULOUS TONGUE: These may lead to an infectious process in the elderly not indicated by temperature elevation. Signs of poor nutritional status, especially pernicious anemia, should be sought.

Throat:

POSITION OF UVULA: Paralysis of the tenth cranial nerve causes the uvula to deviate to the uninvolved side.

Neck:

STIFFNESS: May indicate osteoporosis of spine and normally decreased aging musculature or meningitis.

THYROID ENLARGEMENT: Endocrine disorders impinge on the cerebral metabolic process.

Character and quality of pulses: May indicate cerebrovascular insufficiency.

RADIATION OF MURMURS: Murmurs of mitral regurgitation and other cardiac disorders may radiate to the neck.

LYMPH NODE ENLARGEMENT: Regional lymph nodes often do not enlarge as rapidly in infectious processes in the elderly.

Chest: The physical examination frequently shows no abnormality. Percussion may normally show hyperresonance. Breath sounds may be normally subdued. A prolonged expiratory phase is indicative of emphysema.

Heart: The point of maximal impulse may be normally further to the left because of a usually increasing anteroposterior diameter. An impulse palpable at greater than 2 intercostal spaces indicates ventricular enlargement. A gallop rhythm indicates congestive heart failure, as may pedal edema.

Abdomen: Palpable liver and spleen and ascites may indicate hepatosplenomegaly. Hypertrophy of the kidneys decreases with age.

Rectum: Three positive findings of blood in the stool must be investigated. This yields strong suspicion of gastric carcinoma.

Extremities: Positive findings may indicate compromised blood supply, diabetic neuropathy, or cerebral disease.

Neurologic examination:

CRANIAL NERVES:

CN I: Unilateral loss of smell without nasal disease suggests a frontal lobe lesion.

CN II: Test the visual acuity, determine visual fields, and examine the optic fundi. Suspect increased intracranial pressure from intracranial tumor, brain abscess, benign intracranial hypertension, or meningitis when you detect papilledema. If the papilledema is unilateral, suspect optic neuritis. In the absence of the above conditions, consider malignant hypertension or thrombosis of the central vein of the retina. You may see optic atrophy following a head injury that involves the frontal region or orbit or in a patient with a vascular occlusion lesion of the optic nerve, particularly one with arteriosclerosis, diabetes, or cranial arteritis.

CN III: Suspect complete paralysis of the third nerve if there is complete ptosis of the upper lid and complete internal ophthalmoplegia.

CN III, IV, AND VI: Identify ptosis, nystagmus, and pupillary reactions.

CN V (MOTOR SENSORY): Test temporal and masseter muscles. Test the forehead, cheeks, and jaw on each side for pain sensation. Test for light touch with a wisp of cotton. Test corneal reflex and note tearing and blinking.

CN VII: In lower motor neuron paralysis, such as Bell's palsy, the eye does not close, the eyeball rolls up, there is a flat nasolabial fold, the forehead does not wrinkle, the eyebrow does not raise, and there is paralysis of the lower face. In upper motor neuron paralysis, such as hemiparesis, the eye closes, perhaps with slight weakness, the nasolabial folds are flat, the forehead wrinkles, the eyebrow raises, and there is paralysis of the lower face.

CN VIII: Assess hearing. Ask for tinnitus.

CN IX AND X: Palate and uvula deviate away from the paralyzed side in a lesion of the vagus. Hoarseness may indicate vocal cord paralysis.

CN XI: Suspect lesions in the posterior fossa, posteroinferior cerebellar thrombosis, medullary tumor, motor neuron disease, and poliomyelitis.

CN XII: Fasciculations and atrophy suggest lower motor neuron disease. The tongue deviates toward the paralyzed side.

DECREASED MOTOR FUNCTION, RANGE OF MOTION, AND MUSCLE STRENGTH: Muscle atrophy with fasciculations results from lower motor neuron lesions. Muscle atrophy without fasciculations results often from intrinsic muscle disease.

SENSORY DEFICITS AND STEREOGNOSIS: Symmetric distal sensory loss suggests a peripheral polyneuropathy. Discrimination may be impaired in lesions of the sensory cortex or posterior columns.

DEEP TENDON REFLEX (DTR) AND BABINSKI'S SIGN: Paralysis with loss of DTRs indicates lower motor neuron lesions interrupting the reflex arc. Paralysis with increased DTRs indicates an upper motor neuron lesion. Withdrawal of minor tranquilizers, such as Librium, Valium, and barbiturates, can increase DTRs. Extension of the plantar reflex indicates a lesion of the pyramidal pathways.

ROMBERG'S SIGN: In peripheral neuropathy or diseases affecting the posterior columns, patients only sway with eyes closed. In cerebellar or cerebellar tract disease, the patient sways with eyes open or closed, but the sway is more pronounced with eyes closed. In psychoneurosis the swaying will be back and forth, with reeling or even falling.

FINGER-TO-NOSE AND HEEL-TO-SHIN TESTING: Poor performance in finger-to-nose testing indicates cerebellar disease. Heel-to-shin testing is an unreliable test to use with the elderly.

Mental status questionnaire (MSQ) (see p. 381): Questions 1 and 2 measure learning. Questions 3, 4, 5 measure learning—time. Questions 6, 7, 8 measure memory—recent or remote. Questions 9 and 10 measure general information and memory. In addition, the first four relate to diffuse brain dysfunction or the disoriented type of behavior change. The remaining six questions measure cognitive impairment. Clinically, zero to two errors equal absent or mild chronic brain syndrome. Less than three errors but with poor memory may be an affective disorder. Three to eight errors equal moderate chronic brain syndrome, and nine to ten errors equal severe brain dysfunction.

An error is considered if the answer is incorrect or the question ignored. A nontestable client, who is not uncooperative and suffers no deafness or insuperable language behavior, is to be suspected of severe brain dysfunction.

Face-to-hand test: The initial trials, 1 to 4, are evaluated in the context of further trials. They are almost always correctly reported. The examiner informs or reinforces the response that there were two touches. The 7 to 10 trials are the measurement of the test. Incorrect responses to stimulation are (1) not reported, (2) felt but displaced, or (3) projected or located in space. This is presumptive of brain damage. Erroneous responses include extinction or merely indicating the cheek without mentioning the hand; displacing or localizing the hand touch to the cheek, the knee, or elsewhere; indicating that both cheeks were touched; or projecting, such as pointing to the examiner's hand or displaying exsomesthesia by pointing outside in space. Extinction of the touch to the face is rare and suggests a functional disorder. Assuming that pain and touch are intact, and if you find consistent errors in laterality, there is a lesion of the parietal cortex. If the client is correct in his identification of stimuli on the symmetric trials, but continues to make errors after that, he has an organic mental syndrome. In acute OBS there may be major changes in the score over a relatively short period. In chronic OBS, while there may be variability in the degree of disorientation, memory, and intellectual function, all of these are simultaneously present.

Testing recall: During the interview, tell the client you are going to ask him to remember something and ask him to recall it later. Give him three unrelated things, such as an address, a color, and an object. After about 5 minutes, ask him to repeat the three test items. Normally, all three should be recalled. Individuals without organicity should also be able to recall several presidents and five cities and countries. Of course, education and cultural background must be considered.

Testing basic language skills: It is first necessary to decide if there is a defect of language or of speech production. Impairment of language function is manifest by inappropriate usage of words or a disturbance of appreciation of symbolic values of words. Inappropriate use of words, use of nonsense words, or formulation of sentences in which the word order is unconventional betrays underlying defects. Sensory or receptive aphasia, deafness, or other auditory problems and temporal lobe lesions must be suspected. Impaired ability to read (dyslexia) often results from a lesion in the dominant parietal lobe. Inability to write (dysgraphia) may result from lesions of frontal or parietal lobes. Ill-fitting false teeth commonly cause slurring on consonants. Dysphonia may be a result of respiratory dysfunction, such as inadequate expiratory air flow. Before labeling a person aphasic, exclude motor disturbances; sensory loss, such as blindness, deafness, and diminished touch and position sense, as in peripheral nerve disorders; and general mental impairment. Other causes of language skill difficulties include myopathy, myasthenia gravis, diffuse lesions of the lower brainstem, upper motor neuron lesions, and Parkinson's disease.

Testing attention and concentration: The educational level and recency of calculations must be considered in this test. Ordinarily, serial 7s should be completed in 1½ minutes with no more than four errors. The client should be able to repeat 6 digits forward and 4 digits backward. This ability is lost in Korsakoff's syndrome and senile psychosis. The schizophrenic client may be unable to do these because of lack of concentration. The level of schooling must also be taken into consideration, as well as the anxiety produced by the test itself. Simpler forms of the serial 7 test include counting backward serial 3s or reciting the alphabet.

Testing for abstract reasoning: Oral antidiabetic medications can impair abstraction.

Testing for judgment: Loss of judgment is one of the earliest signs of cortical destruction. It occurs in general paresis, brain tumors, and cerebral arteriosclerosis. In the absence of stupor, coma, catatonia, excitement, severe deafness, marked language difficulty, or other factors that make examination impossible or the results questionable, there is presumptive evidence of brain cell loss or dysfunction.

Testing sensory perception and coordination: Consider hemianopia, perceptual problems, or visual problems. Inability to perform should lead you to suspect cerebellar disease.

Evaluating mood: Alteration of mood is not an uncommon early manifestation of malignancy or metabolic disturbances. The depressed person is downcast in the morning but better as the day goes on. Every depressed person is a suicidal risk. The elderly do commit suicide, more often than not in a less catastrophic, less violent way than younger persons. There may be subintentional suicide through neglect of medical therapy or malnutrition.

Laboratory test rationale

Complete blood count with mean corpuscular volume, mean corpuscular hemoglobin, mean corpuscular hemoglobin concentration, and folic acid and vitamin B_{12} levels: Anemia is not a normal process of aging. Red-cell morphology is necessary to pick up microcytic anemia. Folic acid and vitamin B_{12} are often overlooked as deficiencies in the elderly that can contribute to confusion that may be reversible.

Urinalysis/blood urea nitrogen/creatinine: Uremia and bladder infection is one of the leading causes of reversible confusion in the elderly.

Serum glucose, fasting blood sugar, and 2-hour postprandial: Hypoglycemia can cause early morning confusion. The 2-hour postprandial test is considered a more reliable test for hyper- or hypoglycemia in the elderly because of the high percent of positive glucose tolerance tests after the age of 70.

Electrolytes: The elderly are susceptible to electrolyte imbalances, especially in view of the common medicines they take, such as digitalis preparations in combination with diuretics. The elderly are also susceptible to sodium problems as a result of dehydration.

Thyroid function: Thyroid function disorders are overlooked in the elderly, who often suffer from hypothyroidism and hyperthyroidism.

Liver function: Liver function tests must be carefully evaluated since enzymes are affected by such disease entities as myocardial infarction and osteoporosis.

Fluorescent treponemal antibody absorbtion (FTA) and Venereal Disease Research Laboratories test (VDRL): Positive syphilis tests may explain sensory disturbances and neuropathy.

Serum levels of barbiturates, bromides, and digitalis: Bromism is a cause of delirium in the elderly. Digitalis intoxication can be the cause of weakness, lethargy, nausea, and vomiting.

Chest x-ray: Normally, in the aged, the diaphragms may at times be flattened. The anteroposterior diameter may be somewhat increased. Only when hyperinflation occurs to the point of severe flattening of the diaphragms, with an increased space (more than 2 inches) between the posterior border of the sternum and the anterior margin of the aorta, can you suspect the presence of obstructive pulmonary disease. Decreased peripheral vascularity of lung fields is not present in normal aged persons.

Electrocardiogram: EKG changes with aging are attributable to regressive processes in the myocardium. As a result, the normal EKG reflects a great deal of subclinical disease that may contribute to certain criteria of normality with aging, such as widening of the QRS and P-R intervals. Notching of the P wave becomes so frequent that it is of no diagnostic value. The S-T segment becomes flatter and of greater duration, particularly in the aged female. In the elderly cardiac patient with a marginal coronary arterial circulation, serial electrocardiography often shows unstable S-T segments and T waves unrelated to clinical or laboratory findings, which often disturb the technician more than the patients. Acute cerebral thrombosis may cause transitory symmetric T wave inversions or induce changes of coronary insufficiency.

Electroencephalogram: Most low MSQ scores have abnormal EEGs. A brain syndrome usually is associated with diffuse slowing in all leads. Slowing may be most prominent in one or both temporal lobes. The EEG may reveal such lesions as subdural hematoma, tumor, cerebral infarction, or an epileptic focus. However, a normal EEG does not mean brain damage is not present. Focal abnormalities may be remediable.

Skull x-rays: May be helpful in locating masses and fractures.

Dynamic brain scan, computerized axial tomography, and cisternography: These should be ordered only on the decision of the referring physician. These would not be done on the initial visit. The tests can temporarily increase OBS symptoms. A dynamic brain scan is indicated in acutely ill patients. This test makes it possible to pick up gross deficiencies in blood flow of major arteries. Use it if you suspect metastatic tumor, subdural hematoma, or cerebral infarction. Cisternography is a test for normal pressure hydrocephalus. A radioactive substance is injected into the cerebrospinal fluid within the lumbar subarachnoid space, and the speed of supracortical absorption is measured. Poor absorption is not a clear indication for shunts, especially if the brain syndrome is longstanding. Computerized axial tomography allows a nonintrusive examination of the inside of the skull with pinpointing of lesions.

Acute organic brain syndrome flow sheet

If a majority of the following categories are marked "yes," OBS is probably acute (onset within 1 to 4 weeks). *All of these changes, or parts, occur rapidly.*

Yes	No	Behavior	Yes	No	Behavior
☐	☐	Fluctuating level of awareness	☐	☐	Delusional denial of illness
☐	☐	Recent medical, surgical, and neurologic disease	☐	☐	Inappropriate sexual behavior
			☐	☐	Displacement, such as correct name and wrong address
☐	☐	Recent change in alcohol/drug intake	☐	☐	Anxious when unable to find correct response
☐	☐	Stupor progressing to delirium			
☐	☐	Visual hallucinations	☐	☐	Euphoria/blandness
☐	☐	Misidentification	☐	☐	Inappropriate joking
☐	☐	Great restlessness	☐	☐	Spatial inattention
☐	☐	Febrile, debilitating, or exhausting illness	☐	☐	Disorientation, but with ability to handle cognitive tasks
☐	☐	Dehydration	☐	☐	Paranoia/agitation
☐	☐	Delusional reduplication	☐	☐	Anxiety/depression
			☐	☐	Misnaming

Chronic organic brain syndrome flow sheet

If a majority of the following categories are marked "yes," the OBS is probably chronic. *All or parts of these categories have changed insidiously.*

Yes	No	Behavior	Yes	No	Behavior
☐	☐	Memory impaired and immediate	☐	☐	Nocturnal restlessness
☐	☐	Difficulty in use of names and numbers	☐	☐	Disorientation to person, place, and time
☐	☐	Age greater than 70	☐	☐	Paranoia
☐	☐	Confabulation	☐	☐	Alert facade
☐	☐	Bowel or bladder incontinence	☐	☐	Decreased response to interviewer
☐	☐	Easily distracted			
☐	☐	Intellectual grasp reduced	☐	☐	Caution becomes suspiciousness
☐	☐	Rigidity of response			
☐	☐	Wandering	☐	☐	Compulsive orderliness
☐	☐	Confused by new places or situations	☐	☐	Moodiness and depression
			☐	☐	Poor judgment

DISEASE ENTITIES

Trauma—Subdural hematoma
Suspect if
1. History of head injury followed by inconstant period of normalcy
2. Varying hemiparesis
3. Hemiparesthesia or jacksonian convulsion
4. Fluctuating level of consciousness
5. Change of personality
6. Confusion
7. Forgetfulness
8. Loss of judgment
9. May show gradual deterioration

Objectively
1. Computerized axial tomography or carotid angiography demonstrates mass
2. EEG may show electrically silent area over hematoma
3. Lumbar puncture may show xanthochromia
4. Skull films may show disease area

Action: Refer to physician.

Transient ischemic attacks (T.I.A.)
Suspect if transient attacks of
1. Hemiparesis, hemianesthesia, hemianopia, aphasia, dysarthria, and dysphagia
2. Loss of vision in one eye
3. Vertigo
4. Vomiting
5. Diplopia

Objectively
1. Check hemoglobin
2. Check blood pressure; hindbrain ischemia is more common when hypotension is cause
3. Auscultate neck for bruits
4. Restrict exaggerated neck movements

Action: See T.I.A. protocol.

Diabetes
Suspect if
1. Mild peripheral neuropathy
2. Impaired peripheral circulation
3. Absent tendon reflexes
4. Muscular wasting

5. Peripheral sensory loss with trophic changes
6. Flapping gait
7. Sudden fainting attacks with convulsion or hemiplegia
8. Morning confusion
9. Sudden episodes of irrational behavior

Objectively Obtain glucose tolerance curve.
Action: See diabetes protocol.

Giant cell arteritis

Suspect if
1. Persistent, severe, temporal, or unilateral headache
2. Dimness or loss of visual acuity
3. Accompanying pain in shoulders or hips
4. Temporal arteries tender or without pulsation
5. Temporal arteries stand out as thickened cords under red, hot skin

Objectively
1. Analyze funduscopic examination for retinal hemorrhage or thrombosis of retinal artery or optic atrophy
2. Check for mild fever
3. Check for increased erythrocyte sedimentation rate
4. Check for leukocytosis and occasionally eosinophilia

Action: Refer immediately.

Hypothyroidism

Suspect if
1. Cerebellar ataxia
2. Mental sluggishness
3. Obesity
4. Deepening voice
5. Deafness
6. Bradycardia
7. Peripheral neuropathy

Subjectively (Check for)
1. Constipation
2. Hoarseness
3. Weight gain
4. Facial puffiness
5. Lethargy
6. Dry skin
7. Alopecia
8. History of thyroid surgery
9. History of thyroid problems

Objectively (Check for)
1. DTRs showing slow phase of relaxation
2. Predominant carpal tunnel syndrome
3. Enlarged thyroid and yellow discoloration of skin
4. Cardiac murmurs and gallops; rales in chest if myxedematous
5. T_3, T_4, thyroid-stimulating hormone test results
6. Serum cholesterol equaling 300 mg/100 cc

Action: See hypothyroid protocol.

Vitamin B_{12} deficiency

Suspect if
1. Slowly increasing dementia
2. Forgetfulness
3. Confusion
4. Psychotic reactions, such as paranoia and manic-depressive states
5. History as smoker
6. Peripheral weakness and wasting
7. Pain in legs
8. Paresthesia in hands

Objectively (Check for)
1. Red, raw tongue
2. Fissures at angles of mouth
3. Pigmentation over pressure areas
4. Optic atrophy
5. Low serum vitamin B_{12}, low hemoglobin, high mean corpuscular volume, and low folate levels

Action: See vitamin B_{12} protocol.

Acute onset meningitis

Suspect if
1. Slight headache, fever, and stiffness
2. Disorientation to time and place
3. Lack of desire to get out of bed
4. Increasing drowsiness
5. Loss of interest (may be only symptom)
6. Neck stiffness not a complaint, but present if looked for, affecting flexion but not rotation

7. Vomiting with dehydration, often too late to correct

Objectively
1. Obtain blood culture (to rule out subacute bacterial endocarditis)
2. Check spinal tap
3. Analyze funduscopic examination

Action: Refer immediately.

Drug intoxication

Suspect if
1. Nystagmus
2. Dysarthria
3. Cerebellar ataxia
4. Manual incoordination
5. Loss of balance
6. Feeling of dizziness on looking up
7. Drowsiness
8. Disorientation, particularly of sudden onset
9. Altered behavior
10. Currently taking hypotensive iodides, tranquilizers, or digitalis

Objectively Check serum levels of drugs.

Action
1. Assess need for all drugs the client is taking by asking following questions:
   a. Is the medicine really necessary?
   b. What is its nature?
   c. What does it do?
   d. What are the possible undesirable effects?
   e. What are the side effects?
   f. What are the interactions?
   g. What are the concomitant over-the-counter drugs the client is taking?
   h. Do any of them contribute to malnutrition?
2. Compile listings of drugs, their dosages, and length of time the client has received them
3. Consult with attending physician and discontinue or begin weaning client from all unnecessary medications
4. Note drug categories of particular concern for the elderly:
   a. Antihypertensives
   b. Diuretics
   c. Sedatives
   d. Hypnotics
   e. Salicylates
   f. Tranquilizers

PLAN

The patient is elderly and has been diagnosed as having "chronic organic brain syndrome."

There are several approaches to management of this patient. Consideration should be given to the following points:
1. He is only slightly confused and manages himself well
2. He has no decompensating condition such as heart trouble
3. He is mobile
4. His activities are unrestricted
5. There is a telephone, friend, neighbor, or family close at hand

If these criteria are met, consideration should be given to allowing the patient to live alone if he chooses. It is well known that the elderly do much better in a familiar, constant environment.

Families often desire to care for their elderly relatives. If the following criteria are present, this is a second consideration for management:
1. The family is willing to have the patient live with them, and the patient is willing
2. The family is able to care for the patient emotionally, economically, and environmentally; professional services are available for backup
3. The patient does not need continuous professional care

Environmental considerations include whether or not children will be upset or upsetting to the elderly person and whether any ambulatory aids will necessitate removal of such items as doorsills or doors to bathrooms. If the patient goes to the bathroom alone, the door should be especially distinguished, such as painted white, and the bathroom should be easily accessible and well lighted and should contain safety rails.

The third alternative for the chronic brain syndrome patient is a nursing home. Criteria to be considered in pointing to this alternative include:
1. Inability to live alone
2. Absent or disinterested family
3. Disease entities requiring professional intervention
4. Incontinence
5. Noctural wanderings

In selecting a nursing home, consideration should be given to its locale, such as close to his family or needed medical services, the ratio of professional staff to patients, licensure, the amount of space and time given to recreational and diversional therapy, access to physical therapy, social services, types and amounts of medical/nursing supplies at hand, reality orientation programs, milieu therapy, and advanced preparation of its nursing staff. A good nursing home will have all of these and will also offer other special and helpful services.

BIBLIOGRAPHY
Books

Adams, F. D.: Physical diagnosis, ed. 14, Baltimore, 1958, The Williams & Wilkins Co.
Bates, B.: A guide to physical examination, Philadelphia, 1974, J. B. Lippincott Co., pp. 263-313.
Chinn, A. B., editor: Working with older people, a guide to practice, Public Health Service Publication #1459, vol. IV, Washington, D.C., July 1972, U.S. Government Printing Office.
del Bueno, D. J.: Case studies in pharmacology, Boston, 1976, Little, Brown & Co.
Gatz, A. J.: Manter's essentials of clinical neuroanatomy and neurophysiology, ed. 3, Philadelphia, 1966, F. A. Davis Co.
Gilles, D. A., and Alyn, I. B.: Patient assessment and management by the nurse practitioner, Philadelphia, 1976, W. B. Saunders Co., Chapters 2 and 3.
Gilroy, J., and Meyer J. S.: Medical neurology, Toronto, 1969, The Macmillan Co., Collier-Macmillan Canada, Ltd.
Goldberg, I. K.: Drug therapy in psychiatric disorders of older patients, vol. II, Fort Washington, Pa., 1976, McNeill Laboratories, Inc.
Govoni, L. E., and others: Drugs and nursing implications, New York, 1965, Appleton-Century-Crofts.
Hess, P., and Day, C.: Understanding the aging patient, Bowie, Md., 1977, The Robert J. Brody Co.
Hudak, C. M., and others: Clinical protocols, Philadelphia, 1976, J. B. Lippincott Co.
Keefer, C. S., and Wilkins, R. W., editors: Medicine essentials of clinical practice, Boston, 1970, Little, Brown & Co.
Krupp, M. A., and others: Current medical diagnosis and treatment, Los Altos, Calif., 1974, Lange Medical Publications.
MacLeod, J., editor: Clinical examination, ed. 4, Edinburgh, 1976, Churchill-Livingstone Co.
Prior, J. A., and Silberstein, J. S.: Physical diagnosis, the history and examination of the patient, ed. 4, St. Louis, 1973, The C. V. Mosby Co.
Rossman, I., editor: Clinical geriatrics, Philadelphia, 1971, J. B. Lippincott Co.
Sana, J. M., and Judge, R. D., editors: Physical appraisals methods in nursing practice, Boston, 1975, Little, Brown & Co., Chapter 13 and p. 365.
Smith, W. L., and Phillippus, M. J.: Neuropsychological testing in organic brain dysfunction, Springfield, Ill., 1969, Charles C Thomas, Publisher.
Taylor, C. W., and others: Managing the disturbed elderly patient in family practice, vol. I, Fort Washington, Pa., 1975, McNeill Laboratories, Inc.
Thorn, G. W., and others: Harrison's principles of internal medicine, ed. 8, New York, 1977, McGraw-Hill Book Co.
Wasson, J., and others: The common symptom guide, New York, 1975, McGraw-Hill Book Co., p. 112.

Articles and pamphlets

Dobrin, L., and others: How confused is that elderly patient and why? Patient Care, December 1968, p. 51.
Dobrin, L., and others: Tips on how and when to manage the elderly patient, Patient Care, March 1969, p. 86.
Fink, M., Green, M. A., and Bender, M. B.: The face-hand test as a diagnostic sign of organic mental syndrome, Neurology **2**:48, 1952.
Galton, L.: Drugs and the elderly, Nursing '76 **6**(8):38, 1976.
Lewis, R.: Anemia—a common but never normal concomitant of aging, Geriatrics **31**(12):53, 1976.
Parker, B., and others: Finding medical reasons for psychiatric behavior, Geriatrics **31**(6):53, 1976.
Pearson, L. B.: A protocol for the chief complaint of headache, Nurse Practitioner, September-October 1976, p. 12.
Valenstein, E.: Charting a complete office neurological exam, Patient Care, September 1975.
Valenstein, E.: High use of drugs by elderly merits closer supervision (abstracts), Geriatrics **31**(8):132, 1976.
Valenstein, E.: Drug toxicity is special risk of aged living at home (abstracts) Geriatrics **31**(9):145, 1976.
Valenstein, E.: Making sense of cerebral dominance and syndromes of the non-dominant hemisphere, Geriatrics **31**(11):111, 1976.
Valenstein, E.: Potentially treatable illness often underlies an intellectual decline (abstracts), Geriatrics **31**(11):158, 1976.

APPENDIX

B

EDUCATIONAL PROGRAMS OFFERING SPECIALIZATION IN GERIATRIC/GERONTOLOGIC NURSING

The educational programs designed to prepare registered nurses to work in the expanded role of the nurse are listed below by state and terminal degree or certificate offered.*

California
Master's degree: geriatric nurse practitioner
  California State University at Long Beach
  Department of Nursing
  1250 Belflower Blvd.
  Long Beach, Calif. 90840
    Phone: (213) 498-4464

Colorado
Certificate as geriatric nurse practitioner
  University of Colorado
  School of Nursing
  4200 E. 9th Ave., C287
  Denver, Colo. 30262
    Phone: (303) 394-8581

Florida
Certificate as geriatric nurse practitioner
  University of Miami
  P.O. Box 016960
  Miami, Fla. 33101

Georgia
Certificate as geriatric nurse practitioner
  Emory University
  Nel Hodgson School of Nursing
  Atlanta, Ga. 30322
    Phone (404) 329-6913

Kansas
Certificate as geriatric nurse practitioner
  University of Kansas
  School of Nursing
  39th and Rainbow Blvd.
  Kansas City, Kan. 66103
    Phone: (913) 588-5434

Massachusetts
Master's degree: geriatric nurse practitioner, geriatric nurse clinician
  Boston University
  School of Nursing
  635 Commonwealth Ave.
  Boston, Mass. 02215
    Phone: (617) 738-2206

New Jersey
Master's degree: geriatric nurse practitioner
  Seton Hall University
  College of Nursing
  400 South Orange Ave.
  South Orange, N.J. 07079
    Phone: (201) 648-5060

---

*All information in this section is based on A directory of expanded role programs for registered nurses, 1979, DHEW Pub. No. HRA 79-10, Hyattsville, Md., 1979, Division of Nursing, Bureau of Health Manpower, Department of Health, Education and Welfare.

New York

Master's degree: geriatric nurse practitioner
  Columbia University
  School of Nursing
  630 West 168 St.
  New York, N.Y. 10032
    Phone: (212) 694-3635

Certificate as geriatric nurse practitioner
  Cornell University–New York Hospital
  School of Nursing
  515 East 71st St.
  New York, N.Y. 10021
    Phone: (212) 472-6562

Certificate as geriatric nurse practitioner
  SUNY Upstate Medical Center
  College of Health Related Professions
  750 East Adams St.
  Syracuse, N.Y. 13210.
    Phone: (315) 473-4276

Ohio

Master's degree: gerontologic nurse clinician
  Case Western Reserve University
  School of Nursing
  2121 Abbington Rd.
  Cleveland, Ohio 44106
    Phone: (216) 368-2540, ext. 2180

Pennsylvania

Certificate as gerontologic nurse practitioner
  University of Pittsburgh
  School of Nursing
  Victoria Building
  Pittsburgh, Pa. 15261
    Phone: (412) 624-2400.

MSN in gerontology; nurse clinician program
  University of Pennsylvania
  School of Nursing
  420 Service Dr. SX
  Philadelphia, Pa. 19104

Utah

Master's degree: geriatric nurse practitioner
  University of Utah
  College of Nursing
  2307 Smith Family Living Center
  25 South Medical Dr.
  Salt Lake City, Utah 84112
    Phone: (801) 581-8262

Wisconsin

Certificate as geriatric nurse practitioner
  University of Wisconsin
  School of Nursing
  1402 University Ave.
  Madison, Wis. 53706.
    Phone: (608) 262-4312

National League of Nursing Accredited Masters Programs offers clinical and functional practicums in geriatric/gerontologic nursing.

Arizona

Clinical and functional practicum in geriatric nursing
  University of Arizona
  Tucson, Ariz. 85721

California

Clinical and functional practicum in geriatric health
  California State University at Los Angeles
  5151 State University Dr.
  Los Angeles, Calif. 90032

Clinical and functional practicum in geriatric nursing
  University of California at Los Angeles
  405 Hilgard Ave.
  Los Angeles, Calif. 90024

Illinois

Clinical practicum in geriatric/gerontologic nursing
  Rush University
  1743 West Harrison
  Chicago, Ill. 60612

Maryland

Clinical and functional practicum in gerontology
  University of Maryland
  655 W. Lombard St.
  Baltimore, Md. 21201

Minnesota

Clinical and functional practicum; adult/geriatric nurse associate
  University of Minnesota
  School of Public Health
  1325 Mayo
  Minneapolis, Minn. 55455

New York
Clinical and functional practicum in gerontology
   Adelphi University
   Garden City, N.Y. 11530
Clinical practicum in gerontologic nursing
   University of Rochester
   Rochester, N.Y. 14642

Ohio
Clinical and functional practicum in gerontologic nursing
   Case Western Reserve University
   2121 Abbington Rd.
   Cleveland, Ohio 44106
Clinical and functional practicum in gerontologic and gerontologic mental health nursing
   University of Cincinnati
   Cincinnati, Ohio 45221

Utah
Clinical and functional practicum in gerontologic nursing
   University of Utah
   Salt Lake City, Utah 84112

APPENDIX

C

NURSING ASSESSMENT OF THE GERIATRIC LOWER EXTREMITY

Patricia King

Patient number _____
Date _____
R. N. number _____

Instructions: For each item, circle the response in the appropriate column, unless directed otherwise. Clarification of items appears in the far right column.
1. Mobility (check one): ☐ Walks without assistance ☐ Walks with help of equipment ☐ Does not walk — uses wheelchair ☐ Bedfast
2. Ask the client, "Does the condition of your feet or legs limit your activity in any way?" ☐ Yes ☐ No If *yes*, describe: _____
3. Ask the client to walk approximately 10 feet. Is there any gait disturbance? ☐ Yes ☐ No

Remove the client's shoes and stockings
4. Cleanliness of feet: ☐ Acceptable ☐ Unacceptable
5. Are the stockings a good fit? ☐ Yes ☐ No
6. Does the client usually wear well-fitting, leather (synthetic) shoes that cover his feet completely? ☐ Yes ☐ No If *yes*, are they in good condition? ☐ Yes ☐ No
7. Does the client wear circular garters? ☐ Yes ☐ No

Dermatologic assessment
8. Skin lesions
   a. Fissure between the toes? ☐ Yes ☐ No
   b. Fissure on heel(s)? ☐ Yes ☐ No
   c. Excoriation on legs or feet? ☐ Yes ☐ No
   d. Corn(s)? (Fig. C-1) ☐ Yes ☐ No
   (Corn — painful, circular area of thickened skin, appearing on skin that is normally thin)

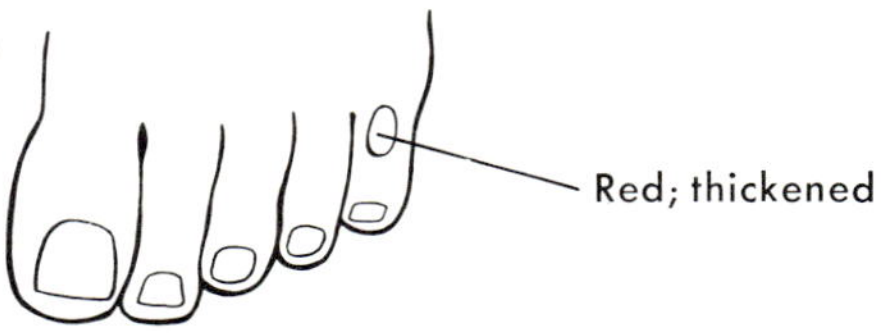

— Red; thickened

Illustrations by Thomas A. King

Fig. C-1. Corn.

e. Callus(es)? ☐ Yes ☐ No
   (Callus — thickened skin, occurring on skin that is normally thick, such as soles)
   f. Plantar wart? ☐ Yes ☐ No
   g. Other? ☐ Yes ☐ No
   Describe: _____
 9. Itching on legs or feet? ☐ Yes ☐ No
10. Rash on legs or feet? ☐ Yes ☐ No
11. Inspect pressure areas on the feet for localized areas of redness. Are any present? ☐ Yes ☐ No If *yes*, which foot? ☐ Right ☐ Left
12. Inspect legs, feet, and toes for localized swelling, warmth, tenderness, and redness. Is any present? ☐ Yes ☐ No Is *yes*, specify location: ☐ Rt. leg ☐ Rt. foot ☐ Lt. leg ☐ Lt. foot
13. Toenails
    a. Ingrown? ☐ Yes ☐ No
       (Ingrown toenail—a sensitive and tender overhanging nail fold)
    b. Overgrown (long)? ☐ Yes ☐ No
    c. Thickened? ☐ Yes ☐ No
    d. Yellow discoloration? ☐ Yes ☐ No
    e. Black discoloration? ☐ Yes ☐ No

Circulatory status
Questions 14 to 18 related to feet only.
14. Do the feet have any red, reddish blue, or bluish discoloration? ☐ Yes ☐ No
15. Is there any brownish discoloration around the ankles? ☐ Yes ☐ No
16. Is the dorsalis pedis present? (Fig. C-2) ☐ Yes ☐ No If *no*, which foot? ☐ Right ☐ Left
17. Is the posterior tibial pulse present? (Fig. C-3) ☐ Yes ☐ No If *no*, which foot? ☐ Right ☐ Left
18. Is the skin dry? ☐ Yes ☐ No

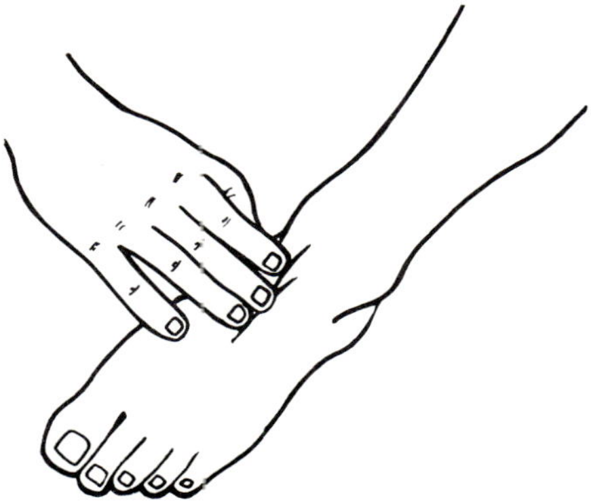

Fig. C-2. Dorsalis pedis pulse. Use three fingers on the dorsum of the foot, usually just lateral to the extensor tendon of the great toe.

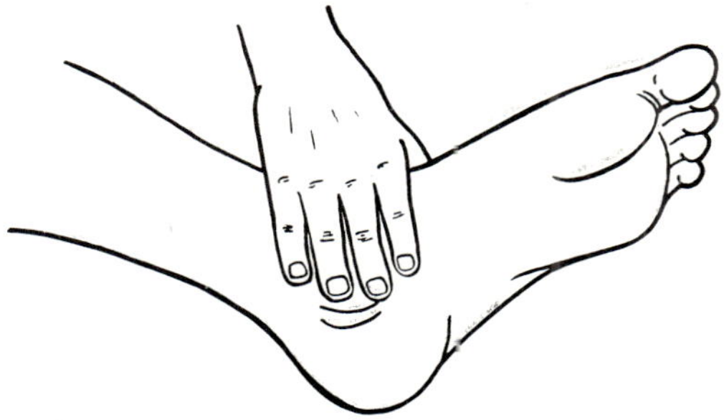

Fig. C-3. Posterior tibial pulse. Curve your fingers behind and slightly below the medial malleolus of the ankle.

Continued

Circulatory status—cont'd
Questions 19-23 relate to both feet and legs.
19. Is edema present? ☐ Yes ☐ No

Check the temperature of the legs and the feet with the backs of your fingers, comparing one extremity with the other

20. Are the feet the same temperature? ☐ Yes ☐ No
21. Are the legs the same temperature? ☐ Yes ☐ No
22. Does the client have any pain in his legs or feet? ☐ Yes ☐ No If *yes*, describe:

Inspect the legs, sides of ankles, soles, and toes for ulceration

23. Is any ulceration present? ☐ Yes ☐ No If *yes*, specify location: ☐ Rt. leg ☐ Rt. foot ☐ Lt. leg ☐ Lt. foot

Structural deformities
24. Hallux valgus (bunion)? (Fig. C-4) ☐ Yes ☐ No
25. Hammer toes? (Fig. C-5) ☐ Yes ☐ No
26. Overlapping digits? ☐ Yes ☐ No

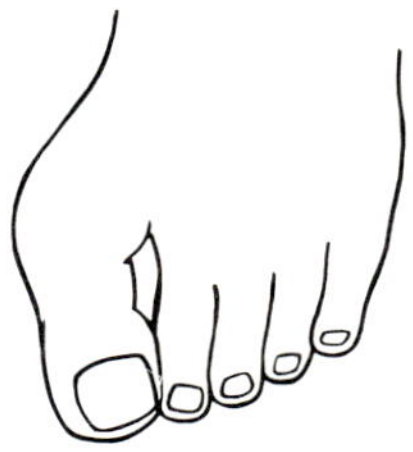

Fig. C-4. Hallux valgus (outward deviation of great toe).

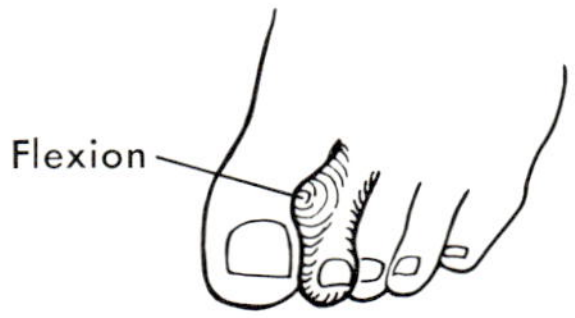

Fig. C-5. Hammer toe.

Ask the client to stand
27. Are the legs the same relative size? ☐ Yes ☐ No
28. Are the legs the same relative length? ☐ Yes ☐ No
29. Are varicosities present? ☐ Yes ☐ No

Additional notes

APPENDIX

D

RELAXATION AS THERAPY FOR THE ELDERLY

Relaxation is an internal state that can be taught by helping a client "feel" his own state of tension, then deliberately relax a tensed muscle group and enjoy the "good" feeling of lack of tension. You and the client should be in a quiet room with a small amount of light. The client should be lying down or partially reclining. If sitting, both feet should be on the floor, the legs uncrossed, and the knees allowed to fall apart as gravity dictates. The hands should be placed in the lap while the arms are supported either by a bed or by the chair arms. You should sit alongside the client, not close enough to invade his territory but near enough to be able to touch certain parts of the body as they are involved in the relaxation technique.

First step: After lying down, the client lies still for a minute and breathes consciously. You say, "Feel yourself breathing, count ten breaths, then take a deep breath and hold it for a count of five, then let go slowly, letting all the air out. Take another ten normal breaths, counting each breath. At the end of the ten breaths take another deep breath and hold for a count of five." Instructions should be given as they are obeyed by the client—*one instruction at a time*.

Second step: Tell the client, "As you take a deep breath, clench your fist for the count of five, then as you let the breath out, slowly relax the fist. Feel the tension of the fist —the muscle should not hurt but may quiver a little when clenched. How did the tension feel? How does the relaxation feel?"

The object is to get the client to receive definite feedback of tension versus relaxation. This should be done several times as a practice session. When the client is fully aware of his feedback, then start the relaxation technique.

Third step: Instruct the client, "Take three slow, deep breaths, and as you let them go, let your whole body sink into the chair (bed). Take ten normal breaths, and while doing this, think of the most pleasant place you have ever been—a mountain valley, a seashore, a quiet lake, or under a wide, spreading tree. Think of this and keep it as your special place where you can relax. Keep the image inside in the space between your chest and your abdomen—your quiet place."

You then touch a muscle group to be tensed and request the client to take a deep breath for a count of five while he tenses it and then to relax the muscle group slowly and breathe normally for ten breaths. The tensing/relaxing should be done three times.

A sequence of muscle groups should be followed—usually the right hand, then the right biceps, then the shoulder muscles shrugged forward. Repeat with left hand and arm and shoulder. The client squeezes

403

the eyelids shut and holds for count of five, then wrinkles the forehead and holds for count of five, relaxes, then makes a grimace. He holds the abdominal muscles for a count of five and relaxes, then holds the buttocks. He tenses the quadriceps muscle of each leg, then pulls the foot up toward the knee (ankle) and then tenses the toes. The client should repeat each tensing three times and relax, then visualize the special image of a pleasant place. *Caution*: some elderly people have a problem with foot cramps when tensing toes and ankles.

The entire procedure will take about 20 minutes. Your voice should be soft, just loud enough to be heard. Total attention should be placed on the procedure, with no distractions allowed. After the procedure the client should be allowed to lie still and enjoy the pleasant sensation of relaxation. However, when time to arise, the client should take a deep breath and stretch. Hypotension often accompanies total relaxation so the client should arise very slowly to avoid a feeling of dizziness. This is imperative in the elderly.

The client should practice twice a day. A cassette tape may be made of the process so the client can use the tape of your voice in his room. After a few practice sessions he may go through the routine without the help of the recording. He should be encouraged to try the technique in a chair, eventually graduating to a chair in a room with other people so he can relax anywhere. He should always be cautioned to get up slowly.

The client should discuss the subjective experience. Some clients who are intensely controlled may complain that they cannot relax "inside." If the procedure is continued over time, this is usually forgotten, but if they continue to complain of being tight inside, you should start at the beginning and slowly and soothingly take the client through the steps, again touching each muscle group. Concentration on muscle groups often brings about the desired state, which allows the client to ignore his internal stimuli.

For the elderly with hearing impairment the soft voice and quiet are unsuitable and demand innovative procedure; use small cards with huge letters for communication. Relaxation cannot be achieved under circumstances of strain, which accompanies difficult communication. Complete explanation beforehand, either by use of earphones with a cassette tape recorder or by written instructions, is necessary. Cards with such words as "squeeze," "relax," and "hold breath" in huge lettering can be used for instruction throughout the sequence of muscle groups. A small light should be placed behind the client, and the card held where the light is focused. Earphones often amplify the sound enough to allow your voice to be used during the learning sessions.

SUGGESTIONS FOR FURTHER READING

Broussard, R.: Relaxation therapy for COPD; Am. J. Nurs. **79**(10):1962-1963, 1979.

Jasmin, S., and Trygstad, L. N.: Behavioral concepts and the nursing process, St. Louis, 1979, The C. V. Mosby Co.

Morris, C. L.: Relation therapy in a clinic; Am. J. Nurs. **79**(10):1958-1959, 1979.

Richter, J. M., and Sloan, R.: The relaxation technique, Am. J. Nurs. **79**(10):1960-1964, 1979.

INDEX

A

Abdomen, evaluating, and organic brain syndrome, 388
Abstract reasoning, testing, and organic brain syndrome, 391
Accidental hypothermia, 29
  assessment of, 130
  causes of, 128, 129
  confusion secondary to, 128-132
  intervention in, 130
  prevention of, 130
  signs and symptoms of, 129, 130
  treatment for, 130-132
Activity(ies)
  assessment of, 70-71
  and sensory alteration, 193
Acute confusion, signs and symptoms of, 101-102
AD-SD complex, 322-326; *see also* Alzheimer's disease
  age of onset, 322
  characteristics of, 322
  etiology of, 324-325
  prognosis of, 322
  symptoms of, 323-324
Adaptation syndrome, general, 281
Adaptations and stress, 32
Adrenal steroids and organic brain syndrome, 387
AGHE; *see* Association of Gerontology in Higher Education
Aging and illness, sensory alteration and, 177-179
Aging condition
  assessing client's relationship to, 284
  and stressors, 278
Aging losses, impact on family system, 355-362
Aging process and the family system, 355-362
Agitation, helping client with, 106
Agnosia
  and communication problems, 94
  progressive, as symptom of AD-SD complex, 323
Air hunger, as symptom of hypoxia, 110-111
Alarm phase, with stressors as source of confusion, 274-278
Alcohol
  -drug interactions, 161
  and hypotension, 144
  and organic brain syndrome, 387

Alcoholism, 30
  and elderly, 159-161
  and loss of brain cells, 34
Aluminum and AD-SD complex, 324
Alzheimer's disease, 35, 36
  in case study, 319-320
  —senile dementia; *see* AD-SD complex
  symposiums on, 321
Ambivalence as experiential concept, 277
American Geriatric Society, 374
Aminopyrine, increased effects of, on elderly, 30
Amphetamines and organic brain syndrome, 387
Anemia(s)
  evaluation, and organic brain syndrome, 386
  hemolytic, confusion secondary to, 116
  iron-deficiency, confusion secondary to, 111-113
  macrocytic, confusion secondary to, 113-116
  pernicious, 30-31
    confusion secondary to, 113-114
Anemic hypoxia
  cause of, 111
  confusion secondary to, 111-113
Anosognosia, 15
Anticoagulants for dementias of aging, 330
Antidepressants and organic brain syndrome, 386-387
Antihypertensives and organic brain syndrome, 387
Anxiety
  of client, and sensory alteration, 194-195, 196
  as experiential concept, 277
  and stress, 32
Aphasia, progressive, as symptom of AD-SD complex, 323
Apraxia, progressive, as symptom of AD-SD complex, 323
Arteriosclerosis, cerebral, 32-33
Arteriosclerotic dementia, 329-330
Arteriosclerotic disease, cerebral, 6
Arteritis, giant cell, diagnosing, and organic brain syndrome, 394
Aspirin and blood loss, 111, 112
Assessment
  of confusion
    related to social interaction, 306
    related to stressors, 304-305
    vs. nonconfusion, 59-60
  of culture, 72-73

405

406 Index

Assessment—cont'd
  holistic; *see* Holistic assessment
  of interaction with environment, 73-75
  of lower extremity, 400-402
  of mental status, 63, 77
  nursing, in nursing process, 48
  of pain, 71-72, 207
  of perceptions, 64-65
  of physiology and structure, 65-72
  place of, in confused client, 66
  of proprioceptive sense, 207
  of senses, 64-65, 78-80
  of sensory alteration
    auditory, 246-248
    in general, 180, 186-187
    tactile, 65
    visual, 227-231
  of stress, 282-288
  total, of confused clients, 75-76
Association of Gerontology in Higher Education, 43
Astereognosis, 208
Atheromatous plaque, 33
Atropine and organic brain syndrome, 387
Attention, testing, and organic brain syndrome, 390
Auditory alteration, assessment for, 246-248
Auditory assessment in confused client, 64-65
Azotemia, 134, 135

B

Barbiturates and organic brain syndrome, 386
Behavior
  disordered (catastrophic), 12, 13-14
  disturbances, evaluating, and organic brain syndrome, 383
  ordered (preferred), 12-13
Belladonna and organic brain syndrome, 387
Bifocals, 226
Biofeedback, 309
Biosphere, 16
Bladder
  inability to empty, 310, 311
  incontinence of, 313-314
Blindness
  and orienting client to environment, 231-234
  and sensory alteration, 177
Blood flow, cerebral, obstruction to, 32-33
Blood-forming components, confusion secondary to, 113-116
Blood loss, gradual, confusion secondary to, 111-113
Blood pressure, assessment of, 68
Body image, 309
  assessment of, in confused client, 65
  helping client maintain a sense of, 105
Body temperature
  and accidental hypothermia, 29
  assessment of, 67
  and hyperthermia, 29
  and hypothermia, 29
  imbalance, confusion secondary to, 127-134
    accidental hypothermia, 128-132
    hyperthermia, 132-134

Bone loss in hypocalcemic patients, 124-125
Boredom and sensory alteration, 193-194
Bowel, incontinence of, 313-314
Bowel function; *see* Elimination
Bowel opening, artificial, 315-316
Brain
  diseases of; *see* Organic brain disease and Organic brain syndrome
  hypoperfusion of; *see* Hypotension
  reticular activating system of, and sensory alteration, 173-174
Brain cells
  death or loss of, 34
  poor perfusion of; *see* Stagnant hypoxia
Brain failure, 8
  causes of, 25
Brain injuries, 33
Brain processes
  mechanical problems in, 32-35
  systemic problems in, 26-32
Brain support
  drug toxicity compromising, 155-164
  glucose imbalance compromising, 152-155
Breathing, assessment of, 67, 68
Breathing problems, evaluating, and organic brain syndrome, 385
Burnout, employee, 373

C

Calcium, 28
  for hypocalcemia, 122-124
  -phosphate relationship, 121
Calcium metabolism, disturbances of, confusion secondary to, 121-127
Cardiac disease, evaluating, and organic brain syndrome, 385
Cardiac failure, confusion secondary to, 139-142
  assessment of, 140
  intervention in, 141-142
  prevention of, 141
  signs and symptoms of, 140, 141
Cardiac patients and sensory alteration, 177-178
Care of client
  whose confusion results from alterations in normal physiologic states, 308-317
  whose confusion results from disruption of pattern and meaning, 268-306
Care managers for confused elderly, 364
Care plan, implementation of, 52
Caregiver(s); *see also* Nurse(s)
  behavioral responses of, when caring for confused elderly, 371-372
  external rewards for, 373-374
  high-risk factors of, and sensory alteration, 180, 184-186
    in relation to hearing, 245-246
    in relation to touch, 205
    in relation to vision, 226-227
  internal rewards for, 372-373
  organizations for, 374

Caregiver(s)—cont'd
  primary, for institutionalized patient with dementia, 341
  urgent needs of, 371-375
Cataracts, senile, 215
Catastrophic behavior, 12, 13-14
Catheter, indwelling, 315
Cerebral arteriosclerosis, 32-33
Cerebral arteriosclerotic disease, 6
Cerebral blood flow, obstruction to, 32-33
Cerebral insufficiency; see Hypotension
Cerebrovascular accident, evaluating, and organic brain syndrome, 385
Cerebrovascular disease, 32-33
Chemotherapy for dementias of aging, 330-331
Chest, evaluating, and organic brain syndrome, 388
Chlorpropamide for diabetes in elderly, 27
Choline for progressive senility, 36
Chvostek's sign and hypocalcemia, 122
Circulatory overload and dehydration, 120
CJD; see Creutzfeldt-Jakob disease
Client(s); see also Patient(s)
  confused; see Confused client(s)
  high-risk factors of, and sensory alteration, 180, 181-183
    in relation to hearing, 239-243
      physiologic manifestations, 239-241
      psychologic manifestations, 241-243
    in relation to touch, 196-203
    in relation to vision, 215-222
Clinics, nursing, as nontraditional nursing setting, 44-45
Cognition, assessing, 60-62
Cognitive decrement, 8; see also Memory, loss of
Cognitive effects, sensory alteration and, 175-176
Cognitive inaccessibility, 4, 5
Coherence, sense of, as personal resource, 274-275
Cohort effect, 22
Color vision, assessment of, 230
Colostomy, 315-316
Coma, hyperosmolar nonketonic, and hyperglycemia, 154, 155
Commands, following, in assessment of confused clients, 61-62
Communication
  with patient with dementia, 343-344
  problems with confused clients, 66
  problems, patient with, 93-94
Concentration, testing, and organic brain syndrome, 390
Conceptual perspectives of confusion, 10-24
Confabulation, 15
Confused client(s)
  acutely, emergency care for, 101-108
  care of
    when confusion results from alterations in normal physiologic states, 308-317
    when confusion results from disruption of pattern and meaning, 268-306
  liabilities of, assessment of, 285

Confused client(s)—cont'd
  personal liabilities of, 275
  personal resources of, 274-275
  resources of, assessment of, 285, 286
Confused elderly
  families of; see Family(ies) of confused elderly
  intervention and treatment approaches for, 362-364
Confusion
  acute, signs and symptoms of, 101-102
  anticipating or predicting, 102-103
  characteristics of, in nursing, 2-3
  conceptual perspectives of, 10-24
  definition of, 2, 8
  drugs and, 157-158
  as label for medical, social, and legal action, 40-41
  medical diagnosis of, 6-8
  at night, helping client deal with, 107
  or nonconfusion, assessing for, 59-60
  nurse's perspectives on, 2-6
  pathophysiology of, 25-36
  predictability of, in high-risk clients, 55-56
  reinforcement of, by nurses, 20-21
  related to social interaction, 306
  related to stressors, 304-305
  resulting from alterations in normal physiologic states, care of client with, 308-317
  resulting from disruption of pattern and meaning, care of client with, 268-306
  secondary to anemic hypoxia, 111-113
  secondary to artificial bowel opening, 315-316
  secondary to changes in elimination, 309-314
  secondary to drug toxicity, 155-164
  secondary to histotoxic hypoxia, 116-136
  secondary to hyperglycemia, 154-155
  secondary to hypoglycemia, 152-154
  secondary to hypoxemic hypoxia, 136-139
  secondary to intubation, 315
  secondary to macrocytic anemia, 113-116
  secondary to pain, 316-317
  secondary to sleeplessness, 316
  secondary to stagnant hypoxia, 139-152
  social interaction and; see Social interaction
  states of, predictors of, 56
  stressors as source of, 270-282; see also Stressors
  variance with physiologic status, 52
  variance with time, 49
Consistency and prevention of sensory alteration, 189-190
Constancy in man, 12-14
Constipation, 312-313
Consultants, nursing care, 45
Continuing education, 374
  in care for elderly, 374
  in geriatric/gerontologic nursing, 44
Coordination, testing, and organic brain syndrome, 391
Council of Nursing Home Nurses, 374
Cranial nerves, evaluating, and organic brain syndrome, 388-389
Creutzfeldt-Jakob disease, 327-328

Crisis, 278-281
 defined, 278
 intervention, 295
 maturational, 280
 resolution process, 279
 situational, 280
 and stressors as source of confusion, 278-281
 symptoms of, 280
Cultural implications and interaction process, 21-24
Cultural lag, 96
Cultural stressors, 274
Culture, assessment of, 72-73
 tool for, 83
Cyanosis as sign of hypoxia, 110

D

Data collection and assessing for confusion, 60-63
 listening phase, 60
 testing phase, 60-63
Daydreaming, excessive, and sensory alteration, 195
Deafness; *see also* Hearing loss
 genetic, 240
 nongenetic, 240-241
Death of spouse, 269-270
Dehydration, 27-28
 confusion secondary to, 116-121
 intervention in, 119-120
 prevention of, 118-119
Deliberative nursing action, 52, 55-56
Delusions, 62
Dementia(s)
 AD-SD complex, 322-326
 of aging, 330-332
 arteriosclerotic, 329-330
 facilitative environment for patient with, 332-345
  guidelines for providing, 332
 multiinfarct, 329-330
 presenile irreversible, 35
 senile; *see* Senile dementias
 stages of
  advanced, 335-336, 346
  early, 333-335, 346
  later, 336-344, 346
  terminal, 344-345, 346
 true, care of patient with, 319-346
Dementia paralytica, 328-329
Depression in patients, 98-99
Deviance in society, 96
Diabetes
 evaluating, and organic brain syndrome, 386
 and hyperglycemia, 154, 155
 and hypoglycemia, 27, 152, 153
 and organic brain syndrome, 393-394
Diagnosis
 medical; *see* Medical diagnosis
 nursing; *see* Nursing diagnosis
Dietary habits, profound changes in, as symptom of AD-SD complex, 323-324
Digitalis toxicity, 158-159
Diplopia
 and aging, 216

Diplopia—cont'd
 assessment of, 229-230
 evaluating, and organic brain syndrome, 384
Diseases and organic brain syndrome, 393-395
Distortion
 and sensory alteration, 194-195
 sound, 244-245
 tactile, 201-203, 204-205
 visual, 222-226
Diuretics and organic brain syndrome, 387
Down's syndrome and AD-SD complex, 324
Dress and the elderly, 23
Drug(s)
 -alcohol interactions, 161
 and confusion, 157-158
 for dementias of aging, 330-331
 misuse and abuse, 159-161
 and organic brain syndrome, 386-387
 taking place of human interaction, 157
Drug intoxications, 30
 and organic brain syndrome, 395
Drug toxicity, confusion secondary to, 155-164
Drug use, assessment of, 71
Dysarthria, 94
Dysphasia and communication problems, 94

E

Ear infections, 240
Ears, evaluating, and organic brain syndrome, 388
Education
 continuing, in care for elderly, 374
 geriatric nursing, at baccalaureate level, 43
 geriatric/gerontologic nursing
  continuing education in, 44
  programs, 397-399
Elderly
 confused; *see* Confused elderly
 dress and, 23
 relaxation as therapy for, 403-404
Electrolyte, fluid and, imbalance, 27-28
 confusion secondary to, 116-121
Elimination
 assessment of, 69-70
 confusion secondary to changes in, 309-314
Emergency care for clients who are acutely confused, 101-108
Emergency treatment for confusion, 103-107
Emotional effects, sensory alteration and, 176-177
Emotional lability of client and sensory alteration, 196
Emotions, loss of, as symptom of AD-SD complex, 323
Endocrine dysfunction, 28-29
Environment
 disruption of pattern and meaning in, leading to confusion, 268-306
 establishing meaning in, for confused client, 103-105
 and hearing problems, 251
 interaction between man and, 16-24
 interaction with, assessment of, 73-75
  tool for, 84-86
 and visual alteration, 231-238

Environmental factors in prevention of sensory alteration, 188, 189, 190, 191, 192, 193
Excitation in man, 12-14
Exercise and sensory alteration, 193
Exotropia
  and aging, 216
  assessment of, 229
Experiential concepts and stressors, 275-277
Extremity(ies)
  evaluating, and organic brain syndrome, 388
  lower, nursing assessment of, 400-402
Eye(s); *see also* Vision
  assessment of, 227-231
  changes in, with aging, 215-222
  evaluating, and organic brain syndrome, 387-388
Eye surgery and sensory alteration, 177

F

Face-hand technique in assessment for touch, 207-208
Face-to-hand test, evaluating, and organic brain syndrome, 390
Falls, history of, evaluating, and organic brain syndrome, 385
Family(ies)
  of confused elderly
    adjustment to aging loss, and confusion, adaptive and maladaptive patterns of, 364-368
    demands on, 353
    intervention and treatment approaches to, 362-364
    therapeutic interaction with, 350-368
  of orientation, 353, 354
  of patient with true dementia
    in advanced stage, 335-336
    in early stage, 333-334
    in later stage, 336-337, 342-343
    in terminal stage, 345
  of procreation, 353
  single-parent, 353-354
Family system
  aging process and impact of aging losses on, 355-362
  development and changes of, 350-355
Fate control, 297
Feeling states and processes experienced by elderly, 276-277
Ferrous sulfate, oral, for iron-deficiency anemia, 112, 113
Fever; *see also* Hyperthermia
  evaluating, and organic brain syndrome, 385
Fluid and electrolyte imbalance, 27-28
  confusion secondary to, 116-121
Folic-acid deficiency, confusion secondary to, 114-116
Foot, assessment of, 70-71, 400-402

G

Gait changes, evaluating, and organic brain syndrome, 384-385
Geriatric clinical nurse specialist, 43
Geriatric nurse clinician, 43
Geriatric nurse practitioner, 42-43
  certification of, 43
Geriatric nurses, organizations for, 374

Geriatric nursing education at baccalaureate level, 43
Geriatric/gerontologic nursing
  continuing education in, 44
  educational programs in, 397-399
Gerontological Society, 374
Gerontology nurse specialist, 43
Giant cell arteritis and organic brain syndrome, 394
Glaucoma and aging, 216
Glucose
  brain requirements for, 26
  imbalance, compromising brain support, 152-155
Grief as experiential concept, 276
Group therapy for institutionalized patient with dementia, 341-343
Growth
  organic, 355
  psychoemotional, 355-357

H

Hallucinations
  evaluating, and organic brain syndrome, 384
  sensory alteration and, 176
Head, evaluating, and organic brain syndrome, 387
Headache, evaluating, and organic brain syndrome, 385
Hearing
  assessment of, 246-248
  sensory alteration in relation to, 239-254
Hearing aids, 243-244, 250-251, 253
Hearing loss; *see also* Deafness
  and aging, 239
  congenital, 240
  delayed, 240-241
  noise and, 240-241
Heart, evaluating, and organic brain syndrome, 388
Heart disease, evaluating, and organic brain syndrome, 385
Heart failure; *see* Cardiac failure, confusion secondary to
Helplessness as experiential concept, 277
Hematoma, subdural, leading to increased intracranial pressure, 146
Hemianopia
  and aging, 216
  tests for, 64, 229
Hemolytic anemias, confusion secondary to, 116
High-risk clients, and prevention of confusion, 55-56
Historic influence on elderly, 22
History, life
  assessment of, 72-73
  tool for, 83
  of client, providing continuity for, 105-106
Histotoxic hypoxia
  cause of, 111
  confusion secondary to, 116-136
    body temperature imbalance, 127-134
    fluid and electrolyte imbalance, 116-121
    renal failure, 134-136
    serum calcium imbalance, 121-127
Holistic assessment
  of client as functioning organism, 63-75

Holistic assessment—cont'd
  confusion or nonconfusion, assessment for, 59-60
  definitions of, 58-59
  process of, 58-86
  sections of, 59-75
Holistic nature of man, 11-14
Home health care as nontraditional nursing setting, 44
Hopelessness as experiential concept, 277
Hormones, brain, discoveries of, 35
Hospital as traditional nursing setting, 44
Humans; see Man
Huntington's chorea, 326-327
Hydration, assessment of, 69
Hydrocephalus, 33
  normal pressure, 328
    confusion secondary to, 148-150
Hyperbaric oxygen for dementias of aging, 331-332
Hypercalcemia, 28
  assessment for, 126
  confusion secondary to, 125-127
  intervention in, 126-127
  prevention of, 126
  signs and symptoms of, 125-126
Hyperglycemia, 27
  confusion secondary to, 154-155
Hypermetamorphosis as symptom of AD-SD complex, 323
Hypernatremia and dehydration, 28
Hyperorality as symptom of AD-SD complex, 323
Hyperosmolar nonketonic coma and hyperglycemia, 154, 155
Hyperosmolarity syndrome, 27
Hypersexuality as symptom of AD-SD complex, 323
Hypertension, 68
  evaluating, and organic brain syndrome, 385-386
Hyperthermia, 29
  confusion secondary to, 132-134
    assessment for, 133
    intervention in, 133
    prevention of, 133
    signs and symptoms of, 132-133
    treatment of, 133-134
Hyperthyroidism, 29
  evaluating, and organic brain syndrome, 386
Hypnotics
  and organic brain syndrome, 386
  sedative, 161-162
Hypocalcemia, 28
  confusion secondary to, 121-125
    assessment of, 122
    intervention in, 124
    prevention of, 122-124
    signs and symptoms of, 121-122
    treatment of, 124-125
Hypoglycemia, 26-27
  confusion secondary to, 152-154
    assessment for, 152
    intervention in, 153
    prevention of, 152-153
    signs and symptoms of, 152
Hypoglycemics, oral, for diabetes in elderly, 27

Hypokalemia and dehydration, 27-28
Hypoperfusion of brain; see Hypotension
Hypoproteinemia and hypothermia, 29
Hypotension, 29-30, 68
  confusion secondary to, 142-146
    assessment for, 143
    intervention in, 144-145
    prevention of, 144
    signs and symptoms of, 143
Hypothermia, accidental; see Accidental hypothermia
Hypothyroidism, 28
  confusion secondary to, 150-152
  evaluating, and organic brain syndrome, 386
  and organic brain syndrome, 394
Hypovolemia and dehydration, 117
Hypoxemia, 26
Hypoxemic hypoxia
  cause of, 111
  confusion secondary to, 136-139
    assessment of, 137
    intervention in, 138-139
    prevention of, 138
    signs and symptoms of, 137
Hypoxia, 26
  anemic; see Anemic hypoxia
  compromising brain support, 110-152
  fourth-level general assessment of, 110
  histotoxic; see Histotoxic hypoxia
  hypoxemic; see Hypoxemic hypoxia
  stagnant (ischemic); see Stagnant hypoxia

I

Ileostomy, 315-316
Illness and aging, sensory alteration and, 177-179
Illusions, helping client deal with, 107
Immobilization and sensory alteration, 177, 178
Immunologic factors and AD-SD complex, 325
Impaction, 312-313
Imprisonment model, 297-301
Inaccessibility, cognitive and social, 4, 5
Incontinence, 313-314
Indwelling catheter, 315
Injuries, evaluating, and organic brain syndrome, 386
Insomnia and sedative hypnotics, 161, 162
Institutionalization
  of patients with dementia, 337-345
  and stressors, 273
Intellectual effects, sensory alteration and, 175-176
Interaction with environment, assessment of, 74-75
  tool for, 84-86
Interaction process between man and environment, 16-24
Intracranial pressure, increased, 33-34
  confusion secondary to, 146-148
    assessment of, 147
    intervention in, 147-148
    prevention of, 147
    signs and symptoms of, 146-147
Intracranial tumors, 34
Intubation, 315
Iron, for iron-deficiency anemia, 112, 113

Iron-deficiency anemia, confusion secondary to, 111-113
Ischemic hypoxia; see Stagnant hypoxia
Isolation, sensory alteration and, 172-177

J

Jakob-Creutzfeldt disease, 35, 327-328
Judgment
   appropriate, assessing, 61
   testing, and organic brain syndrome, 391

K

Knees, assessment of, 70
Knowledge relating to care of elderly, 45

L

L-dopa and slurred speech, 94
Laboratory tests, evaluating, and organic brain syndrome, 391-292
Lacunes in multiinfarct dementia, 329
Language and elderly, 22-23
Language skills, basic, testing, and organic brain syndrome, 390
Legs, assessment of, 70, 400-402
Lethargy, evaluating, and organic brain syndrome, 384
Life history
   assessment of, 72-73
      tool for, 83
   of client, providing continuity for, 105-106
Lips, assessment of, 69
Listening phase of assessment of confused clients, 60
Loneliness as experiential concept, 276
Loss(es)
   aging, 357-362
   of memory; see Memory, loss of
   as stressor, 272
Lower extremity, nursing assessment of, 400-402

M

Macrocytic anemia, confusion secondary to, 113-116
   folic-acid deficiency, 114-116
   hemolytic anemias, 116
   pernicious anemia, 113-114
Man
   in equilibrium, 12-14
   holistic nature of, 11-14
   individual organization in, 14-16
   interaction with environment, 16-24
Massage and tactile alteration, 214-215
Mechanical problems in brain processes, 32-35
Medical diagnosis
   compared to nursing diagnosis, 47-48
   of confusion, 6-8
   nurse's assessment of, 72
Medical history, past, and organic brain syndrome, 385-386
Medications; see also Drug(s)
   and organic brain syndrome, 386-387

Memory
   assessing, 61
   loss of, 8
      as sign of confusion, 3
      and loss of brain cells, 34
   recall and recognition, 61
Meningitis, acute onset, and organic brain syndrome, 394-395
Mental status
   assessment of
      recording, 63
      tool for, 77
   evaluating, and organic brain syndrome, 389-390
Miosis, senile, and aging, 215
Mnemic disturbances, progressive, as symptom of AD-SD complex, 323
Mood, evaluating, and organic brain syndrome, 391
Motor ability, assessment of, 70-71
Mountain States Health Systems, 42
Mouth
   assessment of, 69
   evaluating, and organic brain syndrome, 388
Multiinfarct dementia, 329-330
Muscles, evaluating, and organic brain syndrome, 389
Myxedema; see Hypothyroidism

N

Neck
   assessment of, 71
   evaluating, and organic brain syndrome, 388
Nerves, cranial, evaluating, and organic brain syndrome, 388-389
Neuroleptics and tardive dyskinesia, 162, 163, 164
Neurosyphilis, 328-329
Neurotransmitters and AD-SD complex, 325
Niacin; see Nicotinic acid and pellagra
Nicotinic acid and pellagra, 31
Nicotinic-acid–deficient encephalopathy and pellagra, 31
Night, confusion and screaming at, 107
Noise and hearing loss, 240-241
Nootropic agents for dementias of aging, 331
Normal pressure hydrocephalus, 328
   confusion secondary to, 148-150
Nose, evaluating, and organic brain syndrome, 388
NPH; see Normal pressure hydrocephalus
Numbness, evaluating, and organic brain syndrome, 385
Nurse(s); see also Caregiver(s)
   geriatric clinical nurse specialist, 43
   geriatric nurse clinician, 43
   geriatric nurse practitioner, 42-43
   geriatric nurses, organizations for, 374
   as primary caregiver, 42-45, 66-67
   role of, in care of confused client, 39-46
Nursing
   geriatric/gerontologic, educational programs in, 397-399
   and perspective on confusion, 2-6
Nursing assessment in nursing process, 48
Nursing care consultants, 45

Nursing clinics as nontraditional nursing setting, 44-45
Nursing diagnosis
　compared to medical diagnosis, 47-48
　of confusion
　　connotations of, 88
　　problems with, 88-89
　definition of, 48
　first-level, 52-53
　fourth-level, 54-55
　second-level, 53-54
　taxonomy of, 49-51
　third-level, 54
Nursing education; *see* Education
Nursing failure and problem patients, 91-93
Nursing home as traditional nursing setting, 44
Nursing process, 47-52
Nursing settings, 44-45
Nutritional status, assessment of, 68-69

O

OBD; *see* Organic brain disease
OBS; *see* Organic brain syndrome
Olfactory assessment in confused client, 65
Oral hypoglycemics for diabetes in elderly, 27
Organic brain disease, 6-7
Organic brain syndrome, 6, 7-8
　acute
　　flow sheet, 392
　　vs. chronic, a protocol to determine, 376-396
　chronic
　　flow sheet, 393
　　planning for patient with, 395-396
　reversible and irreversible, 8
Organic growth, 355
Organizational activity for geriatric nurses, 374
Otitis media, 240
Otosclerosis, 240
Ototoxicity, chronic, 240
Overload
　and sensory alteration, 194-195
　sound, 244-245
　tactile, 201-203, 204-205
　visual, 222-226
Oxygen
　for cardiac failure, 141
　hyperbaric, for dementias of aging, 331-332

P

Paget's disease and genetic deafness, 240
Pain
　assessment of, 71-72
　confusion secondary to, 316-317
　sense of, assessment for, 207
　and sensory alteration, 201
Panic of client and sensory alteration, 196
Papilledema and intracranial tumors, 34
Paranoia, evaluating, and organic brain syndrome, 384
Paresis, general, 328-329
Paresthesias, evaluating, and organic brain syndrome, 385
Pathophysiology of confusion, 25-36

Patient(s); *see also* Client(s)
　challenging personal values, 94-97
　with communication problems, 93-94
　depressed, 98-99
　physically unattractive, 97-98
　problem, and nursing failure, 91-93
　troublemakers, 99
　with a true dementia, care of, 319-346
Pellagra, 31
Peptic ulcer disease, evaluating, and organic brain syndrome, 386
Perceptions, assessment of, 64-65
　tool for, 78-80
Perceptual implications and interaction process, 16-18
Pernicious anemia, 30-31
　confusion secondary to, 113-114
Personal liabilities, 275
Personal resources, 274-275
Personal stressors, 272
Personal values of patient vs. those of nurse, 94-97
Phenothiazines and hypothermia, 29
Phosphate-calcium relationship, 121
Physical appearance and judging patients, 96-98
Physiologic states, alterations in, leading to confusion, 308-317
Physiologic status and confusion variance, 52
Physiology and structure, assessment of, 65-72
　tool for, 81-82
Pick's disease, 35, 396
Plaque, atheromatous, 33
Polypharmacy, 155
Potassium for dehydration, 120
Powerlessness
　as experiential concept, 277
　as stressor, 272
Predictability of confusion in high-risk clients, 55-56
Predictors of confusional states, 56
Preferred behavior, 12-13
Presbycusis, 239-240
Presbyopia, 226
　and aging, 215
Presenile dementias, 326-329; *see also* Alzheimer's disease
　irreversible, 35
Pressure and sensory alteration, 201
Primary caregiver; *see also* Caregiver(s)
　for patient with dementia, 341
Prism glasses, 226
Privacy
　for institutionalized patient with dementia, 340
　and prevention of sensory alteration, 188
Proprioceptive sense, assessment for, 207
Pseudosenilities, 8
　diagnosing, importance in, 32
Psychoemotional growth, 355-357
Psychoneurosis, evaluating, and organic brain syndrome, 384
Psychotherapy, individual, for dementias of aging, 331
Psychotropic agents for dementias of aging, 330-331
Pulmonary disease, chronic obstructive, evaluating, and organic brain syndrome, 385

Pulmonary edema and dehydration, 120
Pulse(s)
  assessment of, 67, 68
  evaluating, and organic brain syndrome, 388

R

RAS; *see* Reticular activating system of brain
Reality
  and assessment of confused clients, 62-63
  and holistic assessment, 59
Recall
  and recognition, 61
  testing, and organic brain syndrome, 390
Recognition and recall, 61
Rectum, evaluating, and organic brain syndrome, 388
Rejection
  as experiential concept, 276
  as stressor, 272
Relaxation
  for managing stress, 292
  as therapy for elderly, 403-404
Relocation
  effect on patient with dementia, 337, 340
  and prevention of sensory alteration, 190-191
Renal failure, confusion secondary to, 134-136
  assessment of, 134
  intervention in, 135-136
  prevention of, 135
  signs and symptoms of, 134-135
Renal problems, evaluating, and organic brain syndrome, 386
Research, implications for, 375
Respiration, assessment of, 67, 68
Responsibilities, assignment of and prevention of sensory alteration, 191-192
Restraints as safety measure, 106-107
Reticular activating system of brain, 173-174
Retirement as stressor, 273

S

Safety measures, 107-108
Salicylates and organic brain syndrome, 387
Screaming at night, helping client deal with, 107
Sedative hypnotics, 161-162
Sedatives and organic brain syndrome, 386
Seizures
  in AD-SD complex, 324
  evaluating, and organic brain syndrome, 383-384
Senile dementias, 6, 329-330; *see also* Alzheimer's disease
  and loss of brain cells, 34
  "true," 320-332
    case study of, 319-320
Senility, 8
Sensations, changes in, evaluating, and organic brain syndrome, 384
Senses, assessment of, 64-65
  tool for, 78-80
Sensory alteration(s)
  and cognitive and intellectual effects, 175-176
  effects on sensory function, 175

Sensory alteration(s)—cont'd
  and emotional effects, 176-177
  fourth-level assessment for
    in general, 180, 186-187, 255-257
    in relation to hearing, 246-248, 262
    in relation to touch, 205-208, 258
    in relation to vision, 227-231, 259
  and hallucinations, 176
  and high-risk caregiver factors
    in general, 180, 184-186
    in relation to hearing, 245-246
    in relation to touch, 205
    in relation to vision, 226-227
  and high-risk client factors
    in general, 180, 181-183
    in relation to hearing, 239-243
      physiologic manifestations, 239-241
      psychologic manifestations, 241-243
    in relation to touch, 196-203
    in relation to vision, 215-222
  and high-risk setting factors
    in general, 180, 183-184
    in relation to hearing, 243-245
    in relation to touch, 203-205
    in relation to vision, 222-226
  and illness and aging, 177-179
  implications of, for nursing care of the aged, 179-181
  and intervention
    in general, 181, 193-196, 255-257
    in relation to hearing, 251-254, 262-263
    in relation to touch, 212-215, 258
    in relation to vision, 238, 259
  as isolating experience, 172-177
  model of, 174-175
  prevention of
    in general, 180-181, 188-193, 255-257
    in relation to hearing, 248-251, 262-263
    in relation to touch, 208-212, 258
    in relation to vision, 231-233, 259-261
      for client with severe visual handicaps, 231-234
      for client with specific alterations of sight, 235-238
Sensoriperceptual problems, care of client with, 171-263
Sensory deficits and prevention of sensory alteration, 189
Sensory function, effects on, sensory alteration and, 175
Sensory perception, testing, and organic brain syndrome, 391
Separation as experiential concept, 276
Serum calcium imbalance, confusion secondary to, 121-127
  hypercalcemia, 125-127
  hypocalcemia, 121-125
Setting, high-risk factors of
  in general, 180, 183-184
  in relation to hearing, 243-245
  in relation to touch, 203-205
  in relation to vision, 222-226

Sexual activity for institutionalized patient with dementia, 341
Sign language, 249
Skin, evaluating, and organic brain syndrome, 387
Sleeplessness, confusion secondary to, 316
Slurred speech, 94
Social implications and interaction process, 18-21
Social inaccessibility, 4,5
Social interaction
   and confusion, 296-303
      fourth-level assessment of, 302
      high-risk factors, 301
      prevention and intervention in, 302-303
   confusion related to, 306
Social stressors, 273
Sodium and dehydration, 117, 120
Sound deprivation, 244
Sound overload and distortion, 244-245
Speech, slurred, 94
Spouse, death of, 269-270
Stagnant hypoxia
   cause of, 111
   confusion secondary to, 139-152
      cardiac failure, 139-142
      hypotension, 142-146
      hypothyroidism, 150-152
      increased intracranial pressure, 146-148
      normal pressure hydrocephalus, 148-150
Stenosis of blood vessels to brain, 33
Steroids, adrenal, and organic brain syndrome, 387
Stimulation and prevention of sensory alteration, 188
Stimulus-response situations, 11-12
Stress, 31-32
   chronic, 281-282
Stress incontinence, 313, 314
Stressors
   and client's personal milieu, 269-296
   and confusion, 304-305
      assessment of, 282-288
      intervention in, 292-295
      prevention of, 288-292
   cultural, 274
   defined, 272
   generic, 283
   personal/interpersonal, 272
   social, 273
   as source of confusion, 270-282
Stroke and communication problems, 94
Structure and physiology, assessment of, 65-72
   tool for, 81-82
Stupor, evaluating, and organic brain syndrome, 384
Subdural hematoma
   leading to increased intracranial pressure, 146
   and organic brain syndrome, 393
Suicide
   as response to crisis, 279
   and stress, 283
      assessment of, 286-287
Sundown syndrome, 49
Surgical intervention for dementias of aging, 331
Syphilis, history of, evaluating, and organic brain syndrome, 385
Systemic problems in brain processes, 26-32

T

Tactile assessment in confused client, 65
Tactile deprivation and sensory alteration, 201, 203-204
Tactile overload and distortion, 201-203, 204-205
Tactile senses, deficits in, incidence in aging people, 197-199
Tardive dyskinesia, 162-164
   choline for, 36
Temperature
   body; *see* Body temperature
   sense of, assessment of, 206-207
Tension
   chronic, dealing with, 295
   chronic stress and, 281-282
Terminal drop theory, 31
Terminology, present day, 8
Territoriality for institutionalized patient with dementia, 340
Testing phase of assessment of confused clients, 60-63
Tetany and hypocalcemia, 121
Therapy for elderly, relaxation as, 403-404
Thought(s)
   of client, assessment of, 284-285
   disorganization of, and sensory alteration, 195-196
   slowness of, and sensory alteration, 195
Throat, evaluating, and organic brain syndrome, 388
Thyroid hormones, 28
Thyrotoxicosis, 29
T. I. A.; *see* Transient ischemic attacks
Time
   and assessing confused clients, 62-63
   and confusion variance, 49
Time warp, 18
Tingling, evaluating, and organic brain syndrome, 385
Tolbutamide for diabetes in elderly, 27
Tooth (teeth), assessment of, 69
Touch
   deep and light, assessment of, 207
   need for, in elderly, 199-201
   sensory alteration in relation to, 196-215
Touch blends, 197
Touching, reactions to, 202-203
Tranquilizers
   and organic brain syndrome, 386
   and tardive dyskinesia, 162
Transient ischemic attacks and organic brain syndrome, 393
Trauma and organic brain syndrome, 393
Treatment for confusion, emergency, 103-107
Troublemaker, 99
Tubing in body, client's reactions to, 106
Tumors, intracranial, 34

U

Uremia, confusion secondary to, 134-136
   assessment of, 134
   intervention in, 135-136
   prevention of, 135
   signs and symptoms of, 134-135

Urinary incontinence, 313-314

V

Vasodilators for cementias of aging, 330
Vasopressin for memory failure, 35
Ventilatory problems, confusion secondary to, 136-139
Viral infections and AD-SD complex, 324-325
Vision; *see also* Eye(s)
   assessment of, 227-231
      blurred, evaluating, and organic brain syndrome, 384
   sensory alteration in relation to, 215-238
Visual acuity and aging, 215
Visual assessment in confused client, 64
Visual deprivation, 222
Visual distortion, 222-226
Visual overload, 222-226
Vital signs, assessment of, 57-68
Vitamin B_{12}, for pernicious anemia, 113, 114
Vitamin B_{12} deficiency, and organic brain syndrome, 394
Vomiting, evaluating, and organic brain syndrome, 385

W

Wanderer, patient with dementia as, 341
Weakness, evaluating, and organic brain syndrome, 385
Weight, assessment of, 69
Wheelchair, assessment of client in, 71